FOURTH EDITION

Physical Therapy Clinical Handbook for PTAs

Frances M. Wedge, PT, DScPT, MSc

Board Certified Specialist in Geriatric Physical Therapy (Emeritus)
Certified Exercise Expert for Aging Adults
Former Program Director and Faculty
Physical Therapist Assistant Program
Morton College
Cicero, Illinois

JONES & BARTLETT
LEARNING

World Headquarters
Jones & Bartlett Learning
25 Mall Road
Burlington, MA 01803
978-443-5000
info@jblearning.com
www.jblearning.com

Jones & Bartlett Learning books and products are available through most bookstores and online booksellers. To contact Jones & Bartlett Learning directly, call 800-832-0034, fax 978-443-8000, or visit our website, www.jblearning.com.

Substantial discounts on bulk quantities of Jones & Bartlett Learning publications are available to corporations, professional associations, and other qualified organizations. For details and specific discount information, contact the special sales department at Jones & Bartlett Learning via the above contact information or send an email to specialsales@jblearning.com.

Vice President, Product Management: Marisa R. Urbano
Vice President, Content Strategy and Implementation: Christine Emerton
Director, Content Management: Donna Gridley
Director, Project Management and Content Services: Karen Scott
Director, Product Management: Matthew Kane
Product Manager: Whitney Fekete
Content Strategist: Carol Brewer Guerrero
Manager, Project Management: Kristen Rogers
Project Manager: Belinda Thresher
Digital Project Specialist: Carolyln Downer
Marketing Manager: Mark Adamiak
Content Services Manager: Colleen Lamy
Vice President, Manufacturing and Inventory Control: Therese Connell
Composition: Straive
Project Management: Straive
Cover Design: Kristin E. Parker
Senior Media Development Editor: Troy Liston
Rights & Permissions Manager: John Rusk
Rights Specialist: Benjamin Roy
Cover Image (Title Page, Part Opener, Chapter Opener): © Tuomas A. Lehtinen/Moment/Getty Images
Printing and Binding: LSC Communications

Library of Congress Cataloging-in-Publication Data
Names: Wedge, Frances M., author.
Title: Physical therapy clinical handbook for PTAs / Frances M. Wedge,
    Board Certified Specialist in Geriatric Physical Therapy (Emeritus), Certified Exercise Expert for Aging Adults,
    Former Program Director and Faculty, Physical Therapist Assistant Program, Morton College, Cicero, Illinois.
Description: Fourth edition. | Burlington, Massachusetts : Jones & Bartlett Learning, [2023] | Preceded by Physical therapy
    clinical handbook for PTAs / Kathy Cikulin-Kulinski, PT, DPT, OCS, PTA Instructor, Fox College, Orthopedic
    Clinical Specialist and LSVT BIG Certified Instructor, AthletiCo, Tinley Park, Illinois. Third edition. [2018] | Includes
    bibliographical references and index. | Summary: "This book is a concise and condensed clinical pocket guide
    designed specifically to help physical therapist assistant students and practitioners easily obtain information
    in the areas of physical therapy evidence-based interventions"– Provided by publisher.
Identifiers: LCCN 2021047361 | ISBN 9781284226157 (paperback)
Subjects: LCSH: Physical therapy assistants–Handbooks, manuals, etc. | Physical therapy–Handbooks, manuals, etc.
Classification: LCC RM705 .D75 2023 | DDC 615.8/2–dc23
LC record available at https://lccn.loc.gov/2021047361

6048

Printed in the United States of America
26 25 24 23 22   10 9 8 7 6 5 4 3 2

To my family for their support and patience during this process of editing the "Handbook." To my mentors and colleagues in the physical therapy profession for their guidance and support over the years. I am grateful for the formal and informal knowledge shared by these individuals that has brought me to where I am today.
Thank you.

—Fran Wedge

Brief Contents

PART 1 Physical Therapist Assistant: Roles and Responsibilities 1

PART 2 Safety in the Clinical Environment 27

**PART 6 Neurologic System: Data Collection
and Interventions   277**

PART 7 Cardiopulmonary Interventions   385

Contents

x   Contents

PART 3 **Clinical Documentation** 69

Section 5-5 Basic Clinical Impairments and Activity Limitations Related to Common Musculoskeletal Conditions 233

Section 5-6 Musculoskeletal Intervention Strategies 237

Section 5-7 Physical Therapy Interventions for the Acute, Post-Surgical Orthopedic Patient ...255

Section 5-8 Pharmacology for Musculoskeletal Pathologies.... 267

PART 6 Neurologic System: Data Collection and Interventions 277

Section 6-1 Review of Nervous System Anatomy and Physiology... 281

Section 6-2 Neurologic Data Collection 293

Section 6-3 Types of Neurologic Interventions .317

Section 6-4 Clinical Impairments and Activity Limitations of Neurologic Conditions 337

PART 8 Integumentary Interventions   467

Preface

Welcome to the fourth edition of *Physical Therapy Clinical Handbook for PTAs*.

This text is designed as a reference for a diverse audience including the physical therapist assistant (PTA) graduate, the PTA student, PTA faculty, clinical instructors who mentor PTA students throughout their clinical field work, as well as veteran PTAs who are interested in staying abreast of the most current information and guidelines for treatment.

The fourth edition continues the tradition of embracing the inclusion of evidence-based intervention choices into clinical practice in alignment with the vision of the American Physical Therapy Association (APTA). The role of the PTA and the implications related to interventions provided by the PTA in a variety of clinical settings are considered and incorporated throughout this edition. With the changing healthcare environment, it is imperative that the PTA has the strongest skill set available to make sound clinical judgments while incorporating evidence-based interventions to optimize functional outcomes that are expected in our profession today. This is reinforced throughout the text by use of International Classification of Functioning, Disability and Health (ICF) terminology linking with evidenced-based intervention choices to address impairments related to functional activities and participation restrictions.

The text has been reorganized into 11 parts with two new parts, one that addresses roles and responsibilities of the PTA and a second that consolidates information on general interventions for patient management. The acute care section has also been revised. Orthopedic and neurological acute care interventions are now included in the respective musculoskeletal and neurologic sections of the book for easier reference. In addition, basic laboratory tests and values have been included in the acute care section. The appendices have been revised to include APTA's algorithms for the direction and supervision of the PTA, standardized tests, and examples of acceptable and unacceptable documentation. Finally, revised supplemental slides in PowerPoint format and a test bank on selected topics covered in the Handbook are available to instructors.

Benefits and Additional Resources

This edition strives to maintain and build on the benefits offered by prior editions, including the following:

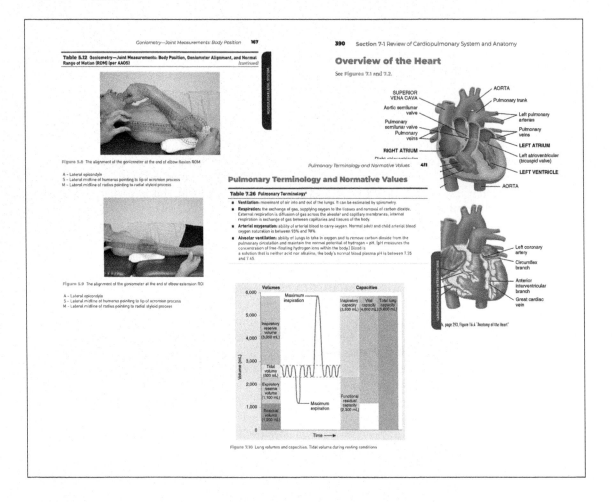

- All new four-color images
- Test bank, available in formats compatible with learning management systems (LMS)
- Tabbed sections for easy referencing
- Easy-to-read tables
- Available as an eBook

108 Section 4-2 Therapeutic Exercises: Indications and Contraindications

Table 4.2 Therapeutic Exercises: Indications and Contraindications¹

Exercises	Indications	Contraindications, Limitations, and Precautions¹
PROM exercises	To demonstrate a movement, to prepare a patient for stretching, to maintain joint connective tissue mobility, to maintain elasticity of muscle, to increase synovial fluid for joint nutrition, to assist circulation, to prevent joint contracture, to decrease pain, to help in the healing process	Contraindication: Disruption of the healing process Limitations: Will not increase muscle strength or endurance, will not prevent or counteract muscle atrophy, will not assist in the blood circulation to the same extent as the active movement
AROM exercises	For weak muscles, to promote bone and soft-tissue integrity, to promote coordination and motor skills, to prevent DVT, to increase blood circulation, for aerobic conditioning, for preparation for functional activities	Contraindications: Disruption of the healing process, harm to recent surgical procedure(s) Limitations: Will not increase strength in muscles that are already strong
AAROM exercises using manual or mechanical assistance (wand, cane, finger ladder, or overhead pulleys)	To increase circulation and prevent DVT; to promote integrity of bone, muscles, ligaments and tendons; to promote coordination and motor abilities; to assist with learning a new movement pattern	Contraindications: Disruption of the healing process, harm to recent surgical procedure(s) Limitations: Will not increase strength in muscles already strong; less effective than AROM exercises
Muscle setting isometric exercises (quadriceps sets; gluteal muscle sets; HS sets)	For very weak muscles, for acute stage of soft-tissue healing, to increase circulation, to promote relaxation, to decrease pain	Precautions: Cardiovascular disease, CVA, Valsalva maneuver (to avoid performing a Valsalva maneuver, the patient can count out loud or sing)
Resisted isometrics exercises (higher intensity than muscle setting): manual or mechanical (door frame or wall)	To increase strength throughout permitted ROM, and when manual or mechanical resistance is painful or harmful	Precautions: Cardiovascular disease, CVA, Valsalva maneuver (to avoid performing a Valsalva maneuver, the patient can count out loud or sing)

(continued)

Slides in PowerPoint format and a test bank are available to instructors. These slides can be used by the director of clinical education for remediation purposes, the clinical instructor as an additional means for assessing a student's understanding, or for the classroom instructor to solidify current concepts. Lastly, the slides can be utilized as a potential adjunct for the hybrid classroom because they can be used as a pre-lecture tool so that classroom time can focus on the interventions associated with the topic presented in the slides.

New to This Edition

The following changes have been incorporated into this edition:

- Part 1, *Physical Therapist Assistant: Roles and Responsibilities*, discusses the role of the PTA and the PT/PTA relationship, with new sections on levels of supervision and clinical decision making. New to Part 1 is a discussion on the healthcare team, including interprofessional practice and a review of ethics and professionalism in physical therapy.
- Part 2, *Safety in the Clinical Environment*, consolidates information on infection control, domestic and family violence, patient safety during interventions, including a review of normal and abnormal values for vital signs, electrolyte imbalance, diabetes, and blood gasses. A new section looks at the issues associated with opioid use and the role of physical therapy in pain management.
- Part 3, *Clinical Documentation*, includes updated information on documentation elements and revisions to the section on the elements of the daily/weekly note.
- Part 4, *Patient Management: General Interventions*, consolidates information on interventions that are applicable for a variety of pathologies, into one chapter. This part includes sections on tissue healing,

therapeutic exercise (including a revised section on exercise topics for the obstetric patient), biophysical agents and modalities, therapeutic massage, and wheelchair management. A new section on interventions for patients with vestibular disorders has been included.

- Part 5, *Musculoskeletal System: Data Collection and Interventions*, has been revised to focus on musculoskeletal data collection and interventions. General exercise interventions, wheelchair management, and mobility are now located in Part 4. New to this part is a discussion on clinical practice guidelines and content on physical therapy interventions in the acute care/post-surgical setting.

- Part 6, *Neurologic System: Data Collection and Interventions*, now includes a discussion on mild traumatic brain injury/concussion and clinical practice guidelines for patients with neurologic pathology. New to this part is content on physical therapy interventions in the acute care setting.

- Part 7, *Cardiopulmonary Interventions*, includes new content on medical cardiac testing and procedures and clinical practice guidelines for cardiovascular and pulmonary pathology. A table has been included for easier reference of lab values for electrolytes, blood, and blood gases. Additionally, a new section on active cycle of breathing technique is included.

- Part 8, *Integumentary Interventions*, now includes color images of the different types and stages of wounds and new images for the rule of nines and Lund Browder charts. Also included in this section are updates to types of grafts used in burn management and a section on wound terminology.

- Part 9, *Geriatric Interventions*, includes revised information on malnutrition, thermal regulation in older adults, and dementia. New content has been added to the section on incontinence to include common types of incontinence and updated interventions. A discussion on clinical practice guidelines for the management of older adults is also included.

- Part 10, *Pediatric Interventions*, includes updates to the pediatric screening tests and revisions to the table on infant reflexes, information on slipped capital femoral epiphyses, and autism spectrum disorder. New sections on juvenile idiopathic arthritis, torticollis, and pediatric clinical practice guidelines have been included.

- Part 11, *Acute Care: Interventions for Select Medical and Surgical Conditions*, includes general guidelines for the PTA working in the acute care setting as well as a new section that presents information on various laboratory tests and implications for the PTA. Acute care orthopaedic management has been integrated into Part 5 of this book and acute care management of patients with neurologic conditions is now located in Part 6.

- Supplemental slides in PowerPoint format designed to augment classroom discussion or topics of interest for the PTA are available:

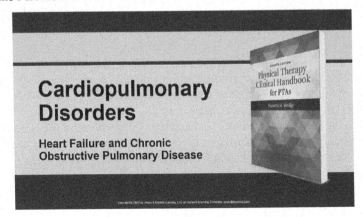

- Balance and Falls Prevention
- Pressure Injuries

- Achilles Tendinopathy
- Parkinson's Disease
- New to this edition: a slide set on Cardiopulmonary Disease has been added!
- New to this edition is a test bank on select topics to support information provided in the Handbook. The test bank is available in LMS-compatible formats.

Acknowledgments

To Olga Dreeben-Irimia for all her hard work and dedication to making the first two editions of this book a valuable resource for PTA students and clinicians alike and for providing such a great foundation to build upon. Thank you.

To my colleague and the author of the third edition of this book, Kathy Cikulin-Kulinski, PT, DPT, OCS, I extend thanks and gratitude. Kathy not only provided invaluable support and encouragement, but she also generously gave of her time reviewing each chapter and providing feedback. I would also like to thank my son, Christopher Wedge PT, DPT, OCS, CSCS, for his help and feedback with the orthopaedic section of this book.

–Fran Wedge

About the Author

Fran Wedge, PT, DScPT, MSc, GCS (Emeritus), CEEAA, graduated from the Royal Orthopedic Hospital School of Physiotherapy, Birmingham, England. Fran obtained her Master of Science degree in professional development from the University of Greenwich, London, and Doctor of Science in Physical Therapy from the University of Alabama at Birmingham. Having worked primarily in geriatrics, Fran became a Board-Certified Specialist in Geriatric Physical Therapy in 2000. Fran recently retired as the program director for the PTA program at Morton College in Cicero, Illinois, and currently works as an educational consultant for developing PT and PTA programs. Nationally, Fran has served as chair of the Academy of Geriatric Physical Therapy task force examining entry-level competencies in geriatric physical therapy for the PTA, has attended item-writing workshops, and served on the TOEFL task force for the FSBPT. Fran is an on-site reviewer for CAPTE. At the state level, Fran has served on ethics, membership, and new careers committees for the Illinois Physical Therapy Association and was a member of the Illinois Department of Professional Regulation Physical Therapy Board from 2015–2022.

Reviewers

Jennifer Ball, PT/ATC, MHR
PTA Program Director, Professor
Oklahoma City Community College
Oklahoma City, Oklahoma

Farica (Ricki) Bialstock, PT, DPT, MS
Professor and Director of Clinical Education,
    Physical Therapist Assistant Program
Nassau Community College
Garden City, New York

LaVonne Couch, PT, DPT, EdD, CSCS
Program Director/Instructor
Rowan College of South Jersey (formerly Rowan
    College at Gloucester County)
Sewell, New Jersey

Julie Feeny, PT, MS
Program Director
Physical Therapy Assistant Program
Illinois Central College
Peoria, Illinois

Betsy Fuller, PT, EdD
Associate Director and Professor, School of
    Physical Therapy
MCPHS University
Worcester, Massachusetts

Suzanne Giuffre
Physical Therapist, EdD in Higher Education
    Administration
Associate Professor and DPT Program Director
Cleveland State University
Cleveland, Ohio

Rhonda Heffner, PTA
Specialty Certification in Orthopedics
Kinesiology Taping Certification
Physical Therapist Assistant Program
Assistant Professor
El Paso Community College
El Paso, Texas

Jacki Klaczak Kopack, PT, DPT
PTA Program Director
Harcum College
Bryn Mawr, Pennsylvania

Deanna Lamb, PhD, PT, MA
PTA Program Director
Professional Skills Institute
Maumee, Ohio

Adeel Haider Rizvi, PT, DPT, PhD
Program Director, Physical Therapist Assistant
Chaffey College
Fontana, California

Wendy L. Smith, PT, DPT, OCS, CLT-LANA
Assistant Professor and Academic Coordinator
    of Clinical Education
Indian River State College
Fort Pierce, Florida

Beth Ann Thorpe, PTA, MS, CSCS
Academic Coordinator of Clinical Education
    and Instructor Physical Therapist Assistant
    Program
Lane Community College
Eugene, Oregon

Jordan Tucker, PT, DPT, EdD
Program Director, Physical Therapist Assistant
    Program
Virginia Western Community College
Roanoke, Virginia

Physical Therapist Assistant: Roles and Responsibilities

SECTION 1-1

Physical Therapist and Physical Therapist Assistant Relationship

The Collaborative Path Between the PT and the PTA[1]

- The physical therapist (PT) performs an initial examination of the patient. The physical therapist assistant (PTA) helps the PT with the initial examination, gathering specific data that the PT requested. The PTA accepts the delegated tasks within the limits of his or her capabilities and considering legal, jurisdictional, and ethical guidelines.
- The PT evaluates the results of data collection and makes a judgment about data value. The PTA does not interpret the results of the initial examination.
- The PT establishes the goals or outcomes to be accomplished by the plan of care and the treatment plan.
- The PT performs the patient's interventions. The PTA performs the patient's selected interventions as directed by the PT.
- The PTA may perform data collection during the course of the patient's interventions to record the patient's progress or lack of progress since the initial examination and evaluation. The PTA may ask the PT for a reexamination.
- The PT performs the reexamination and establishes new outcomes and a new treatment plan.
- The PT performs the patient's new interventions. The PTA performs the selected patient's new interventions as directed by the PT.
- The PT and PTA maintain frequent and ongoing communication regarding patient status.
- Conferences between the PT and PTA regarding patients should be documented.
- The PT performs the discharge examination and evaluation of the patient when the outcomes are met. The PTA can help gather data as requested by the PT.

See Appendix A for supporting algorithms from the American Physical Therapy Association (APTA).

Examples of Communication Between the PT and PTA Relating to Patient Care

Table 1.1 Communication Between PT and PTA[1]

- Discussion of goals and expectations for the patient
- Precautions, contraindications, or other issues related to the interventions
- Information on patient response to physical therapy
- Changes in patient medical status
- Discussion on modifications to the plan of care
- Recommendations for discharge planning
- Communication from other disciplines

PTA Duties (as per the APTA)

Table 1.2 PTA Duties[2]

- Perform selected physical therapy interventions under the direction and at least the general supervision of the PT. The ability of the PTA to perform the selected interventions as directed shall be assessed on an ongoing basis by the supervising PT.
- Make permissible modifications to selected interventions either to progress the patient as directed by the PT or to ensure patient safety and comfort.
- Communicate with the supervising PT when modifications to the established plan of care are needed.
- Document the patient's progress.
- Perform routine operational functions, including direct personal supervision, where allowable by law, of the physical therapy aide and the PTA student and other personnel.

The PTA's Clinical Considerations During Interventions[1]

- The complexity, criticality, acuity, and stability of the patient
- The accessibility to the PT
- The type of setting where services are provided
- Federal and state statutes
- The available PT supervision in the event of an emergency
- The mission of physical therapy services for that specific clinical setting
- The needed frequency of reexamination

Levels of Supervision (per the APTA)[3]

- General Supervision: The PT is not required to be on site but must be available at least by telecommunication.
- Direct Supervision: The PT, or PTA when supervising a student, is physically present and immediately available. The PT or PTA has direct contact with the patient on each date of service.
- Direct Personal Supervision: The PT, or PTA if allowed by law, is physically present and immediately available to direct and supervise tasks related to patient care when performed by the physical therapy aid.
- Telecommunications do not meet the requirements of direct supervision or direct personal supervision.
- Higher levels of supervision may be required by state statutes, reimbursement requirements, or other factors as determined by the PT.

Clinical Decision-Making by the PTA[4] (View Appendix A for *Problem Solving Algorithm* for the PTA)

- The PTA has the ability to gather and use information to help guide decisions about patient care and then implements those decisions clinically.
- PTAs make clinical decisions about treatment progression, assessment of benefit of interventions based on outcomes and progress toward defined goals of treatment.
- Clinical decisions are based on understanding of established goals, understanding of patient and, where applicable, family needs, awareness of the rehabilitation setting, including involvement of the interdisciplinary team, assessment of subjective and objective data, own clinical knowledge, and expertise.
- PTAs must recognize what clinical decisions they can make safely and those that need consultation with the PT.
- The PTA should communicate with the PT when an unexpected response occurs or when expected outcomes are not achieved after several treatments.

The Healthcare Team

The Healthcare Team Members[1]

- Members of various healthcare and related professions who are involved in patient management.
- The patient is always at the core of the healthcare team.
- Family members and caregivers are included in the healthcare team where indicated.

Table 1.3 **Intradisciplinary Team Members**

- Supervising physical therapist (PT)
- Physical therapist assistant (PTA)
- Physical therapy aide or technician—requires direct personal supervision by the PT or PTA if allowed by state law.

Table 1.4 **Professionals of Other Disciplines Who May Interact with the PTA**

- Occupational therapist (OT)
- Certified occupational therapy assistant (COTA)—works under the supervision and direction of the OT
- Speech-language pathologist
- Doctor—may include primary care physician (PCP), surgeon, physiatrist (doctor specializing in physical medicine and rehabilitation), doctor of osteopathic medicine (DO), neurologist
- Physician assistant (PA)
- Nurse—may include registered nurse (RN), licensed practical nurse (LPN), advanced practice nurse (APN), nurse practitioner (NP)
- Certified nursing assistant (CNA)—works under the direction and supervision of the nurse
- Social worker (MSW)
- Orthotist and/or prosthetist

Definitions of Healthcare Teams[1]

- Intradisciplinary team—members of the same discipline working together
- Multidisciplinary team—members of the team work independently within their own disciplines; do not necessarily share a common goal and have limited interaction between disciplines
- Interdisciplinary/Interprofessional team—members from all involved disciplines work together to set goals relevant to the individual patient and work collaboratively on the care plan

Interprofessional Collaboration[5]

- Definition: "When multiple health workers from different professional backgrounds work together with patients, families, caregivers and communities to deliver the highest quality of care"[5]
- Patient centered
- Community and population oriented
- Relationship focused
- Process oriented

Effective Teamwork[5,6]

- Communication, cooperation, coordination, and collaboration
- Interprofessional communication—listening actively, negotiating respectfully, consulting, discussing while attending to verbal and nonverbal parameters
- Awareness of roles and responsibilities of self and other professions
- Maintain mutual respect and shared values when working with other professions

Professional Communication Skills[7]

- Communication issues are identified as one of the top three root causes of untoward events that lead to significant patient harm.
- Common factors lead to poor communication between team members: lack of time, defensiveness, hierarchical structure, conflict, workload, distractions, poor sharing of information, and lack of clarity.
- Improve team function by using effective communication skills.

Table 1.5 Effective Communication Skills[7]

- Listen attentively—be fully present, mindful, not multitasking.
- Provide accurate information that is brief, clear, complete, and timely.
- Use eye contact and address the person by name.
- Express a concern, provide information, and recommend some form of action based on your assessment of the situation.
- Consider use of communication tools, i.e., SBAR (Situation, Background, Assessment, Recommendation). Check backs ensure that the message was received accurately. Hand offs ensure that complete and accurate information is received during transfer of care.
- Provide feedback to others and respond to feedback given by others on the team.

SECTION 1-3

Patient Communication

General Recommendations for Verbal Communication

Table 1.6 **General Recommendations**[1]

- Verbal commands should focus the patient's attention on specifically desired actions for intervention.
- Instructions should remain as simple as possible and must never incorporate confusing medical terminology.
- The general sequence of events should be explained to the patient before initiating the intervention.
- The PTA should ask the patient questions before and during the intervention to establish a rapport with the patient and to provide feedback on the status of the current intervention.
- The PTA should speak clearly in moderate tones and vary his or her tone of voice as required by the situation.
- The PTA should be sensitive to the patient/client's level of understanding and cultural background.

Methods of Effective Patient Communication[1]

- Greet the patient and provide a nonthreatening environment for the patient so that he or she feels welcome and valued.
- Display sensitivity to cultural influences through the careful selection of words and actions.
- When introducing yourself to the patient, position yourself to greet the patient at eye level.
- Be aware of cultural differences when establishing eye contact with the patient because this behavior may not be appropriate in some cultures.
- Introduce yourself by stating your name and title and refer to the patient by his or her last name and title. Avoid using first names and do so only if deemed appropriate by the patient. Ask the patient which name he or she would prefer that you use when addressing the patient to avoid offending and showing disrespect for the patient.
- Explain to the patient your role in the therapeutic relationship.
- Inform the patient what you plan to do initially.
- Advise the patient in regard to options for therapeutic interventions. If more than one option is available, share possibilities and invite the patient's input.
- Obtain informed consent from the patient for the intervention that is to be rendered.
- Advise the patient about the intervention's effects, indications, contraindications, and alternatives.
- Actively involve the patient in the intervention by determining the patient's participation during and after the intervention.
- Respond to the patient's questions and concerns throughout interactions.
- Promote patient autonomy and responsibility throughout interactions.

Informed Consent

Table 1.7 Intervention Elements of Informed Consent for the Patient[1]

- Clear description of the proposed intervention
- Reasonable alternatives to the proposed intervention
- Risks, benefits, and concerns of the proposed intervention
- Assessment of patient understanding
- Patient's acceptance of the intervention

Methods of Effective Listening[1]

- The PTA focuses his or her attention on the patient.
- The PTA helps the patient to feel free to talk by smiling and looking at the patient.
- The PTA pays attention to the patient's nonverbal communication, such as gestures, facial expressions, tone of voice, and body posture.
- The PTA asks the patient to clarify the meaning of words and the feelings involved or to enlarge upon the statement.
- The PTA reflects the patient's message to confirm that he or she understands completely the meaning and the content of the message.
- The PTA takes notes as necessary to help remember or document what was said.
- The PTA uses body language such as nonverbal gestures (nodding the head, keeping eye contact, or keeping hands at side if culturally appropriate) to show involvement in the patient's message.
- The PTA does not abruptly interrupt the patient, giving him or her adequate time to present the full message.
- The PTA empathizes with the patient.

SECTION 1-4

Cultural Competence

General Methods to Increase Cultural Competence

Table 1.8 Methods[1] to Increase Cultural Competence

- Identify personal cultural biases (ethnocentrism) and personal values and beliefs.
- Understand general cultural differences.
- Accept, respect, and value cultural differences.
- Apply cultural understanding.

Guidelines to Cultural Competence

- Provide services that are culturally and linguistically appropriate.
- Provide training to increase cultural awareness, knowledge, and skills.
- Recruit and retain minority staff.
- Provide interpreter services.
- Provide linguistic competency that extends beyond the clinical encounter to the appointment desk, advice lines, medical billing, and other written material.
- Coordinate evaluations and interventions with traditional healers.
- Use community healthcare workers.
- Incorporate culture-specific attitudes and values into health promotion tools.
- Include family and community members in healthcare decision-making.
- Locate clinics in geographic areas that are easily accessible for certain populations.
- Expand hours of operation.

Religious Beliefs and Health Concepts

Table 1.9 Selected Religious Beliefs and Health Concepts[8]

Patients/clients who are members of the Baha'i religious conviction essentially believe that "all healing comes from God." In regard to concepts of health, they have the following beliefs:

- Abortion is forbidden. Birth control is acceptable.
- Alcohol and drugs are forbidden.
- Medications can be used as necessary.
- Healing beliefs are that there is harmony between religion and science. No restrictions are placed on medical healing practices.
- Religious healing practices include prayer. Family and community members assist and support the patient/client.
- Organ donations are permitted.
- Surgical procedures are acceptable.
- Autopsy is not restricted if necessary (from a legal or medical perspective).

(continued)

Table 1.9 **Selected Religious Beliefs and Health Concepts**   *(continued)*

Patients/clients who are members of the Buddhist Churches of America religious conviction essentially believe that "to keep the body in good health is our duty—otherwise we shall not be able to keep our mind strong and clear." In regard to concepts of health, they have the following beliefs:

- Abortion is determined by the patient's condition. Birth control is acceptable.
- Food combinations are restricted, and extremes of diets must be avoided.
- Medications can be used as necessary.
- Healing beliefs are that people should not believe in healing through faith. No restrictions are placed on medical healing practices.
- Family and community members assist and support the patient/client.
- Organ donations are considered an act of mercy, and if there is a hope for recovery, all means may be taken.
- Surgical procedures are acceptable, avoiding the extremes.
- Autopsy is a matter of individual practice.

Patients/clients who are members of the Roman Catholic American religious conviction essentially believe that "the prayer of faith shall heal the sick, and the Lord shall raise him up." In regard to concepts of health, they have the following beliefs:

- Abortion is prohibited. Birth control is unacceptable.
- Food must be eaten in moderation.
- Medications may be taken if the benefits outweigh the risks. Healing beliefs vary depending on the regional religious belief system.
- No restrictions are placed on medical healing practices. Religious healing practices include the sacrament taken by the sick, praying by lighting candles, and having the priest perform a "laying on" of hands.
- Family, friends, the priest, and many outreach programs through the church are ready to assist and support the patient/client.
- Organ donations are permitted if are justifiable.
- Most surgical procedures are acceptable, except for abortion and sterilization.
- Autopsy is permissible.

Patients/clients who are members of the Christian Science religious conviction essentially believe that reliance on consecrated prayer to God, rooted in faith lifted to spiritual perception, is a practical and reliable method to care for all human needs, including health. In regard to concepts of health they have the following beliefs:

- Abortion is generally avoided but as with birth control is a matter of individual judgment.
- There are no food restrictions except for alcohol, tobacco, and sometimes caffeine.
- Medications are generally not used though it is an individual decision. Typically choose spiritual means for the prevention and healing of disease exclusive of medications.
- The church does not dictate individual health care choices. Healing belief includes an acceptance of both physical and moral healing through spiritual means. Religious healing practices may include spiritual healing support by Christian Science practitioners as well as Scriptural and other religious study and quiet prayer.
- Family, friends, and church members assist and support the patient/client. Christian Science Nurses may provide practical nonmedical care to the sick when only spiritual treatment is relied upon.
- Organ donations are left up to the individual's decision.
- Surgical medical procedures are typically avoided.
- Autopsy is not a usual event but may be decided by the individual and the family.

(continued)

Table 1.9 **Selected Religious Beliefs and Health Concepts**   *(continued)*

Patients/clients who are members of the Church of Jesus Christ of Latter Day Saints religious conviction believe the following in regard to concepts of health:

- Abortion is forbidden. Birth control is unacceptable because it conflicts with the Mormon religious belief.
- Alcohol, tea (except for herbal teas), coffee, and tobacco are forbidden. Fasting (24 hours without food and drink) is required once a month.
- Medications are not restricted, but patients/clients may use herbal folk remedies.
- Healing beliefs state that the power of God can bring healing. Medical healing practices are permitted. Religious healing practices include anointing with oil, sealing, prayer, and "laying on of hands."
- Family, friends, church members (such as the Elder and the Sister), and the Relief Society help other church members in case of sickness.
- Organ donations are permitted.
- Surgical medical procedures are permitted, being a matter of individual choice.
- Autopsy is permitted with consent from the next of kin.

Patients/clients who are members of the Hinduism religious conviction essentially believe that "Enricher, Healer of disease, be a good friend to us." In regard to concepts of health, they have the following beliefs:

- There is no policy in regard to abortion. All forms of birth control are acceptable.
- Eating meat is forbidden.
- Medications are acceptable.
- Healing beliefs vary. Some Hindus believe in medical interventions; others believe in faith healing. In terms of the regional religious belief system, no restrictions are placed on medical healing practices.
- Religious healing practice includes a traditional faith healing system. Family, friends, the priest, and the community provide support to the sick.
- Organ donations are permitted.
- Surgical procedures are acceptable. If a member needs an amputation, the loss of the limb is seen as a consequence of sins from a previous life.
- Autopsy is permissible.

Patients/clients who are members of the Islam religious conviction essentially believe that "the Lord of the world created me—and when I am sick, He healeth me." In regard to concepts of health, they have the following beliefs:

- Abortion is not permitted. Birth control is acceptable.
- Foods made with pork and those containing alcohol are forbidden.
- Medications are acceptable, except insulin, which may be refused if it is made from a porcine base (i.e., made from the pancreas of the pig).
- Medical interventions are acceptable. Faith healing generally is not acceptable, although some Muslims use it. In terms of the regional religious belief system, religious healing practices differ. Some Muslims use herbal remedies. Family and friends provide support to the sick.
- Organ donations are permitted.
- Most of the surgical procedures are permitted.
- Autopsy is permissible for medical and legal purposes.

(continued)

Table 1.9 **Selected Religious Beliefs and Health Concepts** *(continued)*

Patients/clients who are members of the Jehovah's Witnesses religious conviction believe the following in regard to concepts of health:

- Abortion is forbidden. Birth control and sterilization are prohibited.
- Tobacco is restricted, and alcohol can be consumed in moderation.
- Medications are acceptable if are not derived from blood or blood products.
- Medical interventions are acceptable if they do not involve blood or blood products. Faith healing is forbidden.
- Religious healing practices involve reading the scriptures to comfort the individual and to lead to mental and spiritual healing. Members of the congregation and Elders pray for the sick.
- Organ donations are forbidden.
- Surgical medical procedures are not opposed, but the administration of blood during surgery is strictly prohibited.
- Autopsy is acceptable if it is required by the law.

Patients/clients who are members of the Judaism religious conviction essentially believe that "O Lord, my God, I cried to Thee for help and Thou has healed me." In regard to concepts of health, they hold the following beliefs:

- Abortion is therapeutically permitted, and some groups accept abortion on demand. Birth control is acceptable, except within Orthodox Judaism.
- Strict dietary laws prohibit mixing of milk and meat. Foods made with pork, meat of predatory animals, fowl, and shellfish are forbidden. Kosher products are required in the diet.
- Medications are not restricted. Medical interventions are expected.
- Religious healing practices include prayers for the sick. Family, friends, the rabbi, and many community services are available to provide support to the sick.
- Organ donations are not permitted, being a very complex issue. Nevertheless, some people of the Judaism conviction practice organ donations.
- Most surgical procedures are permitted.
- Autopsy is permissible under certain circumstances.

Patients/clients who are members of the Mennonite religious conviction believe the following in regard to concepts of health:

- Abortion is acceptable for therapeutic reasons. Birth control is acceptable.
- There are no specific dietary restrictions.
- Medications are not restricted.
- Healing beliefs are considered part of God's work. To pray for the sick is the common practice. Medical interventions are acceptable.
- Religious healing practices include prayers and anointing with oil. Family and the community are available to support the sick.
- Organ donations are acceptable.
- Surgical medical procedures are acceptable.
- Autopsy is acceptable.

(continued)

Table 1.9 **Selected Religious Beliefs and Health Concepts** *(continued)*

Patients/clients who are members of the Seventh-Day Adventists religious conviction believe the following in regard to concepts of health:

- Abortion is acceptable for therapeutic purposes. Birth control is an individual choice.
- A vegetarian diet is encouraged.
- Medications are not restricted.
- Healing beliefs include the concept of divine healing. Medical interventions are permitted. Religious healing practices are anointing with oil and prayer. The family, the pastor, and the Elders pray and anoint the sick person.
- Worldwide, the Seventh-Day Adventist health system includes hospitals and clinics. Organ donations are permitted. Surgical medical procedures are permitted.
- Autopsy is acceptable.

Patients/clients who are members of the Unitarian/Universalist Church religious conviction believe the following in regard to concepts of health:

- Abortion is acceptable, is therapeutic, and can be offered on demand. All types of birth control are acceptable.
- Medications are not restricted. Healing beliefs are that faith healing is superstitious. Medical interventions are permitted.
- Religious healing practices are based on the belief that the use of science facilitates healing. Family, friends, and the church members support the sick. The pastor and the Elders pray and anoint the sick person.
- Organ donations are permitted.
- Surgical medical procedures are permitted.
- Autopsy is acceptable and recommended.

Note: The PTA is urged not to generalize from this guide but to show respect, sensitivity, and understanding to the individual patient/client.

Intervention Strategies Considering Cultural Diversity

Table 1.10 **Intervention Strategies[1] Considering Cultural Diversity**

When providing intervention to **Native American patients**, the therapist needs to recognize the importance of nonverbal communication.

- For example, for Navajo Native Americans, sustained eye contact when speaking directly with someone is rude and possibly confrontational, whereas avoiding eye contact is deemed a sign of respect.
- The therapist needs to focus on positive facial expressions without frowning or negative expression such as the flat affect.
- The therapist needs to address the older member of the family first, rather than the patient.
- Often, Native American patients observe the provider and say very little. They expect the provider to figure out their health problem through instinct rather than through the use of questioning.
- The conversation must be in a very low tone of voice. It is impolite to say, "I beg your pardon" or to imply that the communication was not heard.

(continued)

Table 1.10 **Intervention Strategies Considering Cultural Diversity**   *(continued)*

- The therapist must speak with the patient or the older member of the family in a quiet setting. Note taking is taboo.

- The therapist needs to use memory skills and not record patient's history on a writing pad. If the therapist needs to take patient history, he or she has to use a conversational approach while taking the history.

- Native American patients respond to interventions using silence; at other times, they leave and do not return.

- Consideration must be given to maintaining a very accessible, open schedule for the patient because time orientation is not a priority for Native American patients.

- Native American patients believe that health and wellness exist in a harmonious relationship with all other living things, including spirits.

- Problem solving and decision-making are group experiences. Respected elders or the family have to make decisions about rehabilitation.

When providing interventions or administering tests and measures to **brown- or black-skinned patients**, the therpaist should consider the patient's physiological and integumentary needs.

- For example, to identify pallor, the therapist should determine whether there is an absence of underlying red tones. The skin of the brown-skinned patient with pallor appears yellow-brown, whereas that of the black-skinned patient appears ashen-gray.

- Mucous membranes appear ashen, and the lips and nail beds show similar coloring.

- Erythema (redness) can be hard to detect but palpation reveals the skin is usually warmer in the area and, if edema is present, is tight, and the deeper tissues are hard.

- Cyanosis can be seen by close inspection of lips, tongue, and conjunctiva (of the eyelids). Lips and tongue may be ashen grey. Look for changes to the palms of the hands and the soles of the feet. One method of testing is pressing the palms. Slow blood return indicates cyanosis.

- Ecchymosis (superficial bleeding under the skin) from trauma can be detected by swelling of the skin surface.

- Keloids are scars that form at the site of the wound due to defective remodeling. Keloids are raised, excess scar tissue that continue to enlarge.

When providing interventions to **African American patients**, the therapist should consider the patient's beliefs and potential for practice of traditional healing practices. Physical therapy interventions can be combined with traditional practices as long as they are not antagonistic to each other.

- The patient's background, income, religious practices, and accessibility to health resources also need to be included in the list of considerations. For example, when suggesting an assistive device or an orthosis, the therapist must be familiar with formal and informal sources of help in the African American community.

- Including the patient's family in the rehabilitation process is essential to ensure the patient's motivation and positive outcomes. Because African Americans are verbally expressive, family members should be encouraged to discuss who will take responsibility as the primary caregiver.

- The therapist should keep an open line of communication and be sensitive to the need of African American patients to operate within a family unit.

(continued)

Table 1.10 **Intervention Strategies Considering Cultural Diversity**   (continued)

When providing interventions to **Asian American patients (including Pacific Islanders)**, the therapist should keep in mind the importance of communication and possible difficulties in communication. Many Asian American cultures value silence, such that talking too much can give a negative impression.

- Most East and Southeast Asian cultures emphasize respect and high consideration for authority. Consequently, patients from these cultural backgrounds will never disagree with or contradict the therapists.
- When patients cannot understand specific patient education topics, they may agree to follow through to "save face" and not to embarrass the authority figure (such as the healthcare provider).
- Patients try to avoid being disruptive and will agree to what is said so as not to be offensive.
- An interpreter can be used if the interpreter is able to understand the patient's dialect and regional language differences. Also, the interpreter's gender can be a problem if the interpreter is of the opposite gender and the patient is not comfortable sharing personal or intimate information with a stranger.
- As with any other patient, the therapist needs to establish a partnership with the Asian American patient. Having such a relationship will allow the patient to share information about use of alternative therapies and alert the therapist of any antagonist effects with medications or interventions.
- The therapist needs to help Asian American patients understand that they have a choice in making healthcare decisions. The patient or the patient's family may make decisions based on family needs and not medical needs; also consider financial and/or physical hardships faced by the family.
- In regard to interventions, the therapist should include the patient's extended family and the environmental context in which the patient lives.
- The interventions may have to integrate the Asian American patient's values that differ from Western ideology. These values may include interdependence, social belonging, and agreement with the patient's illness-related conditions.

When providing interventions to **Hispanic American patients**, the therapist should consider the importance of nonverbal communication, the patient's practice of traditional healing practices, language barriers, time orientation issues, and the caregiver's practice of performing self-care or activities of daily living for the patient.

- Important customs include communication strategies such as a smile that expresses warmth and concern, arms relaxed at sides (not crossed), good eye contact (not to members of the opposite sex), shaking hands, and speaking first with the male patient or caregiver.
- The therapist must consider that common traditional healing practices for patients of Puerto Rican and Mexican backgrounds can be found in "botanicas"—stores that sell traditional remedies such as herbs, potions, ointments, amulets, candles, medals, relics, and religious statues.
- A spiritualist may be present in the "botanica" and recommend certain herbs for the patient's illness.
- Other Hispanic American patients may visit a "santeria," a practitioner of Latin American magic who uses spirits to treat illness, or a "curandero," a traditional holistic healer.
- Physical therapy interventions can be combined with traditional healing treatments as long as they are not antagonistic.
- A language barrier, if present, can be remedied by using certified interpreters, who are generally accurate and nonjudgmental.
- The time orientation issue can be accommodated by maintaining an open or "walk-in" schedule.
- The therapist may need to explain to the caregiver the importance of increasing the patient's independence by having the patient take responsibility for activities of daily living and work with the caregiver by showing how to help the patient (without doing all the work for the patient).

Note: The PTA is urged to consider that each patient/client is unique; the strategies described here are simply intended to help maximize use of a culturally competent approach to delivering physical therapy interventions.

SECTION 1-5

Professionalism and Ethics

Professionalism in Physical Therapy

Table 1.11 Elements of Professionalism in Physical Therapy[1]

- Ethical principles and reasoning
- Attitudes of PTs and PTAs
- Decision-making
- Behaviors
- Judgments
- The relationship of PTs and PTAs with other professionals, the public and profession

Core Values for the PT and PTA[9]

The APTA identified one set of Core Values for the PT and PTA in 2019. They are intended to guide the behaviors of PTs and PTAs in providing the highest quality of physical therapy services.

Table 1.12 Core Values for the PT and PTA

- Accountability
- Altruism
- Collaboration
- Compassion and caring
- Duty
- Excellence
- Integrity
- Social responsibility

Integrity in Practice[10]

- Providing ethical and high-quality care
- Promoting evidence-based health care
- Maintaining compliance with documentation, billing coverage, and other regulatory requirements
- Preventing fraud, abuse, and waste in health care

Table 1.13 Examples of Fraud—Intentional Deception Made to Gain an Unentitled Benefit[10]

- Knowingly billing for services not furnished
- Knowingly altering claim forms to increase payment
- Falsifying documentation
- Using unlicensed individuals to provide services

Table 1.14 **Examples of Abuse—Unintentional or Unknowing Misrepresentation of Facts to Gain Payment[10]**

- Misusing codes on a claim
- Excessive charges for services or supplies
- Billing for services not medically necessary
- Billing individual components of an all-inclusive package

Table 1.15 **Waste—Overutilization of Services Resulting in Unnecessary Costs[10]**

- Spending on services that lack evidence of producing better outcomes compared with less expensive alternatives
- Failures of care coordination resulting in unnecessary readmissions, avoidable complications, or declines in functional ability
- Ordering unnecessary tests

Ethics and Professionalism[1]

- Ethical practice examines what is morally good, right, and wrong and involves decision-making.
- Morals are the basis for ethical decision-making and consist of an individual's beliefs, principles, and values.
- Professional ethics consider the ethical duties, obligations, and values of members of that profession.
- Professions develop policies, guidelines, codes of ethics and standards of conduct that must be adhered to by members.
- Ethical standards are not laws, but laws may reflect standards of ethical practice. In this case, a breach of ethical conduct may also result in a violation of the law.

Table 1.16 **Six Fundamental Ethical Principles[1,11]**

- Beneficence—Obligation to do the best for the patient
- Nonmaleficence—Do no harm to the patient
- Justice—Obligation to provide fair and equal treatment to every patient
- Veracity—Obligation for both therapist and patient to be truthful
- Confidentiality—Requirement to not divulge patient information to anyone not involved directly in that patient's care without prior consent
- Autonomy—The patient's right to make choices and decisions over their own care and have those decisions honored

References

1. Barrett C. *Dreeben-Irimia's Introduction to Physical Therapy for Physical Therapist Assistants.* 4th ed. Burlington, MA: Jones & Bartlett Learning; 2020.
2. American Physical Therapy Association. Guide for conduct of the physical therapist assistant. https://www.apta.org/your-practice/ethics-and-professionalism/apta-guide-for-conduct-of-the-physical-therapist-assistant. Accessed December 11, 2020.
3. American Physical Therapy Association. Levels of supervision. https://www.apta.org/apta-and-you/leadership-and-governance/policies/levels-supervision. Accessed December 11, 2020.
4. Skinner SB, McVey C. *Clinical Decision Making for the Physical Therapist Assistant.* Sudbury, MA: Jones and Bartlett LLC; 2011.
5. Interprofessional Education Cooperative. Core competencies for interprofessional collaborative practice: Update 2016. https://www.ipecollaborative.org/core-competencies.html. Accessed April 20, 2020.
6. Bainbridge L, Nasmith L, Orchard C. Competencies for interprofessional collaboration. *J Phys Ther Educ.* 2010;24(1)6–11.
7. Plack MM, Driscoll M. *Teaching and Learning in Physical Therapy: From Classroom to Clinic.* 2nd ed. Thorofare, NJ: Slack Inc.; 2017.
8. Spector RE. *Cultural Diversity in Health and Illness.* 6th ed. Upper Saddle River, NJ: Pearson Prentice Hall; 2004.
9. American Physical Therapy Association. Core values for the physical therapist and physical therapist assistant. https://www.apta.org/apta-and-you/leadership-and-governance/policies/core-values-for-the-physical-therapist-and-physical-therapist-assistant. Accessed December 11, 2020.
10. American Physical Therapy Association. Preventing fraud, abuse and waste: A primer for physical therapists. https://www.apta.org/your-practice/ethics-and-professionalism/preventing-fraud-abuse-and-waste. Accessed December 11, 2020.
11. Swisher LL, Royeen CB. *Rehabilitation Ethics for Interprofessional Practice.* Burlington, MA: Jones and Bartlett Learning; 2020.

Safety in the Clinical Environment

Infection Control

Personal Protective Equipment Overview

Many employers have a standardized policy regarding infection control measures and provide the necessary training and equipment for healthcare workers who are exposed to various bacterial and viral infections throughout the course of their normal workday. It is imperative that healthcare workers comply with these established policies to protect themselves from unavoidable exposure as well as prevent cross contamination from those patients who may be afflicted with a communicable disease. Decreasing risks to exposure of infectious disease processes can be readily achieved by the use of standardized handwashing between patient encounters as well as wearing personal protective equipment.

Personal protective equipment (PPE), according to Siegel and coauthors, is any means or combination of various types of barriers that may be used to protect an individual from an unwanted exposure to some type of infectious agent or contamination.[1]

This protection may include the use of gowns, masks, boots, boot coverings, coveralls, and safety glasses. Masks can come in two forms: surgical masks or respirators. According to the Centers for Disease Control (CDC),[2] Fit testing for a respirator is a practice that may reduce infectious transmission of diseases related to droplet or airborne types of exposure (i.e., coughing, sneezing, and sputum exposure). These diseases may include but not be limited to severe strains of influenza and tuberculosis. Fit testing is typically performed by the Occupational Medical Department of the hospital or skilled nursing facility where the clinician is employed or at the local health department. The benefit of fit testing is that it promotes a tighter seal over the nose and mouth. The respirator has a one-way valve to prevent the pathogen from being breathed in by a clinician who must work in direct contact or within 6 feet of an infected individual.[3]

Use of PPE is not confined to healthcare workers employed in hospitals. Some home health clinicians may also need to be fit tested for a respirator if they will be working with a homebound patient who may have droplet or airborne-related precautions.

CDC's Recommended Standard Precautions[4]

Table 2.1 CDC's Standard Precautions

Practicing Hand Hygiene[5]

Wash hands with soap and water or use an alcohol-based hand sanitizer before and after patient contact and after having direct contact with any substance found in the patient care environment. Alcohol-based hand rubs (gel or foam) kill bacteria more effectively and more quickly than handwashing with soap and water. Alcohol-based hand rub is the preferred method for hand hygiene in *all situations*, except in situations when the hands are visibly dirty or contaminated. Soap and water should also be used before eating and after using the restroom.

Wash hands or use an alcohol-based hand sanitizer immediately:

- Before touching a patient
- Before putting on gloves
- Before performing an invasive procedure or manipulating an invasive device
- After having contact with the patient's skin

(continued)

Table 2.1 **CDC's Standard Precautions**   *(continued)*

- After having contact with blood or bodily fluids or excretions, nonintact skin, a wound dressing, or contaminated items
- After having contact with inanimate objects near a patient
- After removing gloves
- After touching items, surfaces, or physical therapy equipment in the immediate patient care environment (even if the patient was not touched by the physical therapist [PT] or physical therapist assistant [PTA])

Gloves

- Wear gloves when touching blood, body fluids, secretions, excretions, mucous membranes, nonintact skin, and contaminated items/surfaces.
- Put on clean gloves just before touching mucous membranes or nonintact skin. Change gloves between tasks and procedures on the same patient after contact with any material that may contain a high concentration of microorganisms.
- Remove gloves promptly after use, before touching noncontaminated items and environmental surfaces, and before going to another patient. Wash hands immediately to avoid transfer of microorganisms to another patient or environment.
- Do not reuse or wash gloves.
- Perform hand hygiene prior to donning gloves and after removing gloves.

Mask, Eye Protection, Face Shield

- Wear a mask and eye protection or a face shield to protect mucous membranes of the eye, nose, and mouth during procedures and patient care activities that are likely to generate splashes or sprays of blood, body fluids, secretions, or excretions.
- Wear a fit-tested face mask during procedures or encounters that are likely to result in airborne or droplet exposure of highly communicable diseases.

Gown

- Wear a clean, nonsterile gown to protect skin and to prevent soiling of clothing during procedures and patient care activities that are likely to generate splashes or sprays of blood, body fluids, secretions, or excretions.
- Select a gown that is appropriate for the activity and the amount of fluid likely to be encountered.
- Remove a soiled gown as promptly as possible, and wash hands to avoid transfer of microorganisms to other patients or environments.

Patient Care Equipment

- Handle used patient-care equipment that has been soiled with blood, body fluids, secretions, or excretions in a manner that prevents skin and mucous membrane exposures, contamination of clothing, or transfer of microorganisms to other patients or environments.
- Ensure that reusable equipment is not used for the care of another patient until it has been cleaned and reprocessed appropriately.
- Ensure that single-use items are discarded properly.

Environmental Control

- Ensure that the hospital has adequate procedures for the routine care, cleaning, and disinfection of environmental surfaces, beds, bedrails, bedside equipment, and other frequently touched surfaces, and ensure that these procedures are being followed.

(continued)

SAFETY IN THE CLINICAL ENVIRONMENT

Table 2.1 CDC's Standard Precautions   *(continued)*

Linen

■ Handle, transport, and process used linen that has been soiled with blood, body fluids, secretions, and excretions in a manner that prevents skin and mucous membrane exposures and contamination of clothing and avoid transfer of microorganisms to other patients and environments.

Occupational Health and Blood-Borne Pathogens

■ Take care to prevent injuries when using scalpels, needles, and other sharp instruments or devices, when handling sharp instruments after procedures, when cleaning used instruments, and when disposing of used needles.

■ Never recap used needles or otherwise manipulate them by using both hands or any other technique that involves directing the point of a needle toward any part of the body. Instead, use either a one-handed scoop technique or a mechanical device designed for holding the needle sheath.

■ Do not remove used needles from disposable syringes by hand. Do not bend, break, or otherwise manipulate used needles by hand.

■ Place used disposable syringes and needles, scalpel blades, and other sharp items in appropriate puncture-resistant containers, which should be located as close as practical to the area in which the items were used. Place reusable syringes and needles in a puncture-resistant container for transport to the reprocessing area.

■ If you are exposed to infectious blood-borne pathogens, immediately irrigate the exposed area with water and clean any wounds with soap and water or skin disinfectant immediately.

■ Report exposures immediately to your employer and seek medical attention.

Resuscitation

■ Ensure that resuscitation bags or other ventilation devices are readily available where the need for resuscitation is predictable.

Patient Placement

■ Place a patient who contaminates the environment or who does not (or cannot be expected to) assist in maintaining appropriate hygiene or environmental control in a private room.

■ If a private room is not available, consult with infection control professionals regarding patient placement or other alternatives.

CDC Guidelines for Airborne, Droplet, and Contact Transmission-Based Precautions

Table 2.2 Airborne Transmission Guidelines—Infections: Tuberculosis, Measles, and Chickenpox

1. Airborne Infection Isolation Room (AIIR)
2. Mask or fit -test respirator mask when entering the room
3. Limit patient movement out of the room
4. Patient mask when transporting the patient out of the room

Table 2.3 Droplet Transmission Guidelines—Infections: Mumps, Rubella, Pertussis, and Influenza

1. Single patient room
2. Mask when entering the room
3. Limit patient movement out of the room
4. Patient mask when transporting the patient out of the room
5. Patient to maintain at least 3 feet from others
6. Patient to follow respiratory hygiene practices/cough etiquette

Table 2.4 Direct Contact Transmission Guidelines

1. Single patient room
2. Gloves and gown (when touching the patient or the patient's environmental surfaces)
3. Single-patient-use equipment
4. Limit patient movement out of the room
5. Patient to maintain at least 3 feet from others

Occupational Safety and Health Administration's Universal Precautions Recommendations

Table 2.5 Recommendations for Blood-Borne Pathogen and Needlestick Prevention[6]

- Use protective equipment and clothing whenever in contact with bodily fluids.
- Dispose of waste in proper containers and follow the appropriate procedures for handling infectious waste.
- Dispose of sharp instruments and needles in the proper containers.
- Keep the work area and the patient area clean.
- Wash hands immediately after removing gloves and at all times, as required by the agency policy.
- Immediately report any exposure to needlesticks or blood splashes or any personal illness to the direct supervisor and receive instructions about follow-up action.

Asepsis Methods[7]

1. Sterilization of instruments

   - Heat (250°F–270°F/121°C–132°C) and water pressure
   - Ionizing radiation to sterilize medications, plastics, or sutures
   - Flash steam sterilization
   - Low temperature sterilization technologies (ethylene oxide, chlorofluorocarbons ozone)

2. Disinfection (reducing microorganism)

   - Ultraviolet light—for air and surface disinfection
   - Ultrasonic cleaning—for instruments

- Washing with antimicrobial products—for surfaces and hands
- Chemicals such as chlorine and chlorine compounds, iodine solutions, phenolics, quaternary ammonia, hydrogen peroxide
- Hydrotherapy disinfection—includes draining and cleaning tanks, and scrubbing pumps and equipment with a germicidal agent such as chlorine bleach, povidone-iodine, or Chloramine-T
- Antiseptic solutions: alcohol and iodine
- Germicidal soaps
- Antibacterial additives to whirlpools, tubs, tanks, or pools

Types of Nosocomial Infections (Hospital-Acquired Infection)

1. Urinary tract infections
2. Surgical site infections
3. Respiratory tract infections
4. Bloodstream infections
5. Intestinal tract infections
6. Central nervous system infections
7. Nosocomial fungal infections
8. Nosocomial pneumonia such as bacterial pneumonia, Legionnaires' pulmonary aspergillosis, Mycobacterium tuberculosis, viral pneumonias, or influenza
9. Other nosocomial infections by pathogen—*Staphylococcus, Pseudomonas, Escherichia coli*; antibiotic-resistant nosocomial infections such as methicillin-resistant *Staphylococcus aureus,* vancomycin-resistant *Staphylococcus aureus,* vancomycin-resistant enterococci

Infectious Diseases

- Blood-borne pathogens
  - Human Immunodeficiency Virus (HIV)
  - Hepatitis B (HBV)
  - Hepatitis C (HCV)
- Respiratory Disorders
  - Tuberculosis

1. **Acquired immunodeficiency syndrome** (AIDS)[8]: severe phase of the HIV infection; loss of immune system function resulting in the following:
   - Opportunistic infections: *Pneumocystis carinii* pneumonia, esophageal candidiasis, cytomegalovirus infection, Cryptococcus, atypical mycobacteriosis, chronic herpes simplex, toxoplasmosis, or *Mycobacterium* tuberculosis
   - Neurologic dysfunctions: AIDS dementia complex, central nervous system toxoplasmosis, cryptococcal meningitis, encephalopathy, peripheral neuropathy
   - Unusual cancers: Kaposi's sarcoma, non-Hodgkin's lymphoma, primary brain lymphoma

Table 2.6 Possible Transmission of HIV[8]

Direct contact with infected body fluids:

- Blood
- Semen
- Cerebrospinal fluid
- Breast milk
- Vaginal/cervical secretions
- Rectal fluids

Table 2.7 High-Risk Behaviors for HIV[8]

- Unprotected sexual contact
- Needle sharing or injections with contaminated needles
- Maternal–fetal transmission before and during birth or through breastfeeding

Table 2.8 Low-Risk Behaviors for HIV

- Needlesticks
- Casual contacts such as hugging and kissing

Table 2.9 Medical Management of HIV (To Stop HIV Replication)

- Multidrug therapy
- Patient education to prevent the spread of the disease and live a healthy lifestyle
- Supportive care

2. **Hepatitis:**[9] inflammation of the liver commonly caused by viral infection but may also be due to bacterial infection, disease, alcohol, drugs, medication and other toxins. Common types of viral hepatitis:
   - Hepatitis A virus (HAV)—acute infectious hepatitis transmitted through fecal-oral route, contaminated food or water, or close and personal contact with an infected person. A vaccine is available.
   - Hepatitis B virus (HBV)—hepatitis transmitted through contact with infected body fluids or tissues via oral or sexual contact, blood and blood product exposure, birth to an infected mother, and contaminated needles. A vaccine is available.
   - Hepatitis C virus (HCV)—transmitted in the same manner as HBV. It can cause liver damage and liver cancer. There is no vaccine for this type of hepatitis.

Table 2.10 **Prevention of HAV**

- Good hygiene
- Handwashing after using the toilet
- Sanitation
- HAV vaccination
- Healthcare workers wear PPE

Table 2.11 **Medical Management of HAV**

- Intravenous fluids
- Analgesics
- Treatment of acute symptoms

Table 2.12 **Prevention of HBV**

- HBV vaccination
- Education
- Lifestyle changes
- Healthy habits
- Sanitation
- Healthcare workers wear PPE

Remember that the HBV is more contagious than HAV and can survive on a contaminated surface for as long as 7 days.

Table 2.13 **Medical Management of HBV**

- No cure
- Rest, adequate nutrition, and fluids
- Medication for chronic HBV

Table 2.14 **Prevention of HCV**

- Education
- Lifestyle changes
- Sterilization of piercing or tattoo equipment
- Healthcare workers wear PPE
- Patient education to decrease the spread of the disease and to encourage healthy habits

Table 2.15 Medical Management of HCV

- Interferon, Ribavirin or other HCV direct acting antiviral agent
- Treatment of acute illness
- Patient education

3. **Tuberculosis (TB):**[10] highly contagious airborne respiratory infection

- Transmitted through *Mycobacterium* tuberculosis from contact with an infected person
- Spreads from coughing, sneezing, or singing through droplets or sputum

Table 2.16 Medical Management of Acute Tuberculosis

- Airborne precautions
- Isolation until cleared from the contagious stage
- Drug therapy using anti-TB medications for acute illness (e.g., rifampin and isoniazid)

Domestic and Family Violence

Domestic and Family Violence Overview

The American Physical Therapy Association defines family violence as "the intentional intimidation or abuse of children, adults, or elders by a family member, spouse/partner, or caretaker to gain power and control over the victim."[12] The CDC reports that one in four women and one in ten men have experienced some form of intimate partner violence (IPV) during their lifetime. This includes contact sexual violence, physical violence, and stalking. IPV also includes psychological aggression by an intimate partner and more than 43 million women and 38 million men will experience this type of IPV in their lifetime.[13] In 2019, at least one in seven children experienced child abuse and/or neglect. Child abuse claimed the lives of at least 1,770 children in 2018.[14] The CDC reports that elder abuse is common with one in ten community dwelling elders, over 60 years of age, experiencing some form of elder abuse.[15]

Elder Abuse

Elder abuse is defined as "a single, or repeated act, or lack of appropriate action, occurring within any relationship where there is an expectation of trust which causes harm or distress to an older person" and is considered to be underreported globally (World Health Organization, 2020).[16]

In a systematic review by Johannesen and LoGiudice in the journal *Age and Ageing* (2013), elder abuse can be broken into the following five subtypes:[17]

- Emotional or psychological abuse is where the abuser demeans, threatens, causes fear, isolation, deprivation, feelings of shame and powerlessness to the person (see **Table 2.18** for examples).
- Physical abuse may take the form of intentional acts that cause physical pain or injury.
- Sexual abuse includes unwanted sex acts, both physical (fondling, rape) or through exploitative behavior or sexual language that was not consented to by the victim or where consent was garnered in a coercive manner.
- Financial abuse includes gaining control over the victim's finances by illegal use, improper use, or mismanagement of the personal property or financial resources of the victim.
- Neglect occurs when the caregiver does not provide the person with life's necessities or prevents others from providing the necessary and appropriate care.

Child Abuse[14]

Child abuse as described by the CDC is "all types of abuse or neglect inflicted on anyone under the age of 18 by a parent, caregiver, or person assuming a custodial role (coach, teacher, clergy) that results in harm or potential harm." Children under the age of 4 are most vulnerable. The four common types of child abuse are listed below:

- Physical abuse is the use of physical force, such as hitting, kicking, shaking, burning, or other shows of force against a child.
- Sexual abuse involves engaging a child in sexual acts. It includes behaviors such as fondling, penetration, and exposing a child to other sexual activities.
- Emotional abuse refers to behaviors that harm a child's self-worth or emotional well-being. Examples include name-calling, shaming, rejection, withholding love, and threatening.
- Neglect is the failure to meet a child's basic physical and emotional needs. These needs include housing, food, clothing, education, and access to medical care.

Healthcare workers, especially PTs and PTAs, are in a unique position to identify potential abuses that may be occurring in the relationships of those patients that we service during the rehabilitation process just by virtue of the various types of environments in which we work (e.g., hospitals, skilled nursing, home health, school-based/early childhood intervention).

Keen observation skills coupled with exposure to the integumentary system allows PTs and PTAs to recognize the signs and symptoms that often accompany any type of abusive situation. Standard 4F of the American Physical Therapy Association's (APTA) Standards of Ethical Conduct for the PTA endorses the reporting of suspected abuse to the appropriate authority, subject to law.[18] The PTA should be aware of state laws that identify who is considered a mandated reporter. As healthcare workers, PTAs are considered mandated reporters in many states.

Physical therapy providers may be able to intercede through routine screening, including keen observations and active listening, allowing for early identification and intervention for an abusive situation. Community awareness and appropriate referral resources also are responsibilities of the PT and PTA when working with a patient in an abusive situation.

Regardless of the setting, it is important that clinicians realize that any form of abuse warrants action regardless of age, gender, sexual orientation, race, cultural beliefs, or socioeconomic status.

Table 2.17 **PTA Action Steps Related to Suspected Abuse**[13–15,18]

1. Inform supervising PT of suspected abuse and if directed by the supervising PT, you may be asked to contact one of the national call centers.

   - National Child Abuse Hotline: 1-800-4-A-Child (1-800-422-2253)
   - Elder Abuse Helplines and Hotlines: 1-800-677-1116
   - National Domestic Violence Hotline: 1-800-799-SAFE (7233)

2. Always dial 911 or local police during emergencies.

How to Recognize Forms of Domestic and Family Abuse

Table 2-18 **Forms of Domestic and Family Abuse (Sexual, Child, Spousal/Partner/Elder)**[19]

- Using physical violence such as hitting, kicking, or other means of physical force
- Using sexual violence, such as forcing the victim to have sexual intercourse or to engage in other sexual activities against the intimate partner's will
- Using children as pawns, such as accusing the intimate partner of bad parenting, threatening to take the children away, or using the children to relay messages to the partner
- Using denial and blame, such as denying that the abuse occurred or shifting responsibility for the abusive behavior onto the partner
- Using coercion and threats, such as threatening to hurt other family members, pets, children, or self
- Using economic abuse, such as controlling finances, refusing to share money, sabotaging the partner's work performance, making the partner account for money spent, or not allowing the partner to work outside the home
- Using intimidation, such as using certain actions, looks, or gestures to instill fear, and breaking things, abusing pets, or destroying property

(continued)

SAFETY IN THE CLINICAL ENVIRONMENT

Table 2.18 Forms of Domestic and Family Abuse (Sexual, Child, Spousal/Partner/Elder)   *(continued)*

- Using emotional abuse, such as insults, criticism, or name calling
- Using social isolation, limiting the victim's contact with family and friends, requiring the partner to obtain permission to leave the house, not allowing the partner to attend work or school, or controlling the partner's activities and social events
- Using privilege, such as making all major decisions, defining the roles in the relationship, being in charge of the home and social life, or treating the partner as a servant or possession

Difficulties in Identifying and Helping Victims of Domestic and Family Violence[19]

1. Healthcare provider's fears or experiences of exploring the issue of family violence
2. Healthcare provider's lack of knowledge of community resources
3. Healthcare provider's fear of offending the victim and jeopardizing the provider-patient relationship
4. Healthcare provider's lack of time or lack of training
5. Healthcare provider's unresponsiveness, feeling powerless, and not being able to fix the situation
6. Infrequent victim's visits as a patient
7. Victim's unresponsiveness to questions (asked by the healthcare provider)

Methods to Overcome Difficulties in Identifying and Helping Victims of Domestic and Family Violence

Table 2.19 Methods to Overcome Difficulties in Identifying and Helping Victims of Domestic and Family Violence[19]

- Observe the victim for physical and behavioral clues.
- Question the victim and validate the presence of family abuse.
- Respect the victim's privacy and use confidentiality measures.
- If a PTA suspects a patient to be a victim of family abuse, the PTA should immediately report the findings to the PT of record.
- Keep accurate records and precise documentation about the victim's abuse.
- Support and follow up the victim's care.

Signs Indicating a Victim of Domestic or Family Violence[19]

1. The abuser accompanies the victim to all appointments and refuses to allow the victim to be interviewed alone. The abuser uses verbal or nonverbal communication to direct the victim's responses during appointments.

2. The patient is noncompliant with physical therapy treatment regimens and/or frequently misses appointments.
3. The patient makes statements about not being allowed to take or obtain medications (prescription or nonprescription medication).
4. The abuser cancels the victim's appointments or sabotages the victim's efforts to attend appointments (by not providing child care or transportation).
5. The patient engages in therapist hopping.
6. The patient lacks independent transportation, access to finances, or ability to communicate by phone.
7. The abuser tries to explain away the bruising or fracture as the victim's clumsiness.[20]

Domestic and Family Violence Signs Requiring Screening[19]

- The victim's chronic pain
- Injuries during pregnancy
- The victim's repeated and chronic injuries
- Unmanaged gynecological problems
- The victim's exacerbated or poorly controlled chronic illnesses such as asthma, seizure disorders, diabetes, hypertension, or heart disease
- The victim's physical symptoms related to stress, anxiety disorders, or depression; hypervigilant signs such as being easily startled or very guarded; the victim experiencing nightmares or emotional numbing
- The victim's suicide attempts or evidence of self-mutilation
- Eating disorders
- Car accidents in which the victim is the driver or the passenger
- The victim's overuse of prescription pain medications and other drugs

Table 2.20 **Methods to Overcome Difficulties in Identifying and Helping Victims of Child Abuse**

- Observe the victim for physical and behavioral clues.
- Question the victim and validate the presence of abuse.
- Respect the victim's privacy and use confidentiality measures.
- Observe the victim for signs of fear or unwillingness to answer questions with the parent/guardian present.
- Observe the victim looking for approval from the parent/guardian before answering any questions.
- Question answering by the adult/guardian for the child and use of words as "clumsy" to explain away the potential signs of bruising/injury.
- Keep accurate records and precise documentation about the victim's abuse.
- If a PTA suspects a patient to be a victim of child abuse, the PTA should immediately report the findings to the PT of record and to appropriate authorities as mandated by state law.
- Support and follow up the victim's care.

SAFETY IN THE CLINICAL ENVIRONMENT

Patient Safety During Interventions

Normative Values for Vital Signs

Table 2-21 Blood Pressure Normative Values: Adult[21]

Category	Systolic Blood Pressure		Diastolic Blood Pressure
Normal	120 mm Hg or less	and	80 mm Hg or less
Elevated	120–129 mm Hg	and	80 mm Hg or less
Stage I hypertension (HTN)	130–139 mm Hg	or	80–89 mm Hg
Stage II HTN	≥140 mm Hg	or	≥90 mm Hg
Hypertensive crisis	≥180 mm Hg	and/or	≥ 120 mm Hg

Table 2.22 Blood Pressure Normative Values: Infant/Child/Adolescent[22]

Normal blood pressure (BP): infant = 87–105/53–56 mm Hg

Normal BP: child = 97–112/57–71 mm Hg

Normal BP: adolescent = 112–128/66–80 mm Hg

Table 2.23 Heart Rate Normative Values

Normal heart rate (HR): adult = 70 beats per minute (bpm) (range = 60–100)

Abnormal HR: adult = bradycardia = less than 60 bpm

Abnormal HR: adult = tachycardia = more than 100 bpm

Normal HR: infant = 120 bpm (range = 70–170)

Normal HR: child = 125 bpm (range = 75–140)

Normal HR: adolescent = 85 bpm (range = 50–100)

Table 2.24 Temperature and Respiratory Rates

Temperature: Oral	Respiratory Rate (RR)
Normal temperature: adult = 98.6°F (37°C)	Normal RR: adult = 12–18 breaths/min
Normal temperature: adolescent = 98.6°F (37°C)	Normal RR: adolescent = 15–22 breaths/min
Normal temperature: child = 95.9–99.5°F (35.5–37.5°C)	Normal RR: child = 20–40 breaths/min
Normal temperature: infant = 95.9–99.5°F (35.5–37.5°C)	Normal RR: infant = 30–50 breaths/min

Table 2.25 Elements that Increase or Decrease Blood Pressure, Heart Rate, Respiratory Rate, and Temperature

- Increase BP/HR/RR/temperature: infection, anxiety, pain, exercise (only systolic BP and HR), high blood sugar, low blood sugar, and low potassium (only HR), low hematocrit, and hemoglobin (only HR and RR), acute myocardial infarction, coronary artery disease, asthma, and anemia
- Decrease BP/HR/RR/temperature: decreased hemoglobin and hematocrit (only systolic BP and temperature), decreased potassium (only systolic BP), acute myocardial infarction (only HR and systolic BP), narcotics, increased potassium (only HR), decreased blood sugar (only temperature), and anemia (only systolic BP)

Patient Emergency Situations

1. BP = more than 160/100 mm Hg or less than 90/60 mm Hg (may not need to call the emergency medical services; the PTA must take into consideration the patient/client's age, medications, and interventions; may need to stop the interventions, inform the PT, and monitor the patient/client carefully)
2. Resting HR = more than 110 bpm or less than 60 bpm (may not need to call the emergency medical services; the PTA must take into consideration the patient/client's age, medications, and interventions; may need to stop the interventions, inform the PT, and monitor the patient/client carefully)
3. Resting RR = more than 30 breaths/min (may not need to call the emergency medical services; the PTA must take into consideration the patient/client's age, medications, and interventions; may need to stop the interventions, inform the PT, and monitor the patient/client carefully)
4. Absent or decreased breath sounds
5. Sudden cognitive changes
6. Chest discomfort, shortness of breath, sweating, or faintness
7. Sudden severe headache and facial pain
8. Abdominal discomfort, nausea, and/or bloody or dark, tarry stools

General Signs and Symptoms That Warrant Discontinuing Physical Therapy Interventions

Table 2.26 Signs and Symptoms[23] That Warrant Discontinuing Interventions

- Temperature: more than 100°F (37.8°C)
- Systolic BP: more than 250 mm Hg
- Diastolic BP: more than 115 mm Hg
- Fall in systolic BP: more than 10 mm Hg; and a rise in HR: more than 15 bpm
- Resting HR: more than 130 bpm or less than 40 bpm
- Chest pain, palpitations, or irregular pulse
- Oxygen saturation: less than 90%
- Blood glucose: more than 250 mg/dL
- Cyanotic or diaphoretic
- Dizziness or syncope
- Bilateral leg/foot edema

Signs and Symptoms of Hyperglycemia: High Blood Sugar of More Than 200 mg/dL[23]

- Extreme thirst and frequent urination
- Blurred vision and dry skin
- Nausea, vomiting, or abdominal pain
- Fatigue and lethargy
- Dizziness and increased appetite
- Weight loss and infections
- Glucose and ketones in the urine

Table 2.27 **Emergency Treatment: Hyperglycemia and Ketoacidosis**

- Call for medical assistance; monitor the patient until help arrives; inform the PT.
- Hyperglycemia can cause ketoacidosis and ultimately diabetic coma (and death).

Signs and Symptoms of Hypoglycemia: Low Blood Sugar of Less Than 70 mg/dL[23]

- Increased heart rate and lightheadedness
- Sweating, unsteadiness, and weakness
- Headache, fatigue, and impaired vision
- Confusion, pallor, and behavior changes
- Clumsiness and tingling sensation in the mouth

Table 2.28 **Emergency Treatment: Hypoglycemia**

Patient needs fast-acting carbohydrates: half of a cup of orange juice, four or five candies, glucose tablets, or a glass of milk.

Intervention Precautions for Patients with Diabetes

Table 2.29 **Intervention Precautions for Patients with Diabetes[23]**

- Plan the patient's exercises in conjunction with food intake and insulin administration. Ask the patient about his or her nutritional status prior to performing interventions.
- Monitor the patient's glucose levels before exercises. Do not exercise patients with blood glucose ≤70 g/dL or ≥250 mg/dL.
- Monitor the injection site before exercises. Do not exercise at or near the muscles where the injection of insulin was administered. Do not administer interventions such as physical agents at the injection site.
- Exercise at or around the same time of day.
- Do not administer thermal interventions without testing the patient's superficial sensations.

Table 2.29 Intervention Precautions for Patients with Diabetes   *(continued)*

- Do not exercise patients with a high level of ketones in their urine or blood.
- Inform the PT if the patient experienced hypoglycemia or hyperglycemia.
- Educate the patient about avoiding exercising or activities late at night or just before sleep (can cause hypoglycemia at night).
- Educate the patient about diabetic foot care.
- Educate the patient to monitor blood glucose levels before and after exercise and, if exercise is prolonged, during exercise. During or after exercise, hypoglycemia can be managed with a fast-acting carbohydrate (e.g., fruit juice, candy, or honey). Post exercise hypoglycemia may be delayed several hours after exercise. A protein and carbohydrate snack post exercise can help manage this issue.

Signs and Symptoms of Electrolyte Disturbances[23]: Hyperkalemia (High Potassium Level in Blood)

- Reference value (adults): 3.5–5.0 mEq/L. Levels below 3.2 or greater than 5.1 mEq/L may be contraindication for PT
- Muscle weakness and flaccid paralysis
- Initial tachycardia followed by bradycardia and arrhythmia
- Diarrhea and abdominal cramps

Table 2.30 Possible Causes of Hyperkalemia

- High-potassium diet
- Kidney failure
- Addison's disease (hyposecretion of adrenocortical hormones secondary to infections such as tuberculosis or hemorrhage)
- Trauma to muscle
- Decreased aldosterone insulin

Table 2.31 Clinical Safety Measures for Hyperkalemia

- Monitor the patient's cardiopulmonary response to physical therapy interventions.
- Inform the PT.

Signs and Symptoms of Electrolyte Disturbances[23]: Hypokalemia (Low Potassium Level in Blood)

- Muscle fatigue and cramps in the legs
- Slowed reflexes
- Orthostatic hypotension
- Dizziness and arrhythmia

- Irritability and confusion
- Depression
- Respiratory distress
- Nausea, constipation, and vomiting

Table 2.32 **Possible Causes of Hypokalemia**

- Poor nutrition
- Anorexia
- Cushing's disease (hypersecretion of adrenal cortex and excessive production of glucocorticoids secondary to tumor or excessive stimulation of adrenal gland)
- Diuretic medications, steroids
- Dehydration

Table 2.33 **Clinical Safety Measures for Hypokalemia**

- Monitor the patient's cardiopulmonary response to interventions.
- Watch the patient for orthostatic hypotension.
- Inform the PT.

Signs and Symptoms of Electrolyte Disturbances[23]: Hypernatremia (High Sodium Level in Blood)

- Reference value (adults): 135–145 mEq/L
- Weight gain and pitting edema
- Pulmonary edema and dyspnea
- Hypertension and tachycardia
- Restlessness, agitation, and confusion

Table 2.34 **Possible Causes of Hypernatremia**

- Cushing's disease
- Fluid loss (excessive sweating)
- Decreased fluid intake
- Dehydration
- Kidney disease

Table 2.35 **Clinical Safety Measures for Hypernatremia**

- Observe the patient for the signs and symptoms of hypernatremia.
- Monitor the patient's cardiopulmonary response to interventions.
- Inform the PT.

Signs and Symptoms of Electrolyte Disturbances[23]: Hyponatremia (Low Sodium Level in Blood)

- Muscle weakness and muscle twitching
- Hypotension and tachycardia
- Anxiety and headache
- Restlessness and convulsions
- Cyanotic and cold, clammy skin
- Shock

Table 2.36 **Possible Causes of Hyponatremia**

- Addison's disease
- Poor sodium intake
- Excessive fluid retention
- Kidney disease
- Excessive fluid loss (due to sweating, vomiting, diarrhea, or diuretic medications)

Table 2.37 **Clinical Safety Measures for Hyponatremia**

- Observe the patient for the signs and symptoms of hyponatremia.
- Monitor the patient's hypotension.
- Inform the PT.

Signs and Symptoms of Electrolyte Disturbances[23]: Hypercalcemia (High Calcium Level in Blood)

- Reference value (adult): 9–11 mg/dL. Less than 7 results in tetany, greater than 12 leads to coma.
- Generalized weakness and decreased muscle tone
- Weight loss and anorexia
- Bone pain and fractures
- Drowsiness and lethargy
- Headache and confusion
- Hypertension and cardiac arrest

Table 2.38 **Possible Causes of Hypercalcemia**

- Hyperparathyroidism
- Bone cancer
- Multiple fractures
- Osteoporosis
- Excess intake of calcium, vitamin D

Table 2.39 Clinical Safety Measures for Hypercalcemia

- Monitor the patient's cardiopulmonary response to interventions.
- Inform the PT.

Signs and Symptoms of Electrolyte Disturbances[23]: Hypocalcemia (Low Calcium Level in Blood)

- Muscle cramps and spasms and tetany
- Tingling and numbness
- Irritability and anxiety
- Convulsions
- Hypotension and arrhythmia

Table 2.40 Possible Causes of Hypocalcemia

- Renal disease
- Renal failure
- Hyperparathyroidism
- Decreased absorption of calcium in the gastrointestinal system
- Decreased vitamin D
- Hypoparathyroidism

Table 2.41 Clinical Safety Measures for Hypocalcemia

- Monitor the patient's cardiopulmonary system, especially for orthostatic hypotension.
- Inform the PT.

Signs and Symptoms of Respiratory Acidosis[23]: CO_2 Retention and Impaired Alveolar Ventilation

- PH<7.35
- Dyspnea and cyanosis
- Headache and disorientation
- Decreased deep tendon reflexes (DTRs) and possible coma
- Restlessness and anxiety

Table 2.42 Possible Causes of Respiratory Acidosis

- Hypoventilation
- Chronic obstructive pulmonary disease (asthma, bronchitis, pneumonia, and emphysema)
- Guillain-Barré syndrome
- Myasthenia gravis
- Hypermetabolism (in burns or sepsis)
- Drugs and certain medications (sedatives, narcotics)

Table 2.43 Clinical Safety Measures for Respiratory Acidosis

- Observe the patient for the signs and symptoms of respiratory acidosis.
- Monitor the patient's cardiopulmonary system.
- Inform the PT.
- Respiratory acidosis may lead to disorientation, stupor, and coma or death.

Signs and Symptoms of Respiratory Alkalosis: Low CO_2 and Alveolar Hyperventilation

- PH > 7.45
- Tachypnea and anxiety
- Dizziness and paresthesia
- Blurred vision and diaphoresis
- Arrhythmia and numbness and tingling
- Tetany and convulsions

Table 2.44 Possible Causes of Respiratory Alkalosis

- Hypoxemia
- Anxiety attacks and hyperventilation
- Congestive heart failure
- Pulmonary embolism
- Aspirin poisoning
- Stress
- Central nervous system disease
- Scoliosis
- Excessive exercise

Table 2.45 Clinical Safety Measures for Respiratory Alkalosis

- Observe the patient for the signs and symptoms of respiratory alkalosis.
- Monitor the patient's cardiopulmonary system.
- Inform the PT.

Signs and Symptoms of Overhydration: Excess of Body Fluid

- Swelling or edema in the interstitial tissues
- Shortness of breath with activities
- Increased blood pressure and heart rate
- Lethargy and headache
- Muscle cramps and stiffness and twitches
- Weight gain and pitting edema of the extremities

Table 2.46 Possible Causes of Overhydration

- Excessive fluid intake
- Congestive heart failure
- Renal failure
- Cirrhosis

Table 2.47 Clinical Safety Measures for Overhydration

- Observe the patient for the signs and symptoms.
- Monitor the patient's cardiopulmonary system.
- Elevate the extremities.
- Inform the PT.

Signs and Symptoms of Dehydration: Extreme Decrease of Body Fluid

- Poor skin turgor and skin integrity
- Headache and lethargy
- Increased body temperature and muscle cramps
- Vertigo and orthostatic hypotension
- Irritability, confusion, disorientation, and incoordination
- Rapid heart rate and respiratory rate
- Diarrhea and vomiting

Table 2.48 Possible Causes of Dehydration

- Heat
- Emesis
- Diuretics
- Sodium deficiency
- Sweating

Table 2.49 **Clinical Safety Measures for Dehydration**

- Monitor the patient's cardiopulmonary system, especially for orthostatic hypotension.
- Monitor the patient for fainting or fatigue.
- Inform the PT.
- Ensure adequate hydration during exercise

Deep Vein Thrombosis and Pulmonary Embolus

Table 2.50 **Signs and Symptoms of Deep Vein Thrombosis and Pulmonary Embolus**[23]

Deep Vein Thrombosis (DVT)

- Tenderness or leg pain
- Leg or calf swelling (circumferential leg difference of 1.4 cm for men, 1.2 cm for women is significant)
- Warmth
- Subcutaneous venous distention
- Discoloration
- Palpable cord
- Positive findings on the Wells' Clinical Decision Rule (see **Table 2.51**)

Pulmonary Embolus (PE)

- Dyspnea
- Chest pain (pleuritic pain = sharp, localized pain)
- Persistent cough
- Tachypnea
- Tachycardia
- Hemoptysis (bloody sputum)
- Fever
- Anxiety/restlessness

Table 2.51 **Wells' Clinical Decision Rule for DVT**

Predictor	Score
Previous diagnosis of DVT	1
Active malignancy	1
Lower extremity immobilization (recent) or paralysis	1
Bedridden for past 3 days or major surgery in past 4 weeks	1

(continued)

Table 2.51 Wells' Clinical Decision Rule for DVT *(continued)*

Predictor	Score
Local tenderness (center of posterior calf, popliteal space, or along femoral vein in anterior thigh/groin)	1
Entire lower extremity swelling	1
Unilateral pitting edema	1
Calf difference ⩾ 3 cm	1
Vein distention (nonvaricose)	1
Other diagnosis as likely or more likely than DVT (e.g., calf strain, cellulitis)	−2

Interpretation:
Score ⩽ 0 = low probability of DVT (3%)
Score 1–2 = moderate probability of DVT (17%)
Score ⩾ 3 = high probability of DVT (75%)
From: Wells P, Anderson D, Bormanis J, et al. Value of assessment of pretest probability of deep vein thrombosis in clinical management. Lancet. 1997;350(9094):1795–1798.
Fruth S, Fawcett C. *Fundamentals of Tests and Measures for the Physical Therapist Assistant.* Jones and Bartlett Learning; 2020.

Table 2.52 DVT/PE Risk Factors[23]

- Blood stasis (immobilization, prolonged bed rest [i.e., patients with following diagnoses or conditions: burns, comatose, obstetric/gynecologic, paralysis, elderly or obese])
- Endothelial injury (i.e., surgery, trauma, pelvic or lower extremity fractures, peripherally inserted central catheter (PICC) lines)
- Hypercoagulable states (i.e., clotting disorders, cancer)
- Congestive heart failure diagnosis
- Recent surgery (i.e., total hip arthroplasty, total knee arthroplasty, prostate)
- Recent air or long-distance travel (prolonged sitting with hips and knees flexed)
- Age 50 or over
- Previous history of thromboembolism
- Oral contraceptive use
- Post stroke
- Diabetes mellitus

Table 2.53 International Normalized Ratios (INR)[23,24]

- Healthy, uncoagulated individuals = 0.9–1.1
- Mechanical heart valve patients = 2.5–3.5
- Postsurgical patients = 2.0–3.0
- Post CVA patients = 2.0–3.0
- Cardiac/atrial fibrillation patients = 2.0–3.0

*This lab value is associated with warfarin (Coumadin) use for anticoagulation and is a standardized measure that is used globally.

Clinical Safety Measures for Anticoagulation Therapy

Table 2.54 Clinical Safety Measures for Anticoagulation Therapy: Guidelines for Exercise Interventions Related to PT-INR Lab Values[23,24]

- PT-INR between 2.0–3.0: Proceed with treatment.
- PT-INR > 3.0 in nonmechanical heart valve replacement situations: Proceed with caution with exercise/therapeutic activity, check with nurse or medical doctor preceding treatment. Risk of hemarthrosis becomes elevated with an INR >3.0; adverse effects of falls may result in excessive bleeding; the intensity or activity should be limited until the PT-INR is back in the therapeutic range of 2.0–3.0.
- PT-INR between 5.0–6.0: Hold PT; no activity of any kind, as blood thinning may be at critical levels. Hold PT until PT-INR levels return to 2.0–3.0, which is usually in 2–3 days.

**Always check with the nurse or medical doctor to ensure compliance with the protocol of the treating physician regarding limitations for PT-INR levels and physical therapy participation.

Table 2.55 DVT/PE PTA Pearls

- Always check with nurse or medical doctor when the patient is on anticoagulation therapy before working with the patient.
- Provide patient education for DVT prophylaxis (i.e., ankle pumps, walking, avoidance of prolonged bed rest, avoidance of sitting with hips and knees flexed).
- Know norms for acceptable PT-INR levels for cardiovascular conditions and postsurgical conditions.
- Be aware of subtle signs and symptoms of blood thinning (i.e., nose bleeds, blood-shot eyes, complaints of melena, blood in urine, increased bruising).
- Use caution with manual techniques, TheraBand use, stretching techniques, and taking blood pressure with patients on blood-thinning medications to avoid bruising or joint hemarthrosis.

Acute Care Safety

Table 2.56 Acute Care/Subacute Care Safety

- Check with nursing personnel to temporarily remove suction tubes or disconnect tube feedings.
- Do not dislodge peripheral or central lines. Ask for nursing assistance.
- Do not disrupt the setup of vital medical equipment. Endotracheal tubes, nasogastric tubes, and arterial and central venous catheters contribute to the patient's morbidity and mortality. Ask for nursing assistance.
- Before transfer and ambulation, ensure that the patient is properly dressed. Loose clothing and inappropriate footwear (such as slippers, socks without shoes, or sandals) are not safe. Shoes need to be nonslip, to fit snugly, and to have a low, wide heel.

(continued)

Table 2.56 Acute Care/Subacute Care Safety   *(continued)*

- A safety belt should always be used in transfers and ambulation. The transfer surfaces need to be secured by locking the wheelchair (and stabilizing the wheelchair against a wall or using a wooden block under the wheelchair wheels to increase stability). Transfer surfaces should be at the same height or level as possible.

- The therapist should not hold onto the patient's joints or fragile areas.

- During ambulation and transfers, the urinary (Foley) catheter drainage bag must be secured below the patient's bladder and 2 inches above the floor. The bag must be repositioned after interventions.

- Before ambulation and transfers, inspect the Foley catheter. The tubing must be straight and not twisted.

- When working with patients who suffered fractures and are in traction (such as Bryant's traction or external traction), do not bump the bed or disturb the traction devices (weights). Team up with the nursing staff to reposition the patient and prevent decubitus ulcers.

Outpatient Safety

Table 2.57 Outpatient Safety

- Wash hands between patients.
- Use appropriate PPE when exposure to blood-borne pathogens or biohazards is imminent.
- Use proper lifting and body mechanics when working with patients.
- Practice safe clean-up procedures between patients, including wiping tables/equipment down with an approved disinfecting agent per your company's policy.
- Ensure shoelaces are tied and proper footwear is worn by the patients during treatment.
- Avoid dislodgement of any subdermal ports or fistulas when working with patients.
- Know your company's policies for tornado, fire, flood, workplace violence, and bomb threats.
- Know where the exits are in your facility.
- Make sure equipment is certified or calibrated; remove any malfunctioning equipment from use until repairs are completed.

Home Health Safety

Table 2.58 Home Health Safety[25]

- Provide credentials prior to entering the home.
- Call the patient the night before; ask them to secure pets in another area.
- If entering a high crime area, be aware of your surroundings, call the patient to make them aware of your arrival.
- Reschedule the appointment if you are fearful to park and walk up to the patient's home.
- Know your company's policy on securing additional protection when servicing high crime regions.
- Keep your shoes on in unhygienic situations, use surgical booties in cultural situations related to shoe removal upon entering a patient's home.

(continued)

Table 2.58 Home Health Safety   *(continued)*

- Use appropriate PPE to deter exposure to blood-borne pathogens, biological hazards, or chemical exposures.
- Do not place your home health equipment bag on the floor. Place a disposable barrier between your bag and the surface.
- Use good ergonomics when lifting/transferring patients.
- Be mindful of environmental hazards encountered in the home (i.e., icy sidewalks, water on floors, clutter in walking pathways, porches/concrete in disrepair).
- Keep your car maintained and gas tank full.
- Inform someone where you are at all times.

Select Medications and Patients' Adverse Reactions in the Clinic

Table 2.59 Select Medications and Patients' Adverse Reactions in the Clinic[26]

Medication Group	Most Widely Used Brand Names	Adverse Reactions
Nonnarcotic (nonopioid) analgesics	Aspirin (ASA), Ecotrin	ASA: GI distress, GI bleeding, anemia, tinnitus, hearing loss, dizziness, easy bruising, skin rash
Acetaminophen	Anacin 3, Halenol, Liquiprin, Panadol, Tempra, Tylenol	GI distress, dizziness, lethargy, chills, diaphoresis Chronic use: may cause renal damage or renal failure
Other nonsteroidal anti-inflammatory drugs (NSAIDs)	Advil, Aleve, Anaprox, Naproxen, Motrin, Nuprin, Ibuprofen, Daypro, Dolobid, Feldene, Lodine, Nalfon, Actron, Orudis, Tolectin, Voltaren, Relafen, Celebrex, Vioxx	Headache, dizziness, somnolence (Feldene and Relafen), vertigo, lightheadedness, fatigue, drowsiness, confusion, HTN (Advil, Motrin, Nuprin), blurred vision, skin eruptions, pruritus, rash, fluid retention with edema, GI bleeding, nausea, tinnitus, hearing loss
Narcotic (opioid) analgesics	Hycodan (hydrocodone), Vicodin, Tylenol with codeine (Tylenol #3), Paveral (codeine), OxyContin, Roxicodone, Percolone (oxycodone), Darvon	Nausea, vomiting, lethargy, confusion, lightheadedness, drowsiness, dyspnea, bradycardia, orthostatic hypotension and facial flushing, physical and psychological dependence (Tylenol #3, Paveral), dizziness

SAFETY IN THE CLINICAL ENVIRONMENT

(continued)

Table 2.59 **Select Medications and Patients' Adverse Reactions in the Clinic** *(continued)*

Medication Group	Most Widely Used Brand Names	Adverse Reactions
Muscle relaxant	Soma, Lioresal (baclofen), Paraflex, Parafon Forte, Flexeril, Valium (apo-diazepam), Vivol, Marbaxin, Robaxin	Orthostatic hypotension, facial flushing, tachycardia, bradycardia, nausea, vomiting, drowsiness, dizziness, lightheadedness, ataxia, tremor, headache, vertigo, irritability, diplopia, blurred vision, skin rash, fatigue, slurred speech
Antihypertensive and cardiac (CHF): ACE inhibitor	Capoten, Vasotec, Prinivil, Zestril, Monopril, Accupril, Lotensin	Skin rash, cough, headache, dizziness, fatigue, orthostatic hypotension, GI distress, impaired taste
Antihypertensive and cardiac (angina): calcium-channel blocking agent	Cardizem, Dilacor XR, Tiazac, Calan, Isoptin (verapamil), Verelan, Norvasc, Adalat, Procardia	Headache, fatigue, dizziness, lightheadedness, vertigo, drowsiness, nervousness, insomnia, confusion, gait abnormality, tremor, edema, hypotension, palpitations, skin flushing, GI distress, skin rash, dyspnea, peripheral edema
Antihypertensive and cardiac (angina, arrhythmia, acute MI): beta blocker	Apo-propranolol, Inderal, Novo-Pranol, Tenormin (apo-atenolol), Apo-Metoprolol, Lopressor, Toprol	Confusion, agitation, fatigue, vertigo, drowsiness, weakness, insomnia, bradycardia, hypotension, cold extremities, GI distress, paresthesia of hands, dyspnea
Antidepressants	Elavil, Norpramin, Pertofrane, Sinequan, Nardil, Zonalon, Wellbutrin, Zyban, Prozac, Sarafem, Zoloft, Effexor, Paxil	Drowsiness, dizziness, fatigue, headache, orthostatic hypotension, tachycardia, dry mouth, GI distress, urinary retention, tinnitus, blurred vision, skin rash, HTN, and dyspnea (Zoloft)

ASA: acetylsalicylic acid; CHF: congestive heart failure; GI: gastrointestinal; HTN: hypertension; MI: myocardial infarction

Contraindications to and Precautions for Physical Agents and Modalities

Table 2.60 Contraindications to and Precautions for Physical Agents and Modalities[27,28]

Physical Agent or Modality	Contraindications	Precautions
Therapeutic heat (hot packs, fluidotherapy, contrast baths)	DVT and malignant tumors; open wounds; hemorrhage and bleeding; impaired sensation; impaired cognition; inability to communicate; ischemia and immature scar; atrophic and infected skin	Acute injury, inflammation, edema, pregnancy, cardiac insufficiency, metal (i.e., jewelry in the area), creams or ointments in the area, demyelinated nerves; monitor sensory capability of pediatric and geriatric patients.
Whirlpool	Chronic wounds (eschar); nonlocalized infection wounds; clean granulating wounds; epithelializing wounds; migrating epidermal cells; new skin grafts; new tissue flaps; venous ulcers; non-necrotic diabetic ulcers; bleeding; bowel/bladder incontinence Patients with skin infections; unstable blood pressure; severe epilepsy; upper respiratory infections; tuberculosis and cellulitis; edema of the extremities; lethargy; unresponsiveness; wound maceration; febrile conditions; compromised cardiovascular and pulmonary function; acute phlebitis; renal failure; dry gangrene; incontinence (in full-body whirlpool)	Check whirlpool ground-fault circuit interrupter. Check whirlpool water temperature: ■ Limbs = 103°F–110°F (40°C–43.5°C) ■ Full body immersion not to exceed 102°F (39°C) ■ Open wound = 92°F–96°F (33°C–35°C) ■ Multiple sclerosis = 88°F (31°C) ■ Peripheral vascular disease (PVD) = 95°F–100°F (35°C–37.8°C) Insert tank liner for patients with hepatitis, open wounds, burns, and HIV. Impaired thermal sensation, generalized weakness, cardiac medications, pregnancy, multiple sclerosis. Hubbard Tank: Closely monitor patient's physiological responses.
Paraffin bath	Open wounds and allergic rash; skin infections and recent scars and sutures	Wash the patient's hands or feet prior to application of paraffin bath. Temperature range: 126°F–134°F (52°C–57°C)

(continued)

SAFETY IN THE CLINICAL ENVIRONMENT

Table 2.60 Contraindications to and Precautions for Physical Agents and Modalities[27,28]   *(continued)*

Physical Agent or Modality	Contraindications	Precautions
Aquatic therapy	Bowel or bladder incontinence (except patients who are catheterized); urinary tract infection (UTI) and severe epilepsy; unprotected wounds; unstable blood pressure and severe cardiorespiratory dysfunctions	Patients should shower before immersion. Check water temperature: ■ General pool temperature range = 79°F–97°F (26°C–36°C)
Ultraviolet radiation	Skin cancer; pulmonary TB; irradiation of the eyes; systemic lupus erythematosus; cardiac, kidney or liver disease	Antibiotics such as tetracycline or sulfonamides and drugs such as psoralens can increase photosensitivity and combined with UVL can result in burns to the skin. Photosensitivity; recent X-ray therapy
Ultrasound (US)	Malignancy; hemorrhage; healing fractures; TB; thrombophlebitis; epiphysis of growing bones (of young children); over eye, carotid sinuses; cervical ganglia and spinal cord after a laminectomy; reproductive organs; cardiac pacemaker or other implantable cardiac device, joint cement, plastic implants, and pregnant uterus, recent X-ray therapy	Chronic wounds; damaged or at risk skin; acute inflammation/injury (contraindicated with thermal US). Thermal US periosteal pain must be stopped by decreasing intensity; increasing treatment surface area. Thermal US temperature increases at tissue interfaces: bone/ligaments; bone/joint capsule; bone/muscle. US "hot spot" must be stopped by applying more coupling agent, decreasing the intensity, or moving the transducer. Use a plastic container for US in the water.
Diathermy	Young children (younger than 4 years old); PVD and infections; active DVT, thrombophlebitis, applications over metal, cardiac pacemaker, neural stimulators; malignancy; pregnancy, testes; eyes; and epiphyses of growing bones, acute injury/ inflammation, hemorrhage, impaired cognition, local infection, recent X-ray therapy, TB	Cardiac failure Check the patient often during treatment—the treated area is not visible. Nonthermal SWD (short wave diathermy) is safe for use with metal implants.

(continued)

Table 2.60 Contraindications to and Precautions for Physical Agents and Modalities[27,28] *(continued)*

Physical Agent or Modality	Contraindications	Precautions
Therapeutic cold	Impaired circulation and sensation; Raynaud's disease or phenomenon; PVD; sensitivity/allergic reaction to cold; carotid sinuses, prolonged application over superficial nerves (can result in neurapraxia)	Impaired sensation, impaired cognition, open wound, cardiac failure, hypertension. Monitor patients the first time for urticaria = erythema of the skin with wheal formation and severe itching (remove cold); facial flush = eyelids puffiness and respiratory problems (remove cold); anaphylaxis = decreased blood pressure, increased heart rate, syncope (call emergency services). Monitor the patient's normal physiological response to ice: cold, burning, aching, and numbness (CBAN).
Therapeutic massage	Acute inflammation in the treatment area; acute febrile conditions; severe atherosclerosis; severe varicose veins; DVT phlebitis and recent surgery; thrombophlebitis; cardiac arrhythmia; severe rheumatoid arthritis and hemorrhage; edema secondary to kidney dysfunction, heart failure, and venous insufficiency	Therapeutic massage is a passive modality that is typically used for a short period of time as an adjunct, not as a substitute, to active interventions such as therapeutic exercises, activities, and patient education.
Intermittent compression	Acute inflammation; acute DVT and arterial insufficiency; peripheral arterial disease (PAD) and arterial ulcers; obstructed lymphatic channels; cancer and acute pulmonary edema; cardiac insufficiency; edema in patients with CHF; kidney insufficiency and hypertension; local infection; acute trauma; recent fractures; very young and very old patients	Uncontrolled hypertension, impaired sensation or cognition. Check the patient's blood pressure carefully. Place the patient in a comfortable position with the upper or lower extremity abducted between 20 and 70 degrees, and elevated at approximately 40 degrees.
Electrical stimulation	Healing fractures; demand-type pacemaker, implantable defibrillator; areas of active bleeding; thrombophlebitis; pregnancy; malignancy; active tuberculosis; cardiac arrhythmias and heart conduction dysfunction; localized infection; application over carotid sinuses, pharyngeal or laryngeal muscles; eyes; recent X-ray therapy	Obesity and areas of decreased or absent sensation; severe edema and diabetes; patients with thin fragile skin; peripheral neuropathies; denervated muscle, spinal cord injury (can acquire dysreflexia), diminished cognition, impaired sensation, growing epiphysis

(continued)

SAFETY IN THE CLINICAL ENVIRONMENT

Table 2.60 Contraindications to and Precautions for Physical Agents and Modalities[27,28] *(continued)*

Physical Agent or Modality	Contraindications	Precautions
Iontophoresis	The same as for electrical stimulation; previous allergic reactions to medication or to direct current; cuts, bruises or broken skin; metal near treatment area; recent scars	Check for intact skin; no scratches or abrasions in treatment area. Reminder: Use negative medication for the negative (–) electrode and positive medication for the positive (+) electrode. Use low levels of current intensity for the (–) electrode; the (–) electrode must be twice as large as the (+) electrode.
Transcutaneous electrical nerve stimulation (TENS)	The same as for electrical stimulation; do not apply TENS over the eyes, mucosal membranes, laryngeal or pharyngeal muscles, or head and neck following a cerebral vascular accident, on very young or very old patients, or on patients with epilepsy	Patient education for TENS units: not to be used in the shower or when sleeping; electrode placement; skin inspection—skin irritation; checking adherence of electrodes to the skin; accommodation to electrical stimulation (patient to contact PT/PTA—needs modulation).
Traction	Spinal traction contraindicated for meningitis; spinal cancer; spinal cord pressure; spondylolisthesis; rheumatoid arthritis; osteoporosis and recent fracture; hypertension; osteopenia; acute soft-tissue injury; Down's syndrome; joint hypermobility or instability; very young and very old patients; acute whiplash injury, peripheralization of symptoms with traction.	Spinal traction: acute inflammation aggravated by traction; acute strains and sprains; claustrophobia; hiatal hernia; inability to tolerate prone of supine positions; anxiety with traction; pregnancy; temporomandibular joint (TMJ) syndrome (when using a cervical halter). Cervical traction: observe patient for discomfort in the TMJ—adjust the head halter and ensure force is applied to the occipital region. In general, the traction force should not exceed the weight of the patient's head (can start with a force that is 7% of the patient's body weight).

Pain Management[29,30]

Long term use of prescription opioids is appropriate for certain conditions, i.e., cancer treatment, end-of-life care, but evidence does not support long-term opioid use for the management of chronic pain. Evidence is also insufficient to support opioid use for long-term management of low back pain, headache, and fibromyalgia. Potential risks associated with all narcotics are identified in **Table 2.59**. Cognitive behavioral therapy (CBT), exercise therapy, weight loss and nonopioid medications are recommended by the CDC for management of chronic pain.

Table 2.61 Physical Therapy for Pain Management

- Pain related to acute injury, trauma, or infection is short lived and most of the time resolves as the tissues heal and the infection goes away, but in some cases, pain can persist or recur, becoming chronic.
- Pain is always subjective and varies among individuals. Contextual factors may contribute to how individuals experience and process pain.
- PTs and PTAs provide evidence-based pain management that addresses the needs of the patient and includes physical, cognitive, and behavioral approaches to help manage pain and disability.
- Strategies focus on active self-management of the pain by the patient as opposed to only focusing on passive interventions.
- PTs and PTAs use strategies to aide early, but appropriate, return to function and activity.
- Successful pain management may require an interdisciplinary approach for some patients.
- The PTA should be aware of and understand the roles and scope of practice of other disciplines within the pain management team.
- PTs and PTAs should use valid and reliable assessment tools and outcome measures to assess and monitor pain.
- Intervention should consider cultural and societal factors and reflect goals and priorities of the patient.

References

1. Siegel JD, Rhinehart E, Jackson M, Chiarello L, and the Healthcare Infection Control Practices Advisory Committee. 2007 guideline for isolation precautions: Preventing transmission of infectious agents in healthcare settings. https://www.cdc.gov/infectioncontrol/guidelines/isolation/index.html. Accessed July 27, 2020.
2. Centers for Disease Control and Prevention. Healthcare respiratory protection resources. https://www.cdc.gov/niosh/npptl/hospresptoolkit/policies.html. Accessed July 27, 2020.
3. Centers for Disease Control and Prevention. Filtering out confusion: Frequently asked questions about respiratory protection, fit testing. https://www.cdc.gov/niosh/docs/2018-129/default.html. Accessed July 27, 2020.
4. Centers for Disease Control and Prevention. Standard precautions for all patient care. https://www.cdc.gov/infectioncontrol/basics/standard-precautions.html. Accessed July 27, 2020.
5. Centers for Disease Control and Prevention. Hand hygiene in healthcare settings: Healthcare providers. https://www.cdc.gov/handhygiene/providers/index.html. Accessed July 27, 2020.
6. Occupational Safety and Health Administration. Bloodborne pathogen and needlestick prevention. https://www.osha.gov/bloodborne-pathogens. Accessed July 27, 2020.
7. Centers for Disease Control and Prevention. Disinfection and sterilization. https://www.cdc.gov/infectioncontrol/guidelines/disinfection/index.html. Accessed July 27, 2020.
8. Centers for Disease Control and Prevention. HIV. https://www.cdc.gov/hiv/clinicians/index.html. Accessed July 27, 2020.
9. Centers for Disease Control and Prevention. Viral hepatitis. https://www.cdc.gov/hepatitis/index.htm. Accessed July 28, 2020.
10. Centers for Disease Control and Prevention. Tuberculosis. https://www.cdc.gov/tb/. Accessed July 28, 2020.

11. Centers for Disease Control and Prevention. Hepatitis C. http://www.cdc.gov/hepatitis/hcv/hcvfaq.htm. Accessed September 10, 2015.

12. Family Violence. apta.org. http://www.apta.org/uploadedFiles/APTAorg/About_Us/Policies/Health_Social_Environment/FamilyViolence.pdf. Accessed September 25, 2015.

13. Centers for Disease Control and Prevention. Violence prevention: Preventing intimate partner violence. https://www.cdc.gov/violenceprevention/intimatepartnerviolence/fastfact.html. Accessed July 28, 2020.

14. Centers for Disease Control and Prevention. Violence prevention: Child abuse and neglect prevention. https://www.cdc.gov/violenceprevention/childabuseandneglect/index.html. Accessed July 28, 2020.

15. Centers for Disease Control and Prevention. Violence prevention: Preventing elder abuse. https://www.cdc.gov/violenceprevention/elderabuse/fastfact.html. Accessed July 28, 2020.

16. World Health Organization. Elder abuse. https://www.who.int/news-room/fact-sheets/detail/elder-abuse. Accessed July 28, 2020.

17. Johannesen M, LoGiudice D. Elder abuse: A systematic review of risk factors in community-dwelling elders. *Age and Ageing.* 2013 May;42(3):292–298.

18. American Physical Therapy Association Standards of Ethical Conduct for the Physical Therapist Assistant. apta.org. https://www.apta.org/apta-and-you/leadership-and-governance/policies/standards-of-ethical-conduct-for-the-physical-therapist-assistant. Accessed July 29, 2020.

19. Barrett C. *Dreeben Irimia's Introduction to Physical Therapy for Physical Therapist Assistants.* 4th ed. Burlington, MA: Jones & Bartlett Learning; 2020.

20. Potter C. He just bumps into things: Recognizing and reporting signs of child abuse. *Magazine of Phys Ther.* 2000;8(4):52–62.

21. Understanding Blood Pressure Readings. heart.org. https://www.heart.org/en/health-topics/high-blood-pressure/understanding-blood-pressure-readings. Accessed July 29, 2020.

22. University of Iowa Stead Family Children's Hospital. Vital signs: Normal blood pressure. https://uichildrens.org/health-library/vital-signs-normal-blood-pressure-mmhg-picu-chart. Accessed July 29, 2020.

23. Goodman C, Fuller K, Marshall C. *Pathology for the Physical Therapist Assistant.* 2nd ed. St. Louis, MO: Elsevier; 2017.

24. Mayo Clinic. Prothrombin time tests. https://www.mayoclinic.org/tests-procedures/prothrombin-time/about/pac-20384661. Accessed August 4, 2020.

25. Home health care. osha.gov. http://www.osha.gov/SLTC/home_healthcare. Accessed August 4, 2020.

26. Ciccone CD. *Pharmacology in rehabilitation.* 4th ed. Philadelphia, PA: F.A. Davis; 2007.

27. Cameron M. *Physical agents in rehabilitation.* 5th ed. St. Louis, MO: Elsevier; 2018.

28. Canadian Physiotherapy Association. Electrophysical agents contraindications and precautions: An evidence based approach to clinical decision making in physical therapy. *Physiother Can.* 2010;62(5):1–80 doi: 10.3138/ptc.62.5. Epub 2011 Jan 5

29. International Association for the Study of Pain. IASP curriculum outline on pain for physical therapy. https://www.iasp-pain.org/Education/CurriculumDetail.aspx?ItemNumber=2055. Accessed August 10, 2020.

30. Centers for Disease Control and Prevention. Checklist for prescribing opioids for chronic pain. https://stacks.cdc.gov/view/cdc/38025. Accessed August 10, 2020.

SAFETY IN THE CLINICAL ENVIRONMENT

Clinical Documentation

CLINICAL DOCUMENTATION

Documentation Guidelines

General Documentation Guidelines

Table 3.1 General Guidelines[1,2]

- The patient's right to privacy should be respected regarding written information; personal data are included in the examination and evaluation, reexamination, reevaluation, progress note and in the daily note/treatment note. A SOAP (Subjective, Objective, Assessment, Plan) format may be used for documentation, but caution should be applied to ensure that each section is completed accurately and with required detail.
- The release of medical information, including written physical therapy documentation, must be authorized by the patient in writing.
- All inquiries for medical information submitted to the physical therapist assistant (PTA) should be directed to the supervising physical therapist (PT).
- Treatment notes should include the date and time of service and provider signature. Patient cancellations and "no shows" should be documented and date noted.
- Always write on every line in the chart.
- Write using one pen. If the pen runs out of ink in the middle of an entry, indicate in parenthesis that the first pen ran out of ink.
- Do not backdate an omission in the intervention record. Document any omitted prior entry as a new entry.
- Do not write any entries expressing personal feelings about a patient/client, such as "This patient seems to be malingering."
- Do not write any entries expressing disapproval of or denigrating other healthcare providers or personnel.
- When an interpreter is used this should be noted in the treatment record.
- Any pertinent phone calls with the patient should be recorded and supported by date and time of the conversation.
- Written physical therapy records should be kept in a safe and secure place for 7 years. State practice acts may have specific guidelines on how long records should be kept and these should be consulted.

American Physical Therapy Association (APTA) Documentation Guidelines

Table 3.2 APTA Guidelines[1,2]

- The documentation must be consistent with the APTA's Standards of Practice.
- All documentation must be legible and use facility or practice setting approved abbreviations or symbols.
- All documentation should be legible and written in black or blue ink. Errors must be crossed out with a single line through it, initialed, and dated by the PTA.
- Each intervention session must be documented. The patient's name and identification number must appear on each page of the documentation record.
- The form giving informed consent for the interventions must be signed by a competent adult.

(continued)

Table 3.2 APTA Guidelines *(continued)*

- If the adult is not considered competent, the consent form must be signed by the patient/client's legal guardian.
- If the patient is a minor, the consent form must be signed by the parent or an appointed guardian.
- Each document must include date and time of service and signed by the PT/PTA using his or her first and last names and professional designation. Depending on the clinical facility, the professional license number may be included.
- Document at the time of the visit whenever possible.
- All communications with other healthcare providers or healthcare professionals must be recorded.
- The PTA students' notes should be co-signed by the clinical instructor. This may be the supervising PT or, where permissible by law, the PTA.
- Nonlicensed personnel notes should be co-signed by the PT.
- Include functional progress in respect to goals regularly.
- Demonstrate skilled interventions are being performed in relationship to medical necessity.
- Demonstrate planning and progression throughout the entire episode of care until the conclusion of the episode of care.

Table 3.3 Documenting Skilled Care and Medical Necessity [1,3]

Skilled Care	Medical Necessity
■ Is demonstrated by use of clinical reasoning and problem solving by making links between the subjective, objective, and assessments in the note. Provide documentation supporting the complexity of the service that can only be provided by a PT or PTA.	■ Must demonstrate that the services provided will address the nature and severity of the illness, injury, and medical needs of the patient
■ Must make links between problem solving and intervention choices with respect to why the interventions are necessary (rationale for the intervention based on anatomical and physiological principles)	■ Will be illustrated by denoting the services being provided are safe, effective, and specifically meeting the needs of the patient in accordance with the accepted standard of medical practice
■ Interventions must be linked back to the ICF model (e.g., the impairments in body function and structure, activity limitations and/or participation restrictions) with respect to ongoing review of goals in respect to the plan of care	■ Illustrates that skilled interventions are required to maintain or improve function or deter further progression or deterioration of the patient's functional status
■ Reflects any contributing barriers to potential goal achievement such as comorbidities, safety concerns, environmental barriers, or psychosocial considerations	■ Must link back to function rather than general welfare of the patient ■ Good example: to return to navigating stairs without upper extremity support or assistive devices independently for safe return to work ■ Poor example: return to weight lifting fitness workouts
■ The provider of care must be clearly identified with the proper designations (PT, PTA, or both if co-signing is applicable)	■ The provider of care must be clearly identified with the proper designations (PT, PTA, or both if co-signing is applicable)

CLINICAL DOCUMENTATION

Documentation Summary Pearls

To optimize documentation outcomes, consider the following:

- Demonstration of problem-solving ability related to both skilled interventions and medical necessity will optimize documentation outcomes.
- Keep the goals in the plan of care at the forefront of every note and daily review and frequent referencing will show progress.
- Make clear links between the impairments as related to body systems and functions to demonstrate goal driven interventions.
- Make clear links between the impairments and effect on activity limitations and/or participation restrictions to elucidate functional deficits and support medical necessity and the need for continued skilled interventions.
- Reinforce the need for continued treatment based on potential safety concerns, specific techniques utilized by a licensed and trained clinician, along with the use of standardized tools to elucidate the associations between skill and medical necessity.

Telephone Referral Documentation

Table 3.4 Telephone Referral Guidelines[2, 7] for Any Type of Documentation Platform

- Date and time of the call
- Name of the person calling and name of the healthcare provider who referred the patient
- Name of the PTA who took the referral
- Name of the patient and all other details related to the referral
- Date when a written copy of the referral will be sent to physical therapy
- Name of the PT who will be responsible for the referred patient

Documentation Guidelines on Domestic and Family Violence[4]

- The medical records must be written in the regular course of business during the examination or the interview.
- The medical records must be legible.
- The medical records must be properly stored and accessed only by the appropriate staff.
- The medical records should include the following information:
  - A. The date and time of the patient's arrival at the clinic or the treatment site
  - B. The name, address, and the phone number of the person(s) accompanying the patient (Interview the patient alone if possible.)
  - C. Documentation using the patient's own words about the cause of her or his injuries, using quotation marks and phrases such as "patient states" or "patient reports"
  - D. A detailed description (with explanations) of injuries, including the type, number, size, location (a body chart may be helpful), and resolution; a description of a chronology of the violence

asking about the first episode, the most recent episode, and the most serious episode; identifies the person who hurt the patient using the patient's own words in quotation marks

E. Any documentation of inconsistency between the injury and the explanation about the injury, avoiding legalese and no personal conclusions about the situation

F. Documentation recording the clinician's questions about domestic violence and the patient's response

G. A color photograph(s), including the patient's informed consent for the photograph(s); photographs taken from different angles, including the patient's face in at least one picture; two pictures for each major trauma area; marked photographs, including the patient's name, location, and name(s) of the person taking the pictures

H. Observations on the patient's demeanor, i.e., if agitated, angry or upset

I. If police or other agencies were called, documentation about the investigating officer's name, badge number, phone number, and any actions taken, including date and time of reports given to outside agencies

J. Documentation about the name of the PT, PTA, physician, or nurse who treated the patient (if applicable)

CLINICAL DOCUMENTATION

Documentation Elements

Initial Examination and Evaluation Elements[1]

- Performed and written by the PT, but the PT may include data gathered by the PTA
- Referral, including the reason for referral and the specific intervention requested by the referral source
- Data accompanying the referral: primary medical diagnosis (or onset date), secondary medical diagnoses/comorbidities, medical history, medications, other complications or precautions that may impact physical therapy; any diagnostic imaging or testing
- Personal information, including the patient's date of birth, age, gender, occupation, start of care, and primary complaint
- History of present illness: mechanism of injury, sequence and progression of symptoms, date of the initial onset and status prior to the current visit, prior interventions and results, and associated disability, including symptoms associated with the patient's primary problem, such as location of the problem (may use a body chart), severity, nature (such as aching, burning, or tingling), persistence (constant versus intermittent), and whether aggravated by activity versus relieved by rest general health status; medications
- Patient's past history, including prior episodes of the same problem; prior interventions and responses; other affected areas (or body parts); familial, developmental, and congenital disorders; prior physical therapy
- Tests and measures (data collection): the patient's cognition, vision, hearing, vital signs, vascular signs, sensation and proprioception, coordination, balance, posture, pain, edema, active range of motion (AROM), passive range of motion (PROM), strength, bed mobility, transfers, ambulation (level and stairs), wheelchair use, orthotic/prosthetic devices, durable medical equipment used, activity tolerance, special tests, architectural considerations, requirements to return to prior activity level (including work, school, or home), wound description (for wound care, including the incision status)
- Prior level of function: mobility at home and in the community for work and leisure, employment and/or school
- Socioeconomic factors that may impact rehabilitation and recovery
- Physical therapy diagnosis
- Assessment: reason for skilled care
- Problems
- Plan of care: prognosis, specific interventions strategies, frequency, duration, patient instruction/home program, caregiver training, short-term goals (STGs) and dates of achievement, long-term goals (LTGs) and dates of achievement, patient's rehabilitation potential

Progress Report Elements[1]

The progress report contains more detail than a daily or treatment note and highlights important changes in patient's status since the last examination or progress note. Only PTs can write a note that provides assessment of the patient, but the PT may include data gathered by the PTA in the progress note.

- Attendance
- Current patient status: the patient's cognition, vision, hearing, vital signs, vascular signs, sensation and proprioception, coordination, balance (sit and stand), posture, pain, edema, AROM, PROM, strength, bed mobility, transfers, ambulation (level and stairs), wheelchair use, orthotic/prosthetic devices, durable medical equipment used or needed, activity tolerance, special tests, architectural considerations,

requirements to return to prior activity level (including work, school, or home), and wound description (for wound care and including the incision status)
- Physical therapy diagnosis
- Assessment: reason for skilled care
- Problems
- Plan of care: specific interventions and strategies, frequency of interventions, duration of interventions, patient instruction/home program, caregiver training, STGs and dates of achievement, LTGs and dates of achievement, and patient's rehabilitation potential

Daily/Treatment Note

See Section 3-4.

Summary for the Conclusion of an Episode of Physical Therapy: Discharge Summary[1]

Only PTs can write a note that provides assessment of the patient, but the PT may include data gathered by the PTA.

- Attendance
- Current patient status: the patient's cognition, vision, hearing, vital signs, vascular signs, sensation and proprioception, coordination, balance (sit and stand), posture, pain, edema, AROM, PROM, strength, bed mobility, transfers, ambulation (level and stairs), wheelchair use, orthotic/prosthetic devices, durable medical equipment used or needed, activity tolerance, special tests, architectural considerations, requirements to return to prior activity level (including work, school, or home), and wound description (for wound care, including the incision status)
- Physical therapy diagnosis
- Assessment: reason for skilled care
- Problems
- Plan of care: specific recommendations and instruction/home program provided to patient or caregiver where appropriate, and equipment provided. STGs and dates of achievement, LTGs and dates of achievement, rationale for discontinuation of physical therapy if goals have not been met

Possible Indications for the Conclusion of an Episode of Care

Table 3.5 Possible Indications

- Patient's desire to stop treatment
- Patient's inability to progress toward goals because of medical or psychosocial complications or because financial/insurance resources have been expended
- PT's decision that the patient will no longer benefit from physical therapy
- Goals have been met

International Classification of Functioning, Disability, and Health (ICF) Overview

ICF Overview[5]

The ICF model was formally adopted by the World Health Organization (WHO) in 2001 as a revision of previously used disablement models and by the APTA House of Delegates in 2008. The difference between these models is that the ICF model focuses on components of functioning and disability related to a health condition as opposed to the consequences of disease, as was the case with earlier models. The ICF model now focuses on the positive ability aspects of disablement and considers contextual factors such as personal situations and attitudes in conjunction with environmental considerations as contributing factors to overall functional presentation of a patient. These contextual factors can prove to be a motivator for the patient or a potential barrier. For instance, a positive attitude may allow the patient to be a more active and willing participant with treatment compliance. Conversely, a patient who is depressed or does not have a social support system may be more unwilling and less motivated to actively participate with treatment, resulting in participation restrictions with both treatment and social activities. These attitudinal factors may result in barriers to goal achievement.

Table 3.6 Common Definitions of ICF Terms[6,7]

- **Health condition:** pathology or disease process that is affecting the patient
- **Body functions:** physiologic functions of body systems (including psychological functions)
- **Body structures:** anatomic parts of the body such as organs, limbs, and their components
- **Impairments:** problems in body function or structure resulting in some type of deviation (e.g., drop foot, amputation), loss of function (e.g., decreased strength, decreased range of motion)
- **Activity:** execution of a task or action by an individual (e.g., climbing stairs, driving to work)
- **Participation:** involvement in a life situation (e.g., social situations, work, church, family obligations)
- **Activity limitations:** difficulties an individual may have in executing a task (e.g., inability to climb stairs due to alteration in the musculoskeletal system)
- **Participation restrictions:** problems an individual may experience in relationship to life situations (e.g., weak leg musculature results in need for a walker, making going to the doctor's taxing so the patient may experience difficulty obtaining health care)
- **Environmental factors:** (contextual factors): physical (physical barriers limit patient's ability to function well), social (stairs at the patient's destination result in avoiding social gatherings; patient's spouse is unable to help transfer the patient so the patient avoids social situations), attitudinal (e.g., a patient with depression may not be compliant with home exercises because motivation is affected by depression = barrier to goal achievement)

Making Links Between the ICF Components and Documentation

Use of the ICF model embraces the concept of enablement to depict a patient's status rather than using a disablement model. For documentation to illustrate skill and medical necessity, mindfulness to the ICF model needs to be reflected in the plan of care and subsequent documentation.

The PTA must remember that the health condition of the patient needs to be linked back to impairments associated to conditions affecting the body systems and functions. Once these impairments are outlined in the plan of care, then appropriate interventions reflecting skilled care can be implemented by the healthcare team. Since impairments at the body structure and function level often result in activity limitations or participation restrictions, the PTA must be able to recognize the impact of these limitations/restrictions and clearly document the relationship to exhibit the need for skilled intervention that is medically necessary to return the patient to his or her previous level of functioning.

Table 3.7 Examples of Impairments in Body Function and Structure and Related Activity Limitation, or Participation Restriction[5,6]

Impairments Related to Body Structures and Function	Activity Limitation
Weakness in the lower extremity	Knee buckles on heel strike Decreased speed during gait training Decreased safety during transfers and gait training Unable to ambulate on uneven terrain
Incoordination in both upper extremities	Unable to comb hair within tolerable time frame Unable to don clothes without continuous guidance Unable to brush teeth without continuous guidance
Temporomandibular joint (TMJ) dysfunction	Limited bite and chewing Unable to consume full meals without food alteration
Left knee effusion	Unable to ascend/descend 10 steps Unable to ambulate 20 feet in 9 seconds Unable to tolerate 30 minutes of unassisted walking

Considerations for Making Links When Documenting

- **Health condition:** the medical diagnosis of the patient that should be included on all documentation reflecting the timeline of tissue healing when appropriate.
- **Body systems and function:** anatomical and physiological function of the patient. The term "impairment" is used if an abnormality exists (e.g., pain and inflammation, post-surgical muscle atrophy, DVT's, contractures etc.).
- **Activity:** what the patient can do (e.g., transfers with minimum assistance).
- ***Activity limitation:** the patient's inability to perform the activity (pain and inflammation result in need for minimum assistance with transfers).
- **Participation:** to what extent can the patient participate.
- ***Participation restrictions:** result when there is insult at the body systems and functional level inhibiting the patient's ability to participate in the social, physical, or emotional aspect of the activity. Impairments and activity limitations may result in participation restrictions (e.g., pain, inflammation, and weakness in the legs can result in patient's inability to navigate steps to leave the home to go grocery shopping).
- **Environmental factors** (contextual factors): obstacles the patient may encounter in his or her daily life (e.g., stairs, ramps, thick carpeting, cluttered pathways) that contribute to activity limitations or participation restrictions.
- **Personal factors** (contextual factors): psychosocial considerations that may motivate a patient to participate (need to return to work) or perhaps hinder willingness to participate (e.g., depression, obesity, poor self-esteem).

Daily/Weekly SOAP Note Elements

SOAP Note Elements [1,7,8]

The most common format for daily notes is the SOAP (Subjective, Objective, Assessment, Plan) format. It is important to include evidence of skilled treatment and patient response in the daily treatment note. Flow sheets can be used to track intervention parameters, but they cannot provide the detail needed to show delivery of skilled care.

Subjective Data

Table 3.8 **Examples of Subjective Data**

- Patient's complaints of pain with relevance to the patient's condition
- Patient's response to the previous treatment
- Patient's description of functional improvements, such as being able to perform activities of daily living
- Patient's lifestyle situation, such as being able to go out to dinner or entertain friends (as he or she used to do before having this condition)
- Patient's goals, such as to be able to drive his or her car in 2–3 weeks
- Patient's compliance or difficulties with the home exercise program (HEP)

Strategies for Writing Subjective Data

- Do not include irrelevant information; include only information that affects the interventions and goals, describes a change in the patient's condition, and proves the effectiveness or ineffectiveness of interventions.
- Include the patient's pain information in the subjective data.
- Section may include caregiver reports if indicated.

Objective Data

Table 3.9 **Examples of Objective Data**

- The results of the physical therapy measurements and tests, such as manual muscle testing, goniometry, gait assessment, and specific neurological assessments (such as balance, sensation, or proprioception)
- The description of the interventions provided to the patient, such as physical agents and modalities, therapeutic exercises, wound care, functional training (such as gait using assistive devices), patient education/instruction (such as postsurgery precautions), and discussion and coordination with other disciplines (e.g., occupational therapy gave the patient a shoehorn to be able to put his or her shoes on)
- The description of the patient's function, such as performing transfers, gait (with or without assistive devices, on even or uneven surfaces and stairs), or bed mobility (such as turning from supine to side lying to sitting)
- The PTA's objective observations of the patient during interventions (such as the increase in the number of exercise repetitions), tests and measurements (such as compensating for muscular weakness), and patient education/instruction (such as understanding the HEP on the first performance)

Objective Data Guidelines

Table 3.10 Guidelines

- Describe the reason(s) for interventions and the interventions provided to the patient in enough detail that another PT or PTA could read the description and replicate the interventions (improves different therapists' follow-up, quality, and consistency of intervention).
- Describe the patient's response to each intervention; in this way, the most effective intervention response can be found and used during the patient's physical therapy.
- Do not reference the PTA: "PTA applied moist hot pack to lower back, 20 min with patient prone." Instead, document, "Moist hot pack applied to lower back for 20 mins, patient lying prone."
- After repeating tests and measurements that were performed in the initial examination, describe the results by comparing them to the initial results.
- Use reliable and valid tests and measures as directed by supervising PT.
- Use words that describe the patient performing a function so that the reader can visualize the function. Connecting the impairment in body function and structure to activity limitation(s) or participation restrictions.
- Organize the information in a logical manner.
- Use words that portray skilled physical therapy services.
- Include any copy of written information that was given to the patient (such as the home exercise program).
- Describe patient/caregiver understanding of the written information provided to the patient.

Strategies for Writing Objective Data

- The results of tests and measures must be documented, considering the PT's initial evaluation. Do not introduce new tests and measures. Consider the patient's starting and ending positions and points of measurement from the initial evaluation.
- Detail the patient's function by documenting elements such as type of assistive device, type of equipment, distance, speed, time, repetitions, sets, type of gait pattern, amount of assistance, reason for assistance, and the environment.
- Detail the interventions by documenting treatment elements such as type of intervention, type of equipment or machine, position of the patient, description of the treated area, the patient's physiologic response, parameters, i.e., settings, intensity, number of repetitions, number of sets.

Assessment Data

Table 3.11 Examples of Assessment Data

- Patient's overall response to interventions
- Patient's progress toward STGs and LTGs (from the PT's initial evaluation)
- Explanations as to why the interventions are necessary
- Effects of interventions on the patient's impairments and functional limitations

CLINICAL DOCUMENTATION

Strategies for Writing Assessment Data

- Be consistent when relating the information in the assessment with the subjective data and objective data in the daily/weekly SOAP note and the initial evaluation.
- Do not make generalized statements, but rather be specific in describing the patient's progress (or lack of progress) toward the STGs and LTGs.
- Do not introduce new information (such as tests or measures) that is not mentioned in the initial evaluation.
- Indicate why continued therapy is indicated.

Plan Data

Table 3.12 Examples of Plan Data

- Plan for the next intervention session.
- Plan for consultation with another discipline.
- Plan for the frequency of the interventions.
- Plan for reevaluation or discontinuation of physical therapy by the PT.
- Plan to discuss with the PT any changes in patient's condition, introduction of new exercises, or specific patient goals or complaints to the PTA.

Strategies for Writing Plan Data

- Do not forget to include information about working as a team with the PT.
- Write relevant information and suggestions for the next treatment session by considering STGs and LTGs.
- Include the number of remaining intervention sessions.

See Appendix E for examples of SOAP notes.

Patient Education

The PTA's Responsibilities During Patient Education[7]

- To communicate clearly and simply by using everyday words, repeating the information as necessary, and explaining new words
- To gain the learner's attention, motivation, and active participation
- To provide an overview of the learning process such as the objectives, purposes, and nature of the tasks and the procedures to follow
- To stimulate the learner's recall of previous learning
- To relate present learning to past and future learning
- To monitor and control the learning and the environment
- To organize learning units over a period of time
- To break down learning into a series of steps or units
- To determine the best sequence(s) of learning units and experiences such as a sequence from familiar to unfamiliar, simple to complex, or concrete to abstract
- To provide ample opportunity for practice and repetition
- To progress at a comfortable pace for the learner
- To give timely feedback
- To provide accurate knowledge of results
- To recognize successful behaviors
- To reduce conditions that have a negative impact on learning, such as pain or discomfort, anxiety, fear, frustration, feelings of failure, humiliation, embarrassment, boredom, or time pressures

Patient Education for Patients/Clients Who Have Difficulty Reading

Table 3.13 Recommendations[7] for Patients/Clients Having Difficulty Reading

- Materials need to be written in plain language, consistently using the same words.
- Unfamiliar healthcare terms need to be defined, and repetition can be used to reinforce the information.
- Sentences must be short and simple, with each item marked with a bullet point.
- Each list should contain five or six bullet points.
- Attention can be drawn to essential information by making circles or arrows or adding dividers or tabs to the material.
- Use pictures or illustrations whenever possible.

Patient/Client Education for Older Adults

Table 3.14 Recommendations[9] for Older Adults

- Assess how and when the patient (client) is ready to learn by finding out the patient's (client's) interest and level of motivation to learn.
- Tie new information into past experiences.
- Enhance the learning process:
  - Teach the patient (client) in an environment conducive to learning, such as a quiet place.
  - Sit near the patient (client).
  - Speak clearly.
  - Teach in brief sessions.
- Instructions can be taught one step at a time by demonstrating and describing the intervention and encouraging the patient (client) to practice each step.
- Adjust the teaching method to the patient's (client's) learning style and special needs. For example, if the patient (client) is a visual learner, the PTA may need to give the patient (client) a picture of the exercise that he or she learned today. Considering the patient's vision, the PTA should give the patient a large-sized print (type size of at least 16 points) of the exercise picture.
- Find out the patient's (client's) preference for method of learning, such as reading, listening, watching, or doing.
- Encourage the patient (client) to bring a family member or a friend to the teaching session for support and to reinforce and clarify information.

Patient Education for Patients/Clients Who Have Visual Impairments

Table 3.15 Recommendations[9] for Patients/Clients with Visual Impairments

- Introduce yourself and other people present in the room.
- Ask whether the patient (client) wants assistance, and provide directions.
- For a HEP, write the material in large print size (16 points).
- In written materials, use simple fonts. Avoid italics. Write clearly and concisely, or print the information in braille.

Patient Education for Patients/Clients Who Have Hearing Impairments

Table 3.16 Recommendations[9] for Patients/Clients with Hearing Impairments

- Move a chair closer to face the patient (client). Get the patient's (client's) attention by touching him or her; speak clearly and distinctly, not loudly.
- Do not exaggerate pronunciation.
- Reduce distracting and interfering sounds.
- Have adequate light in the room because many patients (clients) with hearing impairments read lip movements when looking at the mouth and further speech read when looking at gestures, expressions, and pantomime actions.

Patient Education for Patients/Clients Who Cannot Speak English

Table 3.17 Recommendations for Patients/Clients Who Cannot Speak English[9]

- Use certified interpreters to communicate key information to the patient (client).
- The patient (client) must be comfortable with the interpreter, especially when embarrassing topics may be discussed.
- Greet the patient (client) in his or her native language. Pronounce the patient's (client's) name correctly.
- Speak clearly and concentrate on the most important message(s) for the patient (client).
- Considering cultural diversity, understand the patient's (client's) values and beliefs, and pay attention to nonverbal communication such as voice volume, postures, gestures, and eye contact.
- Working with the family decision-maker, who may be different from the patient (client), is essential for the success of intervention.
- The intervention has to be creative. Considering patient's cultural background, it may involve having the patient's spiritual advisor help with the intervention (as long as the spiritual healing method is not antagonistic to the intervention).

Basic Requirements for the Home Exercise Program

Table 3.18 Home Exercises Program Basic Requirements[7]

- The HEP should be organized, concise (short), and written in layman terms. The words must make sense to the patient (client) and be consistent with the therapist's verbal explanations and demonstrations.
- When a caregiver is involved, he or she must be involved early in the HEP to allow an easier transition at the conclusion of the physical therapy episode of care.
- The HEP represents an extension of the interventions. The HEP starts on the first day of interventions and continues through the last day of physical therapy. The program should be presented within the context of the total process of patient education and rehabilitation and instructions should be provided on continuing home exercises after the conclusion of the episode of care.
- Exercises and activities should be presented in a simple and clear manner.
- The HEP should contain approximately three to five exercises or activities.
- Instructions for the exercises in the HEP should include the number of repetitions, the number of sets, the length of time to hold positions, the amount of exercise resistance, positions for performing the exercises or activities, the duration of exercises or activities, the frequency, and the method of progression.
- The exercises and activities must be sorted in a logical manner so that the patient (client) does not have to change positions too much.
- The HEP may include diagrams, drawings, pictures, or a video of exercises or activities. Any such graphic elements should be clear and uncomplicated.
- Seek out freely available HEP programs, e.g., APTA's Rehabilitation Reference Center.

(continued)

Table 3.18 **Home Exercises Program Basic Requirements**   *(continued)*

- The HEP should be written in the patient's (client's) primary language.
- Technical terms must be avoided, and short sentences must be used as much as possible. Complex words (such as "inflammation") must be replaced with simple ones (such as "redness").
- Each sentence in the HEP must present only one idea and contain no more than one three-syllable word.
- Lines of copy should be no longer than 5 inches wide, and the type size should be 12 points or larger.
- For patients (clients) with vision impairments, the handouts must have a high contrast between the foreground and the background and include large amounts of blank space on the page.
- The HEP should be written at a fifth- or sixth-grade reading level.

Example of a Home Exercise Program to Improve Upper Body Postural Control

Table 3.19 **Example of HEP: Corner Stretch for Tight Pectoralis Major Muscles (Clavicular Portion)**

- Find a corner of your room.
- Bend both elbows with both arms at shoulder level.
- Place both arms against the wall.
- Lean forward until you feel a stretch.
- Hold for 30 seconds.
- Repeat three times, twice each day.

CLINICAL DOCUMENTATION

Electronic Medical Documentation

Table 3.20 **Electronic Documentation**[2,7,10]

- Documents may be completed on a desktop computer, laptop computer, tablet, or smartphone devices.
- If used within a single healthcare organization, the electronic record is termed an electronic medical record (EMR).
- If used in accordance with nationally recognized standards across multiple healthcare organizations with the intent to share, collaborate, and coordinate care through all spectrums, including billing, quality assurance, risk management, and evidence-based practice, the electronic record is referred to as an electronic health record (EHR).
- APTA endorses the use of the term "EHR" because it supports the physical therapy profession's vision for health information utilization by the consumer across the healthcare settings.

Table 3.21 **Benefits of EHR**[2,7,10]

- Improved clinical decision-making using evidence-based practice (EBP), clinical prediction rules, and researched clinical pathways foster optimal outcomes for patient care.
- Electronic submission of billing results in expedient reimbursement.
- Data mining capabilities may promote research efforts and foster data outcomes analysis to allow for larger databases of proven EBP.
- EHR focuses on patient-centered outcomes due to shared decision-making between insurance companies and the patient.
- It results in improved and timely communication amongst the multiple care settings, the healthcare providers, and the patient.
- It promotes point-of-care documentation by using drop-down menus with click-and-pick options to improve efficiency with documentation.

Table 3.22 **Challenges of EHR**[2,7,10]

- Precreated templates may not be user friendly for every type of rehabilitation discipline.
- Documentation efficiency decreases if the clinician reverts to free texting because the templates are not tailored to the specific patient population being serviced.
- Skilled care and medical necessity cannot be clearly delineated in check-box templates, resulting in the need to free text.
- Cost of software/training/implementation/privacy measures/data back-up systems, and ongoing upgrades may be prohibitive for smaller organizations.
- Concerns exist regarding maintaining security of patient information.

Table 3.23 EHR Documentation Tips [2,7,10]

- Cross reference the patient's name with the note being typed to ensure you are on the correct patient in your daily list.
- Avoid documenting on an electronic device in a public area.
- Both skill and medical necessity need to be regularly reflected in the daily note.
- Avoid using the same click-and-pick boxes or phrases for every visit or every patient.
- Avoid copying notes from one visit to the next.
- Document at the time of the visit.
- Free text when appropriate to demonstrate clinical thinking in respect to skilled care and medical necessity.
- All late entries must be entered as an addendum.
- Follow the security processes and policies that your facility uses for the sharing of personal health information in electronic format.
- Continue to follow general guidelines for documentation content and demonstration of skilled care. See Section 3.1.

Health Insurance Portability and Accountability Act (HIPAA) and Documentation

Table 3.24 HIPAA Documentation Requirements[2,7,10]

- Patient records are considered protected health information (PHI).
- PHI needs to be secured in locked file cabinets or records rooms.
- PHI stored in the computer needs to be secured using additional passwords.
- Electronic PHI needs to be backed up to deter security threats.
- Transmission of PHI must be sent through a secure server to avoid a privacy breach of protected information.
- Safeguards such as an encryption process are beneficial to securely sharing PHI.
- Use of password-protected patient portals may increase secure sharing of PHI.
- In the event of an electronic security breach (e.g., laptop stolen), the patient must be notified as per facility policy.
- In the physical therapy facility, during physical therapy practice, the PT/PTA must take safeguards to limit access to areas where the patient's chart is located by ensuring that the area is supervised, by keeping the chart face down or facing a wall if stored vertically, or by escorting any nonemployees in the area.
- The PT/PTA can share patient information with students (for training purposes). When students return to the academic institution, all identification points should be removed from the patient information before it is shared. Alternatively, the student could obtain an authorization from the patient to use the patient's PHI at the academic institution.
- During customary and necessary healthcare communications and practices, PHI can be used or disclosed if the PT/PTA applies reasonable safeguards and implements the minimum necessary standards. The PT/PTA must make every effort to limit the disclosure to the minimum amount of information necessary to accomplish the intended purpose.

(continued)

CLINICAL DOCUMENTATION

Table 3.24 HIPAA Documentation Requirements   *(continued)*

- The physical therapy facility needs to develop and implement policies and procedures that reasonably minimize the amount of PHI used, disclosed, and requested. The policies and procedures must establish standard protocols for routine or recurring requests and disclosures of PHI. For special requests, the policies and procedures must establish a protocol that the requests will be reviewed individually by the facility's (chief) privacy officer.

- The patient (client) has the right to access his or her PHI that was generated during the 6 years before the date of the request. The patient (client) also has the right to access any piece of information that reflects a decision the provider made regarding the patient (client) and to obtain an accounting of PHI disclosures (including the date of each disclosure, the name of the person who received the PHI, a brief description of the PHI disclosed, and a brief statement of the purpose of the disclosure).

- The patient (client) has the right to examine his or her chart and other records, including records the provider thinks that the patient (client) will never see (such as a letter to a collection agency to collect the copayment).

- The patient (client) has the right, on request, to get a copy of his or her records in 30 days (if the records are on-site) and in 60 days (if the records are off-site). The provider can charge a reasonable copying cost (certain state laws require a certain amount per copy per page).

- A PT/PTA cannot use the PHI in marketing.

- Patient (client) authorization for uses and disclosures of PHI is not needed in the following circumstances: patient (client) seeking his or her PHI; Department of Health and Human Services; uses and disclosures required by laws other than HIPAA (such as vital statistics, communicable diseases, Occupational Safety and Health Administration, related workplace surveillance); victims of domestic violence, child abuse, or elder abuse; judicial and administrative proceedings (such as court of law orders or court of law subpoena); Medicare or Medicaid; law enforcement activities; Secret Service; emergency situations with serious threats to health or safety; worker's compensation (to the extent required by state law).

Patient Confidentiality

APTA Standards of Ethical Conduct and Guide for Conduct of the Physical Therapist Assistant[11]

The APTA, in accordance with its Standards of Ethical Conduct for the Physical Therapist Assistant, have established the following guidelines in respect to patient confidentiality. Patient confidentiality also includes policies and procedures set forth by the employer for the healthcare worker in respect to HIPAA.

Standard 2: Physical therapist assistants shall be trustworthy and compassionate in addressing the rights and needs of patients/clients.

2D. Physical therapist assistants shall protect confidential patient/client information and, in collaboration with the physical therapist, may disclose confidential information to appropriate authorities only when allowed or as required by law.

Significance of Patient Confidentiality

- Professional ethical/legal principles and standards require that patient confidentiality be respected.
- Maintaining patient privacy is essential both during the physical examination and for informed consent.
- The existence of patient confidentiality protections encourages the patient to fully divulge relevant health information needed for proper assessment and treatment.

Situations When the Patient's Written Authorization for Release of Medical Information Is Required

- For the patient's attorney or insurance company
- For the patient's employer (unless a worker's compensation claim is involved)
- For any member of the patient's family (except when a member of the family received durable power of attorney for working with healthcare agencies)
- For the patient's authorization to allow medical information to be used in research studies

References

1. APTA elements of documentation within the patient/client management model. apta.org. https://www.apta.org/your-practice/documentation/defensible-documentation/elements-within-the-patientclient-management-model. Accessed December 2, 2020.
2. APTA documentation: Risk management. apta.org. https://www.apta.org/your-practice/documentation/defensible-documentation/risk-management. Accessed June 17, 2020.
3. Quinn L, Gordon J. *Documentation for Rehabilitation: A Guide to Clinical Decision Making*. 2nd ed. Maryland Heights, MO: Elsevier; 2010.
4. Isaac N, Pualani Enos V. Documenting domestic violence: How health care providers can help victims. National Institute of Justice. https://www.ncjrs.gov/pdffiles1/nij/188564.pdf. Accessed December 2, 2020.
5. American Physical Therapy Association. Guide to physical therapist practice 3.0: Introduction. apta.org. http://guidetoptpractice.apta.org/content/1/SEC1.body. Accessed December 7, 2020.

6. World Health Organization. Towards a common language for functioning, disability and health: ICF. 2002. https://www.who .int/classifications/icf/training/icfbeginnersguide.pdf. Accessed December 7, 2020.

7. Barrett C. *Dreeben Irimia's Introduction to Physical Therapy for Physical Therapist Assistants*. 4th ed. Burlington, MA: Jones & Bartlett Learning; 2020.

8. Bircher, WD. *Lukan's Documentation for Physical Therapist Assistants*. 3rd ed. Philadelphia, PA: F.A. Davis; 2008.

9. Bottomley J. *Geriatric Rehabilitation: A Textbook for the Physical Therapist Assistant*. Thorofare, NJ: Slack, Inc.; 2010.

10. Health information technology and patient privacy. apta.org. https://www.apta.org/your-practice/compliance /health-information-technology-and-patient-privacy. Accessed December 9, 2020.

11. Standards of ethical conduct for the physical therapist assistant. apta.org. https://www.apta.org/apta-and-you/leadership -and-governance/policies/standards-of-ethical-conduct-for-the-physical-therapist-assistant. Accessed December 9, 2020.

CLINICAL DOCUMENTATION

PART 4

Patient Management: General Interventions

PATIENT MANAGEMENT: GENERAL INTERVENTIONS

Phases of Tissue Healing and Clinical Interventions

PATIENT MANAGEMENT: GENERAL INTERVENTIONS

Tissue Healing and Interventions

Table 4.1 Tissue Healing and Interventions[1]

Clinical Signs	Interventions
Inflammatory Phase ■ Begins immediately after injury ■ Lasts 2–4 days ■ Signs: pain (dolor), heat (calor), redness (rubor), swelling (tumor), and loss of function	■ Rest the area: immobilize and protect the affected area; exercise the unaffected areas; NWB or PWB; PROM if applicable; continuous passive motion (CPM) postoperatively ■ Ice: apply ice or cold ■ Compression: taping, bracing, or orthotics ■ Elevation: elevate the part ■ Decrease pain: use physical agents and modalities for pain management and swelling ■ Patient education: educate about avoidance of activities and how to protect the area
Proliferation and Migration Phase ■ Begins immediately after the inflammatory phase at approximately fifth day ■ Lasts up to 3 weeks ■ Signs: lessening of inflammation; may still have pain and weakness	■ Protect the area: bracing or orthotics; progressive WB such as PWB or WBAT ■ Decrease pain: physical agents and modalities for pain management and swelling ■ Increase ROM and function: use scar mobilization techniques; PROM, AAROM, AROM; isometric exercises; stretching exercises (start with light stretching because tissue is delicate in the beginning); CKC if pain and swelling subsided; ADLs ■ Patient education: how to protect the affected area; avoid excessive motion for tissue irritation/destruction
Remodeling and Maturation Phase ■ Lasts from 3 weeks to 6[+] months ■ Signs: inflammation resolved ■ Caution: if scar tissue is irritated or stressed, the fibroblastic activity continues; patient may present with pain, swelling, stiffness, and muscle guarding	■ Increase strength and function to normal: restore stability, mobility, joint arthrokinematics, gradual return to work/school/hobbies ■ Patient education: how to avoid future injury

Therapeutic Exercises: Indications and Contraindications

PATIENT MANAGEMENT: GENERAL INTERVENTIONS

107

Table 4.2 **Therapeutic Exercises: Indications and Contraindications**[1]

Exercises	Indications	Contraindications, Limitations, and Precautions[1]
PROM exercises	To demonstrate a movement, to prepare a patient for stretching, to maintain joint connective tissue mobility, to maintain elasticity of muscle, to increase synovial fluid for joint nutrition, to assist circulation, to prevent joint contracture, to decrease pain, to help in the healing process	Contraindication: Disruption of the healing process Limitations: Will not increase muscle strength or endurance, will not prevent or counteract muscle atrophy, will not assist in the blood circulation to the same extent as the active movement
AROM exercises	For weak muscles, to promote bone and soft-tissue integrity, to promote coordination and motor skills, to prevent DVT, to increase blood circulation, for aerobic conditioning, for preparation for functional activities	Contraindications: Disruption of the healing process, harm to recent surgical procedure(s) Limitations: Will not increase strength in muscles that are already strong
AAROM exercises using manual or mechanical assistance (wand, cane, finger ladder, or overhead pulleys)	To increase circulation and prevent DVT; to promote integrity of bone, muscles, ligaments and tendons; to promote coordination and motor abilities; to assist with learning a new movement pattern	Contraindications: Disruption of the healing process, harm to recent surgical procedure(s) Limitations: Will not increase strength in muscles already strong; less effective than AROM exercises
Muscle setting isometric exercises (quadriceps sets; gluteal muscle sets; HS sets)	For very weak muscles, for acute stage of soft-tissue healing, to increase circulation, to promote relaxation, to decrease pain	Precautions: Cardiovascular disease, CVA, Valsalva maneuver (to avoid performing a Valsalva maneuver, the patient can count out loud or sing)
Resisted isometrics exercises (higher intensity than muscle setting): manual or mechanical (door frame or wall)	To increase strength throughout permitted ROM, and when manual or mechanical resistance is painful or harmful	Precautions: Cardiovascular disease, CVA, Valsalva maneuver (to avoid performing a Valsalva maneuver, the patient can count out loud or sing)

(continued)

Table 4.2 Therapeutic Exercises: Indications and Contraindications[1]   *(continued)*

Exercises	Indications	Contraindications, Limitations, and Precautions[1]
Stabilization exercises (isometrics and rhythmic stabilization; co-contraction)	To develop muscle strength and stability, and to assist with postural control (muscles of trunk)	Precautions: Cardiovascular disease, CVA, Valsalva maneuver (to avoid performing a Valsalva maneuver, the patient can count out loud or sing)
Manual and mechanical resistance exercises: PNF D1 flexion; PNF D1 extension; PNF D2 flexion; PNF D2 extension. For concentric contractions, the resistance must be applied in the opposite direction to the desired motion. For eccentric contractions, the resistance must be applied in the same direction as the desired motion.	Manual resistance: For very weak muscles, for the transition from manual to mechanical resistance, where adjustment of resistance is indicated, when the patient's muscles must work maximally at all points in ROM, when protection of healing tissues is indicated, and when prevention of substitute motion is indicated Mechanical resistance: To increase strength and endurance, for independent training, and in the intermediate and advanced stages of rehabilitation	Contraindications: Acute inflammation, acute diseases/disorders, pain, polio or post-polio syndrome, and Guillain-Barré syndrome. Mechanical resistance is not appropriate for very weak muscles and in the early stages of healing Precautions: Cardiovascular conditions (closely monitor vital signs), Valsalva maneuver, Delayed Onset Muscle Soreness (DOMS)
DeLorme PREs: (1) Determine the patient's 10 RM; (2) the patient performs one set of 10 reps at 50% of the 10 RM; (3) the patient performs a second set of 10 reps at 75% of the 10 RM; (4) the patient performs a final set of 10 reps at the full 10 RM.	To increase strength and endurance	Contraindications: Acute inflammation, acute diseases/disorders, pain, polio or post-polio syndrome, Guillain-Barré syndrome Precautions: Cardiovascular conditions (closely monitor vital signs), Valsalva maneuver, DOMS
Oxford PREs: (1) Determine the patient's 10 RM; (2) the patient performs one set of 10 reps at the full 100% RM; (3) the patient performs a second set of 10 reps at 75% of the 10 RM; (4) the patient performs a final set of 10 reps at 50% of the 10 RM.	To increase strength and endurance	Contraindications: Acute inflammation, acute diseases/disorders, pain, polio or post-polio syndrome, Guillain-Barré syndrome. Precautions: Cardiovascular conditions (closely monitor vital signs), Valsalva maneuver, DOMS

(continued)

Table 4.2 **Therapeutic Exercises: Indications and Contraindications**[1]   *(continued)*

Exercises	Indications	Contraindications, Limitations, and Precautions[1]
DAPRE PREs: (1) Determine the patient's 6 RM; (2) in set 1, the patient performs 10 reps at 50% of the 6 RM; (3) in set 2, the patient performs 6 reps at 75% of the 6 RM; (4) in set 3, the patient performs as many as possible reps at 100% of the 6 RM; (5) in set 4, the patient performs as many as possible reps at 100% of the "working weight" performed during set 3. The number of reps done in set 4 is used to determine the "working weight" for the next day.	To increase strength and endurance	Contraindications: Acute inflammation, acute diseases/disorders, pain, polio or post-polio syndrome, Guillain-Barré syndrome Precautions: Cardiovascular conditions (closely monitor vital signs), Valsalva maneuver, DOMS
Circuit training exercises: Using mechanical resistance for various muscle groups, flexibility exercises, and total-body conditioning	To increase muscular strength, to increase muscular endurance, to increase cardiovascular endurance	Contraindications: Acute inflammation, acute diseases/disorders, pain, polio or post-polio syndrome, Guillain-Barré syndrome Precautions: Cardiovascular conditions (closely monitor vital signs), Valsalva maneuver, DOMS
Isokinetic exercises (use accommodating resistance)	To increase muscular strength and endurance, for later stages of rehabilitation, when the patient has full or partial ROM in a pain-free mode	Contraindications: Acute inflammation, acute diseases/disorders, pain, polio or post-polio syndrome, Guillain-Barré syndrome Precautions: Recent musculotendinous surgeries, cardiovascular diseases or disorders Limitations: Resistance depends entirely on the patient's efforts; exercises do not accommodate all muscle groups; the patient cannot perform exercises independently in his or her environment; exercises are nonfunctional; exercises use specialized and expensive equipment Precautions: Can increase blood pressure
Open kinetic chain (OKC) and closed kinetic chain (CKC) exercises.	OKC: For strengthening of individual muscle groups, and for NWB postures. CKC: For functionality, for WB postures, and to stimulate joint and mechanoreceptors	Precautions: When using resistive OKC while terminal knee extension (TKE); when using CKC between 60° and 90° in nonoperative and operative ACL injuries; when using CKC in postoperative meniscal tears

(continued)

Table 4.2 Therapeutic Exercises: Indications and Contraindications[1] *(continued)*

Exercises	Indications	Contraindications, Limitations, and Precautions[1]
Stretching exercises: Manual passive stretching, self-stretching, prolonged mechanical or positional passive stretching, ballistic stretching (for athletes), cyclic mechanical stretching	To elongate structures, to improve ROM, for hypomobile joints	Contraindications: When a bony block limits joint motion; acute infectious and inflammatory processes; acute sharp pain; recent fracture; hematoma joint hypermobility; when contractures provide stability and functionality Ballistic stretching contraindications: sedentary individuals, older patients, patients with musculoskeletal pathology or chronic contracture Precautions: Do not stretch passively beyond normal ROM. Use care in cases involving newly united fractures, osteoporosis, prolonged immobilization, bone malignancy, or total joint replacements
Aerobic conditioning exercises (cardiopulmonary endurance exercises or total-body endurance exercises): (1) Karvonen formula: total heart rate reserve (THRR) = maximal HR – resting HR (40% to 85%) + resting HR; (2) age-adjusted maximal heart rate formula: THRR = (220 – age) 3 (65–85%); (3) MET method; (4) Borg's rate of perceived exertion (RPE) scale method	To increase coronary arteries' blood flow, to increase the heart wall thickness and muscle mass of the left ventricle, to increase blood cortisol level, to improve thermal regulation capability, to reduce the risk of coronary artery disease, to increase aerobic enzymatic activity, to increase the maximum ventilatory ability	Contraindications: Unstable angina; resting systolic BP more than 200 mm Hg; resting diastolic BP more than 110 mm Hg; orthostatic hypotension; acute systemic illness or fever; tachycardia; thrombophlebitis; recent embolism; severe orthopedic problems; metabolic problems (such as thyroiditis) Precautions: Swimming and cross-country skiing, dancing, basketball, racquetball, and competitive activities should not be used with patients who may have cardiorespiratory symptoms or are very deconditioned
Aquatic exercises	Poor standing balance, for stretching, for relaxation, for strengthening, for aerobic conditioning, for PWB gait training	Contraindications: Bowel and bladder incontinence, UTI, unstable BP, skin infections and water and airborne infections, unprotected open wounds, severe epilepsy, severe kidney disease, severe cardiac and respiratory dysfunction Precautions: Patients who experience fear of water (need prior orientation)

(continued)

Table 4.2 **Therapeutic Exercises: Indications and Contraindications**[1]   *(continued)*

Exercises	Indications	Contraindications, Limitations, and Precautions[1]
Relaxation exercises: (1) Progressive relaxation (teaches voluntary contraction and relaxation of the muscles from distal to proximal); (2) one breathing technique (awareness of diaphragmatic breathing while silently repeating the word "one" with each exhalation)	Chronic pain (tension headache, vascular headache, or chronic neck and back pain) with biofeedback; cardiopulmonary stress or chronic pulmonary problems such as asthma or emphysema	Precautions: Patients with cardiopulmonary disorders performing progressive relaxation (when isometrically contracting the muscles)

Relaxation Exercises

Table 4.3 **Relaxation Exercises**

- Relaxation exercises are performed with active participation from the patient to generate a relaxation response.
- The systemic effects of relaxation include decreased sympathetic nervous system (SNS) activity, respiratory rate, oxygen consumption, blood pressure, skeletal muscle blood flow, and muscle tension.
- Relaxation techniques can be performed singly or incorporated into other exercise sessions such as part of the warm-up or cool-down of the aerobic conditioning exercises.
- The relaxation training is effective if it is acceptable to the patient, is easy to apply in different settings, helps to restore the patient's sense of control, and offers immediate reduction of pain.
- Types of relaxation exercises include autogenic training, progressive relaxation, and Feldenkrais awareness through movement.
  - Autogenic training involves conscious relaxation through autosuggestion and a progression of exercises as well as meditation.
  - Progressive relaxation is one of the most widely used techniques that teaches voluntary contraction and relaxation of the muscles, going from distal to proximal.
  - Feldenkrais awareness through movement combines self-massage, movements of the limbs and trunk, deep breathing, sensory awareness, and conscious relaxation procedures to adjust postural and muscular imbalances and decrease pain and tension.[2]
- Other types of relaxation exercises include "one breathing" technique, eye-movement breathing technique, cognitive relaxation techniques such as listening to audiotapes or watching videotapes with instructions or music for relaxation, guided imagery, hypnosis, and nontraditional psychophysical techniques such as Trager psychophysical integration, Tai Chi Chuan, and Hatha yoga.
  - The "one breathing" technique is a form of meditation that involves passive focusing of awareness on the diaphragmatic breathing cycle while silently repeating the word "one" with each exhalation.[2]
  - The patient or the client is instructed to maintain a passive attitude and allow but not force relaxation to occur at its own pace.
  - The eye-movement breathing technique involves looking up toward the eyebrows (without head movement) during the inspiratory phase of diaphragmatic breathing, then holding the breath for 2 seconds, followed by looking down toward the chin (without head movement) while breathing out very slowly and completely. To promote relaxation, the expiratory phase of diaphragmatic breathing can be extended.

(continued)

Table 4.3 **Relaxation Exercises** *(continued)*

- When applying progressive relaxation exercises, the following procedures are used:
  1. Relaxation training can be performed in a quiet environment with low lighting and soothing music.
  2. The therapist's voice should be soft and soothing.
  3. The patient should be in a comfortable position and free of restrictive clothing.
  4. The procedure must be explained to the patient.
  5. The patient needs to breathe in deeply and in a relaxed manner.
  6. The patient is asked to contract voluntarily for a few seconds the distal muscle of the hands or feet.
  7. The patient is asked to voluntarily relax the distal muscle of the hands or feet for a few seconds.
  8. The patient is asked to try to feel a sense of heaviness in the hands or feet.
  9. The patient is asked to try to feel a sense of warmth in the muscles just relaxed.
  10. The exercises can progress to a more proximal area of the body by asking the patient to voluntarily contract and relax the more proximal musculature for a few seconds.
  11. The patient is asked to voluntarily contract isometrically and relax the entire upper extremity or lower extremity.
  12. At the end of the procedures, the patient is asked to try to feel a sense of relaxation and warmth throughout the entire extremity and eventually throughout the entire body.

- Relaxation exercises can be coupled with heating modalities such as hot packs, paraffin, ultrasound, or massage techniques such as light or deep stroking (effleurage).

Exercise Topics for the Obstetric Patient

Table 4.4 **Guidelines Related to Interventions for the Obstetric Patient**[1]

Pregnancy-Induced Pathology: Diastasis Recti

- Diastasis recti: separation of the rectus abdominis muscles in the midline at the linea alba. Any separation larger than 2 cm or two finger widths is considered significant.

- Diastasis recti is seen frequently in childbearing, but it may also be found in men and women beyond childbearing age. The incidence of diastasis recti during pregnancy increases as the pregnancy progresses, reaching a peak in the third trimester.

- Diastasis recti does not always spontaneously resolve after childbirth and may continue past the 6-week postpartum period.

- Diastasis recti can occur above or at the level of the umbilicus and less frequently below the umbilicus.

Diastasis Recti Test

The diastasis is measured by the number of fingers that can be placed between the rectus abdominis muscle bellies. A diastasis can also present as a longitudinal bulge along the linea alba.

Diastasis Recti Intervention

Perform corrective exercises for diastasis recti exclusive of other abdominal exercise until the separation is decreased to 2 cm or less.

Corrective Exercises for Diastasis Recti[1]: Head Lift Corrective Exercise

- Position of the patient is supine hook-lying with hands crossed over midline at the diastasis to support the area.

- As the patient exhales, the patient lifts only her head off the floor or until the point just before a bulge appears.

(continued)

Table 4.4 **Guidelines Related to Interventions for the Obstetric Patient**   *(continued)*

- The patient's hands should gently pull the rectus muscles toward midline.
- The patient lowers the head slowly and relaxes.

Corrective Exercises for Diastasis Recti[1]: Head Lift with Pelvic Tilt Corrective Exercise

- Patient is positioned supine in hook-lying.
- If diastasis recti is present, the arms are crossed over the diastasis and pulled toward midline.
- The patient slowly lifts her head off the floor while performing a posterior pelvic tilt. She then slowly lowers her head and relaxes.
- All abdominal contractions should be performed during exhalation, to minimize intra-abdominal pressure.

Guidelines for Obstetric Exercise Instruction

- Supine positioning should not exceed 5 minutes at any one time after the fourth month of pregnancy to avoid vena cava compression by the uterus.
- When the patient is supine, a small wedge or rolled towel should be placed under the right hip (to lessen the effects of uterine compression on abdominal vessels and to improve cardiac output by turning the patient slightly toward the left). Left side lying is the best position for pregnancy.
- Obstetric patients will also benefit from exercises and training for posture, trunk stabilization exercises, upper and lower extremity strengthening exercises, and pelvic floor exercises. Exercise interventions should be individualized to meet the needs of the obstetric patient.

Recommendations for Obstetric Aerobic Exercise[1]

- It is preferable that the patient exercise regularly at least three times per week rather than intermittently.
- Non-weight-bearing aerobic exercises such as stationary cycling or swimming should be used to minimize the risk of injury, but if able, the patient may continue activities such as running and aerobic dancing.
- Resumption of prepregnancy exercise routines during the postpartum period should occur gradually.
- Physiologic and morphologic changes of pregnancy continue for at least 4–6 weeks postpartum.

Absolute Contraindications to Exercise During Pregnancy[1]

- Incompetent cervix
- Early dilation of the cervix before the pregnancy is full term
- Vaginal bleeding of any amount
- Placenta previa
- Rupture of membranes (loss of amniotic fluid prior to the onset of labor)
- Premature labor or risk of premature labor
- Maternal heart disease
- Maternal diabetes (Type 1) or hypertension
- Intrauterine growth retardation
- Preeclampsia

(continued)

Table 4.4 **Guidelines Related to Interventions for the Obstetric Patient** *(continued)*

Precautions for Exercises During Pregnancy[1]

■ Multiple gestation

■ Anemia

■ Systemic infection

■ Extreme fatigue

■ Musculoskeletal complaints or pain

■ Overheating

■ Phlebitis

■ Diastasis recti

■ Uterine contractions

Suggested Sequence for Obstetric Aerobic Exercise Class[1]

■ Warm-up activities

■ Gentle selective stretching exercises

■ Aerobic activity for cardiovascular conditioning (15 minutes or less)

■ Upper and lower extremity strengthening

■ Cool-down activities

Interventions for Vestibular Disorders[3,4]

Vestibular and balance impairments for older adults are discussed in Table 9-11. In older adults, benign paroxysmal positional vertigo (BPPV), most often due to degeneration of the vestibular system, is a common form of vestibular dysfunction. Vestibular disorders also occur in people of all ages and causes vary. Some common causes in the general population include the following:

● Acoustic neuroma
● Autoimmune inner ear disease
● BPPV
● Concussion / head trauma
● Labyrinthitis/vestibular neuritis secondary to infection
● Meniere's disease
● Otosclerosis
● Ototoxicity

Interventions for management of vestibular disorders focus on:

1. Habituation—used for the treatment of symptoms brought on by motion and or visual stimuli
2. Gaze stabilization—to improve control of eye movements
3. Balance training

Exercises are customized to each person's specific problems. They often start slowly with speed of movement increasing as tolerated by the patient.

Interventions specific to BPPV include the following:

- Epley or Semont maneuvers (may be PT only)
- Brandt-Daroff exercises
- Performing the Epley or Semont maneuvers as home exercises.

Interventions for general vestibular dysfunction include the following:

- Eye tracking exercises head stable and head moving
- Head moving while tracking a stable then moving object
- Tracking the letter X on an index card while moving head up and down and left to right
- Tracking the letter X on the index card with head movements and movement of card in opposite direction
- Head stable while walking
- Head movement while walking
- Balance training with visual and somatosensory cues
- Performing dual task activities.

Biophysical Agents and Modalities: Indications and Applications

Table 4.5 **Biophysical Agents and Modalities: Indications and Applications**[5,6]

Physical Agent/ Modality	Indications	Applications
Therapeutic heat (hot moist pack [HMP])	Joint stiffness; musculoskeletal pain and muscle spasm; preparation for electrical stimulation and massage; subacute, chronic, and traumatic conditions	The patient's sensation and heat tolerance are assessed. The HMP is placed in a terry cloth cover and wrapped in six to eight layers of dry towels; it is then placed on the patient's treated area. Another towel is placed over the hot pack to minimize heat loss. The HMP must be secured well to the patient using towels, pillows, or straps if necessary. If the patient is lying on the HMP, additional towels (more than eight layers) are necessary. The PTA monitors the patient's treated area after 5–10 minutes of HMP application. The patient receives a call bell to alert the PTA of any sensory changes. Treatment time is 15–20 minutes.
Whirlpool	Postsurgical orthopedic conditions such as for hip, knee, and ankle; subacute and chronic musculoskeletal conditions; rheumatoid arthritis (RA). Decrease pain and muscle spasm, manage edema and increase ROM	The PTA assists the patient in immersing his or her body or body part into the whirlpool tank. The PTA uses towels to pad any pressure points and minimize compression on the tank edges. The PTA adjusts the agitator for position, force, direction, depth, and aeration. The PTA monitors the patient's response and tolerance to treatment. Patients who have most of the body immersed in the whirlpool (such as in a Hubbard tank) need close monitoring. Insert a tank liner for patients with hepatitis and open wounds, burns, and HIV. Hubbard tank: Closely monitor the patient's physiological responses. Temperatures: limbs = 103°F–110°F (39°C–43°C); full body = 97°F–100°F (36°C–39°C); multiple sclerosis = 88°F (31°C).[6]
Paraffin bath	Subacute and chronic inflammatory conditions such as RA, OA, joint stiffness, hand contracture, or scleroderma	Glove method: The PTA washes the patient's hands (or feet) prior to treatment. The PTA inspects the patient's hands (or feet) for infection, wounds, or cuts. The patient's sensation and heat tolerance are assessed. The patient is instructed not to touch the sides or bottom of the paraffin container and to avoid movements that could crack the paraffin. The patient is instructed first to dip the treated part into paraffin, creating a higher first layer of paraffin. Then other layers lower than the first one will follow. The patient is instructed to dip the treated part in paraffin until 6–12 layers have formed. The PTA wraps the treated part in plastic and towels. Treatment time is 15 to 20 minutes.
Aquatic therapy	Relaxation and improvement of circulation; muscle strengthening; ROM; gait training with decreased stress on weight-bearing joints; mobility training for RA, OA, joint replacements, MS, and paraplegia	The patient needs to shower before immersion in the water. Water temperature determined by goals of treatment, type of intervention and patient diagnosis. Cooler temperatures used for higher intensity exercise and warmer temperatures for muscle relaxation, mobility, and flexibility. Cardiovascular training = 79°F–82°F (26°C–28°C). Flexibility, strengthening, gait training and relaxation = 79°F–95°F (26°C–35°C). Acute painful musculoskeletal injury = 91°F (33°C).[1]

(continued)

Table 4.5 Biophysical Agents and Modalities: Indications and Applications[5,6] *(continued)*

Physical Agent/ Modality	Indications	Applications
Ultraviolet (UV) radiation	Acne; subacute and chronic psoriasis; decubitus ulcers; infected wounds	Dose depends on the minimal erythemal dose (MED) test, types of UV lamps and diagnosis. MED = smallest UV exposure time to produce faint erythema 8 hours postexposure. MED subsides within 24 hours. First-degree erythema is 2.5 the MED (appears 6 hours after exposure). It presents with definite redness with desquamation and lasts for 1–3 days. Second-degree erythema is 5.0 times the MED (appears 2 hours after exposure). It presents with intense erythema with edema and peeling, with an appearance similar to that seen with severe sunburn. Third-degree erythema is 10.0 times the MED. It appears after the exposure test as erythema with severe blistering, peeling, and exudation. Treatment time = proportion of the MED. UV is applied to clean skin. Both PTA and patient wear protective goggles to protect eyes from UV light.
Ultrasound (US): continuous US (CUS); pulsed US (PUS); phonophoresis	Continuous US provides predominantly thermal effects to tissues, but nonthermal effects can also occur with this mode of delivery. Thermal US (TUS): joint contractures; muscle spasm; musculoskeletal pain; subacute and chronic traumatic and inflammatory conditions; prior to stretching shortened soft tissue; reduction of pain. Pulsed US: tissue healing of dermal ulcers, surgical skin incisions, tendon injuries, bone fractures (although healing of bone tissue requires use of very low intensity pulsed US and is rarely provided in the clinic); acute conditions (where thermal US is contraindicated)	**Treatment technique:** Can be applied via either direct contact or indirect contact using water (or a balloon). Where direct contact is used, a transmission medium or coupling agent, i.e., gel or lotion, must be applied to the skin (between the US transducer and the skin). The PTA places the transducer parallel to the patient's skin, moving it in a slow circular pattern. The transducer is always in firm contact (but not heavy) with the patient's skin. Use a plastic container for US in the water (the transducer must be 0.5–1 inch from the patient's skin). The transducer must not be held in the air (without skin contact) when the US unit is on. For periosteal pain: Decrease intensity; increase treatment surface area. For TUS "hot spot:" Apply more coupling agent; decrease intensity; keep the transducer moving. **Treatment parameters:** ■ Frequency: Deeper tissues (2.5–5 cm) need 1 MHz frequency. Less deep tissues (1–2.5 cm) need 3 MHz frequency. ■ Intensity: to increase tissue temperature at 1 MHz intensity, between 1.5 and 2.0 W/cm² is effective.[5] At 3 MHz intensity, 0.5 W/cm² is effective.[5] ■ Duty Cycle: 100% duty cycle (continuous US) provides a thermal effect. 20% duty cycle (pulsed US) provides a nonthermal effect. ■ Treatment time: 5–10 minutes per treated area or twice the area of the sound head. Phonophoresis: Applied using direct-contact pulsed-mode US. Apply US gel and the medication. Do not whip medication into US gel (air can be trapped in the mixture, decreasing transmission of US). Phonophoresis intensities: direct-contact pulsed mode (20% duty cycle) = 0.5–1 W/cm² at 3MHz frequency for 5–10 minutes.[5]

(continued)

Table 4.5 **Biophysical Agents and Modalities: Indications and Applications[5,6]**   *(continued)*

Physical Agent/ Modality	Indications	Applications
Fluidotherapy	Subacute and chronic musculoskeletal conditions such as RA, OA, muscular pain, reflex sympathetic dystrophy; any other disorder where it promotes desensitization of hypersensitive tissues	Cover open wounds/lesions with a plastic barrier. Safe to use with patients who have splints, bandages, tape, metal implants, artificial tendons, or plastic joint replacements. Procedure: The PTA places the UE in a sleeve (of the machine) or the LE over the treatment slot. The PTA sets the desired temperature between 100°F –118°F (38°C–48°C) and turns the unit on. The PTA adjusts agitation of the cellulose (or silicone) particles to the desired effect and the patient's tolerance. The PTA instructs the patient in stretching or strengthening exercises during treatment. For desensitization, the PTA monitors the patient's response to treatment. Treatment time = 15–20 minutes.
Diathermy: short wave (SWD); microwave (MWD)	Thermal effects: increased tissue temperature, decrease pain, increase soft tissue extensibility, decrease joint stiffness, used prior to stretching to increase ROM Nonthermal or pulsed SWD: wound care and soft tissue healing, to decrease pain and edema, to increase oxygen to the tissue, and to increase muscle, bone, and nerve tissue repair by stimulation of protein synthesis at the tissue cell level, management of symptoms of OA	Remove jewelry and metal on clothing from the field. Check patient often during treatment—the treated area is not visible. SW diathermy delivers a thermal or pulsed electromagnetic field. Typical SWD frequency = 27.12 MHz. ■ SW diathermy-treated area as part of the electrical circuit method: The patient's body part is placed between two conducting electrodes for 15–30 minutes. ■ SW inductive field method: The patient's body part is placed in a magnetic field of electrodes and current is induced within the patient's body tissues (that are not part of circuit). Tissue resistance to the current produces an increased temperature in the deep body tissues. ■ MW diathermy applied using electromagnetic radiation directed an antenna mounted in the treatment applicator. The applicator is placed perpendicular to the skin. Caution when using MW diathermy: When energy is reflected at fat/ muscle and muscle/bone interfaces, it can increase superficial tissues' temperatures (skin or fat). Treatment time MW diathermy = 15–30 minutes.

(continued)

Table 4.5 Biophysical Agents and Modalities: Indications and Applications[5,6] *(continued)*

Physical Agent/ Modality	Indications	Applications
Therapeutic cold: cold pack (CP); ice pack (IP); ice massage with ice cube (IC)	CP/IP: acute and chronic traumatic and inflammatory conditions; edema; muscle spasm; musculoskeletal pain; thermal burns Ice massage with IC: small areas of muscle guarding; muscle spasm; spasticity in UMN dysfunction; acute injuries to decrease pain, edema, and hemorrhage	Test patient's sensation and cold tolerance. First treatment: Monitor adverse effects (such as urticaria; facial flush; anaphylaxis; call EMS for anaphylaxis). Patient's normal response to ice: cold, burning, aching, and numbness (CBAN). ■ A CP wrapped in a warm moist towel is placed on the area to be treated; place two to three dry towels over the CP. Secure the CP to the patient with elastic bandages or towels. The PTA monitors the patient's treated area visually after 5 minutes. The patient receives a call bell. The patient should not lie on the CP. Treatment time = 10–20 minutes. ■ IP treatment is the same as CP treatment except the IP should be placed in dry towels. ■ The IC for ice massage must be round without sharp edges. It is applied in overlapping circles or overlapping longitudinal strokes, with each stroke covering half of the previous stroke. Treated area = 4 inches by 6 inches. The PTA should not do ice massage over bony area or superficial nerves (such as the peroneal nerve in the lower leg). The PTA uses a towel to wipe the excess water as it melts on the skin. Treatment time = 5–10 minutes.
Contrast bath	Subacute trauma; sprains and strains; edema; pain; improve superficial blood flow; RSD	Check water temperature: Hot (warm) = 100–110°F (38°C –44°C); cold = 55–65°F (10°C–18°C). Select water based on the patient's condition: Prepare two pails of water, one for hot water and one for cold water. The PTA first immerses the patient's treated limb in hot water for 3–10 minutes. The PTA then transfers the patient's treated limb to cold water for 1–3 minutes. The treated limb is returned to the hot water again for 4–10 minutes. This sequence of immersion is continued for 20–30 minutes. For edema or acute sprains/strains, it is beneficial to end in cold water.

(continued)

Table 4.5 Biophysical Agents and Modalities: Indications and Applications[5,6]   *(continued)*

Physical Agent/ Modality	Indications	Applications
Therapeutic massage[7]	Subacute and chronic pain; muscle spasm; superficial scar formation and adhesions from trauma or burns; chronic edema; improve circulation; improve lymphatic flow; as an adjunct to postural drainage/ airway clearance. Deep transverse friction can help to effect collagen fiber orientation in wound healing.	Effleurage: The PTA's hand is molded over the patient's body part and moved slowly, but firmly, in a distal to proximal direction. Pétrissage involves kneading, picking up, wringing, or rolling of the tissues using firm pressure. Deep friction is used to stretch scar tissues and loosen adhesions within connective tissue. Deep transverse friction is a specific cross-fiber friction applied at right angles to the tissue targeted. Tapotement is a series of brisk percussive movements following one another in a rapid, alternating manner (hacking, cupping, beating, and pounding). Cupping is applied to the chest to mobilize bronchial secretions in pulmonary physical therapy. Vibration is an oscillating, trembling motion performed rapidly and repeatedly for postural drainage to loosen adherent secretions.
Intermittent compression	Chronic edema; lymphedema (after mastectomies); venous stasis ulcer; traumatic edema; venous insufficiency; amputation	The PTA takes the patient's BP. The patient is positioned comfortably with the UE or LE abducted between 20° and 70° and elevated at approximately 40°. Remove jewelry and clothing from the area to be treated. Before application of compression sleeve, a stockinette is put on, with the PTA removing all the wrinkles in the fabric. The compression sleeve is applied, and the rubber tubing is attached to the sleeve and the pump. Set three parameters: inflation pressure (to be set below the patient's diastolic BP), inflation and deflation time (to be set at a ratio of 3:1, inflating for 80–100 seconds and deflating for 25–35 seconds), and total treatment time (2–3 hours). For amputation, inflate the sleeve for 40–60 seconds and deflate it for 10–15 seconds (4:1 ratio). Lymphedema requires a treatment time of 2- to 3-hour daily sessions; venous stasis ulcer requires treatment lasting for 2.5 hours, three times per week.

(continued)

Table 4.5 **Biophysical Agents and Modalities: Indications and Applications**[5,6]   *(continued)*

Physical Agent/ Modality	Indications	Applications
Electrical stimulation (ES): HVPC; NMES; FES; IFC[5]	Decrease muscle spasm; increase or maintain joint ROM by decreasing joint pain and edema; increase muscle strength; muscle reeducation; repair of the soft tissue in wound healing; decrease edema; increase circulation; decrease spasticity; elicit contractions in denervated muscle to reduce atrophy Interferential current (IFC): pain relief; muscle relaxation; edema control; increased circulation	General Application of ES ■ PTA checks that all controls are at zero before turning on device. ■ The PTA inspects the skin for abrasions/irritations, cleaning the skin and clipping any hair to ensure good adhesion of electrodes. (Do not shave the area.) ■ The PTA selects two or four electrodes based on size of area to be treated and modality used. The PTA prepares and places the electrodes on the patient's area that needs to be treated. The space between two electrodes must be at least the diameter of one electrode. The PTA secures the electrodes to the patient's treated area. ■ The PTA sets the appropriate frequency, waveform, and modulation rate. The PTA slowly adjusts intensity to achieve optimal treatment effects. ■ After 3–4 minutes of treatment, the PTA needs to slightly increase the intensity due to the patient's accommodation. ■ At the end of the treatment, the PTA slowly decreases the intensity to zero before lifting the electrodes from the treated area. ■ The PTA turns all controls to zero. High-volt pulsed current (HVPC): ■ Acute-stage edema control: frequency of 120 pps, continuous mode, with pulse between 20–100 μs for 30 minutes, up to four times per day. ■ Wound healing: Inflammatory stage of tissue healing/ infected tissue: negative polarity for bactericidal effect frequency 100–105 pps, pulse duration 100 μs, for 45–60 minutes. Proliferation stage of tissue healing: positive polarity for wound closure frequency 100–105 pps, pulse duration 100 μs, for 45–60 minutes. A gauze pad with sterile saline solution is applied first over the wound; a small active electrode is attached to gauze (dressing); a large dispersive electrode is placed ipsilateral, proximal to wound. Neuromuscular electrical stimulation (NMES) ■ Muscle strengthening and reeducation (includes Russian stimulation) achieved using muscular contractions in conjunction with the electrical stimulus: frequency between 30 to 80 pps; duty cycle = 1:5; pulse duration small muscles = 125–200 μs; large muscles = 200–350 μs; treatment time = 10–30 minutes.

(continued)

Table 4.5 **Biophysical Agents and Modalities: Indications and Applications[5,6]**   *(continued)*

Physical Agent/ Modality	Indications	Applications
		■ Edema reduction: frequency between 35-50 pps; duty cycle is 2–5 sec on/2–5 sec off; pulse duration small muscles = 125–200 µs; large muscles = 200–350 µs; treatment time = 30 minutes.
		■ Reduction of muscle spasm: frequency between 35–50 pps; duty cycle is 2–5 sec on/2–5 sec off; pulse duration small muscles = 125–200 µs; large muscles = 200 µs–350 µs; treatment time = 10–30 minutes, two times per day.
		■ Stimulation of denervated muscle requires DC waveform and parameters managed by the clinician.
		Functional electrical stimulation (FES):
		■ Most common use is to control for foot drop.
		■ Ankle dorsiflexors and evertor muscles during the swing phase of gait: frequency of 30–50 pps, on/off times are based on functional needs of the activity.
		Interferential current (IFC)
		■ Pain relief: four electrodes placed diagonally to one another over large areas of treatment; frequency = 80–150 pps.
		■ Circulation and edema control: two-electrode placement over or around small areas of treatment; frequency = 20–40 pps.
		■ For circulation through muscle contraction: frequency of 35–50 pps and pulse duration of 125–200 msec.
Iontophoresis	Neuritis; bursitis; musculoskeletal inflammatory condition; calcific tendonitis; muscular relaxation; softening of scar tissue and adhesions; wound care; reducing calcium deposits; decreasing edema; skin conditions such as ischemic ulcers, hyperhidrosis, and fungal infections	Check for intact skin, no scratches or abrasions. The electrical wave form is low amplitude DC (monophasic, continuous current). The current must be started, terminated, or interrupted slowly, never abruptly. Use negative medication for the (–) electrode and positive medication for the (+) electrode; use low levels of current intensity for the (–) electrode; the (–) electrode must be twice as large as the (+) electrode. Alkaline chemical reactions caused by negative polarity are stronger than acidic reactions. Recommended dosage for the positive electrode is 1.0 mA/cm^2 and for the negative electrode is 0.5 mA/cm^2. The current intensity must be lower than 4.0 mA. The treatment time varies from 10 to 40 minutes, depending on the medication dose. For example, if the current intensity of 4.0 mA is comfortable for the patient and a dosage of 80.0 mA/min of dexamethasone is applied, this dexamethasone dosage can be delivered in 20 min (4 × 20 = 80). The PTA observes the treated area

Table 4.5 Biophysical Agents and Modalities: Indications and Applications[5,6]   *(continued)*

Physical Agent/ Modality	Indications	Applications
		every 3–5 minutes, staying alert to any adverse reactions. Negative medications: dexamethasone, acetic acid, salicylate (DAS). Positive medication most typically used: lidocaine. Zinc (+) has been used for wound management and tap water (=/−) used for hyperhidrosis.
Transcutaneous electrical nerve stimulation (TENS): conventional TENS; strong low-rate TENS; burst-mode TENS	Pain management and pain modulation through activation of the gate control theory and the endogenous opiate theory	Patient education for use of TENS units: Not to be used in shower or when sleeping; electrode placement; skin inspection-skin irritation; checking adherence of electrodes to the skin; accommodation to ES (the patient should contact the PT/PTA-modulation TENS). ■ Conventional TENS (high rate): frequency of 100–150 pps; pulse duration of 50–80 μs; may be worn for 24 hours as needed; uses gate theory mechanism; has fast pain relief; is short-lasting (approximately 1 hour). ■ Strong low-rate TENS: frequency of 2–10 pps; pulse duration of 150–300 μs; for 20–30 minutes; longer lasting pain relief. ■ Burst-mode TENS: frequency of 50–150 pps sent in bursts or packets of 1–10 pps; pulse duration is typically preset on unit; for 20–30 minutes; longer lasting pain relief. Conventional TENS uses gate control theory. Low rate and burst TENS use endogenous opiate theory.
Traction: cervical; lumbar	Spinal nerve root impingement caused by herniated nucleus pulposus (HNP) or spinal stenosis; muscle spasm; spinal hypomobility; subacute joint inflammation	Cervical traction: Observe the patient for discomfort in the TMJ; adjust the head halter and ensure force is applied to the occipital region. When the treated segment is lower than C2, the cervical spine must be positioned in 20°–30° of spinal flexion. For nerve root impingement, the cervical spine must be positioned in 15° of spinal flexion. The force of the traction should not exceed the weight of the patient's head. Start at 8–10 pounds (or 7% of the patient's head weight). Increase the force gradually up to 25–30 pounds. Maximum elongation occurs at 25°–35° of spinal flexion. Treatment time = 5–10 minutes for HNP and 10–30 minutes for other disorders. Initially static force is given, and then intermittent force at 15 seconds on and 15 seconds off. Disc problems: use 60 seconds on and 20 seconds off; muscular spasm: use 5 seconds on and 5 seconds off.

(continued)

Table 4.5 Biophysical Agents and Modalities: Indications and Applications[5,6]   *(continued)*

Physical Agent/ Modality	Indications	Applications
		Lumbar traction: Patient may be positioned in prone or supine. Prone positions for posterior HNP. Supine positions used for facet joint dysfunction. To increase L5–S1 space, use a small bench under the patient's lower legs (45–60° of hip flexion). Start with low-force traction—use a split table and 25% of the patient's body weight. Increase the force gradually to half of the patient's body weight (to effect intervertebral separation). Use of a split table decreases leg/pelvis friction. Treatment time for HNP = 5 minutes at first and then increase to 10 minutes; use 10–30 minutes for others. Initially, begin with static force, and then give intermittent force (joint distraction) of 15 seconds on and 15 seconds off. Muscle spasm: use 5 seconds on and 5 seconds off; disc problems: use 60 seconds on and 20 seconds off.
Electromyographic biofeedback (EMG biofeedback)	EMG is used with other interventions to enhance muscle recruitment and increase muscle strength in patients with peripheral nerve injury, muscle weakness caused by immobilization, joint surgery, pain, deconditioning, muscle spasticity, and reeducation of weak or flaccid muscle. EMG can be used in conjunction with relaxation for chronic pain such as tension headaches, and chronic neck and back pain, where the goal is to decrease muscle activity.	Patients receiving EMG biofeedback must have good vision, good hearing, excellent communication abilities, good comprehension of simple commands, good concentration, and motor planning skills. Bipolar technique: Two active electrodes are applied parallel to the muscle fibers at approximately 15 cm, over or near the motor points of treated muscles; a reference electrode is applied between active electrodes or closer to active electrodes. ■ To increase muscular strength of two or more weak muscles, the PTA places two active electrodes widely spaced. ■ To increase muscular strength of one weak muscle, the PTA places two active electrodes close together. Instrument sensitivity must be high for weak muscles. The PTA instructs the patient to contract the muscle isometrically, holding the contraction for as long as possible (up to 10 seconds) to produce a tall and loud audiovisual signal. As the patient's motor recruitment improves, active electrodes must be placed closer together and instrument sensitivity decreased. ■ For relaxation, the PTA places two active electrodes closely spaced. Instrument sensitivity must be low. The PTA instructs the patient to relax and to lower the audiovisual signal; the PTA applies breathing or imagery exercises. As the patient is able to relax, instrument sensitivity must be increased, and the patient should perform functional activities. Treatment time = first 5 minutes and then 10–30 minutes.

Therapeutic Massage Application

Table 4.6 Application of Therapeutic Massage[7]

1. When applying therapeutic massage to a specific anatomical region of the patient's body, the patient should be comfortable and in a relaxed position.
2. The treatment part should be in a gravity-eliminated position or in a position in which the gravity assists the venous flow.
3. The patient's body part must be draped and well supported.
4. The PTA should start with light effleurage and then advance to deep effleurage and other types of stroking necessary in that specific intervention.
5. When using all forms of massage, deep effleurage is followed by pétrissage, then friction, (tapotement and vibration if indicated) and concluding with light effleurage.
6. Massage should begin in the proximal segments of the lower or upper extremity, move distally, and then return to the proximal region.
7. On the lower or upper extremity, all effleurage movements must be directed in a distal to proximal direction, especially for edema treatment.
8. Therapeutic massage treatment depends on the patient's tolerance and specific intervention.
9. Similar to other physical agents or modalities, therapeutic massage is a passive modality that should be used for a short period of time as an adjunct to—not a substitute for—active interventions such as therapeutic exercises and activities and patient education.

Wheelchair Management

Table 4.7 Wheelchair Measurements[8]

Taken on a firm surface (sitting or supine); hips, knees, and ankles should be positioned at 90°.

Seat Width Measurement

- Measure the widest part of hips and add 2 inches to the measurement.
- Typical seat-width dimensions:
  - Standard adult wheelchair = 18 inches
  - Narrow adult or junior wheelchair = 16 inches
  - Extra-wide adult wheelchair = 22 inches
- Potential problems: extra-wide seat width can cause difficulty reaching; narrow seat width can cause lateral pelvis and thighs discomfort.

Seat Depth Measurement

- Measure from the posterior buttocks on the lateral side of the thigh to the popliteal fossa and subtract 2 inches from the measurement.
- Typical seat depth dimensions for standard adult, narrow adult, junior, and extra-wide adult wheelchairs = 16 inches.
- Potential problems: too-long seat depth can cause circulatory problems to posterior knees, posterior tilt sitting, and kyphotic posture; too-short seat depth can cause inadequate thigh support.

Seat Height Measurement

- Measured relative to the entire wheelchair: 2 inches measurement from the floor to the lowest point on the bottom of the foot plate of the footrest.
- Leg length measurement: Measure from the bottom of the patient's shoe to the posterior popliteal fossa and add 2 inches.
- Typical seat height dimensions:
  - Standard adult, narrow adult, and extra-wide adult wheelchairs = 20 inches
  - Junior wheelchair = 18.5 inches
- Potential problems: too-short leg length can cause excessive weight on ischial seat and decubitus ulcers; too-long leg length can cause sacral sitting and sliding forward in the wheelchair.

Back Height Measurement

- Measure from the seat platform to the lower angle of the patient's scapula, midscapula, or top of the shoulder, depending on the patient's needs.
  - Typical back height = 16–16.5 inches
- If a cushion is used, it must be added to the measurement.

Armrest Height Measurement

- Measure from seat platform to olecranon process with elbow flexed to 90 degrees and add 1 inch.
  - Armrest height in a standard wheelchair = 9 inches above the seat.
- If a cushion is used, it must be added to the measurement calculation.

Table 4.8 Wheelchair's Postural Support System[9]

Solid Insert (Seat Support)

■ Types of solid inserts
  - Padded insert board
  - Reinforcement board inside cushion cover
  - Contoured or flat insert board between cushion and wheelchair

■ Benefits of the solid insert
  - Increases stability
  - Decreases possibility of LE's adduction and IR
  - Decreases possibility of posterior pelvic tilt and slipping forward in the seat
  - Improves pelvic position
  - Encourages neutral pelvic tilt and symmetrical spinal alignment
  - Can promote trunk extension and upper body stability
  - Increases head and UE function
  - Has low cost

■ Limitations of the solid insert
  - Increases seat height
  - Can shift on seat to cause asymmetrical seating

Solid Hook-On Seat (Seat Support)

■ Can be installed using hardware to hook to the seat rails. Has adjustable angle and height to be able to change positions of the seat surface on the wheelchair's frame.

■ Benefits of the solid hook-on seat
  - Creates stable base of support
  - Improves pelvic position
  - Decreases possibility of LE's adduction and IR, posterior pelvic tilt, and slipping forward in wheelchair (by raising the anterior portion of the solid hook-on seat)
  - Encourages neutral pelvic tilt and symmetrical alignment of the spine
  - If posterior portion of the solid hook-on seat is raised, can facilitate trunk co-contraction

■ Limitations of the solid hook-on seat
  - Difficult to remove
  - Adds weight to the wheelchair's frame

Pressure-Relieving Foam (Custom or Premade Contoured Seat Cushion)

■ Can increase surface contact and improve pressure distribution and relief. Has different degrees of firmness, and the generic types work well for symmetrical individuals.

■ Benefits of the pressure-relieving foam
  - Increases surface contact
  - Improves distribution of weight
  - Accommodates moderate and severe postural asymmetry

(continued)

Table 4.8 **Wheelchair's Postural Support System**[9] *(continued)*

- Is low maintenance
- Allows easier positioning and repositioning of the patient (client) for the caregiver
- Limitations of the pressure-relieving foam
  - Is expensive
  - Can interfere with sliding transfers
  - Can cause a feeling of being locked in because the movement on the cushion surface is restricted

Comfort Cushion (Planar or Contoured Seat Cushion)

- Made of layered foam and used for postural control and for limited ROM
- Benefits of the comfort cushion
  - Promotes neutral pelvic position
  - Increases patient's comfort
  - Creates a stable base of support
  - Does not interfere with sliding transfers
  - Is inexpensive
  - Is lightweight
  - Patient can sit anywhere on the cushion without any discomfort
- Limitations of the comfort cushion
  - Does not offer pressure relief
  - Gives minimal support and postural control

Pressure-Relieving Air Cushion (Seat Cushion)

- Responds to patient's weight and increases surface contact to improve distribution of weight and relief (bony prominences feel like floating)
- Benefits of the pressure-relieving air cushion
  - Is very lightweight
  - Offers pressure relief (moderate to significant)
  - Improves moderate to significant postural asymmetry
  - Increases sitting time
  - Prevents decubitus ulcers (especially over bony prominences)
  - Improves postural control for specific body segments (using segmented air cushions)
- Limitations of the pressure-relieving air cushion
  - Is expensive
  - May be unstable for some patients (clients)
  - Decreases UE reach distance (because users keep arms closed to the body for stability)
  - May make transfers difficult because of the unstable base
  - Air pressure needs to be monitored carefully
  - Needs continuous maintenance

(continued)

Table 4.8 **Wheelchair's Postural Support System**[9] *(continued)*

Pressure-Relieving Fluid or Fluid/Foam Combination Cushion (Seat Cushion)

■ Has generic contour or planar surface contour with fluid-filled sac. The bony prominences feel immersed in the fluid (increases surface contact); accommodates limited ROM (by cutting foam base as needed); generic contoured shapes work well with symmetrical individuals.

■ Benefits of the pressure-relieving fluid or fluid/foam combination cushion
  • Provides a stable base of support for proper seating alignment
  • Controls postural alignment (using add-on pieces)
  • Increases comfort and sitting tolerance (especially for oblique pelvis)
  • Improves head and shoulders alignment
  • Can be used for moderate to significant seating needs
  • Increases sitting time; decreases possibility of decubitus ulcers (especially over bony prominences)
  • Increases pelvic stability (especially with gel medium fluid)
  • Is easier to position and reposition (for caregivers)

■ Limitations of the pressure-relieving fluid or fluid/foam combination cushion
  • Is expensive
  • Some maintenance required
  • Heavier than foam or air
  • Can cause a feeling of being locked in because the movement on the cushion surface is restricted

Solid Insert (Back Support)

■ Maintains pelvic alignment and can accommodate back contour and provide postural control (with special foaming)

■ Benefits of the solid insert
  • Maintains pelvic alignment (when interfaced with seat surface)
  • Improves upright seating, trunk, and head alignment
  • Provides some lateral support (with shaped foam)
  • Increases trunk control and distal extremities' function
  • Can be easily removed
  • Adds minimal weight to the wheelchair

■ Limitations of the solid insert
  • May not be stable in the chair
  • Can be easily lost or left behind when folding the wheelchair

Pita Back (Back Support)

■ A solid board (padded or unpadded) that slips into a pocket in the back upholstery of the wheelchair. It provides mild to moderate support and is used for patients (clients) who need a slight reminder to sit upright.

■ Benefits of the pita back
  • Encourages trunk extension
  • Is lightweight

(continued)

Table 4.8   **Wheelchair's Postural Support System**[9]   *(continued)*

- Is easy to put on and to remove
- Limitations of the pita back
  - Provides only a slight degree of support
  - Can be lost or left behind when the wheelchair is folded

Solid Hook-On (Back Support)

- A very stable back support that can be aligned and angled as necessary. It can hold planar, contoured, molded back, or air flotation cushion; can be custom made or manufactured; and mounts using permanent (can strengthen the wheelchair frame) or removable hardware.
- Benefits of the solid hook-on support
  - Improves upright sitting
  - Accommodates patients with limited ROM
  - Accommodates patients with any degree of deformity
  - Increases UE and head control
  - Improves comfort and pressure relief
  - Maintains trunk and pelvis alignment
  - Resists extensor thrusting
  - Allows additional attachments (such as headrests)
- Limitations of the solid hook-on support
  - Increases wheelchair weight
  - Requires manipulation and removal of hardware to fold the wheelchair

Head and Neck Supports (Specialized Supports)

- Used for patients with fair, poor, or absent head control. The hardware can be fixed or removable.
- Benefits of head and neck supports
  - Improve anterior, posterior, or lateral head and neck control
  - Promote neutral cervical spine and head position
  - Eliminate uncontrolled lateral flexion and rotation (which disturb trunk and pelvis alignment)
  - Assist with respiration, feeding, swallowing, and visual interaction
  - Improve safety during the patient's (client's) transportation
- Limitations of head and neck supports
  - May interfere with head movement
  - May trigger extensor thrust
  - May cause skin problems in areas of high pressure

Lateral Trunk Support (Specialized Support)

- Used for weak or spastic trunk muscles. Can be straight or contoured; hardware can be fixed or swing away (for transfers).
- Benefits of the lateral trunk support
  - Improves trunk stability and control
  - Increases pelvic alignment

(continued)

Table 4.8 **Wheelchair's Postural Support System**[9] *(continued)*

- Controls lateral trunk flexion
- Facilitates UE movement
- Improves respiration, feeding, and swallowing
- Increases safety during the patient's movement
- ■ Limitations of the lateral trunk support
  - May interfere with trunk movement
  - Increases the weight of the wheelchair (chair)
  - May interfere with the patient's self-propelling ability when using the UE

Anterior Chest Support (Specialized Support)

- ■ Used for upright trunk posture and shoulder control. Can be maximally or minimally supportive (having additional features such as straps and padded straps).
- ■ Benefits of the anterior chest support
  - Eliminates forward lean
  - Discourages shoulder protraction (as in CVA)
  - Improves trunk control (and, in turn, respiration), eating, swallowing, and visual interaction
  - Improves UE, shoulder (promotes better head posture), and head control
  - Improves trunk upright position
  - Stabilizes the trunk to free up the arms and head for movement
- ■ Limitations of the anterior chest support
  - Restricts trunk movement
  - Long usage may limit trunk control improvements

Lateral Hip Guides (Specialized Supports)

- ■ Used for pelvic alignment. Assist with maintenance of the pelvic position on a contoured seat.
- ■ Benefits of lateral hip guides
  - Improve weight distribution (symmetrical weight bearing) on the pelvis
  - Increase sitting time
  - Increase upper and lower body segments alignment
  - Reduce asymmetries in trunk and LEs
- ■ Limitations of lateral hip guides
  - May interfere with transfers (if not removable)
  - Can cause a feeling of being locked in on the seat
  - Increase the weight of the wheelchair

Lateral Knee Guides (Specialized Supports)

- ■ May be built into the cushion contours or fabricated separately (from padded wood or plastic) and attached to the seat or armrest of the wheelchair. Lateral knee guides should extend to the end of the knee for maximal control.
- ■ Benefits of lateral knee guides
  - Maintain alignment of LE

(continued)

Table 4.8 **Wheelchair's Postural Support System**[9] *(continued)*

- Reduce excessive abduction and ER
- Assist patient in maintaining pelvic alignment
- Improve trunk and UE position and function
- Reduce forward sliding of pelvis on the seat of the wheelchair
- Limitations of lateral knee guides
  - If they are too high (as needed), may interfere with transfers (if they are not removable)
  - Add weight to the wheelchair

Medial Knee Block (Specialized Support)

- May be built into the cushion contours or fabricated separately (or as a removable flip-down block). Medial knee block must be positioned at the distal portion of the limb (between the condyles) for maximal control and should never be used to stabilize the pelvis on the seat by pressing it into the groin. Also, it should never be used to prevent the patient (client) from sliding off the front of the seat.
- Benefits of the medial knee block
  - Prevents LE from moving into adduction
  - Prevents pelvic forward rotation (when used with both LEs oriented to one side, with one LE adducted and the other LE abducted)
  - Maintains broad and stable base of support
  - Decreases spasticity (if wide enough)
  - Maintains LE alignment
- Limitations of the medial knee block
  - May interfere with transfers
  - Increases the weight of the wheelchair

Anterior Knee Block (Specialized Support)

- The most effective way to maintain proper pelvic position on the seat. Needs the physician's approval if the patient's hips are subluxed, dislocated, or not properly formed.
- Benefits of the anterior knee block
  - Helps maintain a broad and stable base of support
  - Improves pelvic alignment and functional use of the upper body
  - May facilitate trunk co-contraction, extension, and improved UE ROM (when used with a forward-sloped seat)
  - Reduces extensor tone
  - Increases stability
- Limitations of the anterior knee block:
  - May impose too much pressure at the hips and over the patella
  - Patient (client) may feel restricted

Mobility Training

Table 4.9 Wheelchair Training Elements[9]

- Patient (client) and/or caregiver education in wheelchair use, safety, and maintenance
- Patient (client) and/or caregiver education in proper alignment and pressure relief activities (e.g., arm push-ups, weight shifting by leaning to one side and then the other side)
- Patient (client) and/or caregiver education in use of wheelchair's postural supports: positioning of supports; benefits and limitations of supports; care and maintenance of supports; schedule of use of supports
- Manual wheelchair propulsion training (using both UEs, using one UE, and using one UE and one LE): forward and backward propulsion on flat surfaces and uneven surfaces; turning by pushing harder with one hand than the other hand and taking sharp turns (by pulling one wheel backward while pushing the opposite wheel forward); negotiating obstacles (such as curbs and thresholds)
- Power wheelchair training: for driving skills and safety; use of switches (on and off and turns); use of joystick; safe stopping
- Management of wheelchair wheel locks: use of footrests and armrests; transfer safety with the wheelchair locked; transfers using removable or swing-away armrests; transfers using removable or swing-away leg rests
- Community mobility using the wheelchair practice: mobility when ascending ramps backward (by moving the center of gravity forward; forward lean of the trunk; using quick and short strokes for propulsion); mobility when descending ramps (by gripping the hand rims loosely; increasing the grip to control the speed of the descent; or/and descending in an advanced wheelie position by keeping the spine against the wheelchair back for steep ramps; using gloves)
- Wheelchair curb negotiation practice
  - How to pop up a wheelie (moving into a wheelie position): patient places one hand posteriorly on the hand rims and pulls the hand rims forward abruptly and forcefully; patient trunk and head are moved forward to keep the wheelchair from tipping backward
  - How to maintain balance in the wheelie position: the wheelchair tips farther back when the wheels are pushed forward; the wheelchair tips into upright position when the wheels are pulled back; the patient to come up onto balance on the rear wheels with the front casters off the ground
- Wheelchair curb ascent practice: patient (client) places front casters up on the curb; patient (client) pushes rear wheels up the curb; patient (client) uses momentum to assist.
- Wheelchair curb descent practice: patient (client) can descend backward with forward head and trunk lean; patient (client) pushes rear wheels up the curb; patient (client) can descend forward in wheelie position.
- Wheelchair ascending and descending stairs practice: using the wheelchair; assisted by buttocks bringing wheelchair behind; advanced techniques
- Patient (client) education and practice in how to fall safely and how to return to the wheelchair
- Patient (client) practice in how to transfer into a car (i.e., placing the wheelchair inside the car by pulling the wheelchair behind the car seat or using a wheelchair lift)
- Routine maintenance of the wheelchair: normal cleaning and upkeep; power-chair battery maintenance

References

1. Kisner C, Colby LA. *Therapeutic Exercise: Foundations and Techniques.* 6th ed. Philadelphia, PA: F.A. Davis; 2012.
2. Tan KC. *Practical Manual of Physical Medicine and Rehabilitation: Diagnostics, Therapeutics, and Basic Problems.* St. Louis, MO: Mosby Yearbook; 1998.
3. VeDA. The Vestibular Disorders Association. https://vestibular.org/. Accessed July 7, 2021.
4. Kauffman TL, Scott R, Bar JO, Moran ML, Wolf SL. *A Comprehensive Guide to Geriatric Rehabilitation.* 3rd ed. St. Louis, MO. Elsevier; 2014.
5. Cameron MH. *Physical Agents in Rehabilitation: An Evidence Based Approach to Practice.* 5th ed. St. Louis, MO. Elsevier; 2018.
6. Hecox B, Tsega AM, Weisberg J, Sanko J. *Integrating Physical Agents in Rehabilitation.* 2nd ed. Upper Saddle River, NJ: Pearson Education; 2006.
7. De Domenico G. *Beard's Massage Principles of Practice of Soft Tissue Manipulation.* 5th ed. St. Louis, MO. Elsevier; 2007.
8. Fairchild SL. *Pierson and Fairchild's Principles and Techniques of Patient Care.* 5th ed. St. Louis, MO: Elsevier; 2013.
9. O'Sullivan SB, Schmitz TJ. *Physical Rehabilitation.* 5th ed. F.A. Philadelphia, PA: Davis; 2007.

PART 5

Musculoskeletal System: Data Collection and Interventions

SECTION 5-1

Bones

Human Skeleton

Bones make up the framework of the human body. The human skeleton has 206 bones, including 80 in the trunk (axial skeleton) and 126 in the limbs (appendicular skeleton) (**Figure 5.1**).

Skull
　Frontal
　Parietal
　Temporal
　Zygomatic
　Maxilla
　Mandible

Thorax
　Sternum
　Ribs

Vertebral column

Pelvic girdle
　Ilium
　Sacrum
　Coccyx
　Ischium
　Pubis

Lower limb
　Femur
　Patella
　Tibia
　Fibula
　Tarsals
　Metatarsals
　Phalanges

Shoulder girdle
　Clavicle
　Scapula

Upper limb
　Humerus
　Radius
　Ulna
　Carpals
　Metacarpals
　Phalanges

ANTERIOR VIEW

Figure 5.1 The human skeleton
From Human Biology: Fifth Edition by Daniel Chiras, 2005, page 217, Figure 12-2 called The Human Skeleton

Carpal Bones

Table 5.1 Carpal Bones

Proximal row	Scaphoid (navicular); lunate; triquetrum; pisiform
Distal row	Trapezium; trapezoid; capitate; hamate

Tarsal Bones

Table 5.2 Tarsal Bones

Calcaneus
Cuboid
First metatarsal
Talus
Navicular
First cuneiform (medial cuneiform)
Second cuneiform (intermediate cuneiform)
Third cuneiform (lateral cuneiform)

Muscles: Function, Nerve, Origin, Insertion, and Palpation

1. Sternocleidomastoid
2. Pectoralis minor
3. Serratus anterior
4. External intercostals
5. Rectus abdominis
6. Tensor fasciae latae
7. Sartorius
8. Gracilis
9. Platysma
10. Deltoid
11. Pectoralis major
12. Biceps brachii
13. External abdominal oblique
14. Brachioradialis
15. Adductor longus
16. Rectus femoris
17. Vastus medialis
18. Vastus lateralis
19. Peroneus longus
20. Tibialis anterior
21. Levaor scapulae
22. Trapezius
23. Deltoid
24. Triceps brachii
25. Extensor carpi radialis longus
26. Adductor magnus
27. Splenius
28. Latissimus dorsi
29. Gluteus maximus
30. Biceps femoris
31. Semitendinosus
32. Gastrocnemius

Figure 5.2 Anterior and posterior superficial muscles
From Anatomy and Physiology: Understanding the Human Body by Robert Clark, page 159, Figure 10.3 called The anterior [left] and posterior [right] superficial muscles

Pelvis and Hip Muscles

Table 5.3 Pelvis and Hip Muscles[1]

Muscle	Function	Nerve	Origin	Insertion	Palpation
Iliopsoas	Hip flexion, adduction, external rotation	Femoral nerve (L2–L3)	Iliac fossa, anterior, and lateral surfaces of T12–L5	Lesser trochanter of the femur	Psoas major can be palpated distal to the inguinal ligament on the medial side of the sartorius
Tensor fascia latae (helps knee to extend)	Combined hip flexion, abduction, internal rotation	Superior gluteal nerve (L4–L5)	Anterior Superior Iliac Spine (ASIS)	Through the iliotibial tract to the lateral condyle of the tibia	Iliotibial tract can be palpated at its insertion into the lateral tibial tubercle of the knee
Sartorius	Hip flexion, abduction, external rotation	Femoral nerve (two branches; L2–L3)	ASIS	Proximal part of the medial surface of the shaft of the tibia (pes anserinus)	Palpated at its origin, slightly inferior to the ASIS
Gluteus maximus (sciatic nerve lies underneath)	Hip extension, hyperextension, external rotation	Inferior gluteal nerve (L1–L5; S1–S2)	Posterior sacrum and ilium	Posterior femur distal to the greater trochanter and to the iliotibial band	Palpated in the prone position, when the buttocks are squeezed together, or when extending the hip and flexing the knee
Gluteus medius (with gluteus minimus and Tensor Fascia Latae (TFL) abducts the thigh at the hip joint)	Hip abduction	Superior gluteal nerve (L4–S1)	Outer surface of ilium	Greater trochanter of the femur (lateral surface)	Origin can be palpated slightly below the iliac crest in a side-lying position, with the leg to be palpated raised in a few degrees of abduction

(continued)

Table 5.3 Pelvis and Hip Muscles[1]

(continued)

Muscle	Function	Nerve	Origin	Insertion	Palpation
Gluteus minimus	Hip abduction, internal rotation	Superior gluteal nerve (L4–S1)	Lateral ilium	Greater trochanter of the femur (anterior border)	Cannot be palpated
Adductor magnus	Hip abduction	Superior gluteal nerve (L4–S1)	Outer surface of the ilium	Entire linea aspera and adductor tubercle	Cannot be palpated individually, only as a group
Adductor brevis	Hip abduction	Obturator nerve (L3–L4)	Outer surface of the inferior ramus of the pubis	Proximal part of the linea aspera and the pectineal line	Cannot be palpated individually, only as a group
Adductor longus	Hip abduction	Obturator nerve (L3–L4)	Outer surface of the inferior ramus of the pubis	Middle one-third of the linea aspera	Cannot be palpated individually, only as a group
Piriformis (muscle spasm can cause tenderness of sciatic nerve)	Hip external rotation	Nerves originating from S1 and S2 nerve root segments	Sacrum	Greater trochanter of the femur (superior border)	Cannot be palpated

Knee Muscles

Table 5.4 Knee Muscles[1]

Muscle	Function	Nerve	Origin	Insertion	Palpation
Rectus femoris (powerful knee joint stabilizer)	Hip flexion, knee extension	Femoral nerve (L2–L4)	Anterior Inferior Iliac Spine (AIIS)	Via the patellar ligament to the tibial tuberosity	Palpated as part of the quadriceps femoris group; for atrophy, measure the circumference of each thigh at 3 inches above the mid-patella
Vastus medialis	Knee extension	Femoral nerve (L2–L4)	Linea aspera	Via the patellar ligament to the tibial tuberosity	Palpated as part of the quadriceps femoris group
Vastus lateralis	Knee extension	Femoral nerve (L2–L4)	Linea aspera	Via the patellar ligament to the tibial tuberosity	Palpated as part of the quadriceps femoris group
Vastus intermedius	Knee extension	Femoral nerve (L2–L4)	Anterior femur	Via the patellar ligament to the tibial tuberosity	Palpated as part of the quadriceps femoris group
Biceps femoris	Knee flexion, hip extension	Sciatic nerve for long head (S1–S3); common peroneal nerve for short head (L5–S2)	Long head: ischial tuberosity; short head: lateral lip of the linea aspera of the femur	Common tendon of the two heads inserts at the head of the fibula	Palpated near its insertion into the head of the fibula when flexing the knee
Semimembranosus	Knee flexion, hip extension	Tibial portion of sciatic nerve (L5–S2)	Ischial tuberosity	Medial condyle of the tibia posterior surface	Hamstrings group palpated from the common origin on the ischium to insertion
Semitendinosus	Knee flexion, hip extension	Sciatic nerve (L5–S2)	Ischial tuberosity	Anteromedial surface of the shaft of the tibia (pes anserinus)	Hamstrings group palpated from the common origin on the ischium to insertion

Ankle and Foot Muscles

Table 5.5 Ankle and Foot Muscles[1]

Muscle	Function	Nerve	Origin	Insertion	Palpation
Gastrocnemius	Ankle plantarflexion, knee flexion	Tibial nerve (S1–S2)	Medial and lateral condyles of the femur	Through the Achilles tendon into the calcaneus	Gastrocnemius and soleus can be observed in action by asking the patient to walk on his or her toes
Soleus	Ankle plantarflexion	Tibial nerve (S1–S2)	Posterior fibula and tibia	Through the Achilles tendon into the calcaneus	Gastrocnemius and soleus can be observed in action by asking the patient to walk on his or her toes
Tibialis anterior	Ankle dorsiflexion, foot inversion	Deep peroneal nerve (L4–S1)	Lateral tibia and interosseous membrane	First cuneiform and metatarsal	Palpated medially at the dorsum of the foot at its insertion onto the first metatarsal and the first cuneiform bones
Tibialis posterior (supports the medial longitudinal arch of the foot)	Foot inversion, ankle plantarflexion	Tibial nerve (L5–S1)	Interosseous membrane, adjacent tibia, and fibula	Navicular and most tarsals and metatarsals	Tendon palpated behind and inferior to the medial malleolus
Peroneus longus (supports the lateral longitudinal arch of the foot)	Foot eversion, ankle plantarflexion	Superficial peroneal nerve (L4–S1)	Lateral proximal fibula and interosseous membrane	Plantar surface of the first cuneiform and metatarsal	Tendon palpated with the peroneus brevis tendon behind the lateral
Peroneus brevis	Foot eversion, ankle plantarflexion	Superficial peroneal nerve (L4–S1)	Lateral two-thirds of the lateral surface of the fibula	Plantar surface of the fifth metatarsal bone	Tendon palpated with the peroneus longus tendon behind the lateral malleolus

(continued)

Table 5.5 Ankle and Foot Muscles[1]

(continued)

Muscle	Function	Nerve	Origin	Insertion	Palpation
Extensor digitorum longus (EDL)	Extension of the four lesser toes, ankle, dorsiflexion foot eversion	Deep peroneal nerve (L4–S1)	Anterior surface of the shaft of the fibula	Distal phalanx of the four lesser toes	EDL tendon palpated lateral to the EHL when the toes are extended
Extensor hallucis longus (EHL)	Extension of the great toe, ankle dorsiflexion, foot inversion	Deep peroneal nerve (L4–S1)	Fibula and interosseous membrane	Distal phalanx of the great toe	EHL tendon palpated lateral to the tibialis anterior when the big toe extends
Flexor digitorum longus (FDL)	Flexion of the four lesser toes, ankle plantarflexion, foot inversion	Tibial nerve (L5–S1)	Posterior tibia	Distal phalanx of the four lesser toes	FDL tendon palpated immediately behind the posterior tibialis, just above the medial malleolus, when the toes are flexed
Flexor hallucis longus (FHL; maintains the medial longitudinal arch of the foot)	Flexion of the great toe, ankle, plantarflexion toe, ankle, plantarflexion, foot inversion	Tibial nerve (L5–S1)	Posterior fibula and interosseous membrane	Distal phalanx of the great toe	Cannot be palpated

Shoulder Muscles

Table 5.6 Shoulder Muscles[1]

Muscle	Function	Nerve	Origin	Insertion	Palpation
Upper trapezius	Scapular elevation, upward rotation	Spinal accessory nerve Cranial Nerve (CN) XI (C3–C4)	Occipital protuberance, nuchal ligament	Outer half of the clavicle, acromion process	Palpated with the middle and lower trapezius from the origin through the clavicle, acromion, and spine of the scapula; for lower angle, continue to the spinous processes of the lower thoracic vertebrae (T12)
Middle trapezius (pulls scapula medially)	Retraction of shoulder girdle	Spinal accessory nerve CN XI (C3–C4)	Spinous processes of C7–T3	Superior lip of the spine of the scapula	Same as above
Lower trapezius (pulls scapula downward)	Scapular depression, upward rotation	Spinal accessory nerve CN XI (C3–C4)	Spinous processes of the middle and lower thoracic vertebrae	Base of the spine of the scapula	Same as above
Serratus anterior (prevents winging of the scapula)	Scapular protraction, upward rotation	Long thoracic nerve (C5–C7)	Lateral surface of the upper eight ribs	Anterior surface of the vertebral border of the scapula	Palpated at the medial wall of the axilla, over the ribs
Rhomboid major and minor (raises the medial border of the scapula)	Scapular retraction, downward rotation	Dorsal scapular nerve (C5)	Nuchal ligament and spinous processes of C7 and T5	Vertebral border of the scapula between the spine and the inferior angle	Palpated under the overlying trapezius; patient must have arm in the back in internal rotation (IR), pushing the hand posteriorly into the physical therapist assistant's (PTA's) hand

(continued)

Table 5.6 Shoulder Muscles[1]

(continued)

Muscle	Function	Nerve	Origin	Insertion	Palpation
Levator scapulae (raises the medial border of the scapula)	Scapular elevation, downward rotation	C3 and C4 nerves, and dorsal scapular nerve (C5)	Transverse processes of C1–C4	Vertebral border of the scapula between the superior angle and the base of the spine	Cannot be palpated
Deltoid (anterior, middle, and posterior)	Shoulder abduction, flexion, extension, hyperextension, internal rotation, external rotation, horizontal adduction	Axillary nerve (C5–C6)	Anterior at the lateral third of the clavicle; middle at the acromion process of the scapula; posterior at the inferior lip of the spine of the scapula	Anterior, middle, and posterior at the deltoid tuberosity of the humerus	Palpated from the acromion to the deltoid tuberosity of the humerus
Pectoralis major and minor (rotates the scapula forward and downward)	Major: shoulder flexion to about 90°, internal rotation, adduction, horizontal adduction Minor: scapular rotation	Major: lateral and medial pectoral nerves (C5–T1) Minor: medial pectoral nerve (C8–T1)	Major: clavicular head at the medial third of the clavicle; sternal head at the anterior surface of the sternum, and costal cartilage of the first six ribs Minor: third, fourth, and fifth ribs	Major: both heads at the lateral lip of the bicipital groove of the humerus (crest of the greater tubercle) Minor: medial border of the coracoid process	Major: palpated bilaterally, mostly toward the medial portion; breast tissue overlies the pectoralis major Minor: cannot be palpated
Latissimus dorsi (assists rotating scapula downward)	Shoulder extension, adduction, internal rotation, hyperextension	Thoracodorsal nerve (C6–C8)	Spinous process of T7–L5, sacrum and iliac crest, and lower three ribs	Bicipital groove of the humerus (floor and medial lip)	Palpated most easily along the posterior wall of the axilla when the patient abducts the arm
Teres major	Shoulder extension, adduction, internal rotation	Subscapular nerve (C5–C6)	Axillary border of the scapula near the inferior angle	Medial lip of the bicipital groove of the humerus (crest of the lesser tubercle)	Palpated on the lateral border of the scapula just below the axilla

Rotator Cuff Muscles

Table 5.7 Rotator Cuff Muscles[1]

Muscle	Function	Nerve	Origin	Insertion	Palpation
Supraspinatus (assists deltoid in abduction)	Shoulder abduction	Suprascapular nerve (C5–C6)	Supraspinous fossa of the scapula	Greater tuberosity of the humerus	Palpated as a group at the greater tuberosity of the humerus when the patient has the shoulder extended passively
Infraspinatus	Shoulder external rotation, horizontal abduction	Suprascapular nerve (C5–C6)	Infraspinous fossa of the scapula	Greater tuberosity of the humerus	Same as above
Teres minor	Shoulder external rotation, horizontal abduction	Axillary nerve (C5–C6)	Axillary border of the scapula	Greater tuberosity of the humerus	Same as above
Subscapularis	Shoulder internal rotation, abduction	Suprascapular nerve (C5–C6)	Subscapular fossa of the scapula	Greater tuberosity of the humerus	Cannot be palpated

Elbow and Forearm Muscles

Table 5.8 Elbow and Forearm Muscles[1]

Muscle	Function	Nerve	Origin	Insertion	Palpation
Biceps brachii (main supinator)	Elbow flexion, forearm supination	Musculocutaneous nerve (C5–C6)	Short head: coracoid process of the scapula Long head: supraglenoid tubercle of the scapula	Bicipital tuberosity of the radius	Palpated distally toward insertion when the patient flexes the elbow
Triceps brachii	Elbow extension	Radial nerve (C7–C8)	Long head: infraglenoid tubercle of the scapula Lateral head: lateral/posterior surfaces of the proximal humerus Medial head: medial/posterior surfaces of the distal humerus	Olecranon process of the ulna	Palpated from the infraglenoid tubercle to just before the olecranon process; the patient must be leaning on a table with the arm slightly abducted and the hand on the table (as if a crutch supported the arm)
Brachialis	Elbow flexion	Musculocutaneous nerve (C5–C6)	Distal part of the anterior surface of the humerus	Ulnar tuberosity and coronoid process of the ulna	Cannot be palpated
Brachioradialis (assists rotating the forearm to the mid-prone position)	Elbow flexion	Radial nerve (C5–C6)	Lateral supracondylar ridge of the humerus	Styloid process of the radius	Palpated on the anterolateral aspect of the arm, when the patient has the elbow flexed at 90° and is making a fist, pushing up under the edge of a table
Supinator	Forearm supination	Radial nerve (C6)	Lateral epicondyle of the humerus and the adjacent ulna	Anterior surface of the proximal radius	Cannot be palpated
Pronator teres	Forearm pronation, elbow flexion	Median nerve (C6–C7)	Medial epicondyle of the humerus, coronoid process of the ulna	Lateral surface of the radius at its midpoint	Palpated as the common tendon of the wrist flexor and pronator muscle group, at the medial epicondyle of the humerus

Wrist, Hand, and Finger Muscles

Table 5.9 Wrist, Hand, and Finger Muscles[1]

Muscle	Function	Nerve	Origin	Insertion	Palpation
Flexor carpi ulnaris (FCU)	Wrist flexion, ulnar deviation	Ulnar nerve (C8–T1)	Medial epicondyle of the humerus	Pisiform and base of the fifth metacarpal	FCU tendon palpated proximal to the pisiform on the ulnar side of the palmaris longus when the patient flexes the wrist against resistance
Flexor carpi radialis (FCR)	Wrist flexion, radial deviation	Median nerve (C6–C7)	Medial epicondyle of the humerus	Base of the second and third metacarpals (palmar surface)	FCR tendon palpated radially to the palmaris longus when the patient flexes the wrist and radially deviates the hand
Extensor carpi ulnaris (ECU)	Wrist extension, ulnar deviation	Radial nerve (C6–C8)	Lateral epicondyle of the humerus	Base of the fifth metacarpal	Palpated starting at the ulnar styloid process and going toward the ECU insertion
Extensor carpi radialis longus (ECRL)	Wrist radial deviation, extension	Radial nerve (C6–C7)	Supracondylar ridge of the humerus	Base of the second metacarpal	Palpated on the radial side of the dorsal radial tubercle when the patient clenches the fist
Extensor carpi radialis brevis (ECRB)	Wrist extension	Radial nerve (C6–C7)	Lateral epicondyle of the humerus	Base of the third metacarpal	Palpated on the radial side of the dorsal radial tubercle when the patient clenches the fist
Flexor digitorum superficialis (FDS)	Finger flexion of proximal interphalangeal (PIP) and meta-carpophalangeal (MCP) joints	Median nerve (C7, C8, T1)	Lateral epicondyle of the humerus, coronoid process, and radius	Sides of the middle phalanx of the four fingers	Can be isolated for a specific finger and tested by holding the nontested fingers in extension while asking the patient to flex the PIP joint of the tested finger
Flexor digitorum profundus (FDP)	Flexion of all three joints of the fingers	Median and ulnar nerves (C8–T1)	Upper three-fourths of the ulna	Distal phalanx of the four fingers	Can be isolated for a specific finger and tested by stabilizing the MCP and interphalangeal (IP) joints of the tested finger in extension while asking the patient to flex only the distal interphalangeal (DIP) joints of the tested finger

(continued)

(continued)

Table 5.9 Wrist, Hand, and Finger Muscles[1]

Muscle	Function	Nerve	Origin	Insertion	Palpation
Extensor digitorum (extensor digitorum communis)	Extension of all three joints of fingers (metacarpophalangeal [MCP], PIP, DIP)	Radial nerve (C6–C8)	Lateral epicondyle of humerus	Base of distal phalanx of fingers two through five	Palpated between carpus and MCP joints when fingers are extended
Extensor digiti minimi (EDM)	Extension of all joints of the fifth finger (MCP, PIP, DIP)	Radial nerve–deep branch (C6–C8)	Lateral epicondyle of humerus	Base of distal phalanx of the fourth finger	Palpated as a slight indentation lateral to the ulnar styloid process when patient's palm is resting on the table and patient raises little finger
Flexor pollicis longus (FPL)	Flexion of all joints of the thumb (IP, MCP, carpometacarpal [CMC])	Median nerve (C8–T1)	Anterior surface of the radius	Distal phalanx of the thumb	Palpated on the palmar side of the thumb by asking the patient to flex and extend the thumb
Extensor pollicis longus (EPL)	Extension of all joints of the thumb (IP, MCP, CMC)	Radial nerve (C6–C8)	Middle posterior ulna and interosseous membrane	Base of the distal phalanx of the thumb, dorsal surface	Palpated on the dorsal side of thumb by asking the patient to extend and flex the thumb
Abductor pollicis longus (APL)	Abduction of the thumb	Radial nerve (C6–C7)	Posterior radius, interosseous membrane, and middle ulna	Base of the first metacarpal	Palpated on the radial palmar side of the thumb
Dorsal interossei	Abduction of the fingers at the MCP joint	Ulnar nerve (C8–T1)	Adjacent metacarpals	Base of the proximal phalanx	Cannot be palpated, except for the first finger––is palpable at the base of the proximal phalanx of the first finger
Palmar interossei	Adduction of the fingers at the MCP joint	Ulnar nerve (C8–T1)	Respective metacarpals	Base of the proximal phalanx as originated	Cannot be palpated

(continued)

Table 5.9 Wrist, Hand, and Finger Muscles[1]

(continued)

Muscle	Function	Nerve	Origin	Insertion	Palpation
Adductor pollicis	Adduction of the thumb	Ulnar nerve (C8–T1)	Capitate, base of the second metacarpal, palmar surface of the third metacarpal	Base of the proximal phalanx of the thumb	Palpated (with difficulty) on the palmar side of the web space of the thumb
Opponens pollicis	Opposition of the thumb	Median nerve (C6, C7)	Trapezium bone and flexor retinaculum	First metacarpal	Palpated along the radial shaft of the first metacarpal; it is lateral to the abductor pollicis brevis
Abductor pollicis brevis	Abduction of the saddle joint of the thumb	Median nerve (C6, C7)	Transverse carpal ligament, tuberosity of the scaphoid, and ridge of the trapezium	Radial side of the base of the proximal phalanx of the thumb	Palpated in the center of the thenar eminence, medial to the opponens pollicis
Flexor digiti minimi	Flexion of the CMC and MCP joints of the fifth finger	Ulnar nerve (C8–T1)	Hook of the hamate and flexor retinaculum	Base of the proximal phalanx of the fourth finger	Palpated on the palmar surface of the little finger when flexing the little finger
Opponens digiti minimi	Opposition of the fifth finger	Ulnar nerve (C8–T1)	Hamate bone and flexor retinaculum	Fifth metacarpal	Palpated on the hypothenar eminence on the radial side of the fifth metacarpal
Abductor digiti minimi	Abduction of the MCP joint of the fifth finger	Ulnar nerve (C8–T1)	Pisiform bone, tendon of the flexor carpi ulnaris	Proximal phalanx of the little finger	Palpated on the ulnar border of the hand

Thenar and Hypothenar Muscles

Table 5.10 Thenar and Hypothenar Muscles[1]

Thenar muscles	Abductor pollicis brevis; opponens pollicis; flexor pollicis brevis
	Thenar area innervation: median nerve
Hypothenar muscles	Abductor digiti minimi; opponens digiti; flexor digiti minimi
	Hypothenar area innervation: ulnar nerve

Neck, Trunk, and Back Muscles

Table 5.11 Neck, Trunk, and Back Muscles[1]

Muscle	Function	Nerve	Origin	Insertion	Palpation
Sternocleidomastoid	Cervical flexion and rotation to the opposite side	Accessory nerve-CN XI (C2, C3)	Sternum and clavicle	Mastoid process	Palpated from the manubrium and clavicle to the mastoid
Scalene (anterior, medius, posterior) unilateral neck lateral	Bilaterally assisting in neck flexion and flexion	Lower cervical nerve	Sternum and clavicle	First and second ribs	Difficult to palpate First rib should be palpated from the posterior aspect by placing hands on upper traps and palpating just below the clavicle Second rib is best accessed posteriorly, directly below the upper trapezius but not on the spine of the scapula

(continued)

Table 5.11 Neck, Trunk, and Back Muscles

Muscle	Function	Nerve	Origin	Insertion	Palpation
Rectus abdominis	Trunk flexion and compression of the abdomen	Seventh through twelfth intercostal nerves [T7–T12]	Pubis	Cartilage of the fifth, sixth, and seventh ribs	Palpated at the midline of the thorax over the linea alba when the patient is performing a sit-up
External oblique	Bilateral trunk forward flexion, unilateral lateral flexion, and rotation to the opposite side	Eighth through twelfth intercostal nerves, iliohypogastric and ilioinguinal nerves	Lower eight ribs laterally	Iliac crest and linea alba	Palpated distally until reaching the anterior superior iliac spine; fibers run from out to in, as if both hands were inserted in the pockets
Internal oblique	Bilateral trunk forward flexion, unilateral lateral flexion, and rotation to the same side	Eighth through twelfth intercostal nerves, iliohypogastric and ilioinguinal nerves	Inguinal ligament, iliac crest, thoracolumbar fascia	Cartilages of the tenth through twelfth ribs and the linea alba	Palpated on the lateral part of the anterior abdominal wall distal to the rib cage; fibers run from in to out, as if both hands were taken out of the pockets
Quadratus lumborum [fixes twelfth rib during inspiration, depresses twelfth rib during forced expiration]	Lateral bending of the trunk [to the same side]	Twelfth thoracic (T12) and first lumbar (L1) nerves	Iliac crest	Transverse processes of L2, L5, and twelfth rib	Cannot be palpated
Erector spinae sacrospinalis, iliocostalis, longissimus dorsi, and spinalis dorsi	Head and vertebral column bilateral extension, unilateral lateral flexion	Spinal nerves	Spinous processes, transverse processes, and ribs from the occiput to the sacrum and ilium	Spinous processes, transverse processes, and ribs from the occiput to the sacrum and ilium	Palpated on both sides of the vertebral column by asking the patient to extend the spine while prone

(continued)

SECTION 5-3

Musculoskeletal Data Collection

Goniometry—Joint Measurements: Body Position, Goniometer Alignment, and Normal Range of Motion Degrees (per American Academy of Orthopaedic Surgeons (AAOS))

Axis = A
Stationary arm = S
Movement arm = M

Table 5.12 Goniometry—Joint Measurements: Body Position, Goniometer Alignment, and Normal Range of Motion (ROM) (per AAOS)[2,3]

Figure 5.3 The alignment of the goniometer at the end of the ROM of glenohumeral (GH) flexion

A – Lateral aspect of greater tubercle
S – Parallel to midaxillary line of thorax
M – Lateral midline of humerus pointing to lateral epicondyle

(continued)

Table 5.12 Goniometry—Joint Measurements: Body Position, Goniometer Alignment, and Normal Range of Motion (ROM) (per AAOS) *(continued)*

Figure 5.4 The alignment of the goniometer at the end of the ROM of GH extension

A – Lateral aspect of greater tubercle
S – Parallel to midaxillary line of thorax
M – Lateral midline of humerus pointing to lateral epicondyle

Figure 5.5 The alignment of the goniometer at the end of the ROM of GH abduction

A – Anterior lip of acromion
S – Parallel to sternum
M – Anterior midline of humerus

(continued)

Table 5.12 Goniometry—Joint Measurements: Body Position, Goniometer Alignment, and Normal Range of Motion (ROM) (per AAOS) *(continued)*

Figure 5.6 The alignment of the goniometer at the end of the IR ROM of the GH joint

A – Olecranon process
S – Perpendicular to the floor
M – Parallel to long axis of ulnar pointing to ulnar styloid process

Figure 5.7 The alignment of the goniometer at the end of the external rotation (ER) ROM of the GH joint

A – Olecranon process
S – Perpendicular to the floor
M – Parallel to long axis of ulnar pointing to ulnar styloid process

(continued)

Table 5.12 **Goniometry—Joint Measurements: Body Position, Goniometer Alignment, and Normal Range of Motion (ROM) (per AAOS)** *(continued)*

Figure 5.8 The alignment of the goniometer at the end of elbow flexion ROM

A – Lateral epicondyle
S – Lateral midline of humerus pointing to tip of acromion process
M – Lateral midline of radius pointing to radial styloid process

Figure 5.9 The alignment of the goniometer at the end of elbow extension ROM

A – Lateral epicondyle
S – Lateral midline of humerus pointing to tip of acromion process
M – Lateral midline of radius pointing to radial styloid process

(continued)

Figure 5.10 The alignment of the goniometer at the end of pronation ROM

A – Lateral and slightly proximal to ulnar styloid process
S – Perpendicular to the floor
M – Across dorsal aspect of forearm

Figure 5.11 The alignment of the goniometer at the end of supination ROM

A – Medial and slightly proximal to ulnar styloid process
S – Perpendicular to the floor
M – Across ventral aspect of forearm

(continued)

Figure 5.12 The alignment of the goniometer at the end of wrist flexion ROM

A – Lateral triquetrum
S – Parallel to long axis of ulna
M – Parallel to long axis of 5th metacarpal

Figure 5.13 The alignment of the goniometer at the end of wrist extension ROM

A – Lateral triquetrum
S – Parallel to long axis of ulna
M – Parallel to long axis of fifth metacarpal

(continued)

Table 5.12 Goniometry—Joint Measurements: Body Position, Goniometer Alignment, and Normal Range of Motion (ROM) (per AAOS) *(continued)*

Figure 5.14 The alignment of the goniometer at the end of radial deviation ROM

A – Dorsal aspect of wrist over capitate
S – Dorsal forearm along midline
M – Dorsal midline of third metacarpal

Figure 5.15 The alignment of the goniometer at the end of ulnar deviation ROM

A – Dorsal aspect of wrist over capitate
S – Dorsal forearm along midline
M – Dorsal midline of third metacarpal

(continued)

Table 5.12 **Goniometry—Joint Measurements: Body Position, Goniometer Alignment, and Normal Range of Motion (ROM) (per AAOS)** *(continued)*

Figure 5.16 The alignment of the goniometer at the end of hip flexion ROM

A – Greater trochanter
S – Lateral midline of trunk
M – Lateral midline of femur toward lateral epicondyle

Figure 5.17 The alignment of the goniometer at the end of hip extension ROM

A – Greater trochanter
S – Lateral midline of trunk
M – Lateral midline of femur

(continued)

Table 5.12 Goniometry—Joint Measurements: Body Position, Goniometer Alignment, and Normal Range of Motion (ROM) (per AAOS) *(continued)*

Figure 5.18 The alignment of the goniometer at the end of hip abduction ROM

A – Ipsilateral ASIS
S – On a line between both ASIS
M – Anterior midline of femur

Figure 5.19 The alignment of the goniometer at the end of hip IR ROM

A – Midpoint of patellar
S – Perpendicular to floor
M – Along anterior midline of tibia

(continued)

Table 5.12 **Goniometry—Joint Measurements: Body Position, Goniometer Alignment, and Normal Range of Motion (ROM) (per AAOS)** *(continued)*

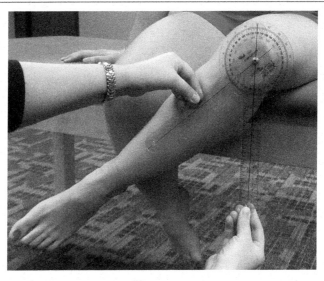

Figure 5.20 The alignment of the goniometer at the end of hip ER ROM

A – Midpoint of patellar
S – Perpendicular to the floor
M – Along anterior midline of tibia

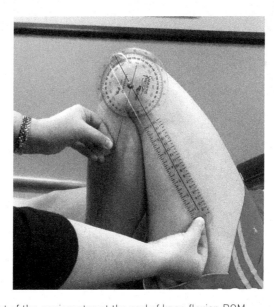

Figure 5.21 The alignment of the goniometer at the end of knee flexion ROM

A – Lateral epicondyle of femur
S – Lateral midline of femur toward greater trochanter
M – Lateral midline of fibula toward lateral malleolus

(continued)

Table 5.12 **Goniometry—Joint Measurements: Body Position, Goniometer Alignment, and Normal Range of Motion (ROM) (per AAOS)** *(continued)*

Figure 5.22 The alignment of the goniometer at the end of knee extension ROM

A – Lateral epicondyle of femur
S – Lateral midline of femur toward greater trochanter
M – Lateral midline of fibula toward lateral malleolus

Figure 5.23 The alignment of the goniometer at the end of dorsiflexion (DF) ROM

A – 1.5 cm inferior tip of lateral malleolus
S – Lateral midline of fibula toward fibular head
M – Parallel to lateral aspect fifth metatarsal

(continued)

Table 5.12 Goniometry—Joint Measurements: Body Position, Goniometer Alignment, and Normal Range of Motion (ROM) (per AAOS) *(continued)*

Figure 5.24 The alignment of the goniometer at the end of plantarflexion (PF) ROM

A – 1.5 cm inferior tip of lateral malleolus
S – Lateral midline of fibula toward fibular head
M – Parallel to lateral aspect fifth metatarsal

Figure 5.25 The alignment of the goniometer at the end of inversion ROM

A – Midpoint between malleoli
S – Anterior midline of tibia toward tibial tuberosity
M – Anterior midline second metatarsal

(continued)

Table 5.12 Goniometry—Joint Measurements: Body Position, Goniometer Alignment, and Normal Range of Motion (ROM) (per AAOS)   *(continued)*

Figure 5.26 The alignment of the goniometer at the end of eversion ROM

A – Midpoint between malleoli
S – Anterior midline of tibia toward tibial tuberosity
M – Anterior midline second metatarsal

(continued)

Table 5.12 Goniometry—Joint Measurements: Body Position, Goniometer Alignment, and Normal Range of Motion (ROM) (per AAOS)

(continued)

Joint	Supine	Prone	Sitting	Goniometer Alignment (Ending Position)	ROM Degrees (AAOS)
Shoulder	Flexion Abduction, IR, ER	Extension		Shoulder flexion (Figure 5-3), Shoulder extension (Figure 5-4), Shoulder abduction (Figure 5-5), Shoulder IR (Figure 5-6), Shoulder ER (Figure 5-7)	Flexion = 180°, Extension = 60°, Abduction = 180°, IR = 70°, IR = 70°, ER = 90°, Horizontal adduction = 135°
Elbow	Extension		Flexion	Elbow flexion (Figure 5-8), Elbow extension (Figure 5-9)	Flexion = 150°, Extension = 0°
Radioulnar (forearm)			Pronation, Supination	Pronation (Figure 5-10), Supination (Figure 5-11)	Pronation = 80°, Supination = 80°
Wrist			Flexion, Extension, Radial deviation, Ulnar deviation	Wrist flexion (Figure 5-12), Wrist extension (Figure 5-13), Radial deviation (Figure 5-14), Ulnar deviation (Figure 5-15)	Flexion = 80°, Extension = 70°, Radial deviation = 20°, Ulnar deviation = 30°
Hip	Flexion abduction, Adduction	Extension	Internal rotation, External rotation	Hip flexion (Figure 5-16), Hip extension (Figure 5-17), Hip abduction/adduction (Figure 5-18), Hip IR (Figure 5-19), Hip ER (Figure 5-20)	Flexion = 120°, Extension = 30°, Abduction = 45°, Adduction = 30°, IR/ER = 45°
Knee	Flexion, Extension			Knee flexion (Figure 5-21), Knee extension (Figure 5-22)	Flexion = 135°, Extension = 0°
Talocrural (ankle)			Dorsiflexion, Plantarflexion	Dorsiflexion (Figure 5-23), Plantarflexion (Figure 5-24)	DF = 20°, PF = 50°
Subtalar (rear foot)			Inversion, Eversion	Inversion (Figure 5-25), Eversion (Figure 5-26)	Inversion = 35°, Eversion = 15°

Cervical and Thoracolumbar Range of Motion Normative Values (per AAOS)

Table 5.13 Cervical and Thoracolumbar ROM Normative Values (per AAOS)[2]

Cervical ROM
Flexion = 45°
Extension = 45°
Left lateral flexion = 45°
Right lateral flexion = 45°
Left rotation = 60°
Right rotation = 60°

Thoracolumbar ROM
Flexion = 80° (tape measure = 4 inches)
Extension = 20° to 30°
Left lateral flexion = 35°
Right lateral flexion = 35°
Left rotation = 45°
Right rotation = 45°

Manual Muscle Testing: Grading System of Hislop and Montgomery

Table 5.14 Grading System of Hislop and Montgomery[4,5]

Grade 5 (normal): completes full ROM against gravity. Maintains end-range position against maximal resistance.

Grade 4 (good): completes full ROM against gravity. Maintains end-range position against moderate resistance. "Yields" (or "gives") at the end-range against maximal resistance.

Grade 3 + (fair +): completes full ROM against gravity. Maintains end-range position against mild resistance and has functional implications.

Grade 3 (fair): completes full ROM against gravity. Unable to maintain end-range position against any resistance.

Grade 2 (poor): completes full ROM in a horizontal plane of motion.

Grade 2 (–) minus (poor minus): completes partial ROM in a horizontal plane of motion.

Grade 1 (trace): examiner visually detects or palpates contractile activity in the muscle(s). There is no movement of the part as a result of contractile activity.

Grade 0 (zero): muscle is quiet, and no activity is detected.

Upper Extremity Manual Muscle Testing

Table 5.15 Manual Muscle Testing: Upper Extremity

Movement, Muscles, and Instructions to the Patient[4,5]	Patient/PTA Positions and Grades
Scapular Abduction and Upward Rotation	
Main muscles: Serratus anterior Others: Pectoralis minor Grades 4 and 5: "Raise your arm forward above your head; don't let me push your arm down." Grade 3: "Raise your arm forward above your head." Grade 2: "Hold your arm in this position (such as above 90°). Let it relax. Hold your arm up again. Let it relax." Grade 1: "Try to hold your arm in this position."	All grades: Patient sitting. Grades 4 and 5: PTA stands at test side and with one hand applies resistance to the patient's arm proximal to elbow. Patient's arm needs to be elevated more than 60° to use the serratus. PTA's other hand palpates edges of the scapula (**Figure 5.27**).

Figure 5.27 Scapular abduction and upward rotation manual muscle testing (MMT)

Scapular Elevation	
Main muscles: Upper trapezius Others: Levator scapulae and rhomboids Grades 4 and 5: "Raise your shoulders toward your ears. Hold it. Don't let me push them down." Grades 1, 2, and 3: "Raise your shoulders toward your ears."	Grades 1 and 2: Patient prone. Grades 3, 4, and 5: Patient, while sitting, elevates the shoulders. Grades 4 and 5: PTA stands behind the patient with both hands over the top of the patient's shoulders and gives resistance in downward direction (**Figure 5.28**).

(continued)

Table 5.15 Manual Muscle Testing: Upper Extremity	(continued)
Movement, Muscles, and Instructions to the Patient[4,5]	**Patient/PTA Positions and Grades**

Figure 5.28 Scapular elevation MMT

Scapular Adduction (Scapular Retraction)

Main muscles: Middle trapezius and rhomboid major Others: Levator scapulae, rhomboid minor and upper and lower trapezius Grades 4 and 5: "Lift your elbow toward the ceiling. Hold it. Don't let me push it down." Grade 3: "Lift your elbow toward the ceiling." Grades 1 and 2: "Try to lift your elbow toward the ceiling."	All grades: Patient prone. Grades 4 and 5: PTA stands at test side and with one hand stabilizes the contralateral scapula. PTA's other hand applies resistance downward toward the floor over the distal humerus (deltoid must be of grade 3 or better) **Figure 5.29**.

Figure 5.29 Scapular adduction MMT

(continued)

Table 5.15 Manual Muscle Testing: Upper Extremity *(continued)*

Movement, Muscles, and Instructions to the Patient[4,5]	Patient/PTA Positions and Grades
Scapular Depression and Adduction	
Main muscles: Lower trapezius Others: Pectoralis and latissimus dorsi Grades 4 and 5: "Raise your arm from the table as high as possible. Hold it. Don't let me push it down." Grade 3: "Raise your arm from the table as high as possible." Grades 1 and 2: "Try to lift your arm from the table past your ear."	All grades: Patient prone. Grades 4 and 5: PTA stands at test side and applies resistance downward toward the floor over the distal humerus (**Figure 5.30**).

Figure 5.30 Scapular depression and adduction MMT

Scapular Adduction and Downward Rotation	
Main muscles: Rhomboids (major and minor) Others: Levator scapulae Grades 4 and 5: "Lift your hand. Hold it. Don't let me push it down." Grade 3: "Lift your hand."	Grades 1 and 2: "Try to move your hand away from your back." Grades 1 and 2: Patient sitting with shoulder in internal rotation and arm extended and adducted behind back. Grades 3, 4, and 5: Patient prone with shoulder in internal rotation and arm adducted across the back. Grades 4 and 5: PTA stands at test side and applies resistance downward and outward over the humerus just above the elbow **Figure 5.31**.

(continued)

Table 5.15 **Manual Muscle Testing: Upper Extremity** *(continued)*

Movement, Muscles, and Instructions to the Patient[4,5]	Patient/PTA Positions and Grades

Figure 5.31 Scapular adduction and downward rotation MMT

Main muscles: Serratus anterior
Grades 4 and 5: "Keeping your elbow straight, try to push your arm up toward the ceiling while I am pushing your arm down."
Grade 3: Keeping your elbow straight, lift your arm up toward the ceiling."
Grades 1 and 2: "Try to push your straight arm toward me."

Grades 1 and 2: Patient sitting facing PTA who is supporting the weight of the limb in a position of shoulder flexion to 90°, slight horizontal adduction (i.e., 15° medial to the sagittal plane), and the elbow extended.
Grades 3, 4, and 5: Patient is supine with the shoulder flexed to 90°, slight horizontal adduction (i.e., 15° medial to the sagittal plane), with the elbow extended.
Grades 4 and 5: PTA stands at the test side and applies resistance to the distal humerus just above the elbow in a downward/posterior direction (**Figure 5.32**).

(continued)

Table 5.15 **Manual Muscle Testing: Upper Extremity**   *(continued)*

Movement, Muscles, and Instructions to the Patient[4,5]	Patient/PTA Positions and Grades

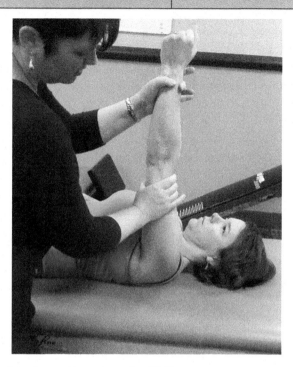

Figure 5.32 Scapular abduction and lateral rotation MMT

Shoulder Flexion

Main muscles: Anterior deltoid and coracobrachialis Others: Pectoralis major, middle deltoid, and serratus anterior Grades 4 and 5: "Raise your arm forward to shoulder height. Hold it. Don't let me push it down." Grade 3: "Raise your arm forward to shoulder height." Grades 1 and 2: "Try to raise your arm."	All grades: Patient sitting. Grades 4 and 5: PTA stands at test side and applies resistance downward over the distal humerus just above the elbow. PTA's other hand stabilizes the shoulder (**Figure 5.33**).

Figure 5.33 Shoulder flexion MMT

(continued)

Table 5.15 Manual Muscle Testing: Upper Extremity   *(continued)*

Movement, Muscles, and Instructions to the Patient[4,5]	Patient/PTA Positions and Grades
Shoulder Extension	
Main muscles: Latissimus dorsi, posterior deltoid, and teres major Other: Triceps brachii (long head) Grades 4 and 5: "Lift your arm as high as you can. Hold it. Don't let me push it down." Grades 2 and 3: "Lift your arm as high as you can." Grade 1: "Lift your arm."	All grades: Patient prone. Grades 4 and 5: PTA stands at test side and applies resistance downward over the posterior arm just above the elbow (**Figure 5.34**).

Figure 5.34 Shoulder extension MMT

Shoulder Scaption	
Main muscles: Anterior and middle deltoid and supraspinatus Grades 4 and 5: "Raise your arm to shoulder height, halfway between straight and to the side. Hold it. Don't let me push it down." Grade 3: "Raise your arm to shoulder height, halfway between straight and to the side." Grades 1 and 2: "Try to raise your arm to shoulder height, halfway between straight and to the side."	All grades: Patient sitting. Grades 4 and 5: PTA stands in front and slightly to the side of the patient and applies resistance downward over the arm above the elbow. Patient elevates arm halfway between flexion and abduction (**Figure 5.35**).

Figure 5.35 Shoulder scaption MMT

(continued)

Table 5.15 **Manual Muscle Testing: Upper Extremity** *(continued)*

Movement, Muscles, and Instructions to the Patient[4,5]	Patient/PTA Positions and Grades
Shoulder Abduction	
Main muscles: Middle deltoid and supraspinatus Grades 4 and 5: "Lift your arm out to the side to shoulder level. Hold it. Don't let me push it down." Grade 3: "Lift your arm out to the side to shoulder level." Grades 1 and 2: "Try to lift your arm out to the side."	All grades: Patient sitting. Grades 4 and 5: PTA stands behind the patient and applies resistance downward over the arm just above the elbow **Figure 5.36**.

Figure 5.36 Shoulder abduction MMT

Movement, Muscles, and Instructions to the Patient[4,5]	Patient/PTA Positions and Grades
Shoulder External Rotation	
Main muscles: Infraspinatus and teres minor Others: Posterior deltoid Grades 4 and 5: "Raise your arm to the level of the table. Hold it. Don't let me push it down." Grade 3: "Raise your arm to the level of the table." Grades 1 and 2: "Turn your palm outward."	All grades: Patient prone. Grades 4 and 5: PTA stands at test side at the level of the patient's waist and applies resistance with two fingers downward at the wrist. PTA's other hand supports the patient's elbow, giving counterpressure at the end of the range (**Figure 5.37**).

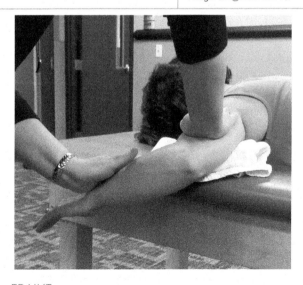

Figure 5.37 Shoulder ER MMT

(continued)

Table 5.15 Manual Muscle Testing: Upper Extremity *(continued)*

Movement, Muscles, and Instructions to the Patient[4,5]	Patient/PTA Positions and Grades
Shoulder Internal Rotation	
Main muscles: Subscapularis, pectoralis major (clavicular and sternal parts), latissimus dorsi, and teres major Others: Anterior deltoid Grades 4 and 5: "Move your forearm up and back. Hold it. Don't let me push it down." Grade 3: "Move your forearm up and back." Grades 1 and 2: "Turn your arm so that the palm faces away from the table."	All grades: Patient prone. Grades 4 and 5: PTA stands at test side and applies downward and forward resistance on the anterior side of the forearm just above the wrist. PTA's other hand applies counterpressure backward and slightly upward (**Figure 5.38**).

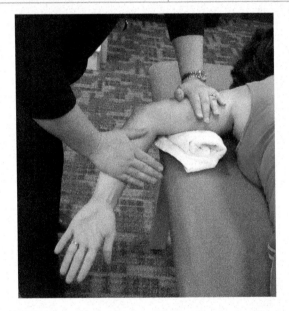

Figure 5.38 Shoulder IR MMT

Elbow Flexion

Main muscles: Biceps brachii (short and long head), brachialis, and brachioradialis Others: Pronator teres, extensor carpi radialis longus, flexor carpi radialis, and flexor carpi ulnaris Grades 4 and 5: "Bend your elbow. Hold it. Don't let me pull it down." Grade 3: "Bend your elbow." Grades 1 and 2: "Try to bend your elbow."	Grades 1 and 2: Patient supine (if cannot sit) with forearm supinated for the biceps, pronated for the brachialis, and in midposition for the brachioradialis, and elbow flexed to 45°. Grades 3, 4, and 5: Patient sitting with arm abducted and forearm supinated for the biceps, pronated for the brachialis, and in midposition for the brachioradialis. Grades 4 and 5: PTA stands in front of the patient and applies resistance over the flexor surface of the forearm proximal to the wrist. PTA's other hand applies counterforce, cupping the palm over the anterior superior surface of the shoulder (**Figure 5.39**).

(continued)

Table 5.15 **Manual Muscle Testing: Upper Extremity**   *(continued)*

Movement, Muscles, and Instructions to the Patient[4,5]	Patient/PTA Positions and Grades

Figure 5.39 Elbow flexion MMT

Elbow Extension

Main muscles: Triceps brachii (long, lateral, and medial heads)
Other: Anconeus
Grades 4 and 5: "Straighten your elbow. Hold it. Don't let me bend it."
Grade 3: "Straighten your elbow."
Grades 1 and 2: "Try to straighten your elbow."

Grades 1 and 2: Patient sitting with arm abducted to 90°, shoulder in neutral rotation, and elbow flexed to about 45°.
Grades 3, 4, and 5: Patient prone with arm in 90° abduction and forearm flexed, hanging over the edge of the table.
Grades 4 and 5: PTA supports the patient's arm above the elbow. PTA applies resistance downward over the dorsal surface of the forearm (**Figure 5.40**).

Figure 5.40 Elbow extension MMT

Table 5.15 **Manual Muscle Testing: Upper Extremity**   *(continued)*

Movement, Muscles, and Instructions to the Patient[4,5]	Patient/PTA Positions and Grades
Forearm Supination	
Main muscles: Supinator Others: Biceps brachii (short and long head) Grades 4 and 5: "Turn your palm up. Hold it. Don't let me turn it down. Keep your wrist and fingers relaxed." Grade 3: "Turn your palm up." Grades 1 and 2: "Turn your palm toward your face."	All grades: Patient sitting. Grades 1 and 2: Patient's shoulder flexed between 45° and 90° and elbow flexed to 90°. Grades 3, 4, and 5: Patient's elbow flexed 90° and forearm in pronation. Patient supinates until the palm faces the ceiling. Grades 4 and 5: PTA stands at the patient's side, supports the elbow, grasps the forearm, and applies resistance to the anterior surface of the forearm at the wrist (**Figure 5.41**).

Figure 5.41 Forearm supination and pronation MMT

Resistance toward pronation = supination MMT.
Resistance toward supination = pronation MMT.

Forearm Pronation	
Main muscles: Pronator teres (humeral and ulnar heads) and pronator quadratus Others: Flexor carpi radialis Grades 4 and 5: "Turn your palm down. Hold it. Don't let me turn it up. Keep your wrist and fingers relaxed." Grade 3: "Turn your palm down." Grades 1 and 2: "Try to turn your palm down."	All grades: Patient sitting. Grades 3, 4, and 5: Patient's arm at side with elbow flexed to 90°and forearm in supination. Patient pronates until the palm faces the floor. Grades 1 and 2: Patient's shoulder flexed between 45° and 90° and elbow flexed to 90°. Forearm in neutral position. Grades 4 and 5: PTA stands at the patient's side and supports the elbow. PTA's other hand grasps the forearm and applies resistance over the posterior surface of the forearm at the wrist (the same as in Figure 5-41 but the forearm is pronated).

(continued)

Table 5.15 Manual Muscle Testing: Upper Extremity *(continued)*

Movement, Muscles, and Instructions to the Patient[4,5]	Patient/PTA Positions and Grades
Wrist Flexion	
Main muscles: Flexor carpi radialis and flexor carpi ulnaris Others: Palmaris longus, flexor digitorum superficialis, flexor digitorum profundus, abductor pollicis longus, and flexor pollicis longus Grades 4 and 5: "Bend your wrist. Hold it. Don't let me pull it down. Keep your fingers relaxed." Grade 3: "Bend your wrist (for all muscles). Bend your wrist leading with the little finger (for FCU). Bend your wrist leading with the thumb side (for FCR)." Grade 2: "Bend your wrist. Keep your fingers relaxed." Grade 1: "Try to bend your wrist. Relax. Bend it again."	All grades: Patient sitting. Grades 3, 4, and 5: Patient's forearm is supinated, posterior side of the forearm is supported on the table (or by the examiner's hand), and wrist is in neutral position. Grade 2: Patient's elbow is supported on the table, and forearm is in midposition with the hand resting on the ulnar side. Grade 1: Patient's fully supinated hand and forearm are resting on the table. Grade 1: PTA supports the patient's wrist in flexion with one hand, while the other hand palpates the appropriate tendon. Grade 2: PTA supports the patient's forearm proximal to the wrist. Grade 3: PTA supports the patient's forearm under the wrist. Grades 4 and 5: PTA stands in front of the patient and supports the patient's forearm under the wrist. PTA's other hand applies resistance to the palm (**Figure 5.42**).

Figure 5.42 Wrist flexion MMT

(continued)

Table 5.15 Manual Muscle Testing: Upper Extremity *(continued)*

Movement, Muscles, and Instructions to the Patient[4,5]	Patient/PTA Positions and Grades
Wrist Extension	
Main muscles: Extensor carpi radialis longus, extensor carpi radialis brevis, and extensor carpi ulnaris Others: Extensor digitorum, extensor digiti minimi, and extensor indicis Grades 4 and 5: "Bring your wrist up. Hold it. Don't let me push it down." Grade 3: "Bring your wrist up." Grade 2: "Bend your wrist back." Grade 1: "Try to bring your wrist back."	All grades: Patient sitting. Grades 3, 4, and 5: Patient's flexed elbow and fully pronated forearm are supported on the table (or by the examiner's hand). Grade 2: Patient's forearm is in neutral position supported on the table. Grade 1: Patient's fully pronated hand and forearm are supported on the table. Grade 1: PTA supports the patient's wrist in extension with one hand, while the other hand palpates the appropriate muscle. Grade 2: PTA supports the patient's wrist in neutral position (elevates it from the table). Grades 3, 4, and 5: PTA stands in front of the patient and supports the patient's forearm under the anterior wrist. PTA's other hand applies resistance to the posterior surface of the metacarpals (**Figure 5.43**).

Figure 5.43 Wrist extension MMT

Finger and Thumb Manual Muscle Testing

Table 5.16 Finger and Thumb Manual Muscle Testing[4]

Finger MCP Flexion

- Tests 1, 2, 3, 4 lumbricals, dorsal interossei, and palmar interossei.
- Grades 3, 4, and 5: Patient sitting with forearm in supination, wrist in neutral position, MCP joints fully extended, and IP joints fully flexed.
- Grades 4 and 5: Patient completes simultaneous MCP flexion and finger extension and holds against maximal or moderate resistance. Resistance is given to fingers individually.

Finger PIP and DIP Flexion

- Tests flexor digitorum superficialis and flexor digitorum profundus.
- Grades 3, 4, and 5: Patient sitting with forearm in supination, wrist in neutral position, and finger to be tested in slight flexion at the MCP joint.
- Grades 4 and 5: Patient completes ROM and holds against maximal or moderate finger resistance.

Finger MCP Extension

- Tests extensor digitorum, extensor indicis, and extensor digiti minimi.
- Grades 3, 4, and 5: Patient sitting with forearm in pronation, wrist in neutral position, and MCP and IP joints relaxed in flexed position.
- Grades 4 and 5: Patient completes active extension ROM with maximal and moderate finger resistance.

Finger Abduction

- Tests dorsal interossei and abductor digiti minimi.
- Grades 3, 4, and 5: Patient sitting with forearm in pronation, fingers in extension and adduction. MCP joints are in neutral positions.
- Grades 4 and 5: Patient completes finger abduction with as much resistance as the uninvolved finger. PTA's resistance depends on the uninvolved patient's finger abduction MMT.

Thumb MCP and IP Flexion

- Tests flexor pollicis brevis and flexor pollicis longus.
- Grades 3, 4, and 5: Patient sitting with forearm in supination, wrist in neutral position. Carpometacarpal (CPM) and IP joints of thumb are at 0°. Thumb is in adduction, lying relaxed by the second metacarpal.
- Grades 4 and 5: Patient completes ROM against maximal and moderate resistance.

Thumb MCP and IP Extension

- Tests extensor pollicis brevis and extensor pollicis longus.
- Grades 3, 4, and 5: Patient sitting with forearm in midposition and wrist in neutral position. CPM and IP joints of thumb are relaxed in slight flexion. MCP joint of thumb is in abduction and flexion.
- Grades 4 and 5: Patient completes ROM with resistance. PTA resistance depends on the uninvolved patient's thumb MP and IP extension MMT.

(continued)

Table 5.16 **Finger and Thumb Manual Muscle Testing** *(continued)*

Thumb Abduction

- Tests mainly abductor pollicis longus and abductor pollicis brevis.
- Grades 3, 4, and 5: Patient sitting with forearm supinated, wrist in neutral, and thumb relaxed in adduction.
- Grades 4 and 5: Patient completes ROM against resistance. PTA resistance is dependent on the patient's uninvolved thumb abduction MMT.

Thumb Adduction

- Tests mainly adductor pollicis.
- Grades 3, 4, and 5: Patient sitting with forearm in pronation, wrist in neutral position, and thumb relaxed and in abduction.
- Grades 4 and 5: Patient completes ROM against maximal and moderate resistance.

Opposition (Thumb to Little Finger)

- Tests mainly opponens pollicis and opponens digiti minimi.
- Grades 3, 4, and 5: Patient sitting with forearm in supination, wrist in neutral position, and thumb in adduction with MCP and IP flexed.
- Grades 4 and 5: Patient completes opposition with resistance at the head of the first metacarpal (in the direction of external rotation, extension, and adduction) for the opponens pollicis and at the palmar surface of the fifth metacarpal (in the direction of internal rotation, flattening the palm) for the opponens digiti minimi.

Lower Extremity Manual Muscle Testing

Table 5.17 **MMT Lower Extremity**

Movement, Muscles, and Instructions to the Patient[4]	Patient/PTA Positions and Grades
Hip flexion	
Main Muscles: Psoas major and iliacus Others: Rectus femoris, sartorius, tensor fasciae latae, pectineus, adductors (brevis, longus, magnus), anterior gluteus medius Grades 4 and 5: "Lift your leg off the table and don't let me push it down." Grade 3: "Lift your leg straight up off the table." Grade 2: "Bring your knee up toward your chest." Grade 1: "Try to bring your knee up to your nose."	Grade 1: Patient lying supine. Grade 2: Patient side lying with tested limb uppermost. Grades 3, 4, and 5: Patient sitting with thighs supported on the table. Grades 4 and 5: PTA standing next to limb to be tested, applies resistance over distal thigh proximal to the knee (**Figure 5.44**).

(continued)

Table 5.17 MMT Lower Extremity *(continued)*

Movement, Muscles, and Instructions to the Patient[4]	Patient/PTA Positions and Grades

Figure 5.44 Hip flexion MMT

Hip extension

Main muscles: Gluteus maximus, semitendinosus, semimembranosus, and long head of biceps femoris Others: Adductor magnus and gluteus medius Grades 3, 4, and 5: "Lift your leg off the table as high as you can. Do not bend your knee." Grade 2: "Bring your leg back toward me. Keep your knee straight." Grade 1: "Try to lift your leg from the table."	Grades 1, 3, 4, and 5: Patient prone. Grade 2: Patient side lying with tested limb uppermost and knee straight. Grades 4 and 5: PTA standing at side of limb to be tested, applies with one hand resistance on posterior leg above the ankle. The other hand stabilizes the pelvis (**Figure 5.45**).

Figure 5.45 Hip extension MMT—examiner showed at opposite side not to obscure activity

(continued)

Table 5.17 MMT Lower Extremity   *(continued)*

Movement, Muscles, and Instructions to the Patient[4]	Patient/PTA Positions and Grades

Hip abduction

| Main muscles: Gluteus medius and gluteus minimus
Others: Gluteus maximus, tensor fasciae latae, obturator internus, gemellus inferior and superior, and sartorius
Grades 4 and 5: "Lift your leg up in the air. Hold it. Don't let me push it down."
Grade 2: "Bring your leg out to the side."
Grade 1: "Try to bring your leg out to the side." | Grades 1 and 2: Patient supine. Grades 3, 4, and 5: Patient side lying with tested limb uppermost and knee straight. Grades 4 and 5: PTA standing behind patient, palpates gluteus medius. PTA other hand applies resistance downward at the lateral surface of knee (**Figure 5.46**). |

Figure 5.46 Hip abduction MMT

Hip adduction

| Main muscles: Adductor magnus, adductor brevis, adductor longus, pectineus, and gracilis
Others: Gluteus maximus and obturator externus
Grades 4 and 5: "Lift your bottom leg up to your top one. Hold it. Don't let me push it down."
Grade 3: "Lift your bottom leg up to your top one. Don't let it drop."
Grade 2: "Bring your leg in toward the other one."
Grade 1: "Try to bring your leg in." | Grades 1 and 2: Patient supine. Grades 3, 4, and 5: Patient side lying with the tested limb lowermost resting on the table. The uppermost limb is in 25° abduction and is supported by PTA. Grades 4 and 5: PTA standing behind patient, cradles the uppermost limb with forearm supporting it on medial knee. PTA other hand applies to lowermost limb resistance on medial distal femur proximal to knee (**Figure 5.47**). |

Figure 5.47 Hip adduction MMT

(continued)

Table 5.17 MMT Lower Extremity *(continued)*

Movement, Muscles, and Instructions to the Patient[a]	Patient/PTA Positions and Grades
Hip external rotation	
Main Muscles: Obturator externus, obturator internus, piriformis, gemelli superior and inferior, quadratus femoris, and gluteus maximus Others: Sartorius, long head biceps femoris, gluteus medius, psoas major, adductor magnus and longus, and popliteus Grades 4 and 5: "Don't let me turn your leg out." Grade 3: "Keep your leg in this position." Grade 2: "Roll your leg out." Grade 1: "Try to roll your leg out."	Grades 1 and 2: Patient supine with tested limb in internal rotation. Grades 3, 4, and 5: Patient sitting. Grades 4 and 5: PTA sitting beside limb to be tested, applies counterpressure to lateral distal thigh above the knee, giving resistance in a medially directed force at the knee. PTA other hand applies resistance in a laterally directed force at the ankle, grasping the ankle above the medial malleolus (**Figure 5.48**).

Figure 5.48 Hip ER MMT

Hip internal rotation	
Main muscles: Gluteus minimus, tensor fasciae latae, and gluteus medius Others: Semitendinosus, semimembranosus, adductor magnus, and adductor longus Grades 4 and 5: "Don't let me turn your leg in." Grade 3: "Keep your leg in this position." Grade 2: "Roll your leg in toward the other." Grade 1: "Try to roll your leg in."	Grades 1 and 2: Patient supine with tested limb in partial external rotation. Grades 3, 4, and 5: Patient sitting. Grades 4 and 5: PTA kneeling in front of tested limb, applies counterpressure to medial distal thigh above the knee giving resistance in a laterally directed force at the knee. PTA other hand applies resistance in a medially directed force at the ankle above the lateral malleolus (**Figure 5.49**).

(continued)

Table 5.17 **MMT Lower Extremity** *(continued)*

Movement, Muscles, and Instructions to the Patient[4]	Patient/PTA Positions and Grades

Figure 5.49 Hip IR MMT

Knee flexion

Main muscles: Long and short heads of biceps femoris, semitendinosus, and semimembranosus Other: Gracilis, tensor fasciae latae, sartorius, popliteus, gastrocnemius, and plantaris Grades 4 and 5: "Bend your knee. Hold it. Don't let me straighten it." Grades 2 and 3: "Bend your knee." Grade 1: "Try to bend your knee."	Grades 1, 3, 4, and 5: Patient prone. Grade 2: Patient side lying with tested limb uppermost. Grades 4 and 5: PTA standing next to limb to be tested (showed here at opposite side not to obscure activity), applies resistance around posterior surface of leg above the ankle. PTA's other hand is placed over the hamstrings on posterior thigh (**Figure 5.50**).

Figure 5.50 Knee flexion MMT

(continued)

Table 5.17 MMT Lower Extremity *(continued)*

Movement, Muscles, and Instructions to the Patient[a]	Patient/PTA Positions and Grades
Knee extension	
Main muscles: Rectus femoris, vastus intermedius, vastus lateralis, vastus medialis longus, and vastus medialis oblique Other: Tensor fasciae latae Grades 4 and 5: "Straighten your knee. Hold it. Don't let me bend it." Grades 2 and 3: "Straighten your knee." Grade 1: "Push the back of your knee down into the table."	Grade 1: Patient supine. Grade 2: Patient side lying with tested limb uppermost. Grades 3, 4, and 5: Patient sitting. Grades 4 and 5: PTA standing at side of tested limb with one hand giving resistance downward over anterior distal leg above ankle. PTA's other hand is under distal thigh not allowing patient to hyperextend the knee (**Figure 5.51**).

Figure 5.51 Knee extension MMT

Movement, Muscles, and Instructions to the Patient	Patient/PTA Positions and Grades
Ankle plantarflexion	
Main muscles: Medial and lateral heads of gastrocnemius and the soleus Others: Posterior tibialis, plantaris, peroneus longus, peroneus brevis, flexor digitorum longus, and flexor hallucis longus Grades 4 and 5: "Stand on your right leg. Go up on your tiptoes. Now go down. Repeat this twenty times." Grade 3: "Stand on your right leg. Go up on your tiptoes. Now go down. Repeat this nine times." Grade 2: "Stand on your right leg. Try to go up on your tiptoes." Grade 1: "Point your toes down."	Grade 1: Patient prone with feet at end of table. Grade 2: Patient standing on limb to be tested with knee extended, with two fingers on the table for balance assist. Grades 2, 3, 4, and 5: PTA standing with lateral view of patient's limb. Grades 3, 4, and 5: Patient standing on limb to be tested with knee extended with two fingers on a table for balance assist (**Figure 5.52**).

(continued)

Table 5.17 MMT Lower Extremity *(continued)*

Movement, Muscles, and Instructions to the Patient[4]	Patient/PTA Positions and Grades

Figure 5.52 Gastrocnemius MMT

Ankle plantarflexion knee bent	
Main muscle: Soleus (best recruited with 45° of knee flexion to place gastrocnemius on slack in attempt to isolate soleus better[7]) Other: Gastrocnemius Grades 3, 4, 5: "Stand on your right leg with your knee bent to 45°, try to raise your heel of the floor as you stand on your tip toes." Grades 2, 1, 0: "Lie on your right side with your top (left) leg bent up towards your chest resting on a pillow to get it out of the way of your right leg", "place your right knee in a flexed position of 45°, now point your toes down." Grade 1: PTA visually detects or palpates a contraction of the muscle, but no actual movement is observed.	Grades 3, 4, and 5: Patient standing with knee flexed to 45°, holding onto a table with two finger support (only if needed for balance), and patient is instructed to perform a heel raise. Grade 5: full heel off the floor more than six repetitions. Grade 4: full heel off the floor three to five repetitions, with subsequent repetitions gradually decreasing in heel distance from the floor. Grade 3: full heel off the floor one or two repetitions only with subsequent repetitions decreasing in heel distance from the floor. Grades 2, 1, 0: PTA stabilizes at the distal ankle and makes ensures that the test leg is flexed 45°at the knee. Grade 2: patient can go through full range of motion without the influence of gravity. Grade 0: no active contraction is observed visually or palpably (**Figure 5.53**).

(continued)

Table 5.17 **MMT Lower Extremity** *(continued)*

Movement, Muscles, and Instructions to the Patient[4]	Patient/PTA Positions and Grades

Figure 5.53 Soleus MMT

Foot dorsiflexion and inversion

Main muscles: Tibialis anterior Others: Peroneus tertius, extensor digitorum longus, and extensor hallucis longus Grades 4 and 5: "Bring your foot up and in. Hold it. Don't let me push it down." Grades 1, 2, and 3: "Bring your foot up and in."	All grades: Patient sitting with heel resting on PTA's thigh. Grades 4 and 5: PTA sitting on stool in front of patient with patient's heel resting on PTA's thigh. One hand is supporting around posterior leg above malleoli. PTA's other hand gives resistance over dorsal and medial aspect of the foot (**Figure 5.54**).

Figure 5.54 Foot DF and inversion MMT

Table 5.17 MMT Lower Extremity   *(continued)*

Movement, Muscles, and Instructions to the Patient[4]	Patient/PTA Positions and Grades
Foot inversion	
Main muscles: Tibialis posterior Other: Tibialis anterior, flexor digitorum longus, flexor hallucis longus, soleus, and extensor hallucis longus Grades 4 and 5: "Turn your foot down and in. Hold it." Grades 2 and 3: "Turn your foot down and in." Grade 1: "Try to turn your foot down and in."	All grades: Patient sitting. Grades 2, 3, 4, and 5: Patient with ankle in slight plantarflexion. Grade 1: PTA palpates tibialis posterior tendon. Grades 4 and 5: PTA sitting on low stool in front of patient. One hand is stabilizing the ankle above malleoli. PTA's other hand gives resistance toward eversion and slight dorsiflexion at the dorsal and medial side of the foot at the metatarsal heads (**Figure 5.55**).

Figure 5.55 Foot inversion MMT

Foot eversion with plantarflexion	
Main muscles: Peroneus longus and brevis Others: Extensor digitorum longus, peroneus tertius, and gastrocnemius Grades 4 and 5: "Turn your foot down and out. Hold it. Don't let me move it in." Grades 2 and 3: "Turn your foot down and out."	All grades: Patient sitting. Grades 2, 3, 4, and 5: Patient with ankle in neutral. Grade 1: PTA palpates main muscle's tendon. Grades 4 and 5: PTA sitting on low stool in front of patient. One hand is stabilizing the ankle above malleoli. PTA's other hand gives resistance toward inversion and slight dorsiflexion at the dorsal and lateral side of the forefoot (**Figure 5.56**).

(continued)

Table 5.17 MMT Lower Extremity *(continued)*

Movement, Muscles, and Instructions to the Patient[4]	Patient/PTA Positions and Grades

Figure 5.56 Foot eversion and plantarflexion

Big Toe and Other Toes Manual Muscle Testing

Table 5.18 Big Toe and Other Toes: Manual Muscle Testing[4]

Hallux and Toe Metatarsophalangeal joint (MTP) Flexion

- Tests lumbricals and flexor hallucis brevis (two heads).
- All grades: Patient sitting with legs hanging over the edge of the table and the ankle in neutral position.
- Grades 4 and 5: Patient completes MTP flexion (for big toe or each lateral toe) and holds against strong or moderate resistance. Resistance is given with the index finger placed beneath the proximal phalanx of the great toe or under the MTP joints of the four lateral toes.

Hallux and Toe DIP and PIP Flexion

- Tests flexor digitorum longus, flexor digitorum brevis, and flexor hallucis longus.
- All grades: Patient sitting with foot on the PTA's lap.
- Grades 4 and 5: Patient completes ROM of toes and the big toe with minimal resistance. Resistance is given under the middle phalanges (for PIP) and under the distal phalanges (for DIP).

Hallux and Toe MTP and IP Extension

- Tests extensor digitorum longus, extensor digitorum brevis, and extensor hallucis longus.
- All grades: Patient sitting with foot on the PTA's lap.
- Grades 4 and 5: Patient extends the big toe or the toes against minimal resistance. Resistance is given by PTA's thumb over the MTP joint or over the IP joint.

Myotomes Testing

Table 5.19 Myotomes Testing[3,6]

- Shoulder shrug: tests upper trapezius muscle and C4 nerve root.
- Shoulder abduction: tests deltoid muscle and C5 nerve root.
- Elbow flexion of supinated arm: tests biceps brachii muscle and nerve roots C5 and C6.
- Elbow flexion of neutral arm: tests brachioradialis muscle and nerve roots C5 and C6.
- Elbow extension: tests triceps brachii muscle and C7 nerve root.
- Radial wrist extension: tests extensor carpi radials longus and brevis muscles and C6 nerve root.
- Wrist flexion: tests FCU, palmaris longus and flexor carpi radialis muscles and C7 nerve roots.
- Thumb extension: tests EPL muscle and C8 nerve roots.
- Fifth digit abduction: tests abductor digiti minimi muscle and C8 nerve root.
- Hip flexion: tests iliopsoas muscles and nerve roots L2, L3.
- Knee extension: tests quadriceps femoris muscles and nerve roots L3 and L4.
- Ankle dorsiflexion: tests anterior tibialis muscle and nerve roots L4 and L5.
- Great toe extension: tests EHL muscle and L5 nerve root.
- Knee flexion: tests hamstring muscles and nerve roots L5 and S1.
- Ankle plantarflexion: tests gastrocnemius muscle and the S1 nerve root.

Pain Rating

Pain is seen as the fifth vital sign and assessment of pain should occur before, during, and after a session of physical therapy. Pain can be assessed many ways, and the PTA should select pain assessment tools that are relevant to patient age and level of understanding.

Table 5.20 Pain Scales: Questions[7,8]

Questions Regarding Pain Location

- "Where is your pain?"
- "Can you point the location?"
- "Has the pain changed its location?"
- "Did the pain go to other areas?"

A body chart may also be used for the patient to mark the location of the pain.

Questions Regarding the Severity of Pain

- "How severe is your pain on a scale of 0 to 10, with 0 meaning no pain and 10 meaning the most severe pain?"
- "Is the pain sharp, dull, or throbbing?"

Can also use a visual analog pain scale with a line 10 cm long on which the patient marks the severity of pain. One example is the Numeric Pain Rating Scale (NPRS).

(continued)

Table 5.20 **Pain Scales: Questions** *(continued)*

The Wong-Baker FACES Pain Scale has been developed for use in children.

A modified Faces Pain Scale can also be used in older adults, including those who have mild cognitive impairment.

Questions Regarding the Type of Pain and Other Signs Involving the Nervous System

- "Do you feel any numbness, tingling, pins and needles, burning sensation, stabbing sensation, or shooting pain?"

Can also use the McGill pain questionnaire, on which the patient marks the type of pain and other signs regarding pain.

Deep Tendon Reflexes (DTR) and Grades

Table 5.21 **Deep Tendon Reflexes and Grades**

DTR Most Tested	DTR Grading
Biceps and brachioradialis: test C5–C6	Absent DTR: grade is 0
Triceps: tests C7–C8	DTR for hyporeflexia: grade is 1+
Quadriceps: tests L2–L4	Normal DTR: grade is 2+
Hamstrings: tests L5–S3	DTR for hyperreflexia: grade is 3+
Achilles tendon: tests S1–S2	DTR for high hyperreflexia (clonus): grade is 4+ or 5+

Orthopedic Special Tests: Shoulder, Elbow, Wrist, and Hand

Table 5.22 **Orthopedic Special Tests: Shoulder, Elbow, Wrist, and Hand**

Area, Test, and Purpose	Interpretation	Procedure
Shoulder: Yergason's for bicipital tendonitis Superior Labrum Anterior Posterior, (SLAP) lesions[6]	Tests: integrity of the transverse humeral ligament (THL) that holds the biceps tendon in the bicipital groove of the humerus. Positive for tendonitis: tenderness (or pain) in the bicipital groove. Positive for THL tear: tendon felt to "pop out" of the groove.	Patient remains seated with elbow flexed to 90° and stabilized against the thorax, forearm pronated. One of the therapist's hands palpates the biceps tendon in the bicipital groove; the other hand resists supination when the patient laterally rotates the arm against resistance.

(continued)

Table 5.22 Orthopedic Special Tests: Shoulder, Elbow, Wrist, and Hand *(continued)*

Area, Test, and Purpose	Interpretation	Procedure
Shoulder: Adson's maneuver for thoracic outlet syndrome (TOS) [9]	Tests: presence of TOS. Positive for TOS: disappearance of the radial pulse when the patient holds a deep breath.	Patient remains seated with head rotated toward the tested shoulder; extends the head while taking a deep breath and holding it. One of the therapist's hands palpates the patient's radial pulse; the other hand rotates and extends the patient's shoulder.
Shoulder: Neer impingement test for injury of the supraspinatus muscle or biceps tendon tear [6]	Tests: overuse injury of the supraspinatus muscle. Positive: patient's face shows pain.	Patient remains seated and the therapist stabilizes the scapula with one hand while forcibly flexing and internally rotating the arm with their other hand. The passive stress causes compression of the greater tuberosity of the humerus against the acromion.
Shoulder: drop arm (Codman's) test for rotator cuff tear [6]	Tests: tear of rotator cuff muscles. Positive: patient drops his or her arm to the side.	Patient remains standing while the therapist abducts the patient's shoulder to 90° and asks the patient to slowly lower his or her arm to the side.
Shoulder: apprehension test for anterior shoulder dislocation [6]	Tests: traumatic instability of the anterior shoulder. Positive: patient complains of pain or apprehensively resists the therapist's hand when moving the patient's arm in external rotation.	Patient remains supine while the therapist abducts the patient's arm to 90° and externally rotates the patient's shoulder slowly.
Elbow: lateral epicondylitis test (Cozen's test) [6]	Tests: inflammation of the lateral epicondyle (tennis elbow). Positive: sudden severe pain in the area.	Patient remains seated with elbow extended, forearm pronated, making a fist. One of the therapist's hands stabilizes the patient's elbow, palpating the lateral epicondyle. The other hand resists the patient's wrist extension and forearm supination.
Elbow: medial epicondylitis test [6]	Tests: inflammation of the medial epicondyle (golfer's elbow). Positive: sudden severe pain in the area.	Patient remains seated with elbow flexed, forearm supinated. One of the therapist's hands stabilizes the patient's elbow, palpating the medial epicondyle. The other hand passively extends and supinates the patient's wrist and forearm.

(continued)

Table 5.22 Orthopedic Special Tests: Shoulder, Elbow, Wrist, and Hand *(continued)*

Area, Test, and Purpose	Interpretation	Procedure
Wrist: Phalen's test for carpal tunnel syndrome[6]	Tests: pressure on median nerve secondary to carpal tunnel syndrome. Positive: tingling sensation in the thumb, index finger, and middle and lateral half of the ring finger.	Patient remains standing. The therapist flexes the patient's wrist, pushing the wrists together and holding them for 1 minute.
Wrist: Tinel's sign for carpal tunnel syndrome[6]	Tests: pressure on median nerve and the rate of regeneration of sensory fibers of the nerve. Positive: tingling and paresthesia into the thumb, index finger, middle and lateral half of ring finger, and distal to the point of pressure. The most distal point felt is the limit of nerve regeneration.	Patient remains seated, with forearm supinated and hand relaxed. The therapist taps over the carpal tunnel.
Thumb: Finkelstein's test for DeQuervain's tenosynovitis[6]	Tests: tendon inflammation of the abductor pollicis longus and extensor pollicis brevis. Positive: pain in the area of these two tendons.	Patient remains seated with elbow extended, making a fist with the thumb inside the fingers. One of the therapist's hands stabilizes the patient's forearm. The other hand moves the patient's wrist toward the ulnar side.

Orthopedic Special Tests: Hip, Knee, and Ankle

Table 5.23 Orthopedic Special Tests: Hip, Knee, Ankle

Area, Test, and Purpose	Interpretation	Procedure
Hip: Ober test for TFL (iliotibial band) contracture[9]	Tests: contracture or tightness (shortness) of the iliotibial band. Positive: tested leg remains abducted while the patient's muscles are relaxed.	Patient remains side lying, with the lower leg flexed at the hip and knee. Patient's tested limb is uppermost, with knee extended. The therapist passively abducts and extends the upper leg, and slowly lowers the limb.
Hip: Thomas test for hip flexion tightness[6,9]	Tests: contracture or tightness (shortness) of hip flexors. Positive: patient's thigh lifts up from the table, bending at the knee.	Patient remains supine. The therapist flexes the unaffected hip, asking the patient to hold his or her knee to his or her chest (flattening the lumbar spine and stabilizing the pelvis). Patient holds the flexed hip against his or her chest.

(continued)

Table 5.23 Orthopedic Special Tests: Hip, Knee, Ankle *(continued)*

Area, Test, and Purpose	Interpretation	Procedure
Hip: Patrick's test (FABER test)[6,9]	Tests: arthritis of the hip or sacroiliac joint dysfunction. Positive: pain in the hip and the tested leg's knee remaining above the opposite knee.	Patient remains supine. The therapist flexes, abducts, and externally rotates the patient's hip until the lateral malleolus rests on the opposite knee above the patella. In this position, the therapist gently pushes the knee downward.
Hip: Supine Straight Leg Raise Test[10]	Test: Hamstring tightness (shortness) Positive: hip flexion range of motion measurement less than 80° suggests hamstring tightness.	Patient remains supine with bilateral lower extremities in extension. The non-test leg should be stabilized. The clinician passively raises the test leg into the straight leg raise position while keeping the knee straight. Hip flexion range of motion measurement is taken to determine if tightness is present.
Knee: Valgus test (abduction test) for medial instability[6]	Tests: instability of the medial collateral ligament (MCL). Positive: pain or excessive gapping of the joint (the tibia moves away from the femur because of gaps on the medial side).	Patient remains supine, with the tested knee first in full extension, then in slight flexion (20°–30°). One of the therapist's hands palpates the knee joint line at the medial side; the other hand at the lateral joint line pushes the knee medially by applying a valgus stress.
Knee: Varus test (adduction test) for lateral instability[6]	Tests: instability of the lateral collateral ligament (LCL). Positive: pain or excessive gapping of the joint (the tibia moves away from the femur because of gaps on the lateral side).	Patient remains supine, with the tested knee first in full extension, then in slight flexion (20°–30°). One of the therapist's hands palpates the knee joint line at the lateral side; the other hand at the medial joint line pushes the knee laterally by applying a varus stress.
Knee: Lachman test for anterior cruciate ligament (ACL) instability[6, 9]	Tests: instability of the ACL. Positive: "mushy" or soft end feel when the tibia is moved forward on the femur. Caution: A false-negative is possible if the femur is not properly stabilized or a meniscal tear is present.	Patient remains supine, with the tested knee in 30° of flexion. One of the therapist's hands stabilizes distal femur; the other hand translates the proximal tibia forward on the femur.

(continued)

Table 5.23 Orthopedic Special Tests: Hip, Knee, Ankle   *(continued)*

Area, Test, and Purpose	Interpretation	Procedure
Knee: McMurray test to identify meniscal pathology[6, 9]	Tests: integrity of the lateral and medial meniscus. Positive: snap or click (or feeling a crepitation) accompanied by pain at the knee suggests damage to the posterior horn of meniscus.	Patient remains supine, with the tested knee completely flexed. One of the therapist's hands grasps the calcaneus, rotating the tibia as the knee is moved into extension. The other hand palpates the knee joint as the knee is extended.
Knee: Thessaly Test for dynamic loading of the knee joint to determine meniscal pathology[9, 11]	Tests the integrity of the medial and lateral meniscus. Positive: medial or lateral joint line discomfort or patient may perceive locking, snapping or catching in the knee joint.	Patient stands on the affected leg while the clinician holds the outstretched hands of the patient for support; patient is instructed to bend the knee slightly (5° knee flexion) and twist on the knee by rotating the body/trunk on the fixed lower extremity for a total of three times. The procedure is repeated with the knee flexed to 20°.
Knee: Thomas Test for rectus femoris tightness[10]	Tests: tightness of rectus femoris. Positive: knee flexion < 80° may suggest rectus femoris tightness.	Patient lies supine. The PTA flexes the unaffected hip, asking the patient to hold that knee to his or her chest (to flatten the lumbar spine and stabilize the pelvis). The PTA passively flexes the affected knee to the limit of motion to assess if the rectus femoris is shortened.
Ankle: Thompson's test for rupture of Achilles tendon[6]	Tests: rupture of Achilles tendon. Positive: absence of plantar flexion when the calf muscles are squeezed.	Patient remains prone, relaxed, with the feet over the edge of the table. The therapist squeezes the calf muscles.

Common Injuries of the Brachial Plexus and Nerves of the Upper Extremity[12,13,14]

The brachial plexus is formed by the anterior rami of C5–T1 nerve roots. The brachial plexus travels through the thoracic outlet and may become entrapped or compressed in this region. Common causes of TOS are identified in **Table 5.24**. The brachial plexus initially divides into three trunks: upper, middle and lower.

Upper plexus injuries (C5, C6) include Erb's Palsy in children and a "stinger" injury in football players.

Middle plexus injuries (C7) are rare in isolation.

Lower plexus injuries (C8, T1) include Klumpke's paralysis.

In addition, complete or whole plexus injuries can occur in children and adults.

Table 5.24 Common Injuries of the Brachial Plexus

Nerve and Its Origin	Motor Innervation	Musculoskeletal Injuries
Median nerve cords: medial and lateral. Divisions: anterior. Trunks: upper, middle, and lower. Origin: nerve roots C6, C7, C8, and T1.	Motor innervation muscles: pronator teres; pronator quadratus; palmaris longus; FCR; FDS; FPL; lateral half of FDP; lumbricals 1 and 2; thenar muscles (abductor pollicis brevis; lateral half of FPB; and opponens pollicis).	Median nerve compression injuries: ■ Thoracic outlet syndrome: presence of a cervical rib or narrowing of the thoracic outlet ■ Pronator teres syndrome: caused by trauma, humeral fracture, hypertrophy of muscle, or repetitive injury (such as using a screwdriver) ■ Anterior interosseus syndrome: caused by fibrous sheaths, thrombosis of vessels, or forearm fractures ■ Carpal tunnel syndrome: caused by hormonal factors in pregnancy, hypothyroidism, congenital bone deformities, rheumatoid arthritis (RA), or overuse syndrome Median nerve trauma injuries: ■ Humeral fractures ■ Wrist lacerations ■ Carpal bones trauma Median nerve lesion deformities: ■ Ape hand: paralysis and atrophy of thenar muscles; opposition is lost; thumb is permanently extended ■ Benediction sign: inability to flex the thumb and second and third digits; they remain in extension because the FDP and FPL are weak; ring and little fingers are flexed while others are extended; cannot make a fist[13]

Table 5.24 Common Injuries of the Brachial Plexus

(continued)

Nerve and Its Origin	Motor Innervation	Musculoskeletal Injuries
Ulnar nerve cord: medial. Division: anterior. Trunk: lower. Origin: nerve roots C8 and T1.	Muscles: FCU; medial half of FDP; palmaris brevis; hand interossei; third and fourth lumbricals; adductor pollicis; medial half of FPB; hypothenar muscles (opponens digiti minimi, abductor digiti minimi, and flexor digiti minimi).	Ulnar nerve compression injuries: ■ Thoracic outlet syndrome: presence of a cervical rib or narrowing of the thoracic outlet ■ Crutches injury: pressure on the axillary region ■ Cubital tunnel syndrome: entrapment at the elbow secondary to trauma, repetitive motion, or inflammatory conditions ■ Guyon's canal (or ulnar tunnel): secondary to RA or trauma (karate) ■ Ulnar nerve lesion deformity: claw hand (hyperextension of the proximal phalanges of the digits and extreme flexion of the middle and distal phalanges; loss of opposition and inability to abduct the little finger)[8]
Radial nerve cord: posterior. Division: posterior. Trunks: upper, middle, lower. Origin: nerve roots C5, C6, C7, C8, and T1.	Muscles: brachioradialis, ECRL, triceps, anconeus, ECRB, supinator, ED, EDM, ECU, abductor pollicis longus, EPL, EPB, extensor indicis.	Radial nerve compression injuries: ■ Spiral groove syndrome (called also Saturday night palsy): caused by falling asleep (inebriated) with the spiral groove of the arm against a hard object or caused by direct trauma ■ Crutches injury: pressure on the axillary region Radial nerve trauma injuries: ■ Radial neck fractures ■ Humeral fractures ■ Shoulder dislocations Radial nerve lesion deformity: upper arm lesions result in weak triceps and decreased ability to push up. Weak wrist extension with reduced ability to make a fist and decreased grip

Common Muscle Substitutions

Table 5.25 **Examples of Common Muscle Substitutions**

- Scapular stabilizers initiate shoulder motion for weak shoulder abductors.
- Lateral trunk muscles or TFL takes over for weak hip abductors.
- Long head of the biceps, coracobrachialis, and anterior deltoid take over for a weak pectoralis major.
- Use of passive finger flexion by contracting wrist extensors for weak finger flexors.
- Use of lower back extensors, adductor magnus, and quadratus lumborum for weak hip extensors.
- Use of lower abdominals, lower obliques, hip adductors, and latissimus dorsi for weak hip flexors.

SECTION 5-4

Types of Musculoskeletal Interventions

Additionally, refer to Part 4 for an overview of general interventions.

Closed Kinetic Chain (CKC) Exercises to Increase Weight-Bearing Control and Stability

Table 5.26 CKC Exercises

CKC Isometric Exercises

- Muscle setting exercises (to facilitate co-contraction of the quadriceps and hamstrings): Patient sits on a chair with the knee extended or slightly flexed and the heel on the floor. Have the patient press the heel against the floor and the thigh against the seat of the chair and concentrate on contracting the quadriceps and hamstrings simultaneously to facilitate co-contraction around the knee joint. Hold the muscle contraction, relax, and repeat rhythmic stabilization.

- Muscle setting exercises (to facilitate contraction of muscles in the ankles, knees, hips and trunk): Patient stands with bilateral weight bearing. Apply manual resistance to the pelvis in several directions as the patient holds the position. This will facilitate isometric contraction of muscles in the ankles, knees, hips, and trunk. Progress to rhythmic stabilization activity by having the patient bear weight only on the involved lower extremity while resistance is applied.

CKC Dynamic Exercises

- Mini-squats (short-arc training): Patient stands and bends both knees up to 30°–45°, and then extends the knees. Progress by using elastic resistance placed under both feet or by holding weights in the hands. Having the knees move anterior to the toes as the hips descend increases the shear forces on the tibia and strains the ACL. Squatting, as if sitting on a chair, in which the tibia remains relatively vertical requires greater trunk flexion to maintain balance and stronger quadriceps contraction to support the load of the pelvis posterior to the knee axis at an angle where patellar compressive loads are great (helping to reduce the stress on the ACL).

- Forward, backward, and lateral step-ups and step-downs: Begin with a low step, 2–3 inches in height, and increase the height as the patient is able. Make sure that the patient keeps the trunk upright. Emphasize control of body weight during concentric (step-up) and eccentric (step-down) quadriceps activity. Instruct the patient that the heel is to be the last to leave the floor and the first to return ("Keep the toes up").

- Standing wall slides: The patient flexes the hips and knees and slides the back down and then up the wall, lifting and lowering the body weight. As control improves, the patient moves into greater knee flexion, up to a maximum of 60°. Knee flexion beyond 60° is not recommended to avoid excessive shear forces on ligamentous structures of the knee and compressive forces on the patellofemoral joint. Wall slides that are performed with a gym ball behind the back decrease stability and require more control.

- Partial and full lunges: Patient assumes a step-forward stance position with weight acceptance on the forward foot. Have the patient rock the body weight forward, allowing the knee to flex slightly, and then rock backward and control knee extension.

Patient Education Topics Related to the Lumbar Spine

Table 5.27 Patient Education for the Lumbar Spine

- When supine, hook lying flexes the spine, while legs extended position extends the spine. A pillow under the head flexes the neck; a small roll under the neck stabilizes a mild lordosis with the head in neutral position.

- When prone, the patient should use a pillow under the abdomen to flex the spine. Without a pillow, this position extends the spine.

- Sitting usually causes spinal flexion, especially if the hips and knees are flexed. To emphasize flexion, the patient should prop the feet up on a small footstool (to increase hip flexion). To emphasize extension, the patient should use a lumbar pillow (or support) in the low back region.

- Standing usually causes spinal extension. To emphasize flexion, the patient should stand with a small stool under one of the feet.

- If tolerated, the patient is taught to perform simple movements while protecting the spine in the functional position.

- Gentle pelvic tilting or chin tucks should be taught in every position tolerated by the patient, including supine, prone, side lying, sitting, and standing.

- Post laminectomy or post diskectomy (in the hospital), the patient is taught:

  1. To use the "log roll" technique to turn from supine to side lying to prone and return
  2. To practice maintaining spinal alignment by keeping the shoulders aligned with the pelvis while rolling the trunk over as a unit (a log) and not twisting the spine
  3. To sit from the supine-lying position by log rolling on to the side, pushing the body up with the hands while bringing the legs forward over the side of the bed
  4. To keep the back in lordosis if there is an extension bias or in flexion if there is a flexion bias
  5. To go from standing to sitting and the reverse with spinal control
  6. To move the trunk as a whole
  7. Not to bend over
  8. Not to lift heavy or moderately heavy objects
  9. Not to twist the back
  10. Not to sit for prolonged periods of time
  11. Not to climb long flights of stairs
  12. To maintain proper body mechanics (to lessen strain and pressure on the spine), including proper body alignment and good posture
  13. To sleep on a firm mattress
  14. To start an exercise program (4–6 weeks postoperatively or when indicated by surgeon) of gradual abdominal muscle strengthening

Abdominal Strengthening Exercises

Table 5.28 Abdominal Muscles Strengthening Exercises[12]

Stabilization exercises

- Drawing-in maneuver: starting in hook lying, have the patient activate the transversus abdominis by drawing the belly button in toward the spine. The abdomen should hollow with minimal to no evidence of substitute movement.
- Abdominal bracing: starting in hook lying, have the patient activate the oblique abdominal muscles by setting the abdominals. There will be some motion of the lateral trunk walls only.
- Pelvic tilt: starting in hook lying, have the patient activate the rectus abdominis by performing a posterior pelvic tilt. The lumbar spine will flatten.
- Activation of the deep muscles of the spine are important before the patient moves to more advanced stabilization exercises and dynamic abdominal strengthening. In addition to activation of abdominal musculature, the patient should also be taught activation of multifidus. One technique to facilitate contraction is to palpate just lateral to the spinous processes of the lumbar spine (L/sp) and have the patient perform the drawing in maneuver.
- The patient should be encouraged to activate the deep muscles throughout the day and in different positions.

Curl-ups

- Position of patient: hook lying, with the lumbar spine flat (posterior pelvic tilt).
- First, have the patient perform the drawing-in maneuver to achieve stabilization of the abdominal muscles, then lift the head off the mat.
- Patient progresses by lifting the shoulders until the scapulae and thorax clear the mat, keeping the arms horizontal. The patient does not come to a full sit-up because after the thorax clears the mat, the rest of the motion is performed by the hip flexor muscles.
- Further progress the difficulty of the curl-up by changing the arm position from horizontal to folded across the chest and then to behind the head.

Diagonal Curl-ups

- To emphasize the external oblique muscles, the patient performs a diagonal curl-up by reaching one hand toward the outside of the opposite knee while curling up, then alternating.
- The patient reverses the muscle action by bringing one knee up toward the opposite shoulder and then repeating with the other knee.

Double Knee to Chest

- To emphasize the lower rectus abdominis and oblique muscles, have the patient set a posterior pelvic tilt, then bring both knees to the chest and return.
- Progress the difficulty by decreasing the angle of the hip and knee flexion.

Pelvic Lifts

- The patient begins with the hips at 90° and knees extended.
- The patient performs a posterior pelvic tilt and lifts the buttocks upward off the mat (small motion; the feet move also upward toward the ceiling).
- The patient should not push against the mat with the hands.

(continued)

Table 5.28 Abdominal Muscles Strengthening Exercises   *(continued)*

Bilateral Straight-Leg Raising (SLR)

- This is a progression in difficulty of the double knee-to-chest exercise (it should be undertaken only if the muscles are strong enough to maintain a posterior pelvic tilt).

- The patient begins with legs extended. The patient first performs a posterior pelvic tilt, then flexes both hips, keeping the knees extended; if the hips are abducted before initiating this exercise, greater stress is placed on the oblique abdominal muscles.

Orthotics

Table 5.29 Orthotics I: Orthopedic Shoes[15]

- For the patient (client) with orthopedic impairments and functional limitations, orthopedic shoes reduce pressure on sensitive deformed structures and are a foundation for ankle-foot orthoses (AFOs) and more extensive bracing.

- The most common orthopedic shoes:
    1. The Blucher lace stay has a separation between anterior margin of the lace stay and the vamp; offers adjustability for edema and is preferred for use with orthotics.
    2. The Balmoral lace stay: the lace stay is continuous with the vamp.
    3. A low quarter-height shoe falls below the malleoli; does not restrict foot or ankle motion.
    4. A high quarter-height shoe covers the malleoli; indicated for rigid pes equinus or to increase stability without an AFO.
    5. Shoes with reinforcements, e.g., toe box to protect toes.
    6. Shoes with special soles e.g., shock absorbent.
    7. Shoes with high heels or low heels e.g., a higher heel puts the ankle in some degree of plantarflexion.

- Foot orthoses: appliances that apply forces to the foot, improve function and relieve pain.
    1. Can be inserts; made of viscoelastic plastics, rubber, rigid plastics, or metal:
        - Longitudinal arch support (LAS): corrects for flat foot—pes planus
        - Scaphoid pad: made of rubber; used under navicular bone
        - UCBL insert: applies medial force to calcaneus and lateral and upward force to medial midfoot
    2. Can be external modifications:
        - Thomas heel: corrects for pronated foot—flexible pes valgus
        - Metatarsal bar: takes pressure off metatarsal heads
        - Rocker bar: improves weight shift on metatarsals; helps in late stance
        - Shoe lifts: for leg-length discrepancy
        - Heel wedges: absorb forces at heel contact; alter alignment of calcaneus

Table 5.30 Orthotics II: Ankle-Foot Orthoses[15]

- Appliances made of a foundation, ankle control, foot control, and a superstructure:
  1. The foundation is made of a shoe and a plastic or metal component. May fix internally with an insert or externally via a stirrup.
  2. The traditional foundation has a steel stirrup that can be solid stirrup (for maximum stability) or split stirrup (eases donning the orthosis).
  3. A plastic or metal insert will fit inside a shoe.
- Types of AFOs:
  1. Solid ankle AFO: limits all foot and ankle motion; used for severe pain and instability; increases stride length and cadence in hemiplegia
  2. Hinged solid ankle AFO: similar to solid ankle AFO; provides slight sagittal motion for foot flat position in early stance; used for spastic diplegia in children
  3. Bi-channel adjustable ankle locks (BiCAALs): an alternative to solid ankle AFO; resists PF and DF
  4. Ypsilon AFO: carbon composite AFO; provides assistance to DF; used for mild to moderate isolated foot drop
  5. Anterior stop AFO: limits ankle DF; prevents excessive knee flexion or "buckling"; helps in late stance of gait
  6. Posterior stop AFO: limits ankle PF; prevents knee hyperextension/recurvatum
  7. Posterior leaf spring AFO: provides DF assistance; used for foot drop
  8. Steel DF spring assist AFO-Klenzak joint: has DF spring assist in each stirrup; provides DF assistance; used for foot drop; bulkier than posterior leaf
  9. Toe off AFO: provides DF assistance; used for mild to severe food drop and instability
  10. Spiral AFO: controls but does not eliminate motion in all planes; fits snugly for maximal control; contraindicated for fluctuating edema
  11. Silicone ankle foot orthosis (SAFO): a contemporary AFO made of silicone for foot drop; provides a flexible dynamic function giving comfort and cosmesis for the foot and ankle; good for heel strike with a smooth transition to toe-off

Table 5.31 Orthotics III: Other Types of Orthoses[15]

- Floor reaction force orthosis: type of solid ankle AFO; resists knee flexion; provides a knee extension moment to control knee flexion in stance.

- Tone-reducing orthosis: plastic AFO designed for spastic cerebral palsy (CP) and spastic hemiplegia (applies constant pressure to plantarflexors and invertors); used for equinovarus and moderate spasticity with varus instability; patients achieve better foot and knee control; contraindicated in fixed deformity.

- Supramalleolar orthosis: used for the ankle to maintain the foot in neutral alignment; allows ankle DF/PF; does not offer knee control; used for spastic diplegia.

- Stabilizing boots AFO: custom-made AFO for paraplegia (used by adults); conforms to the patient's legs and feet; feet angled at 15° PF; legs angled posterior to keep knees extended; patient keeps stability by leaning backward; used with crutches or walker.

Table 5.32 Orthotics IV: Knee–Ankle–Foot Orthoses[15]

- Knee–ankle–foot orthosis (KAFO): appliance made of a shoe, foundation, ankle control, knee control, and superstructure in the form of a thigh band or weightbearing rim if weightbearing is restricted.

- The KAFO may include also foot control.

- The KAFO controls for knee flexion/extension and genu valgum and genu varum. It is used for paralysis or limb deformity.

- The most common knee flexion or extension control of a KAFO is the drop ring lock controlling the knee hinges. In stance, the rings drop, locking the KAFO in extension (may have spring-loaded retention buttons to unlock each upright; the pawl lock with bail release is used for simultaneous locking of uprights). The drop ring lock and pawl lock are contraindicated with knee flexion contracture.

- Sagittal stability of KAFO:
  - Leather kneecap
  - Rigid anterior band: can be suprapatellar or pretibial bands, which do not interfere with sitting; easier to don
  - Electronic stance control mechanism: prevents knee flexion in stance without interfering with knee extension; permits knee flexion in swing

- Frontal plane knee control (for genu varum or genu valgum):
  - Plastic calf shells: semirigid shell for valgum applies lateral force at the knee; semirigid shell for varum applies medial force at the knee
  - Valgum correction strap: knee cap with a fifth strap buckled around lateral upright; less effective than semirigid shells

- Specialized KAFO: KAFO with computer-controlled knee joint.

- Craig Scott KAFO: custom-made KAFO for paraplegia (used by adults). It includes a shoe reinforced with transverse and longitudinal plates.

- BiCAAL AFO set in slight DF; pawl lock with bail release; single thigh band: allows the patient to stand with a backward lean to prevent untoward hip or trunk flexion.

- Walkabout orthosis: custom-made pair of KAFOs permitting hip flexion and extension and restricting hip abduction, adduction, and rotation.

Table 5.33 Orthotics V: Hip-Knee-Ankle-Foot Orthoses, Trunk–Hip–Knee–Ankle–Foot Orthoses, Reciprocating Gait Orthoses, and Standing Frames[15]

- Hip–knee–ankle–foot orthosis (HKAFO): KAFO with added pelvic band and hip joints. The HKAFO controls for hip abduction, adduction, rotation, and flexion. To control flexion, a drop ring lock can be added to the hip joint hinge.

- Trunk–hip–knee–ankle–foot orthosis (THKAFO): HKAFO with a metal band to anchor the trunk. The THKAFO is not widely used because it is difficult to don, the metal band is uncomfortable, and it restricts ambulation in swing to or swing through (when the hip joints are locked).

- Reciprocating gait orthosis (RGO): custom-made THKAFO. The hips are joined by one or two metal cables or rods, the knees are stabilized with knee locks (offset knee joints or pretibial bands), and the feet are stabilized with solid AFOs. The RGO is used for bilateral lower extremities and trunk paralysis. The patient can walk with crutches (using a four- or two-point

(continued)

Table 5.33 **Orthotics V: Hip-Knee-Ankle-Foot Orthoses, Trunk–Hip–Knee–Ankle–Foot Orthoses, Reciprocating Gait Orthoses, and Standing Frames** *(continued)*

gait) by shifting his or her weight to the right, tucking the pelvis (by extending the upper thorax), pressing on the crutches, and allowing the left leg to swing through. The reverse procedure follows for the right leg to swing.

- Standing frame: for standing without crutches. It is used by children and adults.
- Swivel walker: for standing and twirling without crutches. It is used by children and adults. Swivel walkers are similar to standing frames except for the slightly rocking base to enable a swiveling gait.
- Parapodium: for standing and performing activities without crutches; allows sitting. It is used by children and adults. Children can also move from place to place by rotating the upper torso to shift their weight, causing the frame to rock and rotate.

Table 5.34 **Orthotics VI: Corsets, Lumbosacral Orthoses, and Thoracolumbosacral Orthoses**[15]

- Corset: used for low back musculoskeletal disorders, sacroiliac support, and spinal cord injury (SCI) (assists with respiration). The corset increases intra-abdominal pressure but reduces frontal movement. The increase in the intra-abdominal pressure reduces stress on the posterior spinal musculature, diminishing the load on the lumbar intervertebral discs.
- Lumbosacral orthoses (LSOs): control or limit flexion, extension, and lateral motion. The LS flexion extension lateral (FEL) control orthosis (e.g., Knight spinal orthosis) controls flexion, extension, and lateral flexion. An alternative version of LS FEL is used for spondylolisthesis (controls extension). Use of an LS FEL for low back pain is controversial. A plastic LS FEL jacket restricts motion in all directions.
- Thoracolumbosacral orthoses (TLSOs): limit flexion and extension (and gross spinal movement). The amount of movement permitted by a TLSO varies from one person to another. Examples include TLSO flexion/extension devices (e.g., Taylor brace), which may be used for SCI.

Table 5.35 **Orthotics VII: Cervical Orthoses, Orthoses for Scoliosis, and Externally Powered Orthoses**[15]

Cervical Orthoses

- Soft foam-rubber collar: may be used for whiplash; gives minimal support
- Four-poster orthosis: may be used for cervical fracture and SCI; gives moderate support
- Halo orthosis or Minerva orthosis: may be used for cervical fracture and SCI; gives maximal support

Orthoses for Scoliosis

- Cervical thoracic lumbosacral orthosis (CTLSO) such as the Milwaukee orthosis (the oldest orthosis for scoliosis): may be used for all kyphotic and scoliotic curves of 40° or less.
- Boston TLSO: used for midthoracic or lower scoliosis of 40° or less curves; also used for spondylolisthesis and conditions with severe trunk weakness such as muscular dystrophy.
- Wilmington TLSO: has tight contact and fit; is custom made.
- Charleston bending brace and Providence brace: to wear only at night when the effects of gravity are at a minimum; provide overcorrection of the spinal curve.

(continued)

Table 5.35 **Orthotics VII: Cervical Orthoses, Orthoses for Scoliosis, and Externally Powered Orthoses** *(continued)*

Externally Powered Orthoses

- Pneumatic foot control and functional electrical stimulation (FES): enable patients to ambulate in their residences or in the community (in rare cases).
- FES uses electrical stimulation (ES) to the quadriceps and gluteus maximus. The peroneal nerves may also use ES (to initiate DF and reflex hip flexion) if the ankles are not supported by bilateral AFOs.
- To use the FES, the patient (client) needs full passive mobility in all joints and to be able to control the timing and the amount of electrical current to transfer from a chair to the standing position and to walk in different directions.

Orthotic Interventions

Table 5.36 **Orthotic Interventions**[15]

- Patient education for skin inspection, orthosis care, and donning/doffing the orthosis.
- AROM, PROM, and static and dynamic balance and gait training using the orthosis
- Assessments or reassessments:
  - Assessment of the discrepancy of limb length
  - Assessment of sensation
- Functional activities using the orthosis:
  - Traditional MMT for muscle function if permitted
  - In cases of spasticity, functional tests of motor performance
- Assessment and reassessment of gait deviations using the orthosis-examples of common gait deviations and possible causes:
  - Lateral trunk bend in early stance: caused by a too-high medial upright of the KAFO; excessive abduction of the hip joint by the HKAFO; patient requires a cane; insufficient shoe lift; weak gluteus medius; abduction contracture; hip pain; poor balance; short leg
  - Circumduction during swing: caused by knee lock; excessive PF; inadequate PF stop; inadequate DF assist; weak hip flexors; extensor synergy; weak dorsiflexors; pes equinus; knee or ankle ankylosis
  - Hyperextended knee in early stance: caused by inadequate PF stop or knee lock; pes equinus; weak quads; extensor synergy; short contralateral LE; contralateral knee or hip flexion contracture
  - Knee instability in early stance: caused by too much knee flexion; inadequate knee lock; inadequate DF stop; weak quads; knee pain; knee or hip flexion contracture; flexor synergy; short contralateral LE
  - Foot slap in early stance: caused by weak DF; inadequate dorsiflexor assist; inadequate plantarflexion stop
  - Flat foot contact during early stance: caused by inadequate DF stop; inadequate traction from the sole; patient requires a cane; poor balance; pes calcaneus
  - Anterior trunk bending in early stance-leans forward as weight is transferred to LE: caused by inadequate knee lock; weak quads; hip and knee flexion contracture

(continued)

Table 5.36 Orthotic Interventions   *(continued)*

- Posterior trunk bending in early stance-leans backward as weight is transferred to LE: caused by inadequate hip lock; knee lock; weak gluteus maximus; knee ankylosis
- Hip hiking in swing: caused by knee lock; inadequate DF stop; inadequate PF stop; short contralateral LE; weak hip flexors; extensor synergy; weak dorsiflexors; pes equinus; knee or ankle ankylosis
- Vaulting (exaggerated PF of contralateral LE) in swing: caused by knee lock; inadequate DF and PF assist; weak hip flexors; pes equinus; extensor spasticity; short contralateral LE; weak dorsiflexors; knee or ankle ankylosis

Prosthetics: Levels of Amputation

Table 5.37 Levels of Amputation[15]

- Toe disarticulation: amputation at the metatarsal phalangeal joint
- Transmetatarsal: amputation through the midsection of all metatarsals
- Symes ankle disarticulation with attachment of heel pad to distal end of tibia: may include removal of tibial and fibular flares and both malleoli
- Transtibial amputation: below-the-knee amputation (BKA)
  - Short BKA: less than 20% of tibial length
  - Long BKA: more than 50% of tibial length
  - Standard BKA: between 20% and 50% of tibial length
- Knee disarticulation: amputation through the knee joint (femur is intact)
- Transfemoral amputation: above-the-knee amputation (AKA)
  - Short AKA: less than 35% of femoral length
  - Long AKA: more than 60% of femoral length
  - Standard AKA: between 35% and 60% of femoral length
- Hip disarticulation: amputation through the hip joint (pelvis is intact)
- Hemipelvectomy: resection of lower half of pelvis
- Hemicorporectomy: amputation of both lower extremities and pelvis (below L4–L5 level)

Transtibial (Below Knee) Prostheses

Table 5.38 Below-Knee Amputation Prostheses[15]

- Foot and ankle assembly: nonarticulated feet that are light in weight, durable, attractive, and most popular. Types of nonarticulated feet:
  - Solid ankle cushion heel (SACH) foot: simple design; least cost; lowest function; permits PF in early stance; absorbs shock; hyperextends in late stance
  - Stationary attachment flexible endoskeleton (SAFE) foot: good on uneven terrain; permits medial-lateral motion in the rear foot; heavier and more expensive than SACH
- Foot and ankle assembly: articulated feet that have a metal bolt or cable; are shock absorbent; control plantarflexion; have dorsiflexion stop; can loosen over time. Types of articulated feet:

(continued)

Table 5.38 **Below-Knee Amputation Prostheses** *(continued)*

- Single-axis feet: most common; permit PF, DF, and toe break; do not allow medial-lateral or transverse motion; may use rotators-components placed above the prosthetic foot to absorb shock in the transverse plane; rotators used with active individuals who had transfemoral amputations

- Multiple-axis feet: move slightly in all planes for maximum contact with an irregular walking surface; reduce shearing forces on residual limb; heavier and less durable than single-axis or nonarticulated feet

■ Other types of foot and ankle prosthetic componentry:

  - Energy storing, dynamic elastic response

  - Energy storing with multiaxial features

  - Energy storing with vertical shock pylon

■ Energy-storing and dynamic-response feet have internal structures that absorb energy during the stance and release energy at toe-off. They provide a smoother and more energy-efficient gait and are extremely lightweight and durable. Examples of energy-storing dynamic response feet: Flex Foot, Springlite Foot (weighs less than 11 ounces; has shock absorption and smooth transition to midstance and toe-off), Seattle Foot, and Carbon Copy II foot (energy-storing and energy-releasing or dynamic feet; can be used to play basketball or to run).

■ Exoskeletal and endoskeletal shanks-substitutes for human leg:

  - Exoskeletal shank: made of wood or rigid plastic

  - Endoskeletal shank: made of aluminum or rigid plastic pylon covered with foam rubber and a sturdy stocking or similar finish; pylon permits slight adjustment

■ Transtibial socket-plastic receptacle for the amputated foot:

  - BKA requires a patellar tendon-bearing (PTB) socket (has a prominent indentation over patellar tendon). Newer BKA sockets are hypobaric (with total surface bearing; no indentation).

  - Sockets are custom made through computer-aided design (CAD) or computer-aided manufacture (CAM). An electronic sensor transmits a detailed map of the limb to a computerized program consisting of socket-shaped variations. The prosthetist selects the appropriate shape and transmits it to an electronic carver, which creates the model; the plastic is then shaped over the computer-generated model.

  - Sockets have "reliefs," which are concavities over sensitive areas such as bony prominences. Sockets can be unlined, made of thin thermoplastic with removable liners (polyethylene foam liners). "Buildups" are convexities in the socket over pressure-tolerant areas. Transtibial socket usually has a removable polyethylene foam liner. Other sockets made of thin thermoplastic in a rigid frame can be unlined. These types of sockets adhere to the skin better than rigid plastic sockets, improving prosthetic suspension. Plastic sockets or socket liners should be washed to keep them clean, especially in warm climates.

■ Suspension—to hold the prosthesis in place:

  - Supracondylar cuff suspension: consists of a leather strap that fastens around distal thigh and allows the patient (client) to adjust the tightness of the suspension. A suspension cuff with a fork strap or a waist belt is indicated for patients (clients) who climb ladders or perform long-duration activities when the prosthesis is not supported on the ground.

  - Distal attachment: consists of a distal pin mechanism attached to a silicone sheath that is worn next to the skin. The pin inserts into an opening in the socket and locks in place. Provides a secure attachment that prevents slippage during gait.

  - Supracondylar/suprapatellar (SC/SP) suspension: has a high anterior wall that terminates above the patella and medial and lateral walls that extend above the femoral epicondyles, accommodating a short amputated limb. The anterior wall interferes with kneeling and is not cosmetically appealing in sitting.

  - Patients with sensitive skin may need thigh corset suspension. Prolonged use of a thigh corset suspension may produce pressure atrophy of the thigh, and the device is difficult to don.

  - Vacuum-assisted socket suspension promotes fluid exchange, increases proprioception, reduces moisture, and regulates edema fluctuations.

Transfemoral (Above Knee) Prostheses

Table 5.39 Above-Knee Amputation Prostheses[15]

- Foot and ankle assembly: the same as transtibial prostheses. A SACH foot or single-axis foot is used the most.
- Knee unit: allows the user to bend the knee. It is made of an axis (single-axis hinge or polycentric linkage that has better stability), a friction mechanism (can have constant or variable friction), an extension aid (assists with knee extension in the late swing phase of gait; can be external in front of the knee axis and internal within the knee unit), and mechanical stabilizers (manual lock; friction brake).
  - The knee unit can use a constant-friction (remains the same) or variable-friction (friction changes with high friction in the early swing phase of gait, less friction in the midswing phase of gait, and increased friction again in the late swing phase of gait) mechanism. The friction can be applied through sliding of the clamp (least expensive), hydraulically (using oil), or pneumatically (using air).
  - Hydraulic and pneumatic friction units allow symmetrical movements. A newer type of friction knee unit uses computer-programmed electronic sensors that provide almost-instantaneous friction adjustments in gait patterns, accommodating navigation of various terrains and bicycle riding.
  - Knee extension mechanisms: external aids (made of elastic webbing; most simple; may pull knee in extension while sitting) and internal extension aids (elastic strap or coiled spring; keeps knee flexed when sitting; included in pneumatic/hydraulic units).
  - Stabilizing mechanisms: manual lock (when the pin lock is engaged, it prevents knee flexion; most simple; need to disengage pin lock in sitting) and friction brake (one version in clamp sliding allows knee flexion to 25°; another version in hydraulic units stabilizes better).
  - Types of computer-programmed electronic sensors for the knee unit: Rheo Knee (uses a knee's microprocessor to adjust resistance during the stance; maintains knee stability on uneven terrain; uses a lithium battery) and C-Leg (uses computerized sensors and hydraulic pistons; useful for stepping down out of a vehicle and descending curbs, ramps, or stairs).
- Transfemoral socket: quadrilateral socket (with a horizontal posterior shelf for ischial tuberosity and gluteal muscles) and ischial containment socket:
  - Transfemoral sockets are made of flexible plastic (allows for sensory input from external objects) enclosed in a rigid frame that transmits weight to the ground. Concave "reliefs" are made for pressure-sensitive areas and to allow contraction of the gluteus maximus and rectus femoris.
  - An ischial containment socket (also known as a contoured adducted trochanter-controlled alignment method [CAT-CAM] socket) increases the entire transfemoral socket stability. Slight socket flexion allows hip extensors' contraction to reduce lumbar lordosis for equal step length. An example of CAT-CAM is the Comfort Flex Socket System (also called the Hanger Comfort Flex Socket) combined with the Otto Bock C-Leg. This AKA prosthesis uses a microprocessor-controlled hydraulic knee with swing and stance control. It accommodates navigation of uneven surfaces, stairs, slopes, biking, running, dancing, and golfing.
- Suspension:
  - Total suction: provides maximum control of the prosthesis.
  - Partial suction: requires one or more socks or a silicone liner and additional suspension i.e., pelvic band.
  - No suction: has a distal hole; no pressure between inside and outside the socket; requires a pelvic band.

Prosthetics: Pressure-Tolerant and Pressure-Sensitive Areas

Table 5.40 Prosthetics: Pressure-Tolerant and Pressure-Sensitive Areas

Pressure-Tolerant (Buildup) Areas	Pressure-Sensitive (Relief) Areas
Transtibial amputation	**Transtibial amputation**
Patellar tendon	Fibular head and neck
Proximal and medial tibia (at pes anserinus)	Anterior tibial crest
Tibial and fibular shafts	Tibial condyles
Belly of gastrocnemius	Anterior distal tibia
	Medial and lateral hamstring tendons
Transfemoral amputation	**Transfemoral amputation**
Ischial tuberosity	Distolateral end of femur
Gluteals	Pubic symphysis
Lateral sides of residual limb	Perineal area
Distal end (rarely may be sensitive)	Adductor longus tendon

Prosthetic Wearing Schedule Patient Education[16]

Table 5.41 Prosthetics: Wearing Schedule Recommendations

Days 1–2	Half hour in morning, monitor fit, check for excessive areas of pressure.
	Allow some ambulation with prosthesis on.
	Repeat 1/2 hour in the evening, monitoring fit and areas of pressure.
Days 3–4	Increase morning and evening wearing time to 1 hour each session.
	Allow some ambulation.
	Monitor fit and areas of pressure.
Days 5–10	Increase morning and evening wearing time to 2 hours each session.
	Allow some ambulation.
	Monitor fit and areas of pressure.
Days 11–14	Don prosthesis first thing in the morning.
	Check skin for pressure areas before lunch, if no adverse response.

(continued)

Table 5.41 **Prosthetics: Wearing Schedule Recommendations**   *(continued)*

	Continue to wear prosthesis and perform skin check before dinner.
	If no skin concerns, resume wearing the prosthesis until bed time, making sure to check skin for areas of pressure upon removal of prosthesis for the night.
Days 14 +	If no adverse issues have been experienced, the prosthesis may now be worn on a full-time basis.
	Continued monitoring for prosthetic fit and areas of pressure should be done at least once per day by the wearer or a family member to ensure no adverse responses are resulting from prosthetic use.

Interventions for Patients with Lower Extremity (LE) Amputation

Table 5.42 **Interventions for Patients with LE Amputation**[15]

Functional Interventions

- Bed mobility
- Transfers
- Activities of daily living (ADLs)
- Gait training with prosthesis and assistive device (such as crutches or walker for balance deficits)
- Wheelchair training
- Mobility without prosthesis (for use at night)

Residual Limb Care

- Use of removable rigid dressing and temporary prosthesis: both help with early ambulation
- Residual limb wrapping: using elastic bandages and figure-of-eight technique
- Use of shrinker: easier to apply than elastic bandages
- Prevention of contracture: positioning the patient prone as much as possible during the day and attaching a posterior board to the wheelchair in sitting; to avoid knee flexion, and hip flexion, abduction, and ER

Patient Education

- Care of residual limb: including desensitizing activities, hygiene, and bandaging of residual limb
- Care of the uninvolved extremity
- Proper positioning
- Exercises
- Education about edema, pain, and changes in skin color
- Phantom limb: normal
- Phantom pain: abnormal and disabling
- Home exercise program (HEP)

(continued)

Table 5.42 Interventions for Patients with LE Amputation *(continued)*

Therapeutic Exercises

- Individualized
- AROM
- Stretching: for hip and knee extensors
- Strengthening: AKA needs strength in residual hip extensors and abductors mostly; BKA needs strength in residual knee extensors and flexors mostly
- Balance and coordination training

Balance and Coordination Training

- Can start at parallel bars, especially for patients with AKA prostheses (because it is difficult to control the mechanical knee)
  - When using parallel bars, encourage the patient to rest the hand on bars and not to grip or use the parallel bars to pull up into standing.
  - A sturdy mat table can be used to start balance training and for standing posture (equal weight bearing and without excessive lordosis). The PTA should stand near the patient's prosthesis to encourage the patient to shift his or her weight symmetrically and in stepping movements (may use a mirror for visual feedback).
- Static balance training is performed on the amputated side
- The prosthetic tolerance must increase gradually to minimize skin abrasion
- Patient to exercise while standing and performing hip flexion (causes the knee to bend)
- Patient to perform hip extension (stabilizes the knee in stance)
- Patient stepping on a low stool with involved and uninvolved LE (causes to shift weight symmetrically)

Transfer Training

- Patient to start with wheelchair sit to stand transfers. Patient to transfer weight to uninvolved LE first, then to push on armrests to stand.
- Later practice transfers from wheelchair to mat and back, wheelchair to sofa (deep upholstered) and back, wheelchair to low chair and back, wheelchair to toilet and back, and wheelchair to automobile and back (patient to sit sideways with both feet out of the car door, then to pivot on the seat and swing the prosthesis into the car)

Gait Training

- Gait: progression from dynamic balance training
- Proprioceptive neuromuscular facilitation (PNF) exercises for trunk control and LE movement during gait
- Rhythmic counting and walking with music to improve gait symmetry and speed
- For patient who fatigues rapidly: use an assistive device such as a cane (or two canes) or forearm crutches (use caution because the patient may lean on axillary crutches)
- For the patient who is able to ambulate indoors without cane: use the cane when ambulating outdoors to negotiate curbs and on uneven surfaces
- For the patient with generalized weakness: a walker may be needed for maximum stability
  - The patient should not lean too far forward on the walker.
  - In case of a transtibial prosthesis, the patient may use a two-wheeled walker (as opposed to a four-leg walker) to increase speed.

(continued)

Table 5.42 **Interventions for Patients with LE Amputation** *(continued)*

Stairs (with Rails), Ramps, and Curbs Climbing

- Patients with transtibial or Syme's amputations: ascend and descend stairs and inclines with equal step length and normal gait pattern.
- Patients with unilateral transfemoral amputation: ascend by leading with the uninvolved LE and descend by placing the involved LE on the lower step first.
- The techniques are the same for curbs when no rails are available.
- When stairs, ramps, or curbs are too steep, the patient (client) may ascend diagonally or sidestep with the prosthesis on the downhill side.

Prosthetic Gait Deviation Assessment for Patients with Transtibial Amputation[15]

- Excessive knee flexion in early stance: caused by socket too far anterior; high shoe heel; insufficient PF; socket excessively flexed; stiff heel cushion; weak quads; or knee flexion contracture
- Inadequate knee flexion in early stance: caused by socket too far posterior; socket not flexed enough; soft heel cushion; low heel shoe; excessive PF; weak quads; or spastic quads
- Medial thrust at midstance: caused by excessive foot outset
- Lateral thrust at midstance: caused by excessive foot inset
- Premature knee flexion in late stance ("drop-off"): caused by socket too far forward; high shoe heel; insufficient PF; socket flexed too much; DF stop too soft; or knee flexion contracture
- Delayed knee flexion in late stance: caused by socket too far back; socket not flexed enough; DF stop too stiff; excessive PF; low shoe heel; or extensor spasticity

Prosthetic Gait Deviation Assessment for Patients with Transfemoral Amputation[15]

- Circumduction in swing phase: caused by prosthesis too long; locked knee unit; socket too small; loose socket; loose friction; inadequate suspension; foot in PF; or abduction contracture
- Abducted during stance phase: caused by long prosthesis; inadequate lateral wall adduction; high or sharp medial wall; abduction contracture; or weak abductors
- Lateral trunk bending in stance: caused by short prosthesis; low lateral wall; high or sharp medial wall; weak abductors; hip pain; or abduction contracture
- Medial or lateral whip at heel-off: caused by faulty socket contour; knee bolt rotated externally or internally; or foot mal rotated
- Vaulting in swing phase: caused by too-long prosthesis; too-small socket; inadequate suspension; or too little knee flexion
- Forward flexion in stance: caused by unstable knee unit or instability
- High heel rise in swing phase: caused by inadequate friction or too little tension in the extension aid
- Foot slap at heel contact: caused by stiff heel cushion
- Uneven step length: caused by insufficient socket flexion; uncomfortable socket; hip flexion contracture; or instability

Phases of Gait Cycles

Table 5.43 **Phases of Gait Cycles: Traditional Versus Rancho Los Amigos (RLA)[15]**

Traditional	RLA
Heel strike	Initial contact
Heel strike to foot flat	Loading response
Midstance	Midstance
Heel-off	Terminal stance
Toe-off	Preswing
Acceleration	Initial swing
Midswing	Midswing
Deceleration	Terminal swing

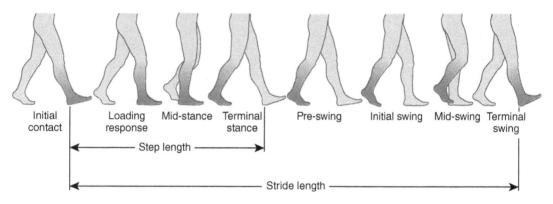

Initial contact   Loading response   Mid-stance   Terminal stance   Pre-swing   Initial swing   Mid-swing   Terminal swing

Step length

Stride length

Figure 5.57 Gait cycle.

Muscle Activation Patterns

Table 5.44 **Muscle Activation Patterns**[15]

Heel Strike

- Person's heel contacts the ground
- Muscles: quadriceps muscles and ankle dorsiflexors muscles (anterior tibialis, extensor hallucis longus, and extensor digitorum longus)

Foot Flat

- Person's sole of the foot makes contact with the ground (immediately after the heel strike)
- Muscles: gastrocnemius and soleus

Midstance

- Person's full body weight is taken by the reference extremity
- Muscles: hip and ankle extensor muscles control the forward motion of the trunk; hip abductors stabilize the pelvis

Heel-Off

- After the midstance, when the person's heel leaves the ground
- Muscles: ankle plantarflexors have peak activity immediately after the heel-off to propel the body forward

Toe-Off

- Person's toe is still in contact with the ground
- Muscles: ankle plantarflexors, quadriceps to control knee flexion and hip flexors

Acceleration

- Starts at the toe-off of the reference extremity until the midswing of the same reference extremity·
- Muscles: hip flexor muscles (iliopsoas) help to accelerate the extremity and propel it forward, dorsiflexors contract to clear toes

Midswing

- Reference extremity moves directly beneath the person's body
- Muscles: hip and knee flexor muscles and ankle dorsiflexors muscles contract to achieve foot clearance of the reference extremity

Deceleration

- Reference extremity is slowing down with the knee extended in preparation for heel strike
- Muscles: hamstrings work hard to decelerate the reference extremity in preparation for the heel strike

Common Gait Deviations: Stance Phase

Table 5.45 Gait Deviations: Stance Phase

- Lateral bending of trunk: weak gluteus medius (Trendelenburg gait)
- Backward leaning of trunk: weak gluteus maximus (difficulty walking stairs/ramps)
- Forward leaning of trunk: weak quadriceps or hip/knee flexion contracture
- Excessive hip flexion: weak hip extensors or tight hip/knee flexors
- Decreased hip flexion: weak hip flexors or tight hip extensors
- Decreased hip extension: tight hip flexors
- Excessive knee flexion: weak quadriceps or knee flexion contracture (difficulty walking stairs/ramps)
- Hyperextension of knee: weak (or tight) quadriceps or contracture of plantarflexors
- Toes contact at heel strike: weak dorsiflexors, tight plantarflexors, shorter leg, or painful heel
- Foot slap (steppage gait): weak dorsiflexors or excessive hip/knee flexion
- Foot flat: weak dorsiflexors (normal for children younger than 2 years of age)
- Excessive dorsiflexion (calcaneus gait): weak plantarflexors
- Excessive plantarflexion (equinus gait): tightness or contracture of plantarflexors
- Varus foot throughout stance: weak peroneal or tight anterior tibialis
- Limited push off: weak plantarflexors or pain in forefoot
- Short stance on involved extremity and uneven gait pattern: pain in ambulation (antalgic gait)

Common Gait Deviations: Swing Phase

Table 5.46 Gait Deviations: Swing Phase

- Limited pelvic retraction (forward rotation of pelvis): weak hip flexors and abdominals
- Limited hip and knee flexion: weak hip and knee flexors
- Circumduction: weak hip and knee flexors
- Hip hiking of quadratus lumborum: weak hip and knee flexors
- Excessive hip and knee flexion (steppage gait): shorter leg, tight plantarflexors, or weak dorsiflexors
- Limited knee flexion: tight quadriceps, weak hamstrings, or knee pain
- Excessive knee flexion: tight hamstrings
- Foot drop (equinus gait): weak dorsiflexors or tight plantarflexors
- Varus or inverted foot: weak peroneals or tight anterior tibialis
- Equinovarus: tight posterior tibialis and gastrocnemius and soleus

Gait Training Points

Table 5.47 Gait Training Points

- Stand on patient's involved or weaker side.
- Key points of control while guarding the patient: patient's shoulder and the safety belt.
- Patient loses balance forward: With one hand, pull the patient back by the safety belt; with the other hand, hold the patient's anterior shoulder and assist the patient to regain balance. If balance cannot be regained and the patient is falling forward, the patient must be instructed to remove the assistive device and reach for the floor while the therapist retards the patient's forward fall by holding the patient by the safety belt. During the fall, the patient can be instructed to cushion the fall by bending the elbows and turning the head to one side.
- Patient loses balance backward: With one hand, hold the patient by the safety belt; with the other hand on the patient's posterior shoulder, assist the patient to regain balance. The therapist's lower extremity is on the patient's involved pelvis to help the patient regain balance. If balance cannot be regained and the patient is falling backward, the patient must be instructed to remove the assistive device while the therapist lowers the patient toward the floor by holding onto the safety belt.

Canes

- Widen base of support (BOS), improve balance (unload forces on involved LE by as much as 30%), and reduce forces acting at the stance hip.
- Canes are not intended for patients with weight-bearing restrictions (such as no weight bearing [NWB] or partial weight bearing [PWB]).
- Canes are used in the hand opposite to the involved lower extremity:
- Widens BOS with decreased lateral shifting of center of mass (COM) compared to when used ipsilaterally
- Approximates a normal reciprocal gait pattern
- Reduces forces created by the abductor muscles acting at the involved hip in the stance phase; creates gravitational moment at the stance hip
- Cane measurement: must be 6 inches from the lateral border of the toes; top of the cane must be at greater trochanter and elbow flexed at about 20°–30°.

Crutches

- Improve lateral stability and balance, and decrease weight bearing on involved LE. (Patient education: Do not lean on axillary crutches because of the potential damage of radial nerve and axillary artery.)
- Crutches are awkward in small and crowded areas.
- Axillary crutches measurement: in standing position from 2 inches (width of two fingers) below the axilla at 2 inches lateral and 6 inches anterior to the foot (can also subtract 16 inches from the patient's height). Elbow must be flexed at about 20°–30° when using crutches.
- Forearm crutches measurement: in standing position, distal end at 2 inches lateral and 6 inches anterior to the foot; elbow must be flexed at about 20°–30°; forearm cuff must be at 1.0–1.5 inches below the elbow.
- Gait patterns for crutches: three-point gait, modified three-point gait; four-point gait; two-point gait; swing to; swing through.

(continued)

Table 5.47 **Gait Training Points** *(continued)*

Walkers

- Widen BOS, decrease weight bearing fully or partially on the involved LE, improve balance, and provide lateral and anterior stability. Walkers offer the greatest stability.
- Walker measurement: the walker handgrip (handle) must be at the greater trochanter, and elbow must be flexed at about 20°–30°.
- Nonrolling walkers can use full weight bearing, PWB, or NWB patterns.

SECTION 5-5

Basic Clinical Impairments and Activity Limitations Related to Common Musculoskeletal Conditions

Clinical Impairments and Activity Limitations of Arthritic Disorders[14]

Table 5.48 Clinical Impairments and Activity Limitations of Arthritic Disorders*

Osteoarthritis: Impairments and Activity Limitations	Rheumatoid Arthritis: Impairments and Activity Limitations
Sensory deficits: decreased proprioception and/or kinesthesia (such as during ambulation and/or ADLs); pain with weight bearing depending on the stages of the disease (or if it involves discal nerve root compromise); aching during sleep; hip pain can be prevalent depending on the stages of the disease; pain upon rising that eases through the morning with movement.	Sensory deficits: sharp pain with certain movements; paresthesia; decreased proprioception and/or kinesthesia.
Motor deficits: decreased muscular strength; decreased muscular endurance; decreased ROM; decreased flexibility (morning stiffness that is eased with movement); sometimes a leg-length discrepancy; decreased balance; deformities such as valgus or varus in the knee joint; joint crepitus; joint swelling (moderate); increased muscular spasms; joint deformity (usually in abduction, flexion, and external rotation); postural deficits (such as increased kyphosis or lordosis); abnormal reflexes. Common in hips, knees, hands and feet.	Motor deficits: decreased flexibility; decreased muscular strength; decreased muscular endurance; decreased flexibility (morning stiffness lasting more than 1 hour); decreased ROM; joint swelling; increased joint laxity; crepitus; increased, joint hypermobility or hypomobility; increased skin and soft-tissue temperature; edema; decreased balance and coordination; joint deformity especially in the second and third MCP and PIP; may have Boutonniere deformity (PIP joint flexion and DIP joint hyperextension); Swan neck deformity (PIP joint hyperextension and MCP and DIP joints flexion); valgus deformity at the knees and ankles; clawed toes deformity. Symmetrical joint involvement affecting any joints.
Functional deficits: antalgic gait pattern; may need assistive device in transfers and ambulation; decreased independence with ADLs (such as dressing) and home management activities; decreased independence with IADLs; inability to ambulate stairs (steps); inability to participate in work/play/school or perform leisure activities.	Functional deficits: decreased independence with ADLs and home management activities; decreased independence with IADLs; inability to ambulate stairs (steps); inability to participate in work/play/school or perform leisure activities; may need assistive devices in transfers and ambulation. Systemic deficits: fatigue (lack of energy). Pulmonary: may have pleural effusion or pleuritis; shallow breathing; chest pain during inspiration. Cardiac: pericarditis, vasculitis, conduction defects; vision, integument and renal changes may also be present.

* These are basic guidelines. The PTA should also consider the findings from the physical therapist's (PT's) initial examination and evaluation and any environmental factors that may be associated with these diagnoses.

Clinical Impairments and Activity Limitations of Other Musculoskeletal Conditions

Table 5.49 Impairments Activity Limitations and Participation Restrictions Related to Tendonitis, Bursitis, Sprains, Strains, Dislocations, and Fractures

- Sensory deficits: pain at rest and with weight bearing; decreased sensation; decreased proprioception and/or kinesthesia.

- When cervical spine is involved (such as with an acceleration injury or cervical sprain of the cervical spine (CSp)), the patient can have neck pain; headaches, vertigo, dysesthesias (numbness, burning, prickling, or tingling) of the face and upper extremities; and changes in vision and hearing.

- In rib fractures, the patient may have pain with deep inspiration. In brachial plexus lesions, the patient may have sharp and burning pain in the upper extremity and numbness and pins and needles in the upper extremity.

- In cervical disk pathology, the patient can have sensory changes in the respective dermatomes. In cervical facet syndrome, the patient can have paresthesia and pain with hyperextension and rotation of the CSp.

- Motor deficits: increased muscular spasms; decreased muscular strength; decreased muscular endurance; decreased ROM; decreased flexibility; localized swelling; joint crepitus with active motion; decreased balance (if the deficit is in the lower extremity); postural deficits; muscular substitutions (stronger muscles compensate for the loss of motion); postural changes (such as forward head kyphosis with cervical sprain).

- Upper and lower extremity fractures can present with edema, ecchymosis, structural deformity and limited ROM.

- Functional deficits: decreased independence with ADLs (such as dressing) and home management activities, decreased independence with instrumental ADLs (IADLs), inability to ambulate stairs or steps (if it is in the lower extremity), and inability to participate in work/play/school or perform leisure activities.

Musculoskeletal Intervention Strategies

APTA's Guide to Physical Therapist Practice[17] Intervention Categories Most Related to the Musculoskeletal System

Table 5.50 Patient or Client Instruction[17]

Provision of information, education, and training regarding the following:

- Health, wellness, and fitness programs
- Impairments in body functions and structures, activity limitations, and participation restrictions
- Pathology or health conditions
- Performance enhancement
- Plan of care
- Psychosocial influences on treatment such as fear–avoidance beliefs, behave change techniques
- Transitions across new settings
- Transitions to new roles

Table 5.51 Assistive Technology: Prescription, Application, and as Appropriate, Fabrication or Modification of Locomotive Aids, Orthotic and Prosthetic Devices[17]

This category of intervention may include any assistance required for the procurement or proper fitting of any durable medical equipment or appliances that may be of benefit for the improved functioning of the patient. Prescription, application, and as appropriate, fabrication of assistive technologies may include but not be limited to the following:

- Assistive devices for locomotion (i.e., crutches, canes, walkers, rollators, manual wheelchairs, power wheelchairs, power-operated vehicles)
- Orthoses (i.e., ankle foot orthoses [AFOs], knee-ankle-foot orthoses [KAFOs], body jackets, wrist splints, shoe inserts)
- Prostheses (i.e., transtibial, transfemoral, upper extremity prosthesis)
- Seating and positioning technologies (i.e., custom-molded seating, removable trunk supports, upper extremity support trays for wheelchairs, sidelyers, prone standers, manual or power reclining systems for wheelchairs)
- Other assistive technologies to improve safety, function, and independence, such as transfer devices (i.e., transfer boards, mechanical lifts/hoists) and adaptive bathroom equipment (i.e., raised toilet commodes, transfer benches, sliders, adaptive shower chairs and commodes)

Table 5.52 Biophysical Agents

Biophysical agents is a very broad category pertaining to many of the modalities that are utilized in the physical therapy setting for the treatment objective of resolving any impairment or activity limitation that is adversely affecting function. For a review of commonly applied biophysical agents, including indications for use, see Table 4-3 of this text.

Table 5.53 **Functional Training in Self-Care and in Domestic Education, Work, Community, Social, and Civic Life**[17]

Functional training in self-care pertains to integration or reintegration back to competent and safe basic ADLs, such as bed mobility, transfers, dressing, grooming, eating, etc.

Functional training in domestic life pertains to more complex return to ADLs and IADLs such as caring for dependents, maintaining a home, shopping, making accommodations for environmental barriers to the home, or travel.

Functional training in education pertains to integration or reintegration for the resumption of roles and functions in an educational environment and may include training to overcome environmental physical barriers, injury prevention, and use of assistive technology in the school environment.

Functional training in work life includes accommodations or modifications of work barriers. Training may include but is not limited to education for injury prevention, workstation ergonomics, lifting /body mechanics, adaptive equipment for work seating/positioning, orthoses or prostheses application, and locomotion aids.

Functional training in community, social, or civic life considers the social or recreational aspect of return to function in a safe and competent manner. Training may include public transportation use, return to banking, shopping, attending community or civic sponsored events (i.e., town hall meetings, church, garden or book club, library activities), and lastly, integration or reintegration into vocational or enjoyable pastimes (i.e., bowling, fitness classes, quilting, stamp collecting).

Functional training may include the following:

- ADL training
  - Bathing
  - Bed mobility and transfer training
  - Dressing
  - Eating
  - Grooming
  - Toileting
- Barrier accommodations or modifications
- Developmental activities
- Device and equipment use and training
  - Assistive and adaptive device or equipment training during IADL
  - Orthotic, protective, or supportive device or equipment training during IADL
  - Prosthetic device or equipment training during IADL
- Functional training programs
  - Back schools
  - Job coaching
  - Simulated environments and tasks
  - Task adaptation
  - Task training
  - Travel training
  - Work conditioning

(continued)

Table 5.53 **Functional Training in Self-Care and in Domestic Education, Work, Community, Social, and Civic Life** *(continued)*

- Work hardening
- IADL training
  - Community service training
  - School and play activities training
  - Work training
- Injury prevention or reduction
  - Injury prevention education during domestic, education, work, community, social, and civic integration or reintegration
  - Injury prevention education with the use of devices and equipment
  - Safety awareness training during work, community, social, and civic life integration or reintegration

Table 5.54 **Manual Therapy Techniques** [17]

Manual therapy techniques may include the following:

- Manual lymphatic drainage
- Manual traction
- Massage
  - Connective tissue massage
  - Therapeutic massage
- Mobilization
  - Soft tissue
  - Peripheral joints
- Neural tissue mobilization
- Passive range of motion
- PNF
- Neuro developmental techniques (NDT)

Table 5.55 **Motor Function Training** [17]

Motor function training activities may include the following:

- Balance training
  - Developmental activities training
  - Motor control training or retraining
  - Neuromuscular education or re-education
  - Perceptual training
  - Standardized, programmatic, and complementary exercise approaches
  - Task-specific performance training
  - Vestibular training

(continued)

Table 5.55 **Motor Function Training**   *(continued)*

- Gait and locomotion training
  - Developmental activities training
  - Implement and device training
  - Perceptual training
  - Standardized, programmatic, and complementary exercise approaches
  - Training of specific components of gait
  - Wheelchair feature and propulsion training (manual and motorized wheelchairs)
- Posture training
  - Developmental activities training
  - Neuromuscular education or re-education
  - Postural awareness training
  - Postural control training
  - Postural stabilization activities
  - Vestibular training

Table 5.56 **Therapeutic Exercises** [17]

Refer to Section 4-2 for a review of basic exercise interventions. In addition, the following therapeutic interventions may be appropriate for the patient with an orthopaedic diagnosis:

- Gait and locomotor training
- Increased workload over time
- Movement efficiency and energy conservation training
- Walking and wheelchair propulsion programs
- Neuromotor development training
- Developmental activities training
- Motor training
- Movement pattern training
- Neuromuscular education or reeducation
- Standardized, programmatic, or complementary exercise approaches
- Task-specific performance training

Clinical Practice Guidelines

Clinical Practice Guidelines (CPGs), developed by APTA sections, other organizations, societies, and health care organizations, are based on a systematic review of the evidence and provide therapists with resources to help guide clinical decision-making.[18] The Academy of Orthopaedic Physical Therapy, a Section of the APTA, provides access to CPGs relevant to the management of patients with orthopaedic diagnoses. Examples of topics addressed by the Academy of Orthopaedic Physical Therapy include plantar fasciitis, achilles tendinopathy, patellofemoral pain, ACL injury prevention, hip OA, low back pain, adhesive capsulitis, neck pain, carpal tunnel syndrome, pelvic girdle pain, concussion/mild traumatic brain injury, and hip fracture.[19] A full listing and links to the published CPGs can be found at https://www.orthopt.org/content/practice/clinical-practice-guidelines.

Arthritic Disorders: Interventions

Table 5.57 Arthritic Disorders: Interventions

Indication	Interventions
Osteoarthritis (OA) or degenerative joint disease (DJD): degeneration of articular cartilage with hypertrophy of the subchondral bone and joint capsule; common in weight-bearing joints but also found in the shoulder, lumbar and cervical spines, and first carpometacarpal joint of hand and first metatarsophalangeal joint of foot.[14]	Pain management and control of inflammation (physical agents and modalities); joint protection and function (splints, orthotics, gait training with assistive devices, and task modifications); measures to increase flexibility and strength (aquatic therapy, ROM, stretching, and strengthening exercises); manual therapy; patient education about joint protection and weight loss (when indicated).
Rheumatoid arthritis: a chronic systemic disease characterized by a symmetric pattern of destruction in synovial tissues and articular cartilages of the joints of the hands, wrists, elbows, shoulders, knees, ankles, and feet. C1 and C2 joints of cervical spine may also be affected. MCP and PIP joints are often affected early with the DIP joints spared. Swan neck, Boutonniere, and ulnar drift are common deformities of the hand.[14]	Pain management and control of inflammation (physical agents and modalities); prevention of deformities and maintenance of ROM (splints and orthotic devices for ADLs); gait training with assistive devices and task modifications; measures to increase flexibility, strength, and endurance using ROM exercises, stretching exercises with caution and strengthening exercises; patient education for joint protection and disease progression. Contraindication: Avoid stretching to joints that are inflamed.[12]
Systemic lupus erythematosus (SLE): progressive systemic inflammatory autoimmune disorder characterized by inflammation of and damage to connective tissue anywhere in the body. The most commonly affected areas include the skin, joints, nervous system, kidneys, lungs, and other organs. Arthritis can affect any joint. SLE presents with a skin rash on exposed areas of the body. (Butterfly rash across cheeks and nose.)[14]	Pain management (physical agents and modalities); measures to increase strength and endurance (aquatic therapy); measures to decrease chronic fatigue (activity pacing and energy conservation); joint protection (gait training with assistive devices); patient education related to postural awareness and daily walking. Precaution: Avoid excessive exposure to sunlight (ultraviolet light).
Ankylosing spondylitis (Marie Strumpell disease): progressive inflammatory disorder that initially affects the spine and the sacroiliac joints. Later, may affect large joints of the extremities as well as organs (e.g., eyes, digestive tract and less commonly the heart, lungs, and kidneys) can be affected. Posture is affected, resulting in kyphosis deformity of CS/TS and a decrease in lumbar lordosis.[14]	Maintenance of proper posture: deep breathing and stretching exercises (hip extension, shoulder flexion) strengthening of trunk extensors, lumbar stabilization exercises; task modifications and ergonomic modifications (workplace); patient education related to posture awareness and proper sleeping patterns (on a firm mattress without pillows). Exercise programs are customized for the individual patient (swimming is preferred). Precaution: Avoid high impact and flexion exercises, and contact/high risk sports.[12,14]

(continued)

Table 5.57 Arthritic Disorders: Interventions   *(continued)*

Indication	Interventions
Psoriatic arthritis: a chronic, erosive inflammatory disorder associated with psoriasis. Erosive degeneration occurs in the joints of the digits (ends of the fingers or toes) as well as the spine.	Joint protection and maintenance of joint mobility (splints and orthotics; gait training using assistive devices; stretching exercises); patient education related to joint protection.
Gout: chronic disease of uric acid metabolism that occurs as an acute, episodic form of arthritis. Familial history of gout increases risk. It is common in the great toe but may also be observed at the ankle, knee, wrist, and elbow joints causing severe to excruciating pain. Kidneys may also be affected.[14]	Pain management and stress reduction (transcutaneous electrical nerve stimulation (TENS) and electromyographic (EMG) biofeedback for relaxation); joint protection and maintenance of joint mobility (braces and orthotics; gait training with assistive devices); patient education related to the disease, relaxation and stress management to control pain, general fitness exercises, and joint protection; HEP for stretching and strengthening exercises (aquatic exercises are also recommended).
Fibromyalgia syndrome (FMS): a widespread disorder of musculoskeletal pain. FMS is considered systemic and presents with multiple tender points on both sides of the body. Conversely myofascial pain syndrome is localized to one or a few muscles and has no systemic involvement. Fibromyalgia causes chronic pain with diffuse aching or burning in the muscles, stiffness, fatigue, disturbed sleep patterns, and depression.[14]	Pain management and promotion of relaxation (TENS, ultrasound (US), moist hot pack (MHP), massage, whirlpool, breathing exercises, EMG biofeedback for relaxation); flexibility improvement using a progressive graded exercise program that includes aerobic conditioning (walking, biking, stationary bicycle, swimming, low-impact aerobics, or water aerobics and resistance exercises if tolerated).

Overuse Syndromes

Overuse syndromes include the following:

- Tendinopathy: Term applied to any tendon problem not involving ruptured tissue
- Tendinitis: Term applied to acute inflammation of the tendon that may be due to a sudden, acute injury, or repeated microtraumas
- Tendinosis: Term applied to noninflammatory, more chronic degeneration of the tendon often the result of repetitive injuries without enough time to heal
- Bursitis: Inflammation of the bursa frequently due to irritation but may also be a result of trauma

Refer to Table 4-1 for overview of interventions based on stages of tissue healing.

Table 5.58 Tendonitis, Tendinosis, Tendinopathy, and Bursitis: Interventions

Indication	Interventions
Subacromial rotator cuff impingement, also called pitcher's shoulder, is a shoulder impingement syndrome; swimmer's shoulder and tennis shoulder: progressive overuse disorder caused mostly by sports. It results from mechanical impingement of the tendons of the rotator cuff under the coracoacromial arch. Supraspinatus tendinitis and infraspinatus tendinitis are common.[20]	Pain management and joint protection using physical agents and modalities such as ice massage, ice pack, ES, US, phonophoresis, and iontophoresis. Patient education: no shoulder elevation above 80° during early rehab; joint protection; modification of ADLs along with workstation ergonomic assessment or biomechanical recommendations to reduce overuse on more chronically injured tissue. Measures to improve flexibility: stretching exercises (posterior capsule). Measures to increase strength: Codman's pendulum exercises (in the beginning), Active assisted range of motion (AAROM); first strengthen scapular stabilizers and then rotator cuff muscles; initial CKC exercise progressing to OKC and eccentric strengthening for shoulder muscles.
Lateral epicondylitis (tennis elbow), medial epicondylitis (golfer's elbow), and medial valgus stress overload (MVSO). Tennis elbow is chronic inflammation of the common wrist extensor tendons, mainly the ECRB and extensor communis tendons. Golfer's elbow is chronic inflammation of the FCU tendon. MVSO is inflammation of the medial ulnar ligament and capsule from repetitive overuse. All are caused by sports or occupations or cumulative trauma from work injuries.	Acute: RICE, US, ES, phonophoresis, iontophoresis, gentle AROM, splint protection (bracing with counterforce brace for tennis elbow), patient education (to avoid repetitive motions and aggravating activities), and multiple angle muscle setting exercises. Subacute: progress with stretching, progressive resistive exercises (PREs) as tolerated and pain free; joint mobilization; cross fiber massage; gradual return to function training; task modifications if needed. For MVSO, avoid exercises in valgus position of elbow.
DeQuervain's tenosynovitis: inflammation of the EPB and abductor pollicis longus tendons at the first dorsal compartment of the hand from repetitive microtrauma.	Acute: RICE, US, phonophoresis, iontophoresis, ES, splint protection, activity modification, friction massage, muscle setting progressing to resistance exercises as tissues heal; stretching exercises, mobilization and patient education for activity modifications.
Carpal tunnel syndrome (CTS): tenosynovitis or inflamed, swollen, tendons producing a compression syndrome of the median nerve. Causes: commonly occupational (carpenters, factory workers, or food processing workers) or during pregnancy (hormonal). May also be associated with arthritis, diabetes, hypothyroidism. Patients may have atrophy of muscles of thenar eminence and first two lumbricals. Sensory impairment in median nerve distribution of hand.[12,20].	Nonoperative: pain management and relief of aggravating factors (physical agents and modalities); patient education related to job/task modifications; joint protection and support (resting splints or night splints in 0°–20° extension); tendon gliding exercises; nerve and joint mobilization; return to function training (ROM, stretching, and strengthening exercises). Postoperative: edema management (physical agents and modalities; soft-tissue mobilization of scar tissue); tendon and nerve gliding exercises; return to function (ROM exercises; ADLs; strengthening exercises of hand such as gripping exercises and UE exercises); desensitization of tissues; patient education related to CTS, scar-tissue massage, and job/task modifications to prevent recurrence.

(continued)

Table 5.58 Tendonitis, Tendinosis, Tendinopathy, and Bursitis: Interventions *(continued)*

Indication	Interventions
Anterior tibial periostitis (shin splints) and medial tibial stress syndrome (MTSS): overuse conditions caused by abnormal biomechanical alignment, muscle imbalance, poor conditioning, or improper training methods. Muscles involved can be the anterior tibialis and EHL for the anterior compartment, or the posterior tibialis for the posterior and medial compartment (MTSS).	Pain management and edema control (physical agents and modalities); activity modifications (orthotics, patient education related to proper training methods and prevention of recurrence); flexibility improvement (stretching exercises-gastrocnemius/soleus frequently tight); strengthening exercises (dorsiflexors and evertors for anterior tibial periostitis and plantar flexors and invertors for MTSS).
Achilles tendinopathy: microtrauma/overloading of the Achilles tendon due to altered foot biomechanics, muscle imbalance, poor footwear, changes in training or running surfaces.[20]	Acute stage: activity modification, pain and inflammation reduction (RICE); heel lift initially, gentle dorsiflexion AROM and stretching as tolerated; US: phonophoresis. Subacute stage: eccentric strengthening, closed and open chain resistance exercises; stretching, foot orthoses, taping.[20]
Plantar fasciitis: Chronic inflammation of plantar aponeurosis (with or without calcaneal heel spur). Causes: Repetitive strain of plantar fascia causing microtears, associated with high arches, flat feet, tight gastrocnemius/soleus muscles; tight plantar fascia. Excessive pronation (most common). Repetitive activities: prolonged walking on hard or irregular surfaces or running, poor footwear.	Increase proper mechanical alignment: eliminate the causes, taping, orthotics. Patient education regarding selection of footwear. Rest, physical agents and modalities for pain and swelling, joint and soft tissue mobilization. Stretching exercises: calf stretching and toe extension stretching exercises. Strengthening exercises after pain and swelling have subsided: intrinsic and extrinsic muscles of the foot. General body conditioning: pool or stationary bicycle to decrease weight-bearing through limb.
Patella femoral pain syndrome (PFPS), also called chondromalacia patella, jumper's knee, fat pad syndrome, anterior knee pain: overuse disorder characterized by pain around the patellar especially with running, jumping, deep squatting, or stair climbing. Symptoms aggravated by faulty mechanics, muscle imbalance, foot or hip deviations.[12,20]	Acute: Rest and modalities to reduce pain and swelling; ROM and flexibility exercises, muscle setting within pain-free range; brace or tape to unload the joint. Subacute: proximal hip stabilization exercises; stretching tight structures; patellar mobilization; balance/joint proprioception exercises (bilateral → unilateral); strengthening exercises hip and knee avoiding CKC knee flexion at 90° or greater, progressing to unilateral strengthening as pain and motor control improve.[12,20]
Bursitis: Subacromial/subdeltoid bursitis and trochanteric bursitis: caused by trauma, chronic overuse, inflammatory arthritis (such as RA), or biomechanical/gait abnormalities (for trochanteric bursitis). Athletes are prone to shoulder bursitis from overuse when the arm is at or above shoulder level. Hip bursitis is often seen in runners or athletes who participate in running-oriented sports such as soccer or football.	Acute: RICE; joint protection (splint or brace); reduction of pain and inflammation (physical agents and modalities); PROM, AAROM in pain-free ranges; muscle setting exercises. Subacute: promotion of functional activities, stretching of tight structures, strengthening exercises; improve neuromuscular control, increase muscle endurance; patient education related to proper usage and recurrence prevention. Shoulder bursitis: Codman's pendulum exercises and AAROM exercises in acute stage; shoulder stabilization and correction of faulty posture. Trochanteric bursitis: US, stretching exercises for Iliotibial band tightness, strengthen quads, hamstrings, hip abductors, extensors.[12,20]

Strains, Sprains, Dislocations, and Fractures: Interventions

Table 5.59 Strains, Sprains, Dislocations, and Fractures: Interventions [12, 20]

Indication	Interventions
Strains	

■ Injuries to muscles and tendon from direct trauma, overstretch, or excessive muscular contraction or overuse.
■ Three grades[20]:
  • First degree: mild injury, tear of few fibers
  • Second degree: moderate injury, tear of about 50% of fibers
  • Third degree: severe injury, tear (rupture) of all fibers
■ Common strains:
  • Rotator cuff tears (RCT): degenerative strain, occurring over time with impingement at the acromion from repetitive use and trauma or falling on to an outstretched hand
  • Hip strain (of HS, iliopsoas, adductors, and rectus femoris)
  • HS strain: most common in runners
  • Lumbar spine strain (from sudden violent contraction or fast stretch of combined extension/rotation)
	Nonoperative:
	■ Small tears - acute:
	  • Pain management: RICE; physical agents and modalities
	  • Patient education for ADL modifications (no overhead activities for RCT) and recurrence prevention
	  • PROM within pain-free range.
	  • Interventions for associated areas as tolerated.
	Small tears - subacute/return to function:
	  • Stretching exercises: shoulder flexibility and abduction for RCT
	  • Strengthening exercises
	  • Improve neuromuscular control, muscle endurance
	  • Progress functional activities
	■ Hip strain:
	  • Gait training with crutches to limit further irritation and allow for tissue healing
	■ For adductor longus strain:
	  • Avoid early aggressive stretching
	  • Large tears may need surgery
	■ For HS strain:
	  • Acute: Patient education to avoid in acute-phase full knee extension combined with forward flexion
	  • Subacute—AROM; aquatic exercises and strength (submaximal isometrics)
	Postoperative (RCT):
	■ Codman's pendulum
	■ Shoulder isometrics
	■ AAROM
	■ Strength exercises
	■ Gradual return to function training

(continued)

Table 5.59 Strains, Sprains, Dislocations, and Fractures: Interventions *(continued)*

Indication	Interventions
Sprains	
<ul><li>Injuries to ligaments from direct or indirect trauma</li><li>Three grades:<ul><li>Grade 1: mild, slight stretching of fibers, joint is stable</li><li>Grade 2: moderate, some fibers torn, increased joint mobility</li><li>Grade 3: severe (may need surgery), complete tear, joint is unstable</li></ul></li><li>Common sprains:<ul><li>AC joint sprain: from direct fall on acromion or indirect from a fall on outstretched arm</li><li>MCP or IP joint sprain</li><li>Skier's thumb: rupture of ulnar collateral ligament of MCP from hyperextension of thumb, common in skiing</li><li>Knee sprains: ACL (most commonly sprained), PCL, MCL, LCL</li><li>Ankle sprains: lateral ligaments (ATF, CF, PTF) or medial ligament (deltoid ligament; rare);</li><li>Meniscal tear (sudden trauma or gradual degeneration)</li><li>Lumbar spine sprain: from sudden violent force or repeated stress</li></ul></li></ul>	Nonoperative:<ul><li>RICE</li><li>Physical agents and modalities</li><li>NWB or WBAT</li><li>Braces, splints, and orthotics for immobilization and weight-bearing reduction</li><li>Isometrics</li><li>PROM, AAROM, AROM; isotonic exercises</li><li>CKC exercises</li><li>Isokinetic and isotonic exercises</li><li>General conditioning program (especially for LS)</li><li>Cycling and stair climbing activities</li><li>Proprioception, balance, and coordination</li><li>Patient education to prevent recurrence (especially for LS for lifting and sitting)</li><li>Return to prior level of function training</li></ul>Postoperative:<ul><li>Follows similar path as nonoperative care, except for WB status and postoperative precautions (such as for ACL reconstruction-no knee extension in final 40° extension and no OKC knee extension with resistance placed distally)</li><li>Meniscal repair: NWB and no knee flexion from 90°–100° for 4–6 weeks; no squats for 3–6 months</li></ul>
Dislocations	
<ul><li>Can occur due to trauma, laxity of tissues surrounding the joint.</li><li>Glenohumeral subluxation (partial dislocation); glenohumeral dislocation: at shoulder joint in abduction, extension, and ER (for anterior dislocation); abduction, flexion, and IR (for posterior dislocation)</li><li>Anterior dislocations are more common; posterior are rare</li><li>Inferior instability can occur as a result of muscle weakness/paralysis i.e., hemiplegia</li></ul>	Nonoperative:<ul><li>Avoid positions that duplicate the mechanism of injury during the acute phase to allow for tissue healing.</li><li>Immobilization (braces, orthotics, slings)</li><li>Physical agents and modalities for pain and swelling</li><li>Strengthening exercises of uninvolved joints and general conditioning</li><li>Patient education for precautions (for anterior lesion-no shoulder abduction and ER) and activity modifications</li><li>Codman's pendulum</li></ul>

(continued)

Table 5.59 **Strains, Sprains, Dislocations, and Fractures: Interventions**   *(continued)*

Indication	Interventions
<ul><li>Common types:<ul><li>Bankart lesion: an avulsion of the capsule and anterior labrum from the glenoid rim with disruption of medial scapular periosteum</li><li>Perthes lesion: similar to Bankart except the medial scapular periosteum remains intact</li><li>Hill-Sachs lesion: a compression fracture from impaction of the posterolateral humeral head against the anterior/inferior glenoid rim (may result in a loose body)</li></ul></li></ul>	<ul><li>Active assistive stretching exercises of tight structures, i.e., posterior structures in anterior dislocation</li><li>Strengthening exercises (isometrics, T-band) of rotator cuff (concentrate on infraspinatus and teres minor), scapular stabilizers and anterior shoulder muscles</li><li>Scapular stabilization</li><li>Precautions when starting isotonic resistive exercises</li><li>Proprioceptive exercises</li><li>CKC exercises</li><li>Joint mobilization</li></ul>Postoperative:<ul><li>Similar to nonoperative care, but varies considering the procedure and the patient</li></ul>

Fractures

<ul><li>Scapular and clavicular fracture: from direct or indirect trauma</li><li>Proximal humerus fracture: of humeral head, lesser or greater tuberosity or humeral shaft</li><li>Supracondylar fracture: transverse fracture distal one-third of humerus, often seen in children</li><li>Intercondylar fracture: of the articular surface of the elbow</li><li>Radial head fracture: from a fall on the outstretched arm</li><li>Olecranon fracture: from a fall on olecranon</li><li>Elbow fracture</li><li>Colles' fracture: from a fall onto an outstretched arm; distal radius displaced dorsal = dinner fork deformity</li><li>Smith's fracture: from a fall onto an outstretched arm with the elbow supinated; the distal radius is displaced ventrally</li><li>Scaphoid fracture: from a fall onto an outstretched arm in a younger person</li><li>Boxer's fracture: neck of fifth metacarpal</li><li>Bennet's fracture: proximal to first metacarpal</li></ul>	Nonoperative:<ul><li>Pain management and swelling reduction: physical agents and modalities; in UEs may use compression pump for lymphedema</li><li>Immobilization: casts, splints, orthotics, or slings</li><li>Activity modification</li><li>Mobility training: transfers; gait training with assistive devices and NWB/PWB or toe touch weight bearing balance training</li><li>Patient education on signs of circulatory problems (especially in wrist fractures) and to prevent recurrence and for safety</li><li>Functional use of extremity: ROM exercises; adaptive equipment</li><li>Functional activities of non-immobilized joints</li><li>Restoration of motion post-immobilization: ROM exercises</li><li>Strengthening exercises after immobilization</li></ul>Postoperative:<ul><li>See Section 5-7 for postoperative physical therapy management of patients with fractures.</li></ul>

(continued)

Table 5.59 **Strains, Sprains, Dislocations, and Fractures: Interventions** *(continued)*

Indication	Interventions
■ Mallet finger: avulsion fracture or tendon injury of the extensor tendon = DIP joint flexion contracture	
■ Patellar fracture	
■ Hip fracture: includes subcapital fracture, femoral neck fracture, intertrochanteric fracture, subtrochanteric fracture; most common in geriatric patients; if untreated, can cause avascular necrosis of the hip	
■ Pelvis and acetabulum fracture	
■ Ankle fracture: unimalleolar, bimalleolar, or trimalleolar	
■ Distal tibia fracture	
■ Calcaneal fracture: from a fall from a height	
■ Talus fracture: from a fall from a height and landing on foot on crouched position	
■ Compression fracture: osteoporosis traumatic events	

Thoracic Outlet Syndrome, Adhesive Capsulitis, Low Back Disorders: Interventions

Table 5.60 Thoracic Outlet Syndrome, Adhesive Capsulitis, Low Back Pain Symptoms: Interventions[12,20]

Indication	Interventions*
Thoracic Outlet Syndrome (TOS)	
■ Compression of the neurovascular bundle (brachial plexus, subclavian artery/vein, vagus and phrenic nerves, sympathetic trunk) in thoracic outlet, between bony and soft tissue structures ■ Causes of TOS: • Compression occurs when the size or shape of the thoracic outlet is altered, i.e., cervical rib, hypertrophy of scalene muscles • Poor or strenuous posture, trauma, or constant muscle tension in shoulder girdle; caused by drooping shoulder and forward head postures, carrying heavy loads, or osteoporosis • Repetitive overhead movements such as in athletes (swimmers, tennis and volleyball players, or baseball pitchers) or occupations (electricians and painters)	■ Pain management: physical agents and modalities ■ Patient education for task modifications (work, play, or sleep) and avoidance of repetitive movements ■ Postural retraining, including postural awareness and correction ■ Stretching exercises of the anterior scalenes and pectoralis minor ■ Strengthening exercises, including scapular stabilization such as scapular retraction and seated rowing exercises with a T-band or tubing ■ Nerve mobilization ■ Joint and soft tissue mobilization ■ Vascular or neurologic TOS may require surgery
Adhesive Capsulitis (Frozen Shoulder)	
■ Restriction in shoulder ROM secondary to inflammation and fibrosis of shoulder capsule, usually following injury or repetitive microtrauma ■ Has a capsular pattern of limitation such as ER, abduction and flexion, and least restricted in IR ■ Primary: idiopathic (occurs spontaneously) ■ Secondary: post trauma or immobilization	Early acute stage: ▪ Cryotherapy ▪ Thermotherapy ▪ US ▪ TENS ▪ EMG biofeedback for muscle relaxation ▪ Codman's pendulum ▪ AAROM with wand and pulleys in pain-free mode ▪ Isometric exercises ▪ Joint mobilization

Indication	Interventions*
	Subacute stage: ■ Restoration of normal scapular motion: stretching exercises; scapular stabilization strengthening exercises ■ Recovery of function: strengthening exercises using isotonic first and then PREs for deltoid, rotator cuff, and upper arm muscles ■ Postural reeducation to avoid shoulder protraction and kyphotic postures
Lumbar Stenosis	

■ Narrowing of spinal canal, nerve root canal or foramen secondary to osteoarthritis, joint swelling, osteophytes, spondylolisthesis, faulty posture
■ Produces pain (from nerve root compression) in LS extension
	■ Precaution for all: extension exercises produce increased symptoms
	■ Interventions depend on symptoms
	■ Stenosis:
	  • William's flexion exercises
	  • Postural reeducation
	  • Patient education for lifting techniques, sitting, and sleeping
	  • Physical conditioning

Lumbar Disc Pathology	
Terminology: ■ Herniation: general term signifying any bulge of the annulus ■ Disc protrusion: nucleus bulges against intact annulus ■ Prolapse: rupture of nucleus into vertebral canal ■ Extruded disc: nucleus extends through annulus but nuclear material is confined by the posterior longitudinal ligament ■ Sequestrated disc: nucleus is free within the spinal canal Signs and symptoms: ■ Radicular signs: with most common posterior/posterolateral disc protrusion patient experiences posterior thigh pain and numbness going down the knee and pain in buttocks radiating down to legs ■ Peripheralization: repeated movements of the spine (most typically flexion) cause symptoms to radiate down the legs ■ Centralization: repeated movements or positions of the spine cause symptoms to move away from the legs toward lumbar spine midline	Nonoperative: ■ Pain modulation: physical agents and modalities; lumbar traction-patient prone for posterior HNP ■ Joint protection: corset or orthosis ■ Measures to increase flexibility: stretching exercises either in flexion or extension, depending on the direction of movement that promotes centralization of symptoms. Patient education about HNP, proper body mechanics, and posture ■ Core stabilization ■ Measures to increase strength: William's flexion or McKenzie extension exercises depending on centralization ■ Measures to increase cardiovascular fitness ■ Task modifications: work, play, or school ■ Postural reeducation ■ Return to function training: ADLs; balance training

(continued)

MUSCULOSKELETAL SYSTEM: DATA COLLECTION AND INTERVENTIONS

Table 5.60 Thoracic Outlet Syndrome, Adhesive Capsulitis, Low Back Pain Symptoms: Interventions *(continued)*

Indication	Interventions*
	Postoperative:
	■ Patient education for postoperative precautions: no bending, lifting, or trunk rotation; no sitting for more than 1 hour at a time; proper posture
	■ Bed mobility and transfers: log-roll technique
	■ Gait training with walker or crutches
	■ LE circulation: ankle pumps
	■ Isometrics: ensure proper breathing; avoid Valsalva maneuver
	■ CKC exercises
	■ ROM and strengthening exercises
	■ General conditioning
	■ Return to function training

Spondylolysis and Spondylolisthesis[20]

■ Spondylosis Causes: Stress fracture or fracture of the pars interarticularis of the posterior aspect of the vertebra

■ Spondylolisthesis Causes: Anterior slippage due to instability of a superior vertebra over an inferior vertebra. Typical causes include congenital deformation of pars interarticularis, mechanical or degenerative changes or trauma involving fracture of vertebral arch.

■ Commonly found at L4–L5 and L5–S1 levels

■ There are five types (I – V) of spondylolistheses which describes the pathology in greater detail

■ There are four grades (determined by radiographic imaging) which indicate the severity of the anterior slippage:

Grade I: 0–25% (least severe)
Graded II: 25–50%
Grade III: 50–75%
Grade IV: 75–100% (most severe)

■ Signs and symptoms:
- Pain at the level of the belt line
- Low back spasming
- Radicular symptoms if nerve root compression occurs

	Nonoperative:
	■ Precautions for both: no extension exercises (may cause more anterior migration of the vertebra)
	■ Pain, inflammation, and/or spasm modulation: biophysical agents and modalities
	■ Interventions: focus on spinal stabilization, abdominal and paravertebral strengthening exercises in neutral spine; stretching exercises of the trunk and lower extremities, body mechanics
	Operative:
	■ No rehabilitation until radiographic confirmation for adequate healing is received from the surgeon
	■ No extension while in the TLSO brace; gradual return to spinal stabilization, abdominal strengthening, lower extremity and trunk flexibility strengthening, lumbar spine ROM, with an emphasis on neutral spine and gradual return to functional activities
	■ Patient education for precautions: no lumbar extension
	■ LE circulation: ankle pumps
	■ Gait training
	■ ROM exercises

Indication	Interventions*
Scoliosis	
■ Lateral curvature of the cervical, thoracic, or lumbar spine	Nonoperative:
■ Causes: idiopathic, bone related or neuromuscular	■ Stretching exercises: tight muscles on concave side
■ Structural: irreversible lateral curvature of spine with fixed vertebral rotation; forward flexion of the trunk will reveal a rib hump	■ Strengthening exercises: all muscles on convex side
	■ Core strengthening
■ Nonstructural: reversible; forward flexion of the trunk of more than 25° decreases the curvature	■ Bracing: Boston or Milwaukee brace for curves less than 40°
	■ Shoe lift: for mild scoliosis
■ Most common nonstructural: "S" curve (right thoracic, left lumbar curve) in adolescent females	■ Postural reeducation: postural awareness
	■ Breathing exercises
■ Surgery is indicated when curve is in excess of 40°	■ Aquatic therapy
	Postoperative:
	■ Postoperative brace: TLSO
	■ Effective cough and pulmonary hygiene postoperatively
	■ Gait training
	■ Activity limitation for several months

SECTION 5-7

Physical Therapy Interventions for the Acute, Post-Surgical Orthopedic Patient

Total Knee Arthroplasty[12,20]

Table 5.61 **Indications for TKA**

- Osteoarthritis, rheumatoid arthritis, or post-traumatic arthritis
- Severe knee pain, especially with weight bearing
- Degeneration of articular cartilage of the knee (mostly on the medial tibiofemoral area)
- Genu varum or genu varus
- Decreased range of motion of the knee joint
- Knee instability
- Revision of a previous surgery

Table 5.62 **Types of TKA Implant Procedures Including Hardware**

- Cemented or uncemented
- Hybrid
- Unicompartmental—either medial or lateral surface replaced
- Bicompartmental—Both femoral and tibial surfaces replaced
- Tricompartmental—femoral, tibial and patellar surfaces replaced
- Metal-backed tibia or metal-backed patella
- All-polyethylene patella
- Metal-backed polyethylene tibial component
- Patella resurfacing
- Posterior cruciate or bicruciate substituting

Table 5.63 **Surgical Approaches Used for TKA**

- Standard or traditional anterior approach
- Minimally invasive
- Quadriceps splitting or quadriceps sparing

Table 5.64 **Prediction of Successful Outcome for Postoperative TKA**

- Patient's functional ability and status preoperatively

Table 5.65 Medical/Physical Therapy Goals Immediately Post TKA[12,15]

- Prevent complications: infection; deep vein thrombosis* (DVT); pulmonary emboli (PE)
- Reduce pain and swelling
- Promote range of motion ROM (CPM may be used during early recovery, but does not replace general ROM exercises)
- Restore patient's safety
- Restore gait
- Restore independence with ADLs

* In case of DVT, stop knee ROM exercises until anticoagulation therapy is completed (as per doctor's orders).

Table 5.66 Standard Types of Physical Therapy Interventions Post TKA

- Physical therapy starts day 1 post surgery.
- The PT or PTA must assist the surgical and nursing team in preventing DVT and PE.
- Discharge planning starts in the initial examination.
- PT protocol: inspect wound for drainage, erythema, and pain; breathing exercises; ankle ROM exercises (e.g., ankle pumps, circumduction, dorsiflexion/plantarflexion; AROM); isometrics (quads, HS, gluteals); knee PROM/AROM; transfers; patient education about weight bearing (depends on the surgeon) and gait status; gait training; ROM exercises; TKEs/SLRs; discharge planning.
- Provide breathing exercises to promote lung function.
- Use active exercises and weight bearing as tolerated (in and out of bed) to prevent DVT and PE.
- Patients can be weight bearing as tolerated using an assistive device (or per doctor's orders).
- Provide active ROM.
- Provide strengthening exercises (and exercises as per doctor-specific protocol).
- In acute care, achieve knee ROM: 0°–90°.

Total Hip Arthroplasty (THA)[12,20]

Table 5.67 Indications for THA

- Osteoarthritis, rheumatoid arthritis, or post-traumatic arthritis
- Severe hip pain with weight bearing and marked limitations of motion secondary to loss of articular cartilage
- Nonunion fracture, instability of hip, or deformity of hip
- Bone tumors
- Failed conservative interventions for hip osteoarthritis or rheumatoid arthritis
- Revision of a previous surgery

Table 5.68 Contraindications for THA

- Systemic infection
- Joint infection (acute)
- Chronic osteomyelitis
- Paralysis of muscles around the hip
- Neuropathic hip joint

Table 5.69 Surgical Approaches to THA and Postoperative Restrictions[12,20]

Cemented or noncemented
Femoral head and acetabulum replaced
May be traditional approach or minimally invasive approach using one or two small incisions for either posterior, anterior, or lateral approaches

Traditional Approaches for THA

Posterior and Posterolateral approach: most frequently used for primary THA (may have hip instability or dislocation postoperatively); may need repair of posterior capsule to reduce risk of dislocation	■ No hip flexion past 80°–90° ■ No hip adduction past midline (past neutral) ■ No internal rotation
Direct lateral approach: requires division of tensor fascia latae; may have a positive Trendelenburg sign post-surgery due to abductor weakness	■ Avoid hip flexion more than 90° ■ No hip extension, adduction with hip external rotation past neutral ■ No combined motion of hip flexion, abduction, and external rotation ■ No antigravity hip abduction until approved by surgeon if gluteus medius impaired due to surgery
Anterolateral approach: incision over the greater trochanter, gluteus med and min impacted during surgery, post-op hip abductor weakness, lower incidence of hip dislocation	■ Avoid hip flexion more than 90° ■ No hip extension, adduction with hip external rotation past neutral ■ No combined motion of hip flexion, abduction, and external rotation ■ No antigravity hip abduction until approved by surgeon if gluteus medius impaired due to surgery
Direct Anterior approach: incision lateral and distal to ASIS, retraction of rectus femoris and sartorius, more rapid post-op recovery	■ Avoid hip flexion more than 90° ■ No hip extension, adduction with hip external rotation past neutral ■ No combined motion of hip flexion, abduction, and external rotation

Table 5.70 **Patient Education: Surgical Approaches to THA and Precautions Related to ADLs**[12]

Posterior/Posterolateral Approach

- Transfer toward the uninvolved extremity.
- Do not cross the legs.
- In sitting, keep the knees slightly lower than the hips, do not sit in low, soft chairs, and use a raised toilet seat.
- While standing up from a chair or sitting down in a chair, do not bend the trunk over the legs.
- Use a shower chair in the bathtub.
- When ascending stairs, lead with the uninvolved leg.
- When descending stairs, lead with the involved leg.
- Pivot on the uninvolved leg.
- While standing, avoid rotating the body toward the involved leg.

Direct Lateral Approach, Anterolateral and Anterior Approaches

- Do not cross legs.
- During acute care physical therapy, step to—but not past—the involved leg (do not over-stretch the involved hip).
- While standing, avoid rotating the body away from the involved hip.

Table 5.71 **Risk Factors Contributing to Postoperative (After THA) Hip Joint Dislocation**[12]

- Patient older than 80 years old
- Patients with dementia or other cognitive disorders
- Patients with rheumatoid arthritis
- Soft-tissue problems due to chronic inflammatory diseases
- Prior hip surgery
- Muscle weakness preoperatively or post-operatively; contractures

Table 5.72 **Standard Physical Therapy Interventions Post-THA**[12]

- Physical therapy starts day 1 post surgery.
- PT protocol: Determine the patient's weight-bearing status prior to the initial examination (the weight-bearing status is dependent on the surgeon). The weight-bearing status may be TDWB (touchdown weight bearing) or PWB.
- The PT or PTA should check positioning, correct use of, abduction pillow/wedge if used.
- Assist the surgical and nursing team with postoperative complication prevention, such as breathing exercises (to promote lung function); use ankle pumps, quadriceps sets, and gluteal sets (to prevent thromboembolic disease).
- Encourage the patient to cough and use an incentive spirometer.
- Use AROM exercises (heel slides, hip abduction, if able, terminal knee extension).
- Resistance exercises for upper extremities and uninvolved lower extremity.

(continued)

Table 5.72 **Standard Physical Therapy Interventions Post-THA**   *(continued)*

- Review THA precautions with the patient; ensure that the patient is repositioned every 2 hours with the hip-abductor pillow in place (if indicated); provide bed mobility training.
- Provide transfer training: from supine to sitting, and from sitting to standing (the patient should use the upper extremity when shifting weight). Be careful that the patient does not pivot on the involved leg.
- Provide gait training with a front-wheeled walker (FWW) for older patients and with crutches for younger patients.
- Provide caregiver education for home discharge.

Total Shoulder Arthroplasty (TSA)[12, 20]

Table 5.73 **Indications for TSA Secondary to Osteoarthritis**

- Pain with activities, pain at rest
- Loss of shoulder range of motion
- Decreased ability to perform ADLs, especially overhead activities
- Rotator cuff arthropathy
- Osteoarthritis
- Rheumatoid arthritis
- Avascular necrosis
- Osteoporosis

Table 5.74 **Surgical Approaches for Shoulder Arthroplasty**

- Total shoulder arthroplasty: both glenoid and humeral surfaces are replaced
- Hemiarthroplasty: replacement of one surface at the glenohumeral joint
- Reverse total shoulder arthroplasty: used when the rotator cuff is severely damaged. ROM will be limited with this approach. The metal ball and plastic socket are reversed. The ball is placed on the glenoid fossa, and the plastic cup is placed on the humerus. Rotator cuff arthropathy usually results in need for this technique. (Longer rehabilitation is needed due to the need for additional rotator cuff repairs.)

Table 5.75 **Common Post-TSA Precautions***

- Passive range of motion restriction for as long as 6 weeks for a hemiarthroplasty or traditional TSA; limited external rotation (30°–40° with the humerus in neutral adduction), no extension past neutral.
- PROM restriction for as long as 12 weeks for a reverse TSA; no extension or IR past neutral, limited external rotation to 20°, no combined extension, adduction, IR.
- Abduction shoulder-pillow used for as long as 8 weeks.
- Placement of the shoulder in a sling to protect soft tissues, removed only for exercise initially.
- No lifting or pushing through upper extremities for 6–12 weeks.*

* Precautions may vary based on approach and surgeon preference.

Table 5.76 **General Acute Care Protocol for TSA**

- Observation of the patient for hypotension and neurologic deficits
- Patient education to avoid lifting, pushing, carrying, or pulling
- Applying ROM of joints proximal/distal to the surgical area (especially the hand and elbow, to decrease edema and maintain strength)
- Applying passive ROM (as per physician protocol in accordance with type of surgical approach)
- Patient education for self-assisted ROM exercises
- Patient education for an HEP, dependent on the surgeon's preference: trunk balance exercises and activities (pendulum exercises into different planes of motion, scapular stabilization exercises, weight bearing on involved tabletop abduction with lateral stepping)

Spinal Surgery Procedures and Precautions[12,20]

Table 5.77 **Spinal Neurosurgical Procedures[12,20]**

- **Discectomy:** decompression of the nerve root by removing intervertebral nuclear disc material; indicated for disc herniation or nerve root impingement
- **Laminectomy:** excision of laminae or posterior vertebral arch; most common approach is performed posteriorly; most frequently performed in combination with a discectomy
- **Microdiscectomy:** decompression of the nerve root and extruded disc material through an incision made in the inferior aspect of the lamina; less invasive than laminectomy
- **Spinal fusion:** union of two or more vertebrae to immobilize specific vertebrae and strengthen the involved vertebral column; bone grafts (taken from the patient's own iliac spine or from cadaver) are inserted between the involved vertebrae; may include screws, rods, and/or plates; can occur in lumbar or cervical areas
- **Vertebroplasty:** injection of cement to repair a compression fracture (to relieve back pain secondary to fracture)[21]
- **Kyphoplasty:** balloon insertion to create space between vertebral bodies followed by injection of cement to deter collapse of the fractured vertebrae (to relieve pain secondary to a compression fracture)[21]

Table 5.78 **Spinal Surgery Postoperative Interventions and Precautions**

Postoperative Interventions

- Transfers and gait training for household distances
- Bed mobility
- Application of Functional tasks and home exercise program orthotic device
- Functional tasks and home exercise program
- LE AAROM or AROM supine: ankle pump, heel slides, SAQ, quad sets

(continued)

Table 5.78 **Spinal Surgery Postoperative Interventions and Precautions** *(continued)*

Postoperative Precautions

- Patient education:
  - Log rolling technique: hips and shoulders roll as a unit
  - Brace application and wearing schedule
- No spinal rotation (no twisting of the spine)
- No excessive trunk flexion when sitting (no bending)
- No excessive trunk extension post laminectomy
- Avoid long periods of sitting
- No lifting
- Stair climbing is not contraindicated
- No fetal position during sleep

Types of Fractures and Surgical Hardware[12,14,20]

Table 5.79 **Major Types of Fractures[12,14]**

- **Open (compound) fracture:** the skin is punctured (can have fragments of bone that protrude through the skin); associated with high-energy injury; has a high risk of infection.
- **Closed fracture:** the skin is not punctured; the skin has no wound.
- **Nondisplaced fracture:** the fracture segments are not displaced relative to each other.
- **Displaced fracture:** the fracture segments are displaced relative to each other.
- **Simple fracture:** typically, two parts are fractured; there is no rupture of ligaments and skin.
- **Comminuted fracture:** typically, three or more parts of the bone are fractured; the bone is splintered into pieces.
- **Transverse or oblique fracture:** typically affects a long bone, which bends and causes failure on the convex side of the bend; the fracture line is at right angles to the long axis of the bone.
- **Greenstick fracture:** fracture of long bone in children. Long bone bends under stress and results in fracture on the convex side of the bone.
- **Spiral fracture:** fracture caused by a twisting force that induces spiral tension and breakage of a long bone.
- **Avulsion fracture:** fracture caused by traction (straight pulling) injury that induces tension and bone breakage from pulling of the ligament(s) or muscle(s).
- **Compression fracture:** caused by a compression-force injury, typically in a cancellous type of bone such as a vertebra; can result from trauma or from osteoporosis (causes loss of bone height).
- **Stress (fatigue) fracture:** can be caused by repetitive or rhythmic trauma or stress on the bone.
- **Pathological fracture:** fracture of a diseased or weakened bone produced by pathology such as osteoporosis, bony tumor, or other disease involving the bone.

Table 5.80 **Types of Fracture-Stabilizer Hardware**[12,14,20]

- **Internal fixation (hardware):** to stabilize fractures; consists of internal wires, screws, or pins applied directly to fractured bone segments.
- **Dynamic hip screw and lateral side plate:** to stabilize intertrochanteric hip fractures; consists of a large screw that includes a side plate and several small screws.
- **Intramedullary hip screw:** to stabilize intertrochanteric hip fractures; consists of an intramedullary rod and a dynamic hip screw.
- **Intermedullary rod (or nail):** to stabilize diaphyseal long bone fractures; consists of a longitudinal rod (or nail) that is placed within the medullary canal (or cavity) of the bone.
- **Percutaneous pin:** to stabilize a bone, fracture, or joint; consists of a pin that is placed through the skin into the affected bone.
- **External fixation (hardware):** to stabilize fractures; consist of devices such as pins and rods that are applied externally to fractured bone segments.
  - It may be intimidating for the patient to see the pins and rods protruding from the skin.
  - The therapist should examine the area for loose hardware (and excessive or purulent drainage); if any is found, the therapist needs to stop the activity and contact the surgical team.

Fractures of the Pelvis[20]

Table 5.81 **Types of Pelvic Fractures: Physical Therapy Interventions**

Stable pelvic fracture: fracture without involvement of the pelvic ring or with minimal displacement of the pelvic ring. Includes avulsion fractures of pelvic structures	<ul><li>The patient may not require surgical external fixation or weight-bearing restrictions (PWB) if the capsular ligaments of the hip were not stretched.</li><li>Depending on the injury, there may be weight-bearing restrictions but just on the side of the injury.</li><li>Bed rest may be indicated for some patients.</li><li>Physical therapy interventions include AROM exercises (for hip and distal joints) and lower extremity strengthening exercises when stable.</li></ul>
Unstable pelvic fracture: may consist of multiple fractures with displacement of the pelvic ring	<ul><li>The patient may undergo surgical repair (with internal or external fixation) or be maintained on extended bedrest.</li><li>The patient may be NWB for up to 8 weeks (as per surgeon). Patient will receive the same preventive precautions as per THA.</li><li>The patient's function may be limited by pain and the inability to achieve a functional sitting position.</li><li>The patient is totally dependent on transfers out of bed; he or she may need a reclining wheelchair with an adjustable back to assist with patient transfers.</li><li>Also, the patient may need a brace for compressive support.</li><li>Physical therapy interventions include active ROM for both upper extremities, ankle pumps, gentle knee, and hip ROM.</li></ul>

Humeral Fractures

Table 5.82 **Humeral Fractures: Physical Therapy Interventions**

- Humeral fractures are splinted or casted and placed in a shoulder sling.
- Patient education: NWB on the involved upper extremity; teach hand, wrist, and elbow range of motion exercises (may have the occupational therapist treat the patient).

Hip Fractures[12,20]

Hip fractures may be addressed with THA or open reduction internal fixation (ORIF). Surgical intervention is based on fracture site and surgeon preference.

Table 5.83 **Types of Hip Fractures**

Nondisplaced (or Minimally Displaced) Femoral Neck Fractures

- The least severe hip fracture injuries.
- In a nondisplaced fracture, the fracture site is typically stable.
- Full weight bearing with AD is typically permitted immediately postsurgery.
- Patient may be treated conservatively with bed rest and / or protected weight bearing

Displaced Femoral Neck Fractures

- Fracture will be managed surgically.
- The vascular supply to the femoral head can be affected.
- The patient's early mobilization is important for prevention of DVT, atelectasis, pneumonia, and decubitus ulcers.
- Typically early full weight bearing with an assistive device (AD) is encouraged.

Intertrochanteric Hip Fractures

- Surgery is indicated.
- Weight bearing post-surgery may range from NWB to TDWB (10%) based on the type of surgery and preference of surgeon.

Subtrochanteric Hip Fractures

- Surgery is indicated.
- Postoperative physical therapy consists of helping the patient to regain control of the proximal hip musculature.
- Weight bearing post-surgery may range from NWB to TDWB (10%) based on the type of surgery and preference of surgeon.
- Healing may take 3 months.

Hip Open-Reduction Internal Fixation[12,20]

Table 5.84 Hip Open-Reduction Internal Fixation: General Acute Care Protocol

- The PT or PTA must take into consideration the patient's emotional reaction, as most individuals are not prepared for this procedure (typically ORIF is an emergency surgery), and the patient's pain level.
- Provide bed mobility training, transfer training.
- Breathing exercises to promote lung function, ankle pumps, etc., to reduce risk of thromboembolic disease.
- Provide isometrics (quadriceps sets; gluteal sets).
- Use A/AROM: hip flexion, extension, abduction, and adduction; heel slides; ankle pumps.
- Resistance exercises for upper extremities and uninvolved lower extremity.
- Provide patient education for safety and mobility training.
- To ambulate, the patient needs good functional quadriceps contraction and the ability to lift the hip against gravity.
- Provide gait training with a FWW (weight-bearing status is assigned by the surgeon and can range from NWB to WBAT) for approximately 200 feet in acute care.
- Provide caregiver training for home discharge.

Foot and Ankle Fractures[20]

Table 5.85 Fractures of the Foot and Ankle: Physical Therapy Interventions

- Fractures of the foot and ankle may involve the metatarsals, tarsals, malleoli, talus, or calcaneus. Stress fractures may also feature in the metatarsals, calcaneus, lateral malleolus, and navicular.
- Fractures of foot and ankle typically require surgical fixation, although some foot fractures may be treated conservatively.
- Post-surgery patient may be NWB (for several months) and placed in a CAM boot for protection.
- As bone healing progresses, physical therapy consists of ROM and strengthening exercises and gait training.
- Patient is educated on NWB gait and transfers.

SECTION 5-8

Pharmacology for Musculoskeletal Pathologies

Table 5.86 Common Medications Used for Musculoskeletal Pathologies[20,22]

*Classes of Drugs	Purpose of Medication	*Common Side Effects	PTA Implications
Antibiotics			
- Penicillin (Amoxil) - Cephalosporins (Keflex) - Tetracyclines (Sumycin) - Sulfonamides (Bactrim) - Quinolones (Cipro, Levaquin) - Other (Vancomycin)	- Prevention of infections prophylactically - Commonly used pre- and post-operatively to inhibit the growth of bacteria - Commonly used after joint surgeries or traumatic injuries/skin trauma - Can be used for skin infections (cellulitis, osteomyelitis, staph infection)	- Nausea/vomiting - Diarrhea - Rashes - Yeast infections /urinary tract infection - Some antibiotics increase sensitivity to ultraviolet light (tetracyclines, sulfonamides)	- Never provide dosing or discontinuation instructions to the patient—defer all medication-related questions to the appropriate healthcare professional. - Some antibiotics affect blood sugar levels. - Some antibiotics affect blood-clotting mechanisms. - Wash hands frequently and between patient encounters. - Use proper personal protective equipment (PPE) and sanitize equipment after working with patients with suspected infection. - Prolonged quinolone use may predispose some individuals to tendinopathies/tendon rupture.

(continued)

*Classes of Drugs	Purpose of Medication	*Common Side Effects	PTA Implications
Analgesics			
Opioid ■ Morphine (Roxanol) ■ Oxycodone (Oxycontin) ■ Oxycodone with acetaminophen (Percocet) ■ Hydrocodone with acetaminophen (Norco, Vicodin) ■ Meperidine (Demerol) ■ Codeine ■ Codeine with acetaminophen (Tylenol #3, #4)	■ Decrease pain by blocking transmission in pain pathways in the central nervous system ■ Creates a feeling of euphoria ■ Often used post-surgically/post-traumatically for acute and chronic pain ■ Treats nociceptive pain	■ Physical dependence ■ Addiction ■ Orthostatic hypotension ■ Dizziness ■ Drowsiness ■ Constipation ■ Impaired judgement ■ Nausea/vomiting ■ Allergic reactions ■ Slowed respiratory rate	■ See Section 2-4 for further discussion. ■ Increased fall risk due to orthostatic hypotension, dizziness, drowsiness. ■ Pain masking may result in over stressing healing tissues. ■ Impaired judgment may result in patient's willingness to do more than they are capable of OR more than they should tolerate (compliance with weight-bearing restrictions, precautions/contraindications)..
Non-Opioid Acetaminophen (Tylenol, Excedrin)	■ Antipyretic ■ Relief of mild to moderate pain ■ No significant anti-inflammatory or anticoagulation effects – frequently used post- surgery ■ Commonly used over-the-counter medications for headaches, menstrual cramps, muscle soreness, fevers, sore throats	■ Liver toxicity (increased risk associated with long-term use or alcohol consumption of more than three beverages/day or patients with hepatic disease)	■ Safe to use with patients taking Coumadin. ■ Signs and symptoms (Sx & Sx) of liver toxicity: jaundice (skin, eyes); right upper belly pain; dark urine color/gray colored or pale stool; extreme nausea and/or diarrhea.

(continued)

Table 5.86 Common Medications Used for Musculoskeletal Pathologies

*Classes of Drugs	Purpose of Medication	*Common Side Effects	PTA Implications
Non–steroidal Anti-Inflammatory			
■ Aspirin (Bayer, Ecotrin)	■ Antipyretic (adults) ■ Anti-inflammatory ■ Relief of mild to moderate acute and chronic pain ■ Commonly used over-the-counter medications for headaches, menstrual cramps, muscle soreness, fevers, sore throats, osteoarthritis, rheumatoid arthritis, sprain, strains, bursitis ■ Sometimes used for anti-coagulation as per physician instruction	■ Reye Syndrome (children/adolescents) ■ Antiplatelet effects ■ Nausea/vomiting ■ Acute kidney injury (especially with dehydration or elderly or patients with known kidney dysfunction) ■ Increased risk of gastrointestinal (GI) bleeding/bleeding if taken with Coumadin ■ Rash ■ Anemia	■ ↑ Risk of bruising/bleeding ■ GI bleeds (prolonged use) ■ Sx & Sx of acute kidney injury: distal edema in bilateral feet and hands ■ Sx & Sx GI bleeds = bloody vomit, coffee ground appearance when vomiting, blood in stool or melena ■ Increased risk of bruising/bleeding during rehabilitation
Nonsteroidal Anti-Inflammatory (NSAIDS)			
■ Ibuprofen (Advil, Motrin) ■ Naproxen (Aleve, Naprosyn) ■ Ketoprofen (Orudis) ■ Diclofenac (Voltaren) ■ Piroxicam (Feldene) ■ Indomethacin (Indocin)	■ Antipyretic ■ Anti-inflammatory ■ Relief of mild to moderate acute and chronic pain ■ Medications commonly used for headaches, menstrual cramps, muscle soreness, fevers, sore throats, osteoarthritis, rheumatoid arthritis, sprain, strains, bursitisSome NSAIDs available over the counter others may require prescription. ■ May sometimes be prescribed by the physician in higher dosages	■ Nausea/vomiting ■ Upset stomach ■ Acute kidney injury (especially with dehydration or elderly or patients with known kidney dysfunction) ■ Increased risk of GI bleeding/bleeding if taken with Coumadin or aspirin products	■ Sx & Sx acute kidney injury: distal edema in bilateral feet and hands ■ Sx & Sx GI bleeds = bloody vomit, coffee ground appearance when vomiting, blood in stool or melena ■ Increased risk of bruising/bleeding during rehabilitation

*Classes of Drugs	Purpose of Medication	*Common Side Effects	PTA Implications
Nonsteroidal Anti-Inflammatory COX-2 (Cyclooxygenase-2 Inhibitors)			
■ Celecoxib (Celebrex)*prescription only	■ Non-inflammatory agent that is safer on the stomach lining ■ Osteoarthritis/rheumatoid arthritis, ankylosing spondylitis, Juvenile idiopathic arthritis ■ Menstrual cramps, muscle soreness, fevers, sore throats, sprain, strains, bursitis	■ Nausea/vomiting ■ Upset stomach ■ Bleeding risk ■ Hypertension ■ Increased risk of GI bleeding/bleeding if taken with Coumadin or aspirin products ■ Acute kidney injury (especially with dehydration or elderly or patients with known kidney dysfunction) ■ Cardiovascular thrombotic risk (myocardial infarction, stroke) in patients with cardiovascular disease	■ Sx & Sx acute kidney injury: distal edema in bilateral feet and hands ■ Sx & Sx GI bleeds = bloody vomit, coffee ground appearance when vomiting, blood in stool or melena ■ Increased risk of bruising/bleeding during rehabilitation
Anti-inflammatory			
Corticosteroids/ glucocorticoids ■ Cortisone ■ Dexamethasone (Decadron) ■ Methylprednisolone (Medrol) ■ Prednisone (Deltasone) ■ Prednisolone (Prelone) ■ Hydrocortisone (Cortef)	■ Suppress and reduce inflammation ■ Commonly used for inflammation associated with RA, joint pain; tendonitis; bursitis, pulmonary dysfunctions or exacerbations of autoimmune diseases ■ Targets nociceptive pain ■ Suppression of immune system	■ Elevated blood glucose levels (diabetic patients and those at high risk for diabetes) ■ ↑ risk of infection ■ ↑ risk of osteoporosis ■ Muscle weakness ■ ↑ risk of glaucoma/ cataracts	■ Monitor glucose reactions in patients undergoing iontophoresis if dexamethasone or another steroid is being used or during therapeutic exercise. ■ Avoid scheduling PT on same day as injection to avoid pain masking with treatment and allow inflammation reduction to occur without additional tissue stressing at the targeted injection region.

(continued)

(continued)

Table 5.86 Common Medications Used for Musculoskeletal Pathologies

*Classes of Drugs	Purpose of Medication	*Common Side Effects	PTA Implications
		■ Stomach ulcers ■ Impaired wound healing ■ Insomnia ■ Mood changes/psychiatric disturbances ■ Abnormal fat distribution to face, abdomen, upper back ■ Edema	■ Wear PPE if the patient is immunocompromised and on steroids. ■ Observe for any mood or personality changes. ■ Observe for osteonecrosis, tendon rupture or skin atrophy at the injection sites especially with long-term use.

Neuropathic Pain Medications

Anticonvulsants ■ Gabapentin (Neurotin) ■ Pregabalin (Lyrica) **Antidepressants** ■ Duloxetine (Cymbalta) ■ Amitriptyline (Elavil)	■ Blocks or slows nerve conduction ■ Indicated more for chronic non-inflammatory pain and neuropathic pain ■ Sometimes may be used with a fast-acting pain reliever for breakthrough pain ■ Used with patients with diabetic neuropathies; trigeminal nerve dysfunction; fibromyalgia, epilepsy, or depression ■ Chronic pain syndromes (Elavil)	■ Dizziness ■ Edema ■ Dry mouth ■ Drowsiness/fatigue ■ Nausea vomiting ■ Ataxia, paresthesia (Neurontin) ■ Angioedema (Lyrica) ■ Confusion ■ Blurred vision ■ Hypertension ■ Bleeding risk (Cymbalta) ■ Elevated glucose levels (Cymbalta) ■ Suicide warning	■ Pain relief effects may not be observed or reported for several weeks after they are prescribed, as these medications are often extended-release, designed to be taken daily as opposed to round-the-clock dosing ■ ↑ fall risk ■ Observe for bilateral distal edema hands and feet = kidney dysfunction ■ Suicidal thoughts/tendencies ■ Sx & Sx of angioedema = swelling of the eyes, lips, bilateral hands and/or feet, and throat (difficulty breathing, swallowing, new onset of hoarseness since taking the medication)

*Classes of Drugs	Purpose of Medication	*Common Side Effects	PTA Implications
Bisphosphonates			
■ Alendronate (Fosamax) ■ Ibandronate (Boniva) ■ Zoledronic Acid (Reclast) ■ Risedronate (Actonel) ■ Etidondrate (Didronel)	■ Prevention and/or treatment of osteoporosis to improve bone density ■ Paget's disease ■ Corticosteroid induced osteoporosis ■ Often taken in conjunction with vitamin D and calcium	■ Back pain ■ Severe joint pain / musculoskeletal pain ■ GERD/esophageal pain if patient does not follow instruction to sit upright for 30 minutes after ingestion ■ Osteonecrosis of jaw (new onset of jaw pain) ■ Abdominal pain, diarrhea	■ Avoid interventions in supine position for at least 30–45 minutes after taking the drug ■ Be aware of any new reports of increasing muscle, bone, joint, jaw pain and inform supervising PT on record
Anticoagulants			
■ Heparin ■ Warfarin (Coumadin) ■ Low Molecular Weight Heparin (Lovenox does not require prothrombin time and international normalized ratio (PT-INR) monitoring)	■ Prevention of DVT, PE, stroke, atrial fibrillation, or other cardiovascular-related conditions	■ Bruising/bleeding ■ Dizziness ■ Anemia ■ Nausea/vomiting ■ Flatulence	■ Check PT-INR levels prior to treatment ■ PT-INR > 3.0 check with nursing or doctor's office before proceeding with treatment ■ PT-INR > 6.0 hold PT ■ Sx & Sx of excessive blood thinning: nosebleeds, blood shot eyes, skin bruising ■ ↑ Fall risk if dizziness occurs

(continued)

Table 5.86 Common Medications Used for Musculoskeletal Pathologies

(continued)

*Classes of Drugs	Purpose of Medication	*Common Side Effects	PTA Implications
Disease-Modifying Antirheumatic Drugs (DMARDs) ■ Etanercept (Enbrel), ■ Infliximab (Remicade), ■ Azathioprine (Imuran), ■ Cyclophosphamide (Cytoxan), ■ Methotrexate (Rheumatrex)	■ RA ■ Influence metabolites and immune responses	■ Fatigue ■ Headache ■ Dizziness ■ Chest pain, hypotension, tachycardia ■ Abdominal pain, nausea and vomiting ■ Diarrhea, constipation ■ Arthralgia, myalgia, back pain ■ Rash ■ Upper respiratory tract infection, cough ■ Hepatic and renal toxicity ■ Paresthesia	■ Assess vital signs during exercise ■ Monitor for signs and symptoms of infection ■ Monitor for any new or increased back or other musculoskeletal pain ■ Monitor for signs and symptoms of liver or kidney disease
Gout Agents ■ Allopurinol (Aloprim) ■ Colchicines ■ Corticosteroids / Glucocorticoids	■ Hyperuricemia (elevated blood uric acid concentration) ■ Local inflammation and acute bouts of arthritic gout pain	■ Drowsiness ■ Hypotension, hypertension, bradycardia ■ Nausea, diarrhea, vomiting ■ Renal insufficiency ■ Allergic reactions ■ Bone marrow depression (such as leucopenia), aplastic anemia	■ Monitor for signs of renal failure ■ Assess blood pressure and other vital signs ■ Assess for signs and symptoms of bone marrow depression (fatigue, fever, chills)

*Classes of Drugs	Purpose of Medication	*Common Side Effects	PTA Implications
Skeletal Muscle Relaxants ■ Diazepam (Valium), ■ Cyclobenzaprine (Flexeril) ■ Carisoprodol (Soma) ■ Orphenadrine Citrate [Norflex]	■ Decrease muscle spasm, ■ Relax the muscles	■ Dizziness ■ Drowsiness, fatigue ■ Confusion ■ Hypotension, headache ■ Arrhythmias ■ Dry mouth ■ Nausea, constipation ■ Ataxia	■ Monitor vital signs ■ Increased risk of falls with dizziness, ataxia ■ Increased risk of dependence with diazepam

* Brand names associated with classes of medications and side effects found within this table are not representative of an all-inclusive list. It is incumbent on the clinician to research an appropriate drug information resource to obtain complete information about medications that patients may use while attending rehabilitation.

References

1. Moore KL. *Clinically Oriented Anatomy*. 3rd ed. Baltimore, MD: Williams and Wilkins; 1992.
2. Norkin CC, White DJ. *Measurements of Joint Motion: A Guide to Goniometry*. 4th ed. Philadelphia, PA: F.A. Davis; 2003.
3. Fruth SJ, Fawcett C. *Fundamentals of Tests and Measures for the Physical Therapist Assistant*. Burlington, MA: Jones and Bartlett Learning; 2020.
4. Hislop HJ, Montgomery J. *Daniels and Worthingham's Muscle Testing: Techniques of Manual Examination*. 8th ed. Philadelphia, PA: W.B. Saunders; 2007.
5. Shirley Ryan Ability Lab. Rehabilitation measures database: Manual muscle test. https://www.sralab.org/rehabilitation-measures/manual-muscle-test. Accessed January 3, 2021.
6. Magee DJ. *Orthopedic Physical Assessment*. 6th ed. Philadelphia, PA: W.B. Saunders; 2014.
7. Wong-Baker FACES Foundation. The Wong-Baker FACES Pain Scale. https://wongbakerfaces.org/. Accessed January 22, 2021.
8. Shirley Ryan Ability Lab. Rehabilitation measures database: Pain. https://www.sralab.org/rehabilitation-measures/database?contains=pain. Accessed January 22, 2021.
9. Gulick D. *Ortho Notes: Clinical Examination Pocket Guide*. Philadelphia, PA: F.A. Davis; 2005.
10. Clarkson H. *Musculoskeletal Assessment: Joint Motion and Muscle Testing*. 3rd ed. Philadelphia, PA: Lippincott Williams & Wilkins; 2013.
11. Karachalios T, Hantes M, Zibis AH, Zachos V, Karantanas AH, Malizos KN. Diagnostic accuracy of a new clinical test (the Thessaly test) for early detection of meniscal tears. *J Bone Joint Surg Am*. 2005 May;87(5):955–962.
12. Kisner C, Colby LA. *Therapeutic exercise: Foundations and Techniques*. 6th ed. Philadelphia, PA: F.A. Davis; 2012.
13. Rothstein JM, Roy SH, Wolf SL, Scalzitti DA. *The Rehabilitation Specialist's Handbook*. 3rd ed. Philadelphia, PA: F.A. Davis; 2005.
14. Goodman CC, Fuller KS. *Pathology for the Physical Therapist Assistant*. 2nd ed. St. Louis, MO. Elsevier; 2017.
15. O'Sullivan SB, Schmitz TJ. *Physical Rehabilitation*. 5th ed. Philadelphia, PA: F.A. Davis; 2007.
16. Seymour, R. *Prosthetics and Orthotics, Lower Limb and Spinal*. Baltimore, MD: Lippincott, Williams and Wilkins; 2002.
17. Interventions. *Guide to Physical Therapist Practice 3.0*. American Physical Therapy Association; 2014. https://guide.apta.org/interventions. Updated August, 1. 2014. Accessed February 3, 2021.
18. APTA. Clinical practice guidelines. https://www.apta.org/patient-care/evidence-based-practice-resources/cpgs. Accessed February 3, 2021.
19. Academy of Orthopaedic Physical Therapy. Clinical practice guidelines. https://www.orthopt.org/content/practice/clinical-practice-guidelines. Accessed February 3, 2021.
20. Manske RC. *Fundamental Orthopedic Management for the Physical Therapist Assistant*. 4th ed. St. Louis, MO: Elsevier; 2016.
21. Kauffman TL, Scott R, Barr J, Moran MJ. *A Comprehensive Guide to Geriatric Rehabilitation*. 3rd ed. St. Louis, MO: Elsevier; 2014.
22. Ciccone CD. *Pharmacology in Rehabilitation*. 4th ed. Philadelphia, PA: F.A. Davis; 2007.

PART 6

Neurologic System: Data Collection and Interventions

Review of Nervous System Anatomy and Physiology

Parts of the Brain and Their Functions

See **Figure 6.1**, **Figure 6.2**, and **Figure 6.3**.

Figure 6.1 Brain stem
Anatomy and Physiology: Understanding the Human Body by Robert K. Clark, page 196, Figure 12.9 "The brainstem consists of the medulla oblongata, pons, and midbrain"

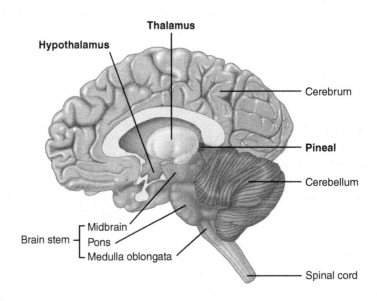

Figure 6.2 Diencephalon
Anatomy and Physiology: Understanding the Human Body by Robert K. Clark, page 197, Figure 12.10 "The thalamus, hypothalamus, and epithalamus represented here by the pineal gland are included in the diencephalon"

Hypothalamus

Cerebrum

Cerebellum

Midbrain

Brain stem — Pons

Medulla oblongata

Spinal cord

Figure 6.3 Cerebrum
Anatomy and Physiology: Understanding the Human Body by Robert K. Clark, page 199, Figure 12.12 "The cerebrum"

Table 6.1 Brain Stem, Diencephalon, Cerebrum, and Cerebellum and Their Functions

Brain Components	Functions
Brain stem: midbrain, pons, medulla oblongata	■ Midbrain: contains ascending and descending tracts and specific cranial nerve nuclei; important for motor control ■ Pons: contains nuclei for regulation of respiration and for cranial nerves V, VI, and VII ■ Medulla oblongata: regulates respiratory, cardiac, and vasomotor centers; contains nuclei for cranial nerves VIII through XII
Diencephalon: thalamus and hypothalamus	■ Thalamus: relays information to specific cortical sensory areas ■ Hypothalamus: controls body temperature, emotions, aggression, eating, drinking, sleep/wake cycles, sexual behaviors, and regulation of the autonomic nervous system
Cerebrum: cerebral hemispheres and basal ganglia	■ Cerebral hemispheres: see functions of each lobe in Table 6.2 ■ Basal ganglia: forms an associated motor system called the extrapyramidal system; important in formation of motor plans and adjustment of movements
Cerebellum: archicerebellum, paleocerebellum, and neocerebellum	■ Archicerebellum: equilibrium and regulation of muscle tone ■ Paleocerebellum: maintenance of posture and control of voluntary movement ■ Neocerebellum: smooth coordination of voluntary movements

Cerebral Hemispheres and Their Functions

See **Figure 6.4** and **Figure 6.5**.

Figure 6.4 Lobes of the cerebrum
Anatomy and Physiology: Understanding the Human Body by Robert K. Clark, page 201, Figure 12.16 "The Lobes of the Cerebrum"

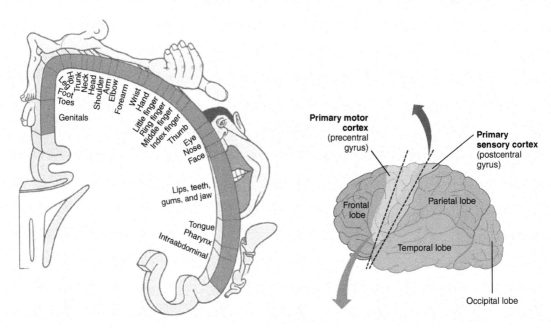

Figure 6.5 Specific functions of the central lobes. **A.** Sensory. **B.** Motor
Anatomy and Physiology: Understanding the Human Body by Robert K. Clark, page 203, Figure 12.19 "Specific Functions of the Central Lobes"

Specific functions of the central lobes	
Lobe	**Function**
Frontal	Motor area, controls skeletal muscle.
Parietal	Sensory area, integrates the senses of touch, pain, etc.
Occipital	Visual area, integrates visual stimuli.
Temporal	Olfactory and auditory areas, integrates sound and smell.

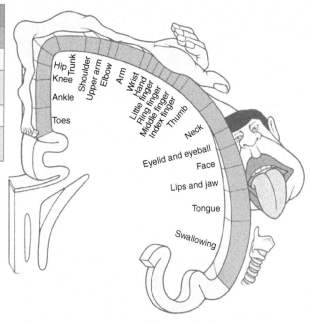

Figure 6.5 *(Continued)*

Table 6.2 Lobes of the Brain and Their Functions

Lobe	Functions
Frontal: precentral gyrus, prefrontal cortex, and Broca's area	■ Precentral gyrus: primary motor cortex for voluntary muscle activation of the contralateral side of the body ■ Prefrontal cortex: controls emotions, abstract thinking, and judgment ■ Broca's area: controls the motor (expressive) aspect of speech for the left hemisphere
Parietal: postcentral gyrus	■ Primary sensory cortex; integrates sensations from the contralateral side of the body for pain and temperature, touch, proprioception, and combined sensations; important for short-term memory
Occipital: primary visual cortex	■ Primary visual cortex: receives and processes visual stimuli and associative visual cortex ■ Associative visual cortex: gives meaning to visual information by processing visual stimuli
Temporal: primary auditory cortex, auditory cortex, and Wernicke's area	■ Primary auditory cortex: receives and associative processes auditory stimuli; important for long-term memory ■ Associative auditory cortex: processes auditory stimuli ■ Wernicke's area: controls the comprehension (receptive) aspect of speech
Limbic: oldest part of the brain	■ Instincts, emotions, preservation of individual, feeding, aggression, and endocrine sexual responses

Spinal Cord

See **Figure 6.6**, **Figure 6.7**, and **Figure 6.8**.

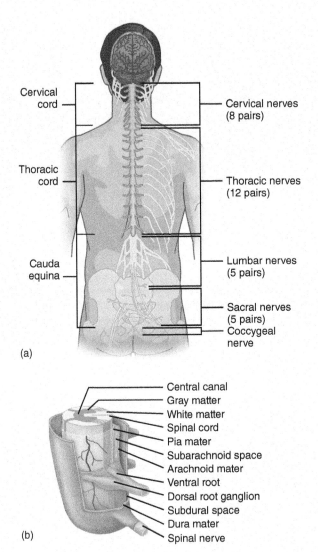

Cervical cord

Thoracic cord

Cauda equina

(a)

Cervical nerves
(8 pairs)

Thoracic nerves
(12 pairs)

Lumbar nerves
(5 pairs)

Sacral nerves
(5 pairs)

Coccygeal nerve

Central canal
Gray matter
White matter
Spinal cord
Pia mater
Subarachnoid space
Arachnoid mater
Ventral root
Dorsal root ganglion
Subdural space
Dura mater
Spinal nerve

(b)

Figure 6.6 Spinal cord and its protective structures
Anatomy and Physiology: Understanding the Human Body by Robert K. Clark, page 214, Figure 12.25 a, b "The spinal cord and its protective structures"

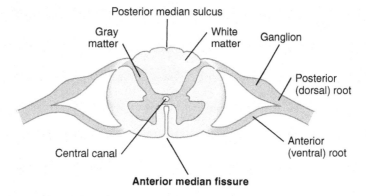

Figure 6.7 Spinal nerve roots
Anatomy and Physiology: Understanding the Human Body by Robert K. Clark, page 215, Figure 12.27 "A transverse section of the spinal cord showing spinal nerve roots"

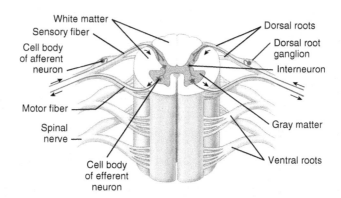

Figure 6.8 Spinal cord and dorsal root ganglia
Human Biology: Fifth Edition by Daniel D. Chiras, page 181, Figure 10-8 "The Spinal Cord and Dorsal Root Ganglia"

Table 6.3 Spinal Cord

- The spinal cord (SC) is a cylindrical mass of nerve tissue that is situated in the vertebral canal it is protected by bone and surrounded by meninges.
- The SC is a continuation of the medulla oblongata. It starts at the foramen magnum in the skull and ends at the conus medullaris (L1–L2).
- The SC contains gray matter (cell bodies and unmyelinated axons) and white matter (myelinated ascending and descending tracts).
- The gray matter is situated in the center of the cord (in shape of letter H) and is made of cell bodies and dendrites of neurons. The white matter is arranged in tracts around the gray matter.
- The gray matter contains two anterior (ventral) horns and two posterior (dorsal) horns. Anterior horns contain efferent (motor) neurons. Posterior horns contain afferent (sensory) neurons.

(continued)

Table 6.3 **Spinal Cord**   *(continued)*

- The SC is divided into thirty-one segments with thirty-one pairs of spinal nerves (SNs): eight cervical, twelve thoracic, five lumbar, five sacral, and one coccygeal. Each SN has an anterior root and a posterior root. The anterior root has motor fibers and posterior root has sensory fibers. There is no posterior root for C1.
- In the cervical spine, the nerve roots exit above the corresponding vertebral body (C8 exits below C7 and above T1). In the thoracic/lumbar spine, the nerve roots exit below the corresponding vertebral body.
- The SC gives rise to the C4–T1 nerve roots (which supply the upper extremities) and the L1–S5 nerve roots (which supply the lower extremities).
- The SC is a pathway for motor impulses from the brain and sensory impulses to the brain.
- The SC mediates the stretch reflexes and the defecation and urination reflexes.

Ascending (Sensory) Tracts

Table 6.4 **Sensory (Afferent) Tracts**

- Dorsal columns convey sensations of proprioception, kinesthesia, vibration, stereognosis, barognosis, graphesthesia, two-point discrimination, and tactile localization.
- Spinothalamic tracts convey sensations of pain and temperature and crude touch.
- Spinocerebellar tracts convey sensations of proprioception (from muscle spindles and GTO), and touch and pressure receptors.
- Spinoreticular tracts convey sensations of deep and chronic pain.

Descending (Motor) Tracts

Table 6.5 **Motor (Efferent) Tracts**

- Corticospinal (or pyramidal) tracts function in voluntary motor control.
- Vestibulospinal tracts control muscle tone, antigravity muscles, and postural reflexes, head stabilization.
- The rubrospinal tract assists in motor function.
- The reticulospinal tracts modifies pain impulses, automatic postural responses.
- The tectospinal tract assists in head turning in response to visual stimuli.

Autonomic Nervous System

Table 6.6 **Sympathetic Nervous System**

- Thoracolumbar division of autonomic nervous system (ANS): prepares the body to cope with stressful situations (fight or flight); has afferent and efferent nerve fibers
- Sympathetic nervous system (SNS) effects: increased heart rate (HR) and blood pressure (BP); constriction of peripheral blood vessels; dilation of the pupils; dilation of the bronchioles; slowing of peristalsis; secretion of epinephrine and norepinephrine by adrenal medulla

Table 6.7 **Parasympathetic Nervous System**

- Craniosacral division of ANS: conserves and restores homeostasis; has afferent and efferent nerve fibers
- Parasympathetic nervous system (PNS) effects: decreased HR and BP; dilation of peripheral blood vessels; constriction of the pupil; constriction of the bronchioles; increasing of peristalsis and glandular activity

Brain Meninges and Ventricles

See **Figure 6.9** and **Figure 6.10**.

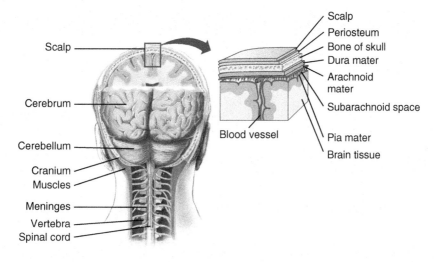

Figure 6.9 Brain meninges

Anatomy and Physiology: Understanding the Human Body by Robert K. Clark, page 190, Figure 12.5 "In addition to the bone, the central nervous system is protected by meninges"

Figure 6.10 Brain ventricles

Anatomy and Physiology: Understanding the Human Body by Robert K. Clark, page 191, Figure 12.6 "The location and flow of cerebrospinal fluid"

Table 6.8 Brain Meninges and Ventricles

Meninges	Ventricles Filled with Cerebrospinal Fluid
Dura mater: outside, tough, and fibrous membrane	Lateral ventricles: large and irregularly shaped; communicate with third ventricle
Arachnoid: middle, delicate, and vascular membrane	Third ventricle: located posterior and deep; communicates with fourth ventricle
Subarachnoid space: contains cerebrospinal fluid (CSF) and major arteries	Fourth ventricle: located in pons and medulla; communicates with subarachnoid space.
Pia mater: inside, thin, and vascular membrane covering the brain surface	

Role of Cerebrospinal Fluid

Table 6.9 Role of Cerebrospinal Fluid (CSF)

- CSF protects the brain and helps in the exchange of nutrients and waste products.
- CSF is produced in the choroid plexus in ventricles.
- CSF normal pressure: 100–180 mm H_2O (9–14 mmHg).
- Total CSF volume: 125–150 mL.

Brain Blood Supply

Table 6.10 Brain Blood Supply

Carotid system: supplies the frontal, parietal, and parts of temporal lobe	The carotid system originates from the aortic arch that becomes the right and left common carotid arteries (which then divide and form the internal and external carotid arteries). The internal carotid artery enters the cranium and forms the anterior and middle cerebral arteries.
Vertebrobasilar system: supplies the brain stem, cerebellum, temporal, occipital lobes, and part of thalamus	The vertebrobasilar system originates from the subclavian artery and vertebral artery (which unite and form the basilar artery). The basilar artery forms the right and left posterior cerebral arteries.
Circle of Willis: connects the carotid and vertebrobasilar systems	The circle of Willis consists of the anterior and posterior communicating arteries.

Muscle Sensory Receptors and Their Functions

Table 6.11 Sensory Receptors and Their Functions

Sensory Receptors	Functions
Muscle spindles: situated in the belly of the muscle and parallel to the muscle fibers	Monitor changes in muscle length and the velocity of these changes; monitor position, movement sense, and motor learning
Golgi tendon organ: situated at the musculotendinous insertion of the muscle	Monitors tension within the muscle; provides a protective mechanism to the muscle

Neurologic Data Collection

Patient Arousal Levels

Table 6.12 Patient's Arousal Levels[1]

Arousal Level	Description
Alert	Patient is aware of his or her environment, paying attention to the therapist and able to cooperate with treatment.
Coma	Patient is totally unresponsive to stimuli and cannot be awakened. Patient is not able to express himself or herself. Patient can be monitored with the Glasgow Coma Scale (includes three activities; eye opening, best motor response, verbal response).
Lethargic	Patient is drowsy and ready to sleep. Patient has difficulty concentrating on tasks and needs stimulation to keep awake.
Obtunded	Patient has diminished arousal and awareness to his or her environment. Patient may require repeated stimulation to notice the therapist.
Stupor (semi-coma)	Patient has decreased responsiveness to his or her environment and cannot interact with the therapist. Patient needs noxious (unpleasant) stimulation to be aroused.

Memory and Amnesia Terms

Table 6.13 Memory and Amnesia Terms[2]

- **Memory:** mental registration, retention and recollection of past experiences, knowledge, ideas, and sensations.
- **Short-term (immediate) memory:** immediate recollection of experiences, knowledge, ideas, and sensations that occurred in the immediate past (seconds to minutes). The capacity of short-term memory is approximately seven items.
- **Long-term memory:** recollection of experiences, knowledge, ideas, and sensations that occurred in the distant past (days, months, years). The capacity of long-term memory is unlimited.
- **Amnesia:** significant loss of memory. It can be caused by cerebral vascular accident (CVA), seizure, trauma, alcoholism, intoxication, senility, or an unknown cause.
- **Anterograde (post-traumatic) amnesia:** amnesia for events that occurred after the onset of amnesia. It involves amnesia of new learned material that was acquired after the causative event. This is a more common type of amnesia.
- **Retrograde amnesia:** amnesia for events that occurred prior to the onset of amnesia. It involves amnesia of prior learned material that was acquired prior to the causative event. This is a less common type of amnesia.

Orientation Terms

Table 6.14 Orientation Terms[1,3]

- Orientation: cognitive adaptation of an individual that is assessed within an unfamiliar environment (e.g., hospital, skilled nursing facility) to determine accurate awareness of person, place, time, and situation.
- Assessed using three or four domains.
- Three domains consist of the individual knowing: person (their name), place (hospital, skilled nursing, rehab unit), and time (day of the week).
- Four domains consist of the individual knowing: person (their name), place (hospital, skilled nursing, rehab unit), time (day of the week), and situation (the condition or event that brought them to the hospital, nursing home, etc.).
- If an individual is NOT oriented to one or more of the domains, it is documented in the medical record as the domains that were correctly identified listed in parentheses, (e.g., "oriented x 2/4 [person, place]").

Ranchos Los Amigos Levels of Cognitive Functioning

Table 6.15 Levels of Cognitive Functioning[3]

I. No response: Patient is unresponsive to any stimuli.

II. Generalized response: Patient responds inconsistently and nonpurposefully to stimuli. Responses such as total-body movements or vocalization may be the same regardless of the stimulus.

III. Localized response: Patient specifically but inconsistently responds to stimuli. Patient may follow uncomplicated commands in an inconsistent, delayed manner such as squeezing the hand or closing the eyes.

IV. Confused—agitated: Patient is in a high level of activity. Patient exhibits bizarre, nonpurposeful behavior relative to stimuli and environment. Patient is unable to cooperate directly with the treatment. Patient exhibits the following cognitive deficits: (1) very limited gross attention span; (2) confabulation; (3) incoherent and inappropriate verbalization; (4) impairment in short- and long-term memory; and (5) inability to discriminate among persons or objects.

V. Confused—inappropriate: Patient is able to respond somewhat consistently to simple commands. Patient responds in a nonpurposeful, random, or fragmented way to complex commands or unstructured activities. Patient exhibits gross attention in regard to the environment but is highly distractible and cannot focus. Patient is able to perform previously learned tasks with structure. Patient's cognitive deficits include (1) difficulty with complex and unstructured activities, (2) inability to learn new information, (3) inability to focus on a specific task, (4) impaired memory, (5) confabulation, and inappropriate verbalization.

VI. Confused—appropriate: Patient demonstrates goal-directed and appropriate behavior but is dependent on external input or instruction. Patient consistently follows simple commands and demonstrates carry over for relearned tasks (such as self-care activities). Patient's cognitive deficits are related to incorrect responses due to memory problems. Past memories have more depth and detail than more recent ones.

(continued)

Table 6.15 **Levels of Cognitive Functioning** *(continued)*

VII. Automatic—appropriate: Patient appears to demonstrate appropriate behavior in familiar settings. Patient is oriented to environment. Patient performs daily routines automatically mostly in a robot-like manner. Patient demonstrates carry over for new learning activities but at times has difficulty remembering them. Patient is able to initiate social and recreational activities but needs organization. Patient's cognitive deficits are minimal confusion and impaired judgment.

VIII. Purposeful—appropriate: Patient recalls and integrates past and recent events. Patient is oriented and reactive to environment. Patient demonstrates independent carryover for new learning. Patient exhibits the following cognitive deficits: (1) decreased abstract reasoning; (2) decreased tolerance to stress; (3) judgment difficulties in emergency or unusual situations; and (4) decreased premorbid abilities.

Terms of Cognitive–Perceptual Deficits

Table 6.16 **Cognitive–Perceptual Deficits**[1]

Agnosia: inability to recognize familiar objects with one sensory modality, although the patient is able to recognize the same object with another sensory modality.

Anosognosia: denial, neglect, and lack of awareness of the presence or severity of a person's own neurologic dysfunction (such as paralysis in stroke).

Apraxia: inability to produce purposeful movements, although there is no sensory or motor loss. Patient has intact sensation, strength, coordination, and comprehension.

Figure–ground discrimination deficit: inability to pick out an object from the background on which it is embedded.

Form constancy deficit: inability to pick out an object from an array of similarly shaped objects.

Homonymous hemianopsia: blindness in the outer half of the visual field of one eye and the inner half of the visual field of the other eye. Patient cannot receive information from either the right or the left of the visual environment.

Ideational apraxia: inability to produce purposeful movements on his or her own or on command.

Ideomotor apraxia: inability to produce purposeful movements on command but can produce them on his or her own.

Position in space deficit: inability to determine and interpret spatial concepts such as up or down, in or out, in front or behind, or under or over.

Right/left discrimination deficit: inability to identify the right and left sides of one's own body or that of the examiner.

Somatognosia: inability to identify own or other person's body parts and the relationship of one body part to another. Somatognosia is also an impairment in the body scheme.

Spatial-relation deficit: inability to perceive the relationship between self and one or more objects.

Topographical orientation deficit: inability to understand and remember the relationship of one place to another.

Unilateral neglect: inability to register and integrate visual stimuli and perceptions from one side of the environment (usually the left side). Patient ignores stimuli occurring in that side of personal space. The deficit is not attributed to any sensory problem.

Speech and Communication Functions and Impairments

Table 6.17 Speech and Communication Functions and Impairments[1]

Speech and Communication Functions	Impairments
Expressive function: assessment of fluency of speech and speech production	■ Broca's aphasia (nonfluent, expressive, or motor aphasia): speech is interrupted, uncoordinated, difficult to produce, and with awkward articulation. It is the result of a lesion involving the third frontal convolution of the left hemisphere. ■ Verbal apraxia: inability to volitionally articulate as a result of a lesion in the cortical dominant hemisphere. ■ Dysarthria: speech production difficulty caused by motor impairments related to respiration, phonation, articulation, and jaw and tongue movements. It is the result of a lesion in the CNS and PNS.
Receptive function: assessment of comprehension	■ Wernicke's aphasia (fluent or receptive aphasia): auditory comprehension is impaired while speech is spontaneous and flowing smoothly. It is the result of a lesion in the posterior first temporal gyrus of the left hemisphere.
Dysfunction of all language modalities	■ Global aphasia: severe aphasia with impairments in comprehension and speech production, reading comprehension, and writing.

Sensory Function: Sensory Receptors

Table 6.18 Sensory Receptors: Function and Testing

Sensory Receptors	Function and Testing
Barognosis (combined cortical sensations)	Function: ability to recognize different gradations of weight in similar size or shape objects Testing: The physical therapy assistant (PTA) places different weights with the same size (shape), one at a time, in the patient's tested hand. The patient, with eyes closed, is asked to indicate if the weight is "heavier" or "lighter" than the previous one (or comparing bilaterally).
Graphesthesia (combined cortical sensations)	Function: ability to recognize numbers, letters, or symbols traced on the skin Testing: The PTA traces (with a pencil) numbers, letters, or symbols on the patient's tested hand. The patient, with eyes closed, is asked to identify the figures drawn on the skin.
Kinesthesia (deep sensations)	Function: sensation and awareness of active or passive movement Testing: The PTA moves the patient's limb. The patient, with eyes closed, is asked to identify the direction of movement (up or down, in or out) while the limb is in motion. The patient, with eyes closed, may also duplicate the movement with the opposite limb.

(continued)

Table 6.18 Speech and Communication Functions and Impairment *(continued)*

Sensory Receptors	Function and Testing
Pain (superficial sensations)	Function: ability to recognize sharp or dull sensation in response to sharp or dull stimuli Testing: The PTA applies a disposable safety pin or a paper clip to patient's skin. The patient, with eyes closed, is asked to indicate when the stimulus is felt.
Proprioception (deep sensations)	Function: position sense and the awareness of the joints at rest Testing: The PTA positions the patient's limb. The patient, with eyes closed, is asked to identify the limb's position (up or down, in or out).
Stereognosis (combined cortical sensations)	Function: ability to recognize by touch or manipulation of the shape of familiar objects Testing: The PTA gives the patient one object (such as a coin, a key, or a pencil). The patient, with eyes closed, is asked to name the object.
Touch (superficial sensations)	Function: ability to differentiate between touch and nontouch in response to slight touch or no touch Testing: The PTA applies a cotton ball (or a piece of tissue) to the patient's tested skin. The patient, with eyes closed, must respond to PTA ("yes" or "no") to indicate when the stimulus was applied.
Two-point discrimination (combined cortical sensations)	Function: ability to differentiate between one or two blunt points applied to the skin simultaneously (the smallest distance between two stimuli) Testing: The PTA applies simultaneously two stimuli (the rounded part of two paper clips) to the patient's tested skin. The patient, with eyes closed, is asked to differentiate between one or two stimuli. When two stimuli are perceived by the patient, the PTA needs to measure the distance between the stimuli. Consideration must be given to acute perception of stimuli in the distal upper extremities (UEs) as compared with lower extremities (LEs).

Sensory Function: Dermatomes

Dermatomes represent sensory distribution of the cutaneous nerves corresponding to the spinal segments providing their innervation. As part of a sensory assessment, dermatomes are evaluated first as superficial sensations, then as deep or combined (cortical) sensations. Dermatome testing is performed in a distal to proximal direction. It is generally not necessary to test every segment of each dermatome; testing of general body areas is sufficient.

Table 6.19 Dermatomes*

Upper-Extremity Dermatomes

C1: top of the head

C2: temple, forehead, occiput

C3: neck, posterior cheek

C4: superior part of chest above axilla (clavicle area)

C5: lateral aspect of the arm, deltoid muscle region

C6: anterior arm, lateral side of hand to thumb, and index finger

(continued)

Table 6.19 Dermatomes   *(continued)*

C7: lateral arm and forearm to index, long, and ring fingers

C8: middle arm and forearm to long, ring, and little fingers

Trunk Dermatomes

T1: medial side of forearm to base of little finger

T2: axillary region

T4: nipple level

T6: xiphoid process level

T10: umbilicus level

T12: anterior superior iliac crest level

Lower-Extremity Dermatomes

L1: lower abdomen and groin region

L2: anterolateral thigh (back and front of thigh to knee)

L3: anteromedial thigh, leg, upper buttock

L4: medial buttock, lateral thigh, medial leg, dorsum of foot, large toe

L5: posterior lateral thigh, lateral leg, dorsum of foot, medial half of sole, first to third toes

S1: lateral plantar surface of foot, posterior thigh and leg

S2: posterior thigh and leg

S3: groin, medial thigh to knee

S4–S5: perineum, genitals, lower sacrum

* For the dermatome chart, see **Figure 6.11**.

NEUROLOGIC SYSTEM: DATA COLLECTION AND INTERVENTIONS

Figure 6.11 Map of dermatomes (specific skin regions to test within each dermatome indicated with an X).

Motor Function: Tonal Abnormalities

Table 6.20 Hypertonia and Hypotonia

- **Clonus:** Cyclical, spasmodic fluctuation of muscle contraction and relaxation in response to a repeated stretch of a spastic muscle. Usually spastic muscles react to a large and quick stretch by increasing their resistance. Clonus is common in plantarflexors and jaw and wrist muscles of upper motor neuron (UMN) lesions.

- **Cogwheel rigidity:** Condition in which tremor coexists with rigidity. It is common in Parkinson's disease. When the PTA moves the patient's extremity passively, it feels like a cogwheel (by letting go, then increasing the resistance to movement).

- **Decerebrate rigidity:** Sustained contraction and posturing of the trunk and extremities in full extension. It indicates a grave condition, in which a lesion is present in the brain stem between the superior colliculi and the vestibular nuclei.

- **Decorticate rigidity:** Sustained contraction and posturing of the trunk and lower extremities in extension and upper extremities in flexion. It is less grave than decerebrate rigidity, with a lesion being present in the corticospinal tract at diencephalon (above superior colliculus).

- **Dystonia:** Prolonged involuntary muscular contractions causing repetitive twisting or writhing of body parts and fluctuations in muscle tone (with increased or decreased muscular tone). This condition can be found in conjunction with CNS lesions (commonly in basal ganglia), neurodegenerative disorders (Wilson's disease or Parkinson's disease), or metabolic disorders (amino acid or lipid). Dystonia can also be found in torticollis, and the primary idiopathic dystonia can be inherited.

- **Flaccidity:** Decreased or absent muscular tone (hypotonia). The extremities are easily moved passively (floppy) without any resistance. This condition is common in conjunction with lower motor neuron (LMN) lesions affecting the anterior horn cell or peripheral nerve and in UMN lesions of the cerebellum or pyramidal tract.

- **Lead-pipe rigidity:** Constant rigidity. It is not dependent on the velocity of passive movement.

- **Rigidity:** Resistance to passive movement involving agonist and antagonist muscles. It is characterized by stiffness and inability to bend or be bent. This condition is caused by a lesion in basal ganglia. It is common in Parkinson's disease.

- **Spasticity**: Increased tone or resistance of muscles. It causes stiff and awkward movements. This condition is a result of an UMN lesion.

Motor Function: Myotatic Reflexes (Stretch Reflexes)

Table 6.21 Stretch Reflexes[4]

Nerve Root	Site and Testing
C5–C6	Biceps: Patient sitting with arm flexed and supported. Tap over the biceps tendon in the cubital fossa. Normal response: elbow flexion.
C7–C8	Triceps: Patient sitting with arm supported in abduction and elbow flexed. Tap over the triceps tendon (above the olecranon). Normal response: elbow extension.

NEUROLOGIC SYSTEM: DATA COLLECTION AND INTERVENTIONS

(continued)

Table 6.21 **Stretch Reflexes** *(continued)*

Nerve Root	Site and Testing
L2–L4	Quadriceps (patellar): Patient sitting with knee flexed (and foot unsupported). Tap over the quadriceps tendon between the patella and tibial tuberosity. Normal response: knee extension.
L5–S2	Medial Hamstrings: Patient prone with knee half-flexed and supported. Tap over the hamstring tendon at the knee. Normal response: knee flexion.
S1–S2	Achilles (ankle): Patient prone with foot over the end of the table. Tap the tendon above its insertion on the calcaneus. Normal response: foot plantarflexion.

Motor Function: Grading Scale for Muscle Stretch Reflex

Table 6.22 **Grading Scale for Muscle Stretch Reflex**[1,4]

0 Absent: no visible muscle contraction.

1+ Hyporeflexia: slight muscle contraction with little or no joint movement.

2+ Normal: slight muscle contraction with slight joint movement.

3+ Hyperreflexia: brisk (visible) muscle contraction with moderate joint movement.

4+ Abnormal: strong muscle contraction. Patient (client) can have clonus and/or the reflex can spread to the contralateral side.

Motor Function: Babinski's Reflex

Table 6.23 **Babinski's Reflex Testing**[1,4]

Normal response (negative Babinski sign): no reaction or flexion (plantarflexion) of the great toe when the lateral border of the sole of the foot is stimulated (stroked).

Abnormal response (positive Babinski sign): extension (dorsiflexion) of the great toe, and fanning of the other toes, when the lateral border of the sole of the foot is stimulated (stroked). An abnormal response indicates a lesion of the corticospinal (pyramidal) tract. It is a normal reflex in infants younger than the age of 6 months.

Motor Function: Cranial Nerve Functions and Impairments

Table 6.24 Cranial Nerves: Functions and Impairments

Cranial Nerve (CN)	Functions and Impairments
CN I: olfactory (sensory)	Function: smell Impairment: anosmia (loss of the sense of smell)
CN II: optic (sensory)	Function: vision and pupillary reflexes Impairments: blindness and absence of pupillary reflexes (when shining the light in the eye)
CN III: oculomotor (motor and sensory) Muscles: medial, superior, and inferior rectus; inferior oblique; levator palpebrae superioris	Function: elevates upper eyelids; constricts pupil; moves eyes up/down Impairments: ophthalmoplegia (paralysis of ocular muscles with eye deviation); severe ptosis (difficulty raising the eyelids); mydriasis (abnormal pupil dilation)
CN IV: trochlear (motor and sensory) Muscle: superior oblique	Function: depresses the adducted eye Impairments: weakness in depression of ipsilateral adducted eye; diplopia (double vision)
CN V: trigeminal (motor and sensory) Muscles: masseter; temporalis; pterygoids; mylohyoid; tensor tympani; palatini; anterior belly of digastric	Function: sensation from face, cornea, and muscles of mastication Impairments: loss of facial sensation and corneal reflex; weakness and atrophy of muscles of mastication; deviation of open jaw to ipsilateral side
CN VI: abducent (motor and sensory) Muscle: lateral rectus	Function: abduction of the eye Impairments: diplopia; convergent strabismus (the eye deviates by turning inward); paralysis of ipsilateral eye muscle
CN VII: facial (motor and sensory) Muscles: buccinator; stapedius; stylohyoid; platysma; occipitalis; posterior belly of digastric	Function: facial expression; articulation; winking; food and drink ingestion; nasal and lacrimal secretions; salivary secretions; taste Impairments: paralysis of ipsilateral upper and lower facial muscles; loss of lacrimation; dry mouth and decreased salivation; loss of taste ipsilateral in the anterior two thirds of the tongue
CN VIII: vestibulocochlear (sensory)	Function: hearing; equilibrium Impairments: nerve deafness; disequilibrium; vertigo (sensation of having objects moving around the person); nystagmus (involuntary cyclical movements of the eyes)

(continued)

NEUROLOGIC SYSTEM: DATA COLLECTION AND INTERVENTIONS

Table 6.24 Cranial Nerves: Functions and Impairments *(continued)*

Cranial Nerve (CN)	Functions and Impairments
CN IX: glossopharyngeal (motor and sensory) Muscles: stylopharyngeus; superior pharyngeal constrictor	Function: elevates the pharynx; salivary secretions; taste; sensations in the root of the tongue, tonsils, uvula, and soft palate Impairments: minimal dysphagia (difficulty swallowing); partial dry mouth; loss of taste ipsilateral in the posterior third of the tongue; loss of gag reflex; anesthesia in the tonsillar region
CN X: Vagus (motor and sensory) Muscles: palate; pharyngeal constrictors; laryngeal intrinsics	Function: taste; swallowing; phonation; slowing of the heart rate; constriction of bronchioles; increased peristalsis; digestive secretions; sensations to auditory meatus; sensations to pharynx and larynx; visceral sensations Impairments: dysphagia; hoarseness; paralysis of soft palate with deviation of velum and uvula to the contralateral side; anesthesia of pharynx and larynx on the ipsilateral side; anesthesia of ipsilateral auditory meatus
CN XI: spinal accessory (motor and sensory) Muscles: SCM; trapezius	Function: swallowing; phonation; movements of head and shoulder Impairments: muscular weakness in shrugging the shoulders on the ipsilateral side; muscular weakness in turning the head to the opposite side
CN XII: hypoglossal (motor and sensory) Muscles: styloglossus; hyoglossus; genioglossus; tongue intrinsics	Function: movements of the tongue Impairments: atrophy of the ipsilateral muscles of the tongue; tongue deviation to the ipsilateral side on protrusion

Motor Function: Cerebellar Dysfunction Characteristics

Table 6.25 Cerebellar Dysfunction Characteristics[1]

Cerebellar Dysfunction	Characteristics
Ataxia: uncoordinated movements; a combination of cerebellar and sensory dysfunction	Can be observed in the patient's gait, posture, and patterns of movement such as dysmetria and movement decomposition.
Dysarthria: speech articulation dysfunction (also called scanning speech)	Speech is hesitant and slow, with inappropriate pauses and lengthened syllables. The melodic quality of speech is distorted. The patient demonstrates normal word selection and grammar.

(continued)

Table 6.25 **Cerebellar Dysfunction Characteristics** *(continued)*

Cerebellar Dysfunction	Characteristics
Dysdiadochokinesia: impaired ability to perform rapid alternating movements	The patient is unable to perform rapid forearm supination and pronation. As speed increases, the patient's movements become irregular with rhythm and range deficits.
Dysmetria: inability to judge the distance or range of a movement	The patient is unable to reach an object because of either overestimating or underestimating the distance where the object is located.
Hypotonia: decrease in muscle tone due to cerebellar dysfunction	The patient demonstrates reduced resistance to passive movement. The patient's muscles are soft and flaccid.
Intention (kinetic) tremor: involuntary oscillatory movement of a limb during voluntary motion; intention tremor absent at rest	The patient demonstrates involuntary tremor when trying to reach a target. The tremor increases when the limb is close to the target or when the movement speed increases.
Movement decomposition (dyssynergia): inability to perform a smooth movement at once.	When asked to complete a movement, the patient performs a series of component parts of the movement.
Postural (static) tremor: involuntary oscillatory movement of the body during standing (static) posture	The patient demonstrates involuntary postural tremor back and forth when trying to maintain a standing posture. This tremor may also be observed in a limb held against gravity.

Motor Function: Basal Ganglia Dysfunction Characteristics

Table 6.26 **Basal Ganglia Dysfunction Characteristics**[1]

Basic ganglia Dysfunction	Characteristics
Akinesia: inability to initiate movement	The patient is unable to start any movement. The patient needs a large amount of concentration and effort to start any limb movement. Akinesia can be found in the late stages of Parkinsonism.
Athetosis; slow, involuntary, twisting movements	The patient demonstrates slow and involuntary twisting or writhing in the upper extremities (mostly hands), neck, tongue, face, and trunk. These movements can be present in combination with spasticity. Athetosis can be found in the athetoid type of cerebral palsy.
Bradykinesia: decrease in size and speed of a movement	The patient demonstrates a slow, shuffling gait, decreased movement, difficulty initiating the movement, or difficulty changing the direction of movement. The patient may also demonstrate decreased arm swing in gait and difficulty stopping when the movement is started. Bradykinesia can be found in Parkinson's disease.

(continued)

Table 6.26 Basal Ganglia Dysfunction Characteristics *(continued)*

Basic ganglia Dysfunction	Characteristics
Chorea: involuntary, rapid, and jerky movements	The patient demonstrates involuntary, rapid, jerky irregular movements of the extremities or facial muscles. Chronic (hereditary) chorea is characteristic of Huntington's disease.
Resting tremor: involuntary, rhythmic, oscillatory movement occurring at rest	The patient demonstrates involuntary tremor in the hands in the form of "pill-rolling" movements (seems as though the patient is rolling a pill between the thumb and the first two fingers). The patient also may have involuntary pronation and supination of the forearm and jaw tremor. Resting tremor is characteristic of Parkinson's disease.
Rigidity: increased muscular tone (see **Table 6.20**)	The patient demonstrates stiffness and ability to bend tone or be bent. Cogwheel rigidity: alternate giving and increased resistance to passive movement. Lead-pipe rigidity: constant resistance to movement. Both are observed in basal ganglia disorders.

Motor Function: Characteristics of Upper Motor Neuron and Lower Motor Neuron Lesions

Table 6.27 UMN Versus LMN[1]

UMN Characteristics (CNS Lesions: Cortex, brainstem, corticospinal tracts, spinal cord)	LMN Characteristics (Cranial nerves and PNS Lesions: anterior horn cell, spinal roots, peripheral nerves)
Typical Pathologies: SCI; CVA; TBI; CP; MS; hydrocephalus	**Typical Pathologies**: polio; tumor of peripheral nerves; peripheral nerve trauma; muscular dystrophy; Guillain-Barré syndrome; Bell's palsy; trigeminal neuralgia
Hypertonicity (dependent on velocity); spasticity (especially in the anti-gravity muscles); contractures; abnormal posturing; deformity	Hypotonicity; flaccidity; proximal weakness (myopathy); distal weakness (neuropathy)
Involuntary muscle spasms in the flexor or extensor muscles	Fibrillation potentials (spontaneous depolarization of muscle fibers not visible through the skin); fasciculations (visible, spontaneous twitching of muscle groups)
Paralysis; paresis	Paralysis
Disuse atrophy (variable and widespread)	Neurogenic atrophy (rapid and severe)
Hyperreflexia; clonus; positive Babinski's sign	Hyporeflexia with diminished or absent deep tendon reflexes; floppy limbs
Dyssynergic patterns of voluntary movements	Weak or absent voluntary movements

Motor Function: Coordination Tests and Scoring

Table 6.28 Coordination Tests and Scoring[1]

Gross motor coordination tests: finger to nose; finger to therapist's finger; finger to finger; forearm supination and pronation; clapping; alternately touch nose to finger; heel on shin; foot tapping; alternate heel to knee; alternate heel to toe

Fine motor coordination tests: thumb to finger opposition; grasp and release test; standardized tests (i.e., Pegboard test, Hand Tool Dexterity Test)

Coordination Scoring

0 = unable

1 = severe impairment

2 = moderate impairment

3 = minimal impairment

4 = normal performance

Motor Function: Balance Tests and Scoring

Table 6.29 Balance Tests and Scoring[4]

- Standing static balance test (eyes open to eyes closed): patient stands in double limb stance; patient stands in single limb stance. Double and single limb stance can also be tested on less stable positions, i.e., foam square, pillows.
- Romberg static balance test (eyes open to eyes closed): patient stands with feet in normal stance position. This test can detect ataxia.
- Sharpened Romberg static balance test (eyes open to eyes closed): patient stands in a tandem heel to toe position. This test is more sensitive than the Romberg static balance test.
- Dynamic balance tests: patient stands, walks, turns, and stops; patient demonstrates tandem walking (placing the heel of one foot directly in front of the toe of the opposite foot); patient demonstrates walking sideways, backward, and cross-stepping. Additional activities can be added to assess ability to maintain balance while moving, i.e., carrying an object, counting, stepping over objects.
- Functional balance tests (See Appendix B for detail on each test.)
  1. Berg Balance Scale: measures skill on fourteen functional activities
  2. Functional reach test: patient stands without support and reaches forward as far as possible with shoulder at 90° flexion, elbow extended, and hand fisted without losing balance
  3. Tinetti POMA mobility test: measures skill on six functional activities such as sitting balance, standing on one leg, turning, ambulation, stepping over obstacles
  4. Timed get up and go test

Balance Scoring

Normal = patient maintains steady static balance without support and for dynamic balance can shift weight in all directions

(continued)

Table 6.29 **Balance Tests and Scoring**   *(continued)*

Good = patient maintains static balance without support and for dynamic balance can pick objects off the floor

Fair = patient maintains static balance with handhold and for dynamic balance can maintain balance while turning the head and trunk

Poor = in static balance patient requires handhold and support and dynamically is unable to accept any challenge or to move without loss of balance

Motor Deficits Associated with Cerebral Vascular Accident: Abnormal Synergy Patterns

Table 6.30 **CVA Synergy Patterns**

- Upper-extremity flexion synergy: scapular retraction and elevation or hyperextension; shoulder abduction and external rotation; elbow flexion (strong component); forearm supination; wrist and finger flexion
- Upper-extremity extension synergy: scapular protraction; shoulder adduction (strong component) and internal rotation; elbow extension; forearm pronation (strong component); wrist and finger flexion
- Lower-extremity flexion synergy: hip flexion (strong component), abduction, and external rotation; knee flexion; ankle dorsiflexion and inversion; toe dorsiflexion
- Lower-extremity extension synergy: hip extension, adduction (strong component), and internal rotation; knee extension (strong component); ankle plantarflexion (strong component) and inversion; toe plantarflexion

Brunnstrom's Spasticity Patterns

Table 6.31 **Brunnstrom's Spasticity Patterns**

- Head rotation to the unaffected side and lateral flexion to the affected (hemi) side
- Shoulder adduction and internal rotation
- Scapula retraction and depression
- Elbow flexion and forearm pronation (can also be supination)
- Wrist flexion and ulnar deviation and fingers/thumb flexion and adduction
- Pelvis elevation and backward rotation
- Hip extension, adduction, and internal rotation
- Knee extension and foot plantarflexion and inversion
- Toes flexion and adduction

Motor Deficits Associated with Cerebral Vascular Accident: Brunnstrom's Stages of Recovery

Table 6.32 Brunnstrom's Six Stages of Recovery

Stage 1: Patient starts to recover from hemiplegia. Patient exhibits the following: flaccidity; hyporeflexia; no voluntary movement of the affected upper and lower extremities.

Stage 2: Patient exhibits the following: beginning of spasticity; hyperreflexia; strong synergy patterns of the affected upper and lower extremities; minimal voluntary movement of the affected areas (including upper and lower extremities).

Stage 3: Patient exhibits the following: severe spasticity; voluntary movement of the affected upper and lower extremities only in synergy patterns.

Stage 4: Patient exhibits the following: spasticity begins to decrease; synergy begins to decrease; beginning of voluntary movement without synergy.

Stage 5: Patient has the capability to progress in the recovery process. If progress continues, patient exhibits the following: minimal synergy patterns; more complicated learned movement (motor) patterns without synergy; coordination deficits.

Stage 6: Patient has the capability to progress to normal. If progress continues, patient exhibits no spasticity, and motor control and coordination are restored to normal.

Cerebral Vascular Accident: Gait Deficits

Table 6.33 CVA Gait Deficits

Hip

- Retraction (caused by trunk and limb spasticity)
- Hiking (caused by weak abdominals)
- Trendelenburg limp (caused by weak abductors)
- Circumduction (caused by hamstrings spasticity, foot drop, and/or decreased ROM in hip/knee flexion)
- Scissoring (caused by adductors spasticity)
- Poor proprioception
- Exaggerated hip flexion (because of the flexor synergy)

Knee

- Increased flexion in stance (caused by hamstrings spasticity and/or weak quadriceps)
- Hyperextension in stance (caused by plantarflexion contracture and/or weak quadriceps)
- Inadequate knee flexion (caused by inadequate hip flexion and/or spastic quadriceps)
- Inadequate knee extension (caused by spastic hamstrings)
- Poor proprioception

NEUROLOGIC SYSTEM: DATA COLLECTION AND INTERVENTIONS

(continued)

Table 6.33 CVA Gait Deficits   *(continued)*

Ankle and Foot

- Equinus gait when the heel does not touch the ground (caused by spasticity or contracture of gastrocnemius and soleus)
- Foot drop (paralysis of dorsiflexors)
- Unequal step length (caused by spastic toe flexors and pain on flexed toes)
- Equinovarus (caused by spastic posterior tibialis and/or gastrocnemius and soleus)
- Exaggerated dorsiflexion (caused by flexor synergy)

Traumatic Spinal Cord Injury: Mechanisms of Injury

Table 6.34 Traumatic SCI: Mechanisms of Injury

- *Flexion injury* is the most common mechanism of injury in SCI, causing high percentages of lumbar or cervical SCI at levels T12 to L2 and C4 to C7. Flexion injuries can cause the following: fractures of the anterior vertebral body, spinal processes, pedicles, and laminae; tearing of the posterior spinal ligaments; disk disruptions; and dislocation of the anterior vertebral body.
- *Flexion–rotation injury* can cause the following: fractures of the posterior pedicles, laminae, and articular facets; dislocations or subluxations of faucet joints; and tearing of the posterior and interspinous ligaments.
- *Compression injury* can cause the following: concave fractures of the spinal endplates; comminuted fractures; teardrop fractures; ruptures of the intervertebral disk.
- *Hyperextension injury* can cause the following: fractures of the spinous processes, faucets, and laminae; avulsion fractures of anterior aspect of vertebrae; tearing of the anterior longitudinal ligament; disk rupture.

* Spinal areas of greatest frequency of injury: C5–C7 and T12–L2

Spinal Cord Injury Syndromes

Table 6.35 SCI Syndromes

- *Anterior cord syndrome* (ACS) can produce the following: loss of motor function below the level of lesion (caused by damage to the corticospinal tract); loss of the sense of pain and temperature below the level of lesion (caused by damage to the spinothalamic tract); and preservation of the proprioception, kinesthesia, and vibratory senses below the level of lesion. ACS can be caused by flexion injury of cervical region with damage of the anterior spinal cord and/or anterior spinal artery.
- *Brown-Sequard syndrome* can produce the following: ipsilateral loss of sensation of the dermatome corresponding to the level of lesion; contralateral loss of the sense of pain and temperature of several dermatomes below the level of lesion; and ipsilateral loss of motor function (characterized by decreased DTRs, clonus, and positive Babinski sign), proprioception, kinesthesia, and vibratory sense. Brown-Sequard syndrome can be caused by hemisection of the spinal cord with damage on one side of spinal cord (from gunshots or stabbing attacks).

(continued)

Table 6.35 SCI Syndromes *(continued)*

- *Cauda equina injury* (lower motor neuron injury) typically produces an incomplete lesion with a potential for regeneration.
- *Central cord syndrome* (CCS) can produce the following: severe motor loss in the upper extremities; less severe motor loss in the lower extremities; mild and varying degrees of sensory impairments; and preservation of sacral tracts and bowel, bladder, and sexual functions. Patients may be able to ambulate with some distal upper-extremity weakness (especially after surgeries to relieve cervical compression). CCS can be caused by hyperextension injury of the cervical spine (from motor vehicle accidents) or congenital narrowing of the spinal canal.
- *Posterior cord syndrome* (PCS) can produce the following: loss of proprioception, two-point discrimination, and stereognosis below the level of lesion; and preservation of motor function, sense of pain, and light touch. PCS can be caused by tabes dorsalis due to late-stage syphilis. PCS is very rare.
- *Sacral sparing* can produce the following: incomplete lesion with varying innervation from the intact sacral segments; preserved perianal sensation; and preserved contraction of the external anal sphincter.

Classification of Spinal Cord Injury

Table 6.36 SCI Classification[3,5]

The American Spinal Injury Association[3,5] classifies SCI injuries as follows:

1. Tetraplegia: complete paralysis of all upper and lower extremities and trunk, including the respiratory muscles due to lesion of the cervical spinal cord
2. Paraplegia: complete paralysis of both lower extremities and part of the trunk due to lesion of the thoracic or lumbar spinal cord or cauda equina

SCI is also classified by the American Spinal Injury Association into the following categories:

1. ASIA A: Complete with no sensory or motor function in the lowest sacral segments (S4 and S5)
2. ASIA B: Incomplete with sensory function but not motor function preserved below the neurologic level (including sacral segments S4 and S5)
3. ASIA C: Incomplete with motor function preserved below the neurologic level, and more than half of key muscles below the neurological level have a muscle grade less than 3
4. ASIA D: Incomplete with motor function preserved below the neurological level, and at least half of key muscles below the neurological level have a muscle grade of 3 or more
5. ASIA E: Normal with normal motor and sensory functions

Levels of lesion are also classified as follows:

1. Neurologic level of lesion: the most caudal segment of the spinal cord with normal motor and sensory function on the right and left sides of the body
2. Motor or sensory level of lesion: the most caudal segment of spinal cord with bilateral motor and sensory normal function
3. Motor level: determined by MMT testing of a key muscle (on right or left) at a myotome adjacent to the suspected level of impairment
4. Sensory level: determined by testing light touch and pin prick (on right or left) at a key dermatome

Data from Umphred D, Lazaro RT. Neurorehabilitation for the Physical Therapist Assistant (2nd ed). Thorofare: SLACK Incorporated; 2014. American Spinal Injury Association. Standard neurological classification of spinal cord injury. Available at: http://asia-spialinjury.org/wp-content/uploads/2016/02/International_Stds_Diagram_Worksheet. pdf. Accessed March 2016.

Traumatic Spinal Cord Injury: Functional Capabilities and Assistance

Table 6.37 SCI Functional Capabilities and Assistance[1,3]

Most Distal Nerve Root Segments Innervated: C1, C2, C3 Levels

- Requirements: full-time attendant; mechanical ventilator or phrenic nerve stimulator during the day; environmental control units to activate light switches, call buttons, and electrical appliances, to turn pages of books, and for speaker phone
- Patient function and assistance: totally dependent on assistance with activities of daily living (ADLs) and transfers; independent when using a power wheelchair (with an electrically controlled reclining back or tilt in space) that has a portable mechanical ventilator, and a mouthstick or sip-and-puff controls; has wheelchair and bed skills
- Key muscles: face and neck muscles and cranial innervation
- Available movements: talking, sipping, blowing, and mastication

Most Distal Nerve Root Segment Innervated: C4 Level

- Requirements: full-time attendant; power tilt-in-space wheelchair (for pressure relief); arm supports (orthotics, flexor hinge hand splint) and adapted eating equipment for a small degree of self-feeding; environmental control units to activate light switches, call buttons, and electrical appliances to turn pages of books and for speaker phone
- Patient function and assistance: totally dependent on assistance with ADLs, transfers, coughing, glossopharyngeal breathing, and skin inspection; can use head or mouth stick (or sip-and-puff, or hand splint) for typing on the computer keyboard and is able to play table games (such as cards or checkers), paint, or draw; independent when using a power wheelchair with head, mouth, chin, or sip-and-puff controls; has wheelchair and bed skills
- Key muscles: diaphragm and trapezius
- Available movements: respiration and elevation of scapula

Most Distal Nerve Root Segment Innervated: C5 Level

- Requirements: part-time attendant; equipment setup; mobile arm supports, deltoid aid, and adapted utensils and splints for self-feeding; adapted equipment for limited self-care activities such as grooming and washing; hand splints or typing sticks for typing on the computer keyboard; power tilt-in-space wheelchair for pressure relief; sliding board
- Patient function and assistance: dependent on some assistance and setup for ADLs, dressing, transfers with sliding board and overhead swivel bar, skin inspection, and coughing with manual pressure to diaphragm; can drive a van with hand controls; has bed and wheelchair skills; independent when using a manual wheelchair with hand-rim projections and a power wheelchair with arm controls; can self-feed and can do pressure relief
- Key muscles: biceps, brachialis, brachioradialis, deltoid, infraspinatus, rhomboids, and supinator
- Available movements: elbow flexion and supination, shoulder abduction to 90° and external rotation, and limited shoulder flexion

Most Distal Nerve Root Segment Innervated: C6 Level

- Requirements: side rails on the bed; universal cuff and adapted utensils for self-feeding; adaptive equipment for dressing and grooming (button hook, zipper pulls); adaptive equipment for bowel and bladder and self-care (in the shower); hand controls and U-shaped cuff for steering wheels; adaptive equipment for self-preparation of occasional light meals

(continued)

Table 6.37 SCI Functional Capabilities and Assistance   *(continued)*

- Patient function and assistance: dependent on very little assistance for ADLs; can independently (with adaptive equipment) self-feed, dress (uses momentum), perform self-care and bowel and bladder care, transfer (with sliding board), do skin inspection, cough (with pressure to abdomen), drive, prepare light meals, and play wheelchair sports; cannot tie shoes; has bed and wheelchair skills; can use the manual wheelchair with hand-rim projections all the time, and the power wheelchair for long distances and in the community

- Key muscles: ECR, infraspinatus, latissimus dorsi, pectoralis major (clavicular portion), pronator teres, serratus anterior, and teres minor

- Available movements: shoulder flexion, adduction, extension, and internal rotation, abduction and upward rotation of scapula, forearm pronation, and wrist extension (tenodesis grasp)

Most Distal Nerve Root Segment Innervated: C7 Level

- Requirements: adaptive equipment for dressing (button hook) and self-care (shower chair, hand-held shower nozzle, and bathroom handles); bowel and bladder care adaptive equipment (digital stimulator, raised toilet seat, urinary drainage device); sliding board; wheelchair-accessible kitchen; hand controls for the car; adaptive kitchen tools

- Patient function and assistance: independent with ADLs, self-feeding, dressing, self-care, transfers (with or without sliding board), bowel and bladder care, manual coughing, light housekeeping, and driving; is able to get in and out of the car; has bed and wheelchair skills; independent when using a manual wheelchair with friction surface hand rims

- Key muscles: EPL, EPB, FCR, triceps, and extrinsic finger extensors

- Available movements: elbow extension, finger extension, and wrist flexion

Most Distal Nerve Root Segments Innervated: C8 to T1 Levels

- Requirements: some adaptive equipment for self-care (tub seat, grab bars); adaptive equipment for housekeeping; hand controls for the car

- Patient function and assistance: independent with ADLs, light housekeeping, meal preparation, transfers, and driving; can work (in an architectural-barriers free environment); has bed and wheelchair skills; independent with a manual wheelchair with standard hand rims

- Key muscles: FCU, FPL, FPB, and intrinsic and extrinsic muscles of finger flexors

- Available movements: all movements of the muscles of the upper extremities, fine coordination, and strong grasp

Most Distal Nerve Root Segments Innervated: T4 to T6 Levels

- Requirements: standing table or standing frame; bilateral knee ankle foot orthoses (KAFOs), reciprocating gait orthoses (RGOs) for limited ambulation

- Patient function and assistance: independent with bed skills, ADLs, wheelchair skills, transfers, and routine housekeeping; can negotiate curbs and perform the "wheelie" in a manual wheelchair; can participate in wheelchair sports; can perform physiological standing at a standing table (standing frame) using KAFOs; may ambulate for short distance with KAFOs or RGOs

- Key muscles: long muscles of the back (sacrospinalis and semispinalis) and the top half of the intercostal muscles

- Available movements: stronger trunk control musculature, pectoral muscles improvement (for lifting), and increased respiratory reserve musculature

(continued)

NEUROLOGIC SYSTEM: DATA COLLECTION AND INTERVENTIONS

Table 6.37 SCI Functional Capabilities and Assistance   *(continued)*

Most Distal Nerve Root Segments Innervated: T9 to T12 Levels

- Requirements: bilateral KAFOs, RGOs, crutches, or walker
- Patient function and assistance: independent with household ambulation when using bilateral KAFOs or RGOs and crutches (or walker); uses wheelchair only for energy conservation
- Key muscles: intercostal and lower abdominal
- Available movements: improvement with trunk control and endurance

Most Distal Nerve Root Segments Innervated: L2, L3, and L4 Levels

- Requirements: bilateral KAFOs or AFOs (L3-L4) and crutches
- Patient function and assistance: able to perform independently functional ambulation when using bilateral KAFOs and crutches; uses wheelchair only for energy conservation
- Key muscles: iliopsoas, quadratus lumborum, rectus femoris, gracilis, and sartorius
- Available movements: hip adduction and flexion, and knee extension

Most Distal Nerve Root Segments Innervated: L4 and L5 Levels

- Requirements: bilateral AFOs and crutches (or canes)
- Patient function and assistance: able to perform independently functional ambulation when using bilateral AFOs and crutches (or canes); uses wheelchair only for convenience and energy conservation
- Key muscles: extensor digitorum, lower back musculature, quadriceps, medial hamstrings (weak), and anterior and posterior tibialis
- Available movements: very good trunk control, hip flexion and knee extension, and weak knee flexion

Classification of Multiple Sclerosis

Table 6.38 MS Categories[1,3]

- Relapsing-remitting MS: the most common type of MS; periods of relapses with acute worsening of the disease and periods of remission with partial or complete disappearance of the disease
- Secondary-progressive MS: starts as relapsing-remitting MS and then progresses with or without relapses and remissions
- Progressive-relapsing MS: commonly seen in patients who develop the disease after 40 years of age; steady progressive type that starts with acute, clear signs and symptoms that steadily worsen; may or may not have episodes or remission
- Primary-progressive MS: a rare form of MS with late onset (after age 40), which progresses constantly without periods of remission

Classification of Amyotrophic Lateral Sclerosis

Table 6.39 ALS Categories[3]

- ALS is a rapidly progressing neurodegenerative disease process that affects the respiratory system, which results in death due to respiratory compromise. This progressive decline typically occurs within 2–5 years after initial diagnosis.
- There are three phases with a total of six stages (see **Box 6-1**).
- Rehabilitation focus initially is on preservation of the cardiovascular system and musculoskeletal system. In the end stages, caregiver training focuses on transfers, respiratory care, and integumentary checks as the patient becomes more confined to bed.

BOX 6-1 Amyotrophic lateral sclerosis stages summary
ALS—Summary of the Stages

Phase I: Independent

    Stage 1: Patient presents with mild weakness without limitations in function.

    Stage 2: Patient exhibits definite weakness in some muscle groups.

    Stage 3: Patient's muscle weakness affects ADLs, especially in the extremities, although independence is still demonstrated and compensation is observed. Respiratory function is beginning to be compromised.

Phase II: Partially Independent

    Stage 4: Patient able to perform most ADLs with adaptations but fatigues quickly. Mobility is primarily through the use of a wheelchair.

    Stage 5: Both upper and lower extremities demonstrate severe weakness, limiting the individual's ability to function independently.

Phase III: Dependent Final Stage

    Stage 6: Patient is bed dependent and requires maximum assistance for all activities.

Reproduced from Neurorehabilitation for the PTA by Darcy A. Umphred and Roland T. Lazaro, page 380; Box 13-1 "Summary of the Stages of ALS."

Classification of Disability Associated with Parkinson's Disease

Table 6.40 Hoehn and Yahr Classification[1]

Stage	Character of Disability
I	Mild symptoms: unilateral disease
II	Bilateral involvement. Balance not impaired.

(continued)

Table 6.40 Hoehn and Yahr Classification   *(continued)*

Stage	Character of Disability
III	Mild to moderate bilateral disease with some postural instability. Some activities restricted, but patient can live independently and continue some forms of employment.
IV	Severe disability. Able to stand and walk unassisted.
V	Confined to bed or wheelchair unless aided.

Types of Neurologic Interventions

Motor Function Interventions: Postural Strategies to Regain Balance

Table 6.41 Balance Strategies[1]

Ankle Strategy: response to small perturbations

Muscles are activated in a distal to proximal sequence. Patient maintains balance by using the ankle musculature (dorsiflexors and plantarflexors). Patient shifts the center of mass forward or backward while keeping the lower extremities relatively rigid. If loss of balance is in a forward direction gastrocnemius is activated followed by the hamstrings and finally the paraspinals. If loss of balance is in a backward direction the anterior tibials are activated followed by the quads and abdominal muscles.

Hip Strategy: response to a rapid or large perturbation

Muscles are activated in a proximal to distal sequence. Patient maintains balance by using the hip and lower trunk musculature. If loss of balance occurs in a forward direction the abdominals are activated first followed by the quads. If loss of balance occurs in a posterior direction the paraspinals are activated first followed by the hamstrings.

Stepping Strategy: response to a large force

Results in center of mass moving outside limits of stability. Patient takes a step (forward, backward, or to the side) to realign the center of mass within the base of support and regain balance.

Motor Function Interventions: Developmental Motor Skills (Essential Functional Skills)

Table 6.42 Developmental Motor Skills[1]

Mobility: ability to move from one position to another. Examples include rolling, supine to side lying and back, side lying to sit and back, sitting to standing and back.

Stability (or static postural control): ability to maintain static postural stability and orientation. It is also the same as static balance (or equilibrium)—the ability to maintain the center of mass over the base of support without any motion. Examples include prone on elbows, half-kneeling, kneeling, quadruped, plantigrade, and standing.

Controlled mobility (or dynamic postural control): ability to maintain dynamic postural stability and orientation. It is also the same as dynamic balance (or equilibrium)—the ability to maintain the center of mass over the base of support during motion. Examples include weight shifting while the body is in motion and reaching while the body is in motion.

Skill: ability to consistently perform coordinated movement sequences while interacting with others or for functional activities in the home, community, and work. Patients with skill deficits have poorly coordinated movements and lack of control, precision, and consistency. Examples include reaching and manipulation using upper extremities as well as walking and talking.

Motor Function Interventions: Restore Movement and Functional Mobility (Using Developmental Sequence Postures)

Table 6.43 Interventions Using the Developmental Sequence Postures[1]

Prone on Elbows Posture (Figure 6.12)

- Places weight bearing throughout the shoulders and elbows
- Improves control of the upper trunk, upper extremity, neck, and head
- Increases strength in shoulder stabilizers musculature
- Increases range of motion (ROM) into spinal extension
- Produces a wide base of support and a low center of gravity

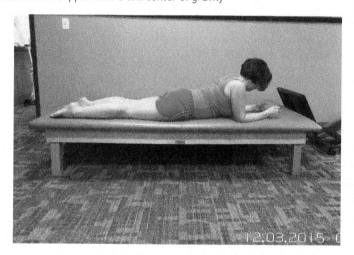

Figure 6.12 Prone on elbows

Quadruped Posture (Figure 6.13)

- Places weight bearing throughout the shoulders, elbows, wrists, knees, and hips
- Improves control of the upper trunk, lower trunk, upper and lower extremities, neck, and head
- Increases strength in the shoulders and hip stabilizers
- Decreases extensor tone at the knees
- Increases ROM in extension at the wrists and fingers
- Produces a wide base of support and a low center of gravity

(continued)

Table 6.43 **Interventions Using the Developmental Sequence Postures** *(continued)*

Figure 6.13 Quadruped

Kneeling and Half-Kneeling Posture (Figures 6.14, 6.15, 6.16)

- Places weight bearing throughout the knees and hips and ankles (in half-kneeling)
- Improves control of the upper/lower trunk, lower extremity, head, and neck
- Increases strength in hip stabilizers
- Decreases extensor tone at the knees
- Improves balance reactions
- Produces a narrow base of support and a high center of gravity in kneeling
- Produces a wide base of support and a high center of gravity in half-kneeling

Figure 6.14 Short kneeling

(continued)

Table 6.43 Interventions Using the Developmental Sequence Postures   *(continued)*

Figure 6.15 Tall kneeling

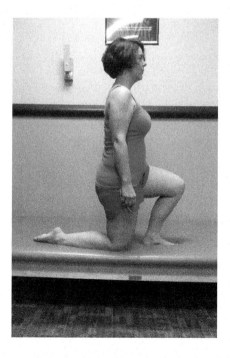

Figure 6.16 Half-kneeling

(continued)

Table 6.43 **Interventions Using the Developmental Sequence Postures** *(continued)*

Bridging Posture (Figure 6.17)

- Places weight bearing throughout the feet and ankles
- Improves control of the lower extremities (if bilateral) and trunk
- Increases strength in the hip stabilizers
- Is a lead-up activity for bed mobility
- Produces a wide base of support and a low center of gravity

Figure 6.17 Bridging

Sitting Posture (Figure 6.18)

- Places weight bearing throughout the upper extremities
- Improves control of the head, neck, upper and lower trunk, and lower extremities
- Improves balance reactions
- Is a functional posture
- Produces a medium base of support and center of gravity

(continued)

Table 6.43 Interventions Using the Developmental Sequence Postures　*(continued)*

Figure 6.18 Sitting

Modified Plantigrade Posture (Figure 6.19)

- Places weight bearing throughout the joints in the upper and lower extremities
- Improves control of the head, neck, upper and lower trunk, and upper and lower extremities
- Improves balance reactions
- Increases ROM in extension at the wrists and fingers
- Is a functional posture
- Produces a wide base of support and a high center of gravity

(continued)

Table 6.43 Interventions Using the Developmental Sequence Postures *(continued)*

Figure 6.19 Plantigrade

Standing Posture (Figure 6.20)

- Places weight bearing throughout the lower extremities
- Improves control of the head, neck, upper and lower trunk, and lower extremities
- Improves balance reactions
- Is a functional posture
- Produces a narrow base of support and a high center of gravity

(continued)

Table 6.43 **Interventions Using the Developmental Sequence Postures**   *(continued)*

Figure 6.20 Standing

Motor Function Interventions: Basic Motor Learning Strategies

Table 6.44 **Basic Motor Learning Strategies**[1]

Cognitive ("What to Do" Decision) Stage of Learning the Skill

The PTA can do the following:

- Explain the purpose of the skill.
- Demonstrate the skill, accentuating the correct performance.
- Ask the patient to explain the task, its components, and its requirements.
- Point out the similarities of the learned task to other tasks.
- Use knowledge of performance feedback by focusing on errors as they become consistent. (PTA does not concentrate on large numbers of random errors.)
- Use knowledge of results feedback by focusing on successful performance.
- For feedback, ask the patient to watch the correct movement.

(continued)

Table 6.44 Basic Motor Learning Strategies *(continued)*

- Ask the patient to evaluate his or her performance.
- Use feedback after each trial in the early learning.
- Use variable feedback later.
- Organize the initial practice of the task.
- Stress controlled movement.
- Provide adequate rest periods.
- Use manual guidance (physically assisting the learner to perform the task; does not overuse assistance in later stages).
- Break complex tasks into simple components.
- Use repeated practice of the same task.
- Use serial or random practice (when a variety of tasks are practiced randomly across trials) of related skills.
- Use mental practice.
- Avoid stressors and mental fatigue.
- Structure the environment by reducing extraneous stimuli and distractors.
- Emphasize a closed environment before moving the patient into an open environment.

Associative ("How to Do" Decision) Stage of Learning the Skill

The PTA can do the following:

- Use knowledge of performance feedback by focusing on errors as they become consistent. (PTA does not concentrate on large numbers of random errors.)
- Use knowledge of results feedback by focusing on successful performance and stressing the relevance of the task to the function.
- Emphasize proprioceptive feedback (the patient's own feeling of the movement).
- Assist the learner to improve self-evaluation and decision-making skills.
- Encourage the patient to self-assess achievements.
- Use variable feedback: summed feedback—feedback use after a set number of trials; faded feedback—feedback given at first after every trial and then less frequently; bandwidth feedback—feedback given when the performance is outside a given error range.
- Avoid excessive augmented feedback.
- Encourage consistency of performance.
- Focus on variable practice order of related skills.
- Progress toward an open environment.
- Change the environment.
- Prepare the learner for the home, community, and work environments.

Autonomous ("How to Succeed" Decision) Stage of Learning the Skill

The PTA can assess need for conscious attention and automaticity of movements:

- Select appropriate feedback: the learner demonstrates appropriate self-evaluation and decision-making skills; when errors are evident, use occasional knowledge of performance feedback or knowledge of results feedback.

(continued)

Table 6.44 Basic Motor Learning Strategies *(continued)*

- Organize practice: stress consistency in variable environments; practice in open environments; use massed practice when the rest time is much less than the practice time.
- Structure the environment: vary environments; help the patient to be ready for the home, community, and work environments; focus on competitive aspects of the task.

Neurologic Facilitation Techniques

Table 6.45 Neurologic Facilitation Interventions[1]

- **Agonist reversals (AR):** slow, resisted concentric contraction of agonist muscles moving through the range, followed by a holding contraction in the range position and then an eccentric contraction while moving slowly back to the initial starting position. AR is a proprioceptive neuromuscular facilitation (PNF) technique.

- **Approximation (AP):** compression of joint surfaces to facilitate extensor muscular contractions and provide joint stability. It can be applied manually, during upright positions, in weight-bearing positions, and in PNF extensor patterns. AP can be applied mechanically using weights, belts, or weighted vests, or while bouncing on a Swiss ball. AP can also be applied to the shoulders or pelvis in upright weight-bearing positions such as in sitting, standing, or kneeling. AP is contraindicated in inflamed joints. AP is a PNF technique.

- **Contract–relax (CR):** strong, isotonic contraction (rotation) of the antagonists (restricting muscles) in a limited ROM, followed by an isometric contraction that is held for 5–8 seconds. Next, voluntary relaxation takes place, followed by active contraction of the agonist muscles into the newly acquired ROM. CR is a PNF technique.

- **Hold–relax (HR):** strong, isometric contraction of the antagonists (restricting muscles) in the limited ROM, followed by a voluntary relaxation and passive range of motion (PROM) of the agonists into the newly gained range. HR is a PNF technique.

- **Hold–relax active contraction (HRAC):** strong, isometric contraction of the antagonists (restricting muscles) in the limited ROM, followed by a voluntary relaxation and active range of motion (AROM) of the agonists into the newly gained range. HRAC is a PNF technique.

- **Joint traction (JT):** manual distraction (or mechanical distraction using ankle or wrist cuffs) to facilitate joint motion and enhance joint awareness. JT can be used in PNF flexor extremity patterns with pulling movements. This technique is contraindicated in patients with hypermobile or unstable joints. JT is a proprioceptive facilitation technique.

- **Manual contacts (MCs):** manual contacts with deep pressure (grip) over the muscles to facilitate muscular contraction. MCs are applied in the direction opposite to the desired motion. MCs guide the direction of movement, provide sensory awareness, and are cues to movement. MC is a proprioceptive facilitation technique.

- **Maximal resistance (MR):** the maximum resistance tolerated by the patient applied in PNF patterns to stronger muscles to create an overflow pattern of the weaker muscles. The overflow is the spread of muscular response from the stronger muscles to the weaker ones. MR is a PNF technique.

- **Muscle positioning (MP):** performed in the midrange for greatest muscular tension; in short ranges for weak contractile force; and in the lengthened range for strong muscular contraction that is enhanced by the stretch mechanism. MP is a PNF technique.

- **Quick stretch (QS):** short stretch applied to a weak muscle in the lengthened range using the diagonal PNF patterns to facilitate the agonist muscular contraction. An example of QS is tapping over the muscle belly or the tendon. QS is a proprioceptive facilitation technique.

(continued)

Table 6.45 Neurologic Facilitation Interventions   *(continued)*

- **Repeated contractions (RCs):** repeated isotonic contractions with quick stretches and resistance performed through the range or part of the range at a point of weakness. RC is a PNF technique.

- **Resistance:** resistance applied to weak muscles. Resistance can be manual (graded); body weight and gravity using upright positions; mechanical (weights, cuffs, vests); or isokinetic. Resistance is a proprioceptive facilitation technique.

- **Resisted progression (RP):** stretching, approximation, and tracking light resistance applied manually (or using a T-band) to the patient's pelvis during locomotion. This technique should not disrupt the patient's coordination, momentum, and velocity. Indications for RP are improved timing and control of the lower trunk or pelvis muscles during locomotion and increased endurance. RP is a PNF technique.

- **Rhythmic initiation (RI):** voluntary muscular relaxation, followed by passive movements, active assisted and active resistive movements (using light resistance), and finally active movements. Indications for RI: spasticity, rigidity (as in PD), difficulty initiating movement (as in PD), aphasia, and inability to relax. RI is a PNF technique.

- **Rhythmic stabilization (RS):** alternating resisted isometric contractions of first the agonist and then the antagonist muscles without any motion allowed. Indications for RS are to increase muscular strength and coordination. RS is a PNF technique.

- **Slow reversals (SRs):** isotonic contractions of first the agonist muscles and then the antagonist muscles using graded resistance. The resistance is applied first to the stronger muscles, progressing to the weaker muscles. At the end, the limb is moved through the full ROM. SR is a PNF technique.

- **Timing for emphasis (TE):** resistive (strong) isometric contractions causing overflow from strong to weak muscles within a synergistic pattern. Motion is allowed only in the weaker muscles. TE is a PNF technique.

Proprioceptive Neuromuscular Facilitation Diagonal Patterns

Table 6.46 Description and Performance of PNF Terminal Positions (Shoulder, Forearm, Wrist, Fingers, Hip, Knee, Ankle)

UE D1 extension: extension, abduction, internal rotation (scapular depression, abduction, and downward rotation); pronation; ulnar extension of wrist; and abduction and extension of fingers including thumb abduction

Figure 6.21 UE D1 extension

(continued)

Table 6.46 Description and Performance of PNF Terminal Positions (Shoulder, Forearm, Wrist, Fingers, Hip, Knee, Ankle *(continued)*

UE D1 flexion: flexion, adduction, external rotation (scapular elevation, abduction, and upward rotation); supination; wrist radial flexion; and fingers flexion and adduction including thumb adduction

Figure 6.22 UE D1 flexion

UE D2 extension: extension, adduction, internal rotation (scapular depression, abduction, and downward rotation); pronation; ulnar extension of wrist, and flexion and adduction of fingers including thumb opposition

Figure 6.23 UE D2 extension

(continued)

Table 6.46 Description and Performance of PNF Terminal Positions (Shoulder, Forearm, Wrist, Fingers, Hip, Knee, Ankle *(continued)*

UE D2 flexion: flexion, abduction, external rotation (scapular elevation, adduction, and upward rotation); supination; radial extension of wrist; and fingers abduction and extension including thumb extension

Figure 6.24 UE D2 flexion

LE D1 extension: extension, abduction, internal rotation (posterior rotation of pelvis); knee extension; and ankle plantarflexion and eversion

Figure 6.25 LE D1 extension

(continued)

Table 6.46 **Description and Performance of PNF Terminal Positions (Shoulder, Forearm, Wrist, Fingers, Hip, Knee, Ankle** *(continued)*

LE D1 flexion: flexion, adduction, external rotation (anterior rotation of pelvis); knee flexion; and ankle dorsiflexion and inversion

Figure 6.26 LE D1 flexion

LE D2 extension: extension, adduction, external rotation (depression of pelvis); knee extension; and ankle plantarflexion and inversion

Figure 6.27 LE D2 extension

(continued)

NEUROLOGIC SYSTEM: DATA COLLECTION AND INTERVENTIONS

Table 6.46 Description and Performance of PNF Terminal Positions (Shoulder, Forearm, Wrist, Fingers, Hip, Knee, Ankle *(continued)*

LE D2 flexion: flexion, abduction, internal rotation (elevation of pelvis); knee flexion; and ankle plantarflexion (or ankle dorsiflexion) and eversion

Figure 6.28 LE D2 flexion

Neurologic Inhibition Techniques

Table 6.47 Inhibition Interventions[1]

Firm Manual Contacts (FMCs)

- Applied to midline abdomen, back, palms, lips, or soles of feet.
- Indications: patients with paresthesia or peripheral nerve injury; TBI.
- FMC is a sensory stimulation technique producing inhibition.

Inhibitory Pressure (IP)

- Deep maintained pressure to tendons.
- Prolonged positioning in extreme lengthened range: prolonged weight-bearing quadruped or kneeling position; prolonged weight bearing on extended wrists, arms, or fingers; modified plantigrade positioning; pressure over calcaneus to decrease plantarflexion tone; tactile deep maintained pressure over acupressure points to decrease pain; firm, maintained pressure using cones in the hands or inhibitory splints or casts for lower leg or wrists.
- IP inhibits muscular tone. It can also be used in combination with relaxation techniques (deep breathing or relaxing environment). IP is a sensory stimulation technique producing inhibition.

(continued)

Table 6.47 Inhibition Interventions

(continued)

Neutral Warmth (NW)

- Wrapping body or body parts using Ace wraps or towel wrap; applying snug-fitting clothes such as gloves, socks, and/or tights; using tepid baths; using air splints. NW is used to decrease muscular tone, reduce pain, and produce relaxation and a calming effect.
- Indications for NW: patients with increased sympathetic activity; patients with high arousal levels; spasticity.
- Precaution for NW: Do not overheat (can increase tone).
- NW is a sensory stimulation technique producing inhibition.

Prolonged Icing (PI)

- Immersion in cold water or ice chips; ice towel wraps or ice packs; ice massage. PI is used to decrease muscular tone, reduce muscular spasms, and decrease metabolism of the tissue.
- Precaution for PI: Monitor the patient carefully for SNS effects such as increased arousal, fight or flight response, or protective withdrawal mechanism.
- PI is a sensory stimulation technique producing inhibition.

Prolonged Stretch (PS)

- Slow, maintained stretch applied at the maximum available lengthened range to inhibit muscular contraction and tone.
- Can be applied using positioning, inhibitory splinting, and/or casting; traction; or mechanical low-load weights.
- PS is a proprioceptive facilitation technique producing inhibition.

Rhythmic Rotation (RRo)

- Relaxation is achieved with slow, repeated rotation movements (either passive or active) of a limb at the point of limitation. As muscular relaxation is obtained, the limb is moved slowly into the new range. When tension is observed, more rhythmic rotation movements are necessary.
- RRo is a PNF technique producing inhibition.

Slow Stroking (SS)

- Applied to paravertebral spinal region; causes generalized inhibition and a calming effect. SS is applied by alternating firm strokes (using a flat hand) downward on the paravertebral muscles for 3–5 minutes while the patient is lying prone (or sitting and resting forward on a tabletop).
- Indications for SS: increased SNS activity; increased arousal.
- Precaution for SS: Patients with large amounts of body hair can be less responsive to the calming effect and may become irritated.
- SS is a sensory stimulation technique producing inhibition.

Slow Vestibular Stimulation (SVS)

- Slow repetitive rolling or rocking movements applied through passive or active-assisted techniques. Examples of SVS include sitting and rocking; rolling side lying; using a rocking chair; using the therapy ball, a bolster, equilibrium board, or a swing; riding a wheelchair.

(continued)

Table 6.47 Inhibition Interventions (continued)

- Indications for SVS: patients with hypertonia or hyperactivity; high arousal; combative-stage TBI. SVS can be combined with deep breathing exercises, imagery relaxation techniques, and quiet environment.
- SVS is a vestibular stimulation technique producing inhibition.

Vestibular Stimulation (VS) of Head and Body

- Use of fast spinning in a chair; spinning in a hammock; prone on a scooter board; or equilibrium board, wobble boards, or therapy ball.
- Indications for VS: hypotonia; children with hyperactivity; coordination problems; akinesia and bradykinesia (in PD).
- VS is a vestibular stimulation technique producing inhibition.

Locomotion Training

Table 6.48 Locomotion Training Sequence[1]

A. Activities to prepare for locomotion using instruction and training
  1. Bridging (focus on lower trunk, hip and pelvis, and LEs)
  2. Quadruped (focus on the trunk, proximal and intermediate UEs, and proximal LEs)
  3. Sitting (focus on upper trunk, pelvis, and proximal and intermediate UEs)
  4. Sit to stand
  5. Kneeling/half-kneeling (focus on trunk, pelvis, proximal and distal LEs, and reciprocal control of LEs)
  6. Modified plantigrade (focus on trunk, UEs, and proximal, intermediate, and distal control of LEs)
  7. Standing (focus on trunk and LEs)
B. Activities at the parallel bars using instruction and training
  1. Moving from sitting to standing and back
  2. Standing balance training
  3. Stepping, sidestepping, and cross-stepping
  4. Training in an appropriate gait pattern
  5. Using the appropriate gait pattern to ambulate forward and to turn
  6. Training to transfer with the assistive device from sitting to standing and back
  7. Standing and weight-shifting balance training with assistive device
  8. Gait training with the appropriate assistive device: forward and turning
C. Indoor locomotion activities using instruction and training
  1. Walking forward and backward
  2. Resisted progression
  3. Sidestepping and cross-stepping
  4. Braiding
  5. Stair climbing
  6. Falling techniques for patients who ambulate independently with assistive devices for the long term
D. Outdoor locomotion activities using instruction and training
  1. Opening doors and passing through thresholds that go outdoors
  2. Climbing curbs
  3. Negotiating ramps, stairs, and sloped surfaces
  4. Walking on even and uneven surfaces
  5. Walking and crossing at stoplights
  6. Entering and exiting buildings in the community
  7. Entering and exiting vehicles
  8. Using elevators and revolving doors

Constraint-Induced Movement Therapy as a Form of Functional Training

---

Table 6.49 **Constraint-Induced Movement Therapy (CIMT) as a Form of Functional Training**

CIMT[6] forces the use of the affected extremity by restraining the unaffected extremity. For example, for a patient having hemiplegia of the right (involved) upper extremity, the therapist constrains the patient's left (uninvolved) upper extremity in a sling. Then the patient uses his or her right (involved) upper extremity repetitively and intensively for 2 weeks.

- CIMT is becoming more widely used in the United States. It was developed by Dr. Edward Taub[7] (a professor of psychology) at the University of Alabama in Birmingham. Taub developed CIMT on the principle of "learned non-use." His idea of "learned non-use" includes three principles[7–9]: constraining the unaffected limb, forced use of the affected limb, and massed practice.

- To start CIMT, a patient (client) needs to be able to extend his or her wrist and move his or her arm and fingers. In addition, patients (clients) need to demonstrate basic head and trunk stability during upright positioning.

- Research has shown that CIMT helps patients (clients) by improving functional use of their affected extremity much more than the regular therapy.[6–9] The results of a 2003 study proved that plastic changes occurred in the motor cortex of patients with TBI who received CIMT intensively (7 hours daily) for 2 weeks.[7] Other studies have shown that CIMT can produce a use-dependent cortical reorganization of the brain in patients (clients) who had CNS injury-related paresis of the upper limb (including chronic hemiparesis from stroke).[8–10]

- CIMT has been found to help children with cerebral palsy use their affected (hemiparetic) upper extremities. These studies[8, 9] suggested that CIMT leads to recruitment of a large number of neurons adjacent to those originally involved in the control of the stroke-affected limb. The research conclusion supports the effectiveness of CIMT in a clinical setting by providing a neurophysiological basis[7, 8] for the therapy-induced effects on the brain's neural network.

- CIMT is a form of "functional training" or "task-oriented training" therapy. It can be applied to patients (clients) who have experienced CVA, TBI, and CP. Tasks considered significant for daily function, such as standing, walking, grasping, and releasing, are emphasized with this technique. Motor learning strategies are used to enhance function.

- Physical therapy goals using functional training based on CIMT may consider the following issues:
  - Training the patient early to avoid learned non-use
  - Considering the patient's history, health status, age, and experience when designing stimulating and interesting activities
  - Involving patient in goal setting and decision-making
  - Structuring the practice using task-related training
  - Structuring the patient's practice as context specific
  - Maintaining focus on the therapist's role as training coach (minimizing hands-on therapy)
  - Monitoring recovery closely
  - Documenting progress using valid and reliable functional outcome measures
  - Being cautious about timetables and predictions (because the recovery may be longer)

Clinical Impairments and Activity Limitations of Neurologic Conditions

Clinical Impairments and Activity Limitations: Cerebral Vascular Accident

---

Table 6.50 (Cerebral Vascular Accident) CVA Impairments and Activity Limitations*

Sensory Deficits

- Impaired sensation in the contralateral upper and lower extremity
- Impaired proprioception
- Loss of superficial touch and pain and temperature
- Numbness
- Thalamic pain syndrome (continuous and severe pain contralaterally; pain can be triggered by noise, bright lights, or light touch)
- Homonymous hemianopsia
- Left hemisphere lesion has right-side hemisensory loss
- Right hemisphere lesion has left-side hemisensory loss

Motor Deficits

- Flaccidity and hyporeflexia (immediately after CVA; does not last long)
- Spasticity (on the opposite side of the lesion)
- Hyperreflexia (such as clonus and positive Babinski sign)
- Synergies
- Primitive reflex patterns (STNR, ATNR, STLR, TLR)
- Associated reactions: Souques—elevation of hemi UE elicits fingers' extension and abduction; Raimiste—resistance to abduction or adduction in noninvolved UE or LE elicits abduction or adduction response in the opposite UE/LE
- Paresis or weakness: in Middle Cerebral Artery (MCA) syndrome, UE is more affected than LE; in Anterior Cerebral Artery (ACA) syndrome, LE is more affected than UE
- Incoordination and balance deficits
- Apraxia (ideomotor and ideational)
- Left hemisphere lesion: difficulty planning and sequencing movements; apraxia (ideational or ideomotor)
- Right hemisphere lesion: difficulty sustaining a movement

Gait Deficits

- Trendelenburg gait (weak abductors)
- Scissoring (spastic adductors)
- Insufficient pelvic rotation during swing
- Circumduction (weak hip flexors during swing)
- Backward leaning of trunk
- Exaggerated hip flexion synergy
- Excessive knee flexion during stance (weak knee extensors)
- Knee in hyperextension as a compensation for weak knee extensors or spastic quads
- Foot drop

(continued)

Table 6.50 (Cerebral Vascular Accident) CVA Impairments and Activity Limitations *(continued)*

- Equinus gait (heel does not touch down)
- Varus foot (weight is borne on the lateral side of the foot)
- Unequal step length (hemi leg does not advance through the end of stance into toe-off)
- Decreased cadence and uneven timing

Communication Deficits

- Broca's or expressive aphasia: speech is impaired; left frontal lobe lesion
- Wernicke's or receptive aphasia: auditory comprehension is impaired; left lateral temporal lobe
- Global aphasia: speech and comprehension are impaired; typical of large left hemisphere lesion
- Dysarthria: motor speech deficit caused by impairments of respiration, articulation, phonation, or sensory feedback
- Left hemisphere lesion has the following: speech and language impairments for the dominant hemisphere (right-handed patients); nonfluent or Broca's aphasia; fluent or Wernicke's aphasia; global aphasia; memory impairments related to language

Perceptual Deficits

- Unilateral neglect: ignores stimuli from the left side
- Anosognosia: denial of dysfunction
- Somatoagnosia: cannot comprehend relationship of one body part to another
- Right and left discrimination: cannot identify right and left sides of body
- Pusher syndrome: lateral lean toward the hemiplegic side
- Right hemisphere lesion has the following: visual perceptual impairments; left-side unilateral neglect; agnosia; visual–spatial impairments; disturbances of body image and body scheme; memory impairments related to spatial–perceptual information

General Cognitive Deficits

- Attention: deficits in areas of sustained attention, divided attention, selective attention, and alternating attention
- Memory: short- and long-term memory
- Confabulation: use of inappropriate words or fabricated stories
- Perseveration: continued repetition of words, thoughts, or acts unrelated to current activity
- Dementia: general decline in higher brain functions such as in judgment, memory, consciousness, communication, and behavior

Left Hemisphere Lesion Cognitive Deficits

Patient may be as follows:

- Slow
- Hesitant
- Cautious
- Insecure
- Fearful

(continued)

Table 6.50 **(Cerebral Vascular Accident) CVA Impairments and Activity Limitations** *(continued)*

- Aware of impairments
- Disorganized in problem solving
- Anxious about his or her poor performance
- Having difficulty with processing delays
- Having difficulty with expression of positive emotions
- Having memory impairments typically related to language
- Having difficulty processing verbal cues and verbal commands.

Right Hemisphere Lesion Cognitive Deficits

Patient may be as follows:

- Impulsive
- Indifferent
- Quick
- Having poor judgment
- Underestimating the problems
- Overestimating the abilities
- Experiencing difficulty grasping the overall organization or pattern, problem solving, and synthesizing information
- Unaware of impairments
- Unable to self-correct
- At risk for safety
- Having rigidity of thought
- Having difficulty with abstract reasoning
- Having difficulty with perception of emotions and expression of negative emotions
- Having difficulty processing visual cues
- Having memory impairments related to spatial–perceptual information

Affective Deficits

- Emotional lability: pathological crying and laughing; changing easily and quickly from laughing to crying
- Irritability
- Agitation
- Increased frustration
- Depression: not psychological, but rather stemming from a direct impairment caused by CVA

Bladder and Bowel Deficits

- Urinary incontinence (due to bladder hyperreflexia or hyporeflexia)
- Bowel incontinence
- Diarrhea
- Constipation
- Bowel impaction

(continued)

Table 6.50 (Cerebral Vascular Accident) CVA Impairments and Activity Limitations *(continued)*

Indirect Impairments

- Deep venous thrombosis (DVT)
- Pressure sores (decubitus ulcers)
- Decreased ROM
- Contracture
- Deformity
- Shoulder subluxation and pain
- Chronic regional pain syndrome (CRPS)
- Deconditioning

* This is a basic guide; the PTA should also consider the results of the physical therapist's (PT's) initial examination and evaluation.

Clinical Impairments and Activity Limitations: Parkinson's Disease

Table 6.51 Parkinson's Disease (PD) Impairments and Activity Limitations

- Rigidity: cogwheel rigidity (jerky resistance to passive movement); lead-pipe rigidity (constant, uniform resistance to passive movement)
- Akinesia (difficulty initiating movement); bradykinesia (difficulty maintaining movement; slowness); hypokinesia (movements reduced in speed, amplitude, and range); freezing episodes (sudden stop during movement); micrographia (abnormally small handwriting)
- Resting tremor: pill-rolling tremor (hand tremor at rest); postural tremor (tremor in sitting or standing against gravity)
- Postural instability (weak trunk extensor muscles cause a flexed, stooped posture with increased neck, trunk, hips, and knees flexion); back pain (as a result of stooped posture)
- Communication and swallowing deficits: dysarthria (decreased voice volume, monotone speech, distorted articulation, and uncontrolled rate of speech); mutism (not speaking or speaking in whispers); sialorrhea (excessive drooling due to increased salivation and decreased swallowing); dysphagia (impaired swallowing; can cause choking or aspiration pneumonia)
- Gait deficits: loss of reciprocal arm swing and decreased stride length; festinating gait (progressive increase in speed with shortening of stride); propulsive festinating gait (increase in speed forward; most common); retropulsive festinating gait (increase in speed backward; less common); plantarflexion contracture gait (with narrow base of support)
- Visual deficits: blurred vision; difficulty reading (cannot be corrected by glasses); decreased blinking (can produce irritation of the eyes)
- Cognitive deficits: bradyphrenia (slowing of thought processes); deficits in learning new skills; deficits in reasoning, abstract thinking, memory, and judgment; dementia (may occur in patients with PD who are 80 years or older)
- Indirect impairments: fatigue (weakness and lethargy); masked face (infrequent blinking and lack of facial expression); kyphosis (caused by contractures in hip and knee flexors, hip rotators, adductors, plantarflexors, neck flexors, shoulder adductors, internal rotators, and elbow flexors); scoliosis (caused by leaning to one side); orthostatic hypotension (caused by Levodopa side effects); pulmonary deficits (airway obstruction due to decreased respiratory movements; may be caused by kyphosis)

Clinical Impairments and Activity Limitations: Multiple Sclerosis

Table 6.52   Multiple Sclerosis (MS) Impairments and Activity Limitations

Motor Deficits

- UMN deficits: spasticity (can be mild to severe)
- Paresis
- Brisk deep tendon (stretch) reflex (DTR)
- Clonus
- Positive Babinski sign
- Involuntary spasm of flexor and extensor musculature
- Exaggerated cutaneous reflexes
- Flexion/extension synergy patterns

Other Motor Deficits

- Slow and stiff movements
- Weak musculature
- Balance and coordination deficits such as asthenia, ataxia, dysmetria, dyssynergia, dysdiadochokinesia, dizziness, intention tremor, and trunk musculature weakness (all with cerebellar involvement)
- Fatigue
- Difficulty walking
- Staggering gait with loss of balance
- Dysarthria (slurred or unarticulated speech)
- Dysphonia (harsh or hoarse speech)
- Dysphagia (difficulty swallowing)

Sensory Deficits

- Paresthesia (pins and needles or numbness)
- Acute, intense, or burning pain (such as trigeminal neuralgia and headache)
- Lhermitte's sign for MS symptoms (flexion of the neck produces a sudden electric shock running down the spine and lower extremities)
- Chronic pain
- Optic neuritis (inflammation of optic nerve)
- Scotoma (dark spot in the center of the visual field)
- Nystagmus
- Lateral gaze palsy (incomplete eye adduction)
- Diplopia (double vision)

Cognitive and Affective Deficits

- Impaired memory, attention, and concentration
- Decreased problem solving and judgment
- Depression

(continued)

Table 6.52 **Multiple Sclerosis (MS) Impairments and Activity Limitations** *(continued)*

- Anxiety
- Emotional lability
- Euphoria
- Bipolar affective disorder (alternative periods of depression and mania)

ANS Deficits

- Bowel deficits (such as constipation, bowel impaction, incontinence, or diarrhea)
- Bladder deficits (such as incontinence, urinary frequency and urgency, urinary hesitancy, excessive and frequent urination at night)
- Sexual deficits (such as impotence, vaginal dryness, or loss of libido)

Clinical Impairments and Activity Limitations: Traumatic Brain Injury

Table 6.53 **Traumatic Brain Injury (TBI) Impairments and Activity Limitations**

Motor Deficits

- Hemiparesis
- Quadriparesis (tetraparesis)
- Abnormal DTRs
- Clonus
- Positive Babinski sign
- Ataxia, hypotonia, coordination and balance deficits (with cerebellar involvement; patient may have bilateral deficits)
- Flaccidity
- Spasticity
- Hypertonicity
- Rigidity (can be decorticate and/or decerebrate rigidity)
- Muscular atrophy, decreased muscular power and/or endurance
- Abnormal synergy patterns

Sensory Deficits

- Sharp and dull discrimination
- Temperature
- Light touch
- Pressure
- Kinesthesia
- Proprioception
- Stereognosis
- Barognosis
- Tactile localization
- Dysphagia

(continued)

Table 6.53 Traumatic Brain Injury (TBI) Impairments and Activity Limitations   *(continued)*

Perceptual Deficits

- Homonymous hemianopsia
- Somatognosia
- Right and left discrimination
- Anosognosia
- Figure–ground discrimination
- Position in space deficit
- Agnosia
- Apraxia (ideomotor or ideational)

Integumentary Deficits

- Postures that aggravate or relieve pain
- Pressure areas

Arousal, Mentation, and Cognition Deficits

- Anterograde (post-traumatic) amnesia
- Retrograde amnesia
- Emotional lability
- Decreased level of consciousness (coma, vegetative state, or persistent vegetative state)
- Attention deficits
- Memory loss
- Altered orientation
- Impaired safety awareness
- Decreased problem solving, reasoning, and judgment
- Perseveration
- Disinhibition
- Impulsiveness
- Aggressiveness
- Irritability
- Apathy
- Sexual inappropriateness
- Egocentricity

Speech and Communication Deficits

- Broca's or Wernicke's aphasia
- Global aphasia
- Dysarthria
- Impaired reading comprehension
- Impaired written expression

Clinical Impairments with Mild Traumatic Brain Injury or Concussion

Table 6.54 Mild TBI or Concussion[11,12]

- Most TBIs that occur each year are mild TBIs or concussions.
- Symptoms might appear within hours or may be delayed. Most symptoms occur within 7–10 days and resolve within a few weeks, although in some cases can last up to 3 months.
- Repeated mild TBIs or mild concussions lead to longer recovery periods and potential for long-term problems.

Physical Symptoms

- Dizziness
- Headache
- Nausea, vomiting
- Visual disturbance
- Fatigue
- Problems with bright lights
- Slurring of speech

Cognition

- Disorientation
- Short- or long-term memory problems
- Deficits in attention and focus on tasks
- Slowed information processing

Social and Emotional Problems

- Anxiety
- Irritability
- Easily distracted
- Emotional lability
- Personality changes

Sleep Disturbances

- Sleeping more or less than usual
- Difficulty falling asleep

Clinical Impairments and Activity Limitations: Traumatic Spinal Cord Injury

Table 6.55 Spinal Cord Injury (SCI) Impairments and Activity Limitations

- *Areflexia* (spinal shock) occurs immediately after injury. It is characterized by absence of motor function, appearance of flaccidity, loss of sensation and reflex activity below the level of lesion, delayed plantar reflex, loss of DTRs, and loss of bulbocavernous and cremasteric reflexes. It can last from several days to several weeks. Areflexia is resolved when the bulbocavernous reflex returns.

- *Motor and sensory impairments* depend on the type of clinical syndrome and the level of lesion (see also **Tables 6.34** and **6.35**). Motor impairments can include the following: hypotonia; flaccidity; spasticity; decreased muscular strength, power, and endurance; hypertonia; muscular substitution; gait and balance deficits; functional deficits; and community and work dysfunctions. Sensory impairments can include the following: loss or decreased superficial, deep, and combined sensations; and pain (traumatic pain after traumatic injury; nerve root pain caused by damage to nerve roots; spinal cord dysesthesia with painful sensations below the level of the lesion; musculoskeletal pain above the level of lesion, most commonly in the shoulder).

- *Autonomic dysreflexia* (hyperreflexia) can occur mostly in lesions above the T6 level in patients having tetraplegia and high-level paraplegia. It is a medical emergency. The PTA needs to take the following steps:

  1. Bring the patient to a sitting position.
  2. Call EMS or a nurse (in hospital/skilled nursing facility).
  3. Examine the bladder drainage system (catheter) for internal/external blockage.
  4. Release the clamped catheter.
  5. Examine the patient for bowel impaction.
  6. Look for other possible causes and manage if indicated.

- Symptoms of autonomic dysreflexia include the following: sudden and marked increase in systolic and diastolic BP; bradycardia; headache; profuse sweating; increased spasticity; restlessness; constricted pupils; flushing above the level of the lesion; blurred vision; constriction below the level of the lesion; nasal congestion; and piloerection (goose bumps). Causes may include bladder distension due to urinary retention (most common), bladder infection or irritation, kidney stones, kidney dysfunction, bowel distension, pressure sores, noxious cutaneous stimuli i.e., tight clothing, sharp objects, and environmental temperature changes.

- *Postural hypotension* (orthostatic hypotension) is a decrease in blood pressure while the patient is trying to assume an erect position. The cause is prolonged immobilization, especially with cervical and upper thoracic SCI. Symptoms include dizziness and a feeling of fainting. A related problem with postural hypotension in SCI is pitting edema of the feet, ankles, and legs.

- *SNS deficit* is impaired temperature control due to damage to the spinal cord. Because of hypothalamic dysfunction, the patient loses the ability to sweat or shiver. Symptoms include the following: diaphoresis (excessive sweating as a compensatory mechanism); spotty areas of localized sweating below the level of lesion; and body temperature dependent on the environmental temperature.

- *Respiratory deficit* depends on the level of lesion and the residual respiratory muscle function. Respiratory impairment is life threatening to the patient with SCI. The effects of respiratory deficit can include decreased ability to cough, altered breathing pattern, and patient's vulnerability to increased secretions, atelectasis (collapsed lungs), and pulmonary infections.

- *Bladder and bowel deficits* can cause the following: urinary tract infections (UTIs); reflexive or spastic bladder (can empty only to a certain fullness pressure) occurring in UMN lesions at the T11–T12 level or higher; flaccid or nonreflexive bladder (can empty only by compressing the lower abdomen) occurring in LMN lesions at the T12 level or lower; reflexive or spastic bowel occurring with UMN lesions; and flaccid or nonreflexive bowel occurring with LMN lesions.

(continued)

Table 6.55 **Spinal Cord Injury (SCI) Impairments and Activity Limitations**   *(continued)*

- *Sexual deficits* can cause the following: decreased erectile capacity mostly with LMN and complete SCI lesions; decreased ejaculation mostly with UMN lesion, higher-level cord lesions, and complete SCI lesions; decreased female sexual response in LMN lesions (and intact response in UMN lesions); and unimpaired fertility. Patients with UMN and incomplete SCI lesions have greater erectile capacity than LMN and complete lesions. Patients with LMN, lower-level cord, and complete lesions have a higher incidence of ejaculation compared to patients with UMN, higher-level cord, and incomplete lesions.

- *Indirect impairments* may include the following: atelectasis and pneumonia (patients with paralyzed or weak muscles of inspiration); decubitus ulcers; DVT; contractures (most common: hip flexion—adduction and internal rotation contractures; shoulder flexion/extension—internal rotation and adduction contractures); heterotopic ossification (abnormal bone formation in the tendons, connective tissue between muscle, aponeurosis, or peripheral part of the muscle; commonly affects areas close to the hips and knees); osteoporosis (below the level of the lesion); and renal calculi.

Clinical Impairments and Activity Limitations: Guillain-Barré Syndrome (Polyneuritis)

Table 6.56 **Guillain-Barré Syndrome Impairments and Activity Limitations**

Motor Deficits

- Paresis or paralysis: symmetrical distribution; progresses from lower extremities to upper extremities, and from distal to proximal; can produce tetraplegia with respiratory failure
- Flaccidity: LMN lesion; demyelination of cranial and peripheral nerves
- Decreased muscular strength, power, and endurance

Sensory Deficits

- Paresthesia (tingling and burning sensations)
- Anesthesia (of distal extremities in a long gloves and stocking pattern)
- Hyperesthesia
- Pain (muscular ache)
- Burning pain

Functional Deficits

- Impaired gait and balance
- Decreased ADLs
- Decreased home or work management and integration in the community

Autonomic Deficits

- Tachycardia
- Blood pressure fluctuations
- Arrhythmia

Clinical Impairments and Activity Limitations: Amyotrophic Lateral Sclerosis

Table 6.57 Amyotrophic Lateral Sclerosis (ALS) Impairments and Activity Limitations

Motor Deficits

- Muscular weakness
- Hyporeflexia
- Hypotonicity
- Atrophy
- Fasciculations
- Muscle cramps
- Spasticity
- Hyperreflexia
- Cervical extensor weakness
- Dysarthria
- Anarthria (loss of motor power to speak distinctly)
- Dysphagia
- Sialorrhea (excess secretion of saliva)

Sensory Deficits

- Spared for the most part
- Some patients may have paresthesia or focal pain in the limbs

Functional Deficits

- Decreased walking ability
- Decreased ADLs
- Deconditioning
- Impaired postural control and balance
- Decreased home or work management and integration in the community

Respiratory Deficits

- Respiratory muscle weakness
- Dyspnea on exertion first and then at rest
- Fatigue
- Recurrent sighing
- Morning headache due to hypoxia
- Difficulty sleeping in supine position
- Weak cough

Cognitive Deficits

- Depression
- Anxiety
- Dementia (frontotemporal dementia)

Neurologic Interventions

American Physical Therapy Association (APTA) Guide to Physical Therapist Practice: Suggested Neuromuscular Interventions

Table 6.58 Therapeutic Interventions[13]

Refer to Section 4.2 for a review of basic exercise interventions. See Section 6-3 for detail on therapeutic interventions specific to patients with neurologic diagnoses.

- Balance, coordination, and agility training: perceptual training; posture awareness training; standardized, programmatic, complementary exercise approaches task-specific performance training; sensory training or retraining; task specific performance training; vestibular training
- Body mechanics and postural stabilization: body mechanics training; postural control training; postural stabilization activities, standing frame and tilt table
- Gait and locomotion training: developmental activities training; gait training; implement and device training; perceptual training; standardized, programmatic, complementary exercise approaches for wheelchair training
- Neuromotor development training: developmental activities training; motor training, motor control, motor learning; movement pattern training; neuromuscular education or reeducation, inhibitory and facilitatory techniques

Table 6.59 Functional Training in Self-Care and Home Management Including ADL and IADL[13]

- ADL training: bathing; bed mobility and transfer training; developmental activities; dressing; eating; grooming; toileting
- Devices and equipment use and training: assistive and adaptive device and equipment training during ADLs and IADLs; orthotic, protective, or supportive device or equipment training during ADLs and IADLs
- Functional training programs: simulated environments and tasks; task adaptation; travel training
- IADL training: caring for dependents; home maintenance; household chores; shopping; structured play for infants and children; yard work
- Injury prevention or reduction: injury prevention education during self-care and home management; injury prevention or reduction with use of devices and equipment; safety awareness training during self-care and home management

Table 6.60 Prescription, Application, and (as Appropriate) Fabrication of Devices and Equipment: Adaptive, Assistive, Orthotic, Protective, Supportive, and Prosthetic[13]

- Adaptive devices: environmental controls; hospital beds; raised toilet seats; seating systems
- Assistive devices: canes; crutches; long-handled reachers; walkers; power devices; static and dynamic splints; wheelchairs (refer to Section 4-5 for wheelchair management and mobility training)
- Orthotic devices: braces; casts; splints; shoe inserts
- Protective devices: braces; cushions; helmets; protective taping
- Supportive devices: compression garments; corsets; elastic wraps; neck collars; serial casts; slings; supplemental oxygen; supportive taping

Table 6.61 **Functional Training in Self-Care and in Domestic Education, Work, Community, Social and Civic Life**[13]

- Devices and equipment use and training: assistive and adaptive device and equipment training during IADLs; orthotic, protective, or supportive device or equipment training during IADLs
- Functional training programs: simulated environments and tasks; task adaptation; task training; travel training
- IADL training: community service training involving instruments; school and play activities training including tools and instruments; work training with tools
- Injury prevention or reduction: injury prevention education during work at job, school, or play; community and leisure integration or reintegration; injury prevention or reduction with use of devices and equipment; safety awareness training during work at job, school, or play; community and leisure integration and reintegration
- Leisure and play activities and training

Table 6.62 **Manual Therapy Techniques**[13]

- Manual traction
- PROM
- Massage: therapeutic massage
- Soft tissue mobilization

Table 6.63 **Biophysical Agents and Modalities**[13]

Biophysical and Modalities

For a review of commonly applied biophysical agents, including indication for use, see Table 4.3 of this text.

Table 6.64 **Patient/Client-Related Instruction**[13]

- Instruction, education, and training of patients/clients and caregivers regarding current condition: pathology; pathophysiology—disease, disorder, or condition; impairments, functional limitations, or disabilities
- Enhancement of performance
- Health, wellness, and fitness
- Plan of care
- Risk factors for pathology; pathophysiology—disease, disorder, or condition; and impairments, functional limitations, or disabilities
- Transitions across settings
- Transitions to new roles

Table 6.65 Airway Clearance Techniques[13]

Breathing Strategies

- Active cycle of breathing or forced expiratory techniques
- Assisted cough/huff techniques
- Autogenic drainage
- Paced breathing
- Pursed lip breathing
- Techniques to maximize ventilation: maximum inspiratory hold
- Staircase breathing
- Manual hyperinflation

Positioning

- Positioning to alter work of breathing
- Positioning to maximize ventilation and perfusion
- Pulmonary postural drainage

Manual and Mechanical Techniques

- Assistive devices
- Chest percussion, vibration, and shaking
- Chest wall manipulation
- Suctioning
- Ventilatory aids

Clinical Practice Guidelines—Neurological Disorders

Clinical Practice Guidelines (CPGs), developed by APTA sections, other organizations, societies, and health care organizations, are based on a systematic review of the evidence and provide therapists with resources to help guide clinical decision-making.[14] The Academy of Neurologic Physical Therapy, a Section of the APTA, provides access to CPGs relevant to the management of patients with neurologic diagnoses. Examples of topics addressed by the Academy of Neurologic Physical Therapy include Vestibular Hypofunction; Locomotion – Chronic CVA, SCI, TBI; Use of AFOs and FES post stroke; Concussion[15]. A full listing and links to the published CPGs can be found at https://www.neuropt.org/practice-resources/anpt-clinical-practice-guidelines.

Cerebral Vascular Accident Interventions

Table 6.66 CVA Intervention Strategies[1,16]

Interventions to Improve Sensory Function

1. Encourage the patient to use the affected extremity.
2. Use sensory stimulation techniques (such as stroking, approximation, superficial, and deep pressure) for functional training.
3. Use feedback and encouragement with the stimulation techniques.

(continued)

Table 6.66 **CVA Intervention Strategies** *(continued)*

4. Use stimulation techniques encouraging the patient's extremities to cross the midline (reaching, PNF).
5. Provide visual, tactile, or proprioceptive stimuli on the affected side (maximizes the patient's attention to the affected side).
6. Do not use intense stimulation to produce withdrawal effects; use pressure splints for deep pressure and joint sensation sensory stimulations.
7. Use the patient and patient's family education for protection of the affected extremity (to prevent trauma to the affected side).

Interventions to Improve Flexibility and Joint Integrity

1. Use daily PROM and AROM exercises in all motions (the PT can also apply joint mobilization) to prevent contractures.
2. Use positioning (with resting splints).
3. Place the affected scapula in protraction and upward rotation to prevent impingement with overhead activities (do not use overhead pulleys).
4. Provide patient education for self-ROM (using the affected UE to horizontally abduct/adduct the unaffected UE to 90°; sitting and leaning forward toward the floor with bilateral UEs).
5. Use weight-shifting activities forward in a modified plantigrade position to stretch the affected plantarflexors.
6. Position the patient supine at the edge of the mat with the affected hip in abduction and extension, knee flexion, and foot placed flat on the floor (or stool) to break the scissoring synergy pattern.

Interventions to Improve Muscular Strength

1. Use strengthening exercises starting with gravity-eliminated powder boards or aquatics (for very weak patients) and continuing with free weights, elastic bands, and isokinetics.
2. Use functional activities and resistive exercises such as step-ups and stair climbing with ankle weights.
3. Use exercise precautions (Valsalva maneuver) with HTN and patients with cardiopulmonary dysfunctions.
4. Use eccentric exercises to decrease cardiovascular stress; use exercises in upright sitting position for HTN.
5. Use safety precautions for patients taking medications (see the safety precautions in Part I).
6. Decrease the risk of injury for older adults with CVA who have been immobilized for long periods of time by starting with concentric low-intensity exercises (instead of eccentric and high-intensity exercises), allowing enough rest periods, and monitoring for fatigue and delayed onset muscle soreness (DOMS).

Interventions to Decrease Spasticity

1. Use appropriate positioning (see the following positioning techniques).
2. Use rhythmic rotation and prolonged stretch.
3. Use slow rocking movements (rocking the patient's body over the elongated limb).
4. Use weight-bearing positioning in kneeling and quadruped positions.
5. Use rotational upper trunk movements in PNF diagonal patterns.
6. Ask the patient to perform side sitting on the affected side to stretch the spastic flexor muscles.
7. Use reciprocal inhibition to reduce tone in the agonist muscles.
8. Use ice wraps or ice packs to decrease neural firing rates.
9. Use relaxation techniques.
10. Use air splints for the affected upper extremity with the patient in a quadruped position with elbow extended.

(continued)

Table 6.66 CVA Intervention Strategies *(continued)*

Interventions to Improve Postural Control and Functional Mobility

1. Rolling: Focus on rolling toward the unaffected side to challenge the affected side. Use the hands' "prayer position" to assist the movement.
2. Supine to sit and back: Focus on rising from the affected side.
3. Sitting: Focus on achieving a symmetrical posture of spine and pelvis and feet flat. Provide verbal and tactile cues to help symmetry. Use the upper extremities in front or at the sides for support in early sitting. Use gentle bouncing on a therapy ball to promote pelvic and trunk alignment. Focus on lateral weight shifts to the affected side to challenge the patient. Scooting-in sitting helps with putting pants on. Coming to the end of the seat to place the feet back under the body helps with transitional movements.
4. Bridging: to develop trunk and hip extensor control for bedpan, pressure relief, scooting, and sit to stand transfers. Include weight shifts and placing hips to the side while bridging. In the beginning, stabilize the foot to achieve the affected left extremity hook-lying position. Use more difficult tasks, such as the patient placing the unaffected foot on a ball while bridging.
5. Sit to stand and sitting down transfers: Ask the patient to use momentum to shift the body forward. Have the patient's feet well back to allow ankle dorsiflexion and assist with forward rotation. Have the patient's hands in prayer position or place the hands in a clasp together on a therapy ball while the patient is moving forward. In the beginning, elevate the patient's seat to decrease hip/knee extension; later lower the seat. Practice small-range movements such as partial squats with the patient against a wall.
6. Standing modified plantigrade: early standing posture to develop postural and extremity control, thereby assisting the quads in extension.
7. Standing: first using a high table or wall support for stabilization, then weight shifting in all positions, and finally reaching in all directions and stepping.
8. Transfers: to both sides, focusing on the affected side. Use different surfaces and heights.

Interventions to Improve Upper-Extremity Function

1. Extended-arm weight-bearing with the hand placed on a support surface: promotes stabilization and decreases flexion synergy.
2. Approximation: for stimulation of the shoulder and scapula stabilizers and elbow extensors.
3. Quadruped position: offers maximal challenge.
4. Reaching: to improve scapular protraction, upward rotation, and elbow, wrist, and finger extension. Beginning reaching starts in side-lying position; advanced reaching includes independently lifting and reaching forward and standing and reaching to pick an object from a shelf.
5. Grasp and manipulation: begins with voluntary gross grasp and release. Voluntary release is more difficult than grasp. The patient needs positioning, stretching, and inhibitory techniques to decrease flexion and increase extension. Use task training such as reaching for an object off a shelf; practice advanced wrist and finger extension with activities such as using utensils to eat, writing, drinking from a cup, or picking up coins.

Interventions to Improve Lower-Extremity Function

1. To activate hip extensors and abductors, dorsiflexors, and knee extensors: Use PNF LE D1 extension; use supine PNF LE D1 flexion; sitting, crossing, and uncrossing the affected LE; standing; step ups; bridging to promote hip extension with knee flexion; lower trunk rotation in side-lying, kneeling, or standing position to decrease retraction and elevation for pelvic control; pelvic shifts while sitting on a therapy ball; hip abduction in hook-lying, supine, side-lying, modified plantigrade, and standing positions.
2. To break up knee hyperextension in standing position: Use foot slides in supine hook-lying position and in sitting; use partial squats.

(continued)

Table 6.66 CVA Intervention Strategies
(continued)

Interventions to Improve Balance

1. Weight shifts first in sitting, then in standing; symmetrical weight bearing in sitting and standing.
2. Shifting toward the affected side in sitting and standing.
3. Weight bearing on the affected hip in sitting and on the affected foot in standing with prohibited unaffected lower-extremity movement or weight bearing.
4. Decrease base of support: sitting—lower extremity uncrossed to crossed; standing—from wide to narrow and tandem; standing on one lower extremity.
5. Change support surfaces: sitting on mat to therapy ball; standing on floor to dense foam.
6. Use sensory inputs: feet on firm surface or foam.
7. Use upper-extremity position and support.
8. Use upper-extremity movements.
9. Use lower-extremity movements.
10. Use trunk movements.
11. Use destabilizing functional activities.
12. Perform dual task training.
13. Change environments: open and closed.
14. Use postural strategies: ankle, hip, medial lateral hip.
15. Use stepping strategies.

Interventions to Improve Locomotion

1. Gait training: Progress the patient from parallel bars and use of assistive devices to no assistive devices; may use an overhead harness and partial body weight support. Maintain the natural rhythm of walking and speed. Encourage the patient to take even steps using verbal cues and/or foot markers placed on the floor. The patient should progress from smaller steps to longer steps, increased distance, and faster speeds. The patient should walk in different environments.
2. Analysis of gait abnormalities.
3. Practice of functional locomotion skills: walking forward, backward, sideward; sidestepping, braiding, step up, step down, lateral step up; stair climbing, step over step; walking on ramps, curbs, uneven terrain, over and around obstacles; crossing the street; stepping on and off an elevator and escalator.
4. Dual-task activities: carrying a tray while walking; walking and talking; bouncing a ball while walking; holding a ball while walking.
5. Treadmill, cycle ergometer, and isokinetic training.
6. Use of orthotics to improve safety. Use the dorsiflexor assist on a temporary basis in the early stages. Use a posterior leaf spring Ankle foot orthosis (AFO) to control for foot drop. Use a solid ankle AFO for maximum stabilization. An AFO set in 5° dorsiflexion limits knee hyperextension; an AFO set in 5° PF stabilizes the knee during midstance.

Interventions to Improve Motor Learning

1. The patient learns the skill in the cognitive stage. The therapist gives simple, clear, verbal instructions, trying not to overload the patient; the patient practices the learned skill or learned component parts of the skill. During this process, correct performance is reinforced, with interventions being provided for errors. Patient's active participation is important. The patient practices skills first on the unaffected side, then on the affected side. The patient can also use mental practice. The patient examines his or her performance; if the patient cannot examine himself or herself accurately, the therapist helps the patient in proper decision making.

(continued)

Table 6.66 CVA Intervention Strategies *(continued)*

2. Feedback may be either intrinsic, occurring naturally as part of the movement response, or extrinsic, as provided by the therapist. Visual inputs, such as patient looking at the movement, are important in early interventions. Proprioception stimulations such as manual contacts, tapping, stretching, antigravity postures, and vibration are important in later learning to enhance the learned skill. In later training, the therapist limits immediate feedback and provides increased sensory stimulations. Pain and fatigue should always be avoided.
3. The patient needs constant practice and repetition for motor learning and recovery. In the beginning, in the hospital, the patient needs adequate rest periods due to decreased endurance. Later, the patient needs variable practice using random practice order to improve performance and for better retention. The learning environment is important, with a closed environment with reduced distractions being offered in the beginning and an open environment with interferences toward the end. Patient motivation needs to be considered by making the therapy session a positive experience and having the patient and family become involved in goal setting.

Table 6.67 Strategies for Right CVA

- Use verbal cues.
- Do not use demonstration or gestures.
- Give frequent feedback.
- Focus on slowing down and controlling movements.
- Focus on the patient's safety.
- Avoid environmental and spatial clutter.
- Do not overestimate the patient's ability to learn.

Table 6.68 Strategies for Left CVA

- Develop an appropriate communication base using words, gestures, and demonstration.
- Assess the patient's level of understanding.
- Give frequent feedback and support.
- Do not underestimate the patient's ability to learn.

Table 6.69 Intervention Strategies for Flaccid, Spastic, and Relative Recovery Stages

Flaccid Stage

The PTA must concentrate on the following interventions:

- Bed mobility turning from supine to side lying and sitting and back
- Pressure splints to provide sensory input and stabilization of the affected extremity and decrease edema
- Use of arm slings / cuff to prevent shoulder subluxation and improve shoulder function
- Use of an arm board or lap tray to provide support for the upper extremity
- Preparation for sitting up

(continued)

Table 6.69 Intervention Strategies for Flaccid, Spastic, and Relative Recovery Stages   *(continued)*

- Preparation for standing up (focus on lower-extremity control)
- Trunk balance
- Stimulation and facilitation techniques to increase tone and voluntary movements

Spasticity Stage

The PTA must concentrate on the following interventions:

- Rehabilitation of patient in the sitting and standing positions as much as possible
- Some treatments started in the flaccid stage in supine position continue in the sitting and standing positions
- Inhibition techniques to decrease spasticity
- Weight bearing on the involved extremity
- Sitting
- Standing
- Progression to treatment in prone lying and kneeling positions
- Gait training with an assistive device
- Working for independent control of affected extremity
- Facilitation techniques for voluntary movement

Relative Recovery Stage

The PTA must concentrate on the following interventions:

- Treatments to improve the patient's gait, balance, and coordination
- Dissociation of mass patterns of movement
- ADLs

Table 6.70 CVA Positioning Techniques

Position the Patient with CVA in Supine Position

- Trunk in midline with head and neck in neutral and symmetrical positions
- A small pillow or towel under the scapula to assist with scapular protraction
- Affected upper limb positioned (on a pillow) in external rotation and abduction with the elbow extended, wrist neutral, and fingers extended
- Hip forward (pelvis protracted) and in neutral position (in regard to rotation), with a small towel under the knee to prevent hyperextension
- Foot and ankle in neutral position (if there is PF, use a splint)
- Nothing placed against the soles of the feet

Position the Patient with CVA in Side-Lying Position on the Unaffected Side

- Head/neck in neutral and symmetrical position; trunk straight in midline position
- Small pillow placed under the unaffected rib cage to elongate the affected side

(continued)

Table 6.70 CVA Positioning Techniques   *(continued)*

- Affected scapula protracted and affected shoulder placed well forward on a supporting pillow
- Elbow extended, wrist neutral, and fingers extended
- Thumb abducted
- Affected hip forward and pelvis protracted
- Affected knee flexed and supported on a pillow

Position the Patient with CVA in Side-Lying Position on the Affected Side

- Head/neck in neutral and symmetrical position; trunk straight in midline position
- Affected upper scapula protracted
- Affected shoulder well forward with elbow extended
- Forearm supinated; wrist neutral
- Fingers extended; thumb abducted
- Affected hip in extension
- Affected knee flexed (another position may be hip and knee in slight flexion with protraction of pelvis)

Position the Patient with CVA Sitting in the Wheelchair (or Chair)

- Head and neck in neutral and symmetrical position
- Spine in extension and aligned in midline position
- Equal weight bearing on both buttocks
- Affected shoulder protracted and forward with elbow supported on a lapboard (or a trough)
- Wrist in neutral position with finger extended and thumb abducted
- Both lower extremities flexed to 90° and in neutral position with regard to rotation

Parkinson's Disease Interventions

Table 6.71 PD Intervention Patterns[1,16]

Interventions to Improve Motor Learning

1. Structured instruction: task-specific learning; structured activities; simple tasks; many repetitions of one activity until learning is achieved; do not overload the patient with new tasks until the initial task is learned
2. Visual cues: brightly colored floor markings during gait training; improve stride length and velocity; decrease shuffling gait
3. Rhythmic auditory stimulation: music or a metronome to increase gait cadence; music for marching in place

Interventions to Improve Relaxation

1. Slow rhythmic rotational movements of the extremities and trunk: PNF diagonal patterns to incorporate rotation; gentle trunk rocking to reduce rigidity; hook-lying position, lower trunk rotation, and rolling in side-lying position; rhythmic initiation; diaphragmatic breathing during PNF diagonal patterns such as PNF D2 flexion and PNF D2 extension
2. Interventions to improve flexibility: PROM and AROM exercises

(continued)

Table 6.71 PD Intervention Patterns *(continued)*

3. PNF diagonal patterns: PNF D2 for bilateral upper-extremity flexion to improve trunk extension and decrease thoracic kyphosis; PNF D1 LE extension to decrease lower-extremity flexed and adducted positions
4. PNF hold–relax or contract–relax technique
5. Light and gentle stretching: hip and knee flexors, ankle plantarflexors, and elbow flexors
6. Prone daily positioning to prevent contracture (early in the disease)
7. Weights to stretch hip and knee flexion contractures (later in the disease)

Interventions to Strengthen Muscles

1. Aquatic exercises: walking pool program; supervised aerobic pool program
2. Aerobic training exercise program: individualized; established by the PT
3. Strength training that focuses on antigravity muscles
4. HEP of daily exercises with moderate duration and intensity: standing corner–wall stretches are effective for kyphotic and forward head posture; overhead flexion and abduction with a cane; modified plantigrade exercises holding lightly at the kitchen countertop; group exercises to increase patient's motivation; patient should not overdo activities and become fatigued
5. Functional training exercises: rhythmic initiation for strengthening exercises; segmental rotation of upper and lower trunk during bed mobility activities; PNF D1 upper-extremity and lower-extremity flexion patterns for movement initiation; anterior and posterior pelvic tilts on a therapy ball to improve pelvic mobility; weight shifting; PNF D2 flexion and D2 extension of upper extremity to increase upper trunk extension; modified wall squats to strengthen hip and knee extensors; modified plantigrade with upper limbs extended on a wall; lateral side stepping; quadruped creeping to teach the patient how to get up from falling; half-kneeling and kneeling as transitional activities

Interventions to Improve Gait

1. Gait training techniques to increase speed, broaden base of support, lengthen stride, improve stepping, facilitate heel to toe pattern, and improve trunk rotation and arm swing
2. Techniques to decrease kyphotic and forward head posture during gait: gait training with an overhead harness instead of an assistive device; walking on a motorized treadmill using an overhead harness
3. Visual (e.g., floor markings) and auditory cues: to walk faster, take larger steps, or swing arms
4. Marching in place with music techniques: to improve step height and increase speed
5. Highlighting of lower trunk rotation during gait: braiding technique of side stepping with alternate crossed stepping
6. Use of different gait training surfaces and techniques: from tile flooring to carpet and outside grass; from eyes open to eyes closed; from closed environment to open environments; from straight flooring to curbs, ramps, and stairs
7. Reduction of freezing episodes during gait: encourage rotational movements or stepping over obstacles

Interventions to Improve Balance

1. Dynamic stability training: weight shifting, reaching, trunk rotation combined with reaching, sitting on a therapy ball
2. Balance-challenging techniques: arms to side, arms folded across chest, feet together, feet apart, arms overhead, single leg raises, stepping, marching in place, functional reach; change the support surface by adding foam or asking the patient to close his or her eyes; as a safety precaution do not use manual displacement because it can cause increased rigidity

(continued)

NEUROLOGIC SYSTEM: DATA COLLECTION AND INTERVENTIONS

Table 6.71 **PD Intervention Patterns** *(continued)*

3. Standing exercises: toe-offs, heel rises, chair rises, modified wall squats, single-limb stance with side kicks, marching in place; as a safety precaution allow the patient to maintain light touch support during standing exercises

Interventions to Improve Cardiopulmonary Function

1. Diaphragmatic breathing exercises
2. Deep breathing training to increase vital capacity
3. Upper-extremity exercises: wrist cuff weights, ergometer, PNF UE bilateral D2 flexion and extension
4. Lower-extremity resistance exercises: ergometer and/or daily walking program; aquatic therapy
5. The PT's individualized aerobic exercise program (based on ACSM guidelines for frequency, intensity, duration, and progression)

Interventions to Promote Patient, Family, and Caregiver Education

1. One-on-one instruction
2. Group sessions
3. Printed materials
4. Computer or video presentations
5. Supportive and positive attitude
6. Support groups

Multiple Sclerosis Interventions

Table 6.72 **MS Intervention Strategies**[1,16]

Interventions to Increase Muscular Strength

1. Use the PT's individualized exercise program for each patient: PT considers the frequency, intensity, type, and time duration of exercise.
2. Avoid exercise fatigue in the patient.
3. Have the patient perform exercises in the morning.
4. Use moderate exercise intensity.
5. Use resistance exercises: free weights, elastic bands, and weight and isokinetic machines.
6. Use circuit training: different stations alternating upper- and lower-extremities exercises.
7. Provide adequate rest periods between exercises.
8. Use slow progression of exercises.
9. Avoid overworking of the patient.
10. Have the patient exercise in a cool environment: prevent overheating; use cooling suits or vests; use aquatic exercises.
11. Do not use free weights with patients having proprioception, incoordination, or tremors.
12. Use written instructions or diagrams with patients having cognitive or memory deficits.
13. Include functional strengthening activities: closed-chain exercises and balance training.
14. Use group exercises to improve the patient's motivation.

Interventions to Increase Flexibility

Use stretching and ROM exercises:
1. Stretch the pectoralis and latissimus dorsi for forward posture deficits.

(continued)

Table 6.72 MS Intervention Strategies   *(continued)*

2. Stretch hip flexors, adductors, hamstrings, and heel cords for patients confined to a wheelchair.
3. Stretch hip and knee extensors and plantarflexors for patients confined to bed.

Interventions to Improve Cardiopulmonary Function[1]

1. Use the PT's individualized aerobic exercise program. The PT needs to test the patient prior to exercise; be cautious with medications' effects and the patient's fatigue.
2. The individualized aerobic exercise program is recommended three times per week, 10-minute sessions, at 50–75% or 50–65% peak VO_2. Recommended exercises are cycling, walking, swimming, water aerobics, or circuit training. Patient education is important for understanding, self-monitoring, safety, and modifications of exercise program.

Interventions to Improve Sensory Deficits

1. Instruct the patient to use adequate lighting all of the time to compensate for visual deficits: use bright light at night; reduce clutter.
2. Give the patient an eye patch for one eye for a double-vision deficit. The eye patch should be used when driving, watching television, or reading; it should not be used all the time.
3. Instruct the patient in skin care, protection, and pressure relief for superficial sensations deficits to prevent decubitus ulcers. The patient should keep the skin clean and dry, inspect the skin daily, and wear comfortable clothes that are soft and not tight. He or she should do push-ups in the chair every 15 minutes and be repositioned in bed every 2 hours. Pressure-relieving devices such as special mattresses, cushions, cuffs, or boots may also be used. The patient should avoid activities that can traumatize skin during transfers, avoid skin contact with hot water or hot objects, and be aware of and seek immediate medical attention for skin blisters or open sores.

Interventions to Decrease Spasticity

1. Use cold packs, ice packs, or cool wraps. Use caution with patients with intact sensations who may develop ANS responses such as increased heart and respiratory rate and nausea.
2. Use ROM exercises early in the disease process.
3. Use stretching exercises: intermittent static stretching for 30–60 seconds for 5–10 repetitions. Use serial casts or air splints. Use stretching as a HEP for the patient and caregiver; teach the patient and caregiver proper stretching techniques. Prevent ballistic stretching. Emphasize stretching the quadriceps, adductors, and plantarflexors, and hamstrings and hip flexors for patients in a wheelchair.
4. Reduce extensor tone. Use lower trunk rotation in side-lying or hook-lying position. The patient may be placed in a hook-lying position, with a therapy ball under the lower legs, and the PTA gently rocking the ball back and forth; the patient may also move from quadruped to side-sitting position.
5. Reduce hypertonicity using inhibitory techniques.
6. Use a positioning schedule for a patient confined to bed or a wheelchair.

Interventions to Decrease Pain

1. Instruct the patient in daily stretching exercises to decrease pain.
2. Use massage and ultrasound to relieve pain.
3. Use postural retraining exercises and orthotic and adaptive devices to decrease pain.
4. Use a soft collar to limit neck flexion for Lhermitte's sign pain.
5. Use aquatic therapy (cooler water) for pain from dysesthesia.
6. Have the patient wear stockings and gloves (neutral warmth technique) for chronic pain relief; be careful that patient is not hot.

(continued)

Table 6.72 MS Intervention Strategies *(continued)*

Interventions to Decrease Fatigue

1. Instruct the patient to avoid heat caused by strenuous activities or environmentally.
2. Use energy conservation: modification of tasks or the environment; use of crutches, walkers, or orthotics; breaking down difficult activities into small parts.
3. Use activity pacing. An activity can be interspaced throughout the day with periodic rest periods. The patient needs to set priorities and limit activities to the most important and enjoyable ones.
4. The PTA should work with the rehabilitation team to help the patient.

Interventions to Increase Balance and Coordination (Especially for Patients with Ataxia)

1. Increase postural stability: joint approximation for shoulders, hips, head, and spine; rhythmic stabilization technique.
2. Promote dynamic postural control: weight shifting, reaching, and stepping activities; aquatic therapy in 85°F water.
3. Promote functional activities: bridging, sit to stand, and scooting activities; real-life functional tasks such as reaching, turning, or bending while sitting or standing; practice transfers from sit to stand and back.
4. Use challenging balance activities: change balance surfaces; decrease base of support; eyes open and eyes closed; use platform training.
5. Stabilize movements. Use light-weight cuffs for ankles or wrists to reduce tremors of limbs and trunk in ambulation; use weighted canes or walkers in ambulation; use a soft collar for head and neck tremors. Take care not to fatigue the patient.
6. Use Frenkel's exercises.

Interventions to Improve Ambulation

1. Use stretching and strengthening exercises: stretch iliopsoas and hamstrings regularly especially if sitting in wheelchair; strengthen mostly hip flexors, ankle dorsiflexors, quadriceps, and hip abductors.
2. Use aquatic exercises, which can reduce tone and fatigue and control ataxia.
3. Use the motorized treadmill (and an overhead harness).
4. Use orthotic devices as necessary: AFO for foot drop and knee hyperextension control; rocker shoes for ankle mobility.
5. Use assistive devices as necessary: walker or crutches to help with fatigue, strength, sensory deficits, and balance.
6. Use wheeled mobility devices for later in the disease: three- or four-wheeled scooters; manual or power wheelchair for postural support and fatigue. Prevent sacral sitting with kyphosis; use gel-cushioned seating, footrests, lap belt, and heel loops.
7. Teach transfers and wheelchair mobility (use transfer board or hydraulic lift).

Interventions to Improve Functionality

1. Use functional mobility training: bed mobility, transfers, gait training.
2. Work with Occupational therapist (OT)/ Certified occupational therapist assistant (COTA) in ADLs.
3. Use adaptive equipment training: raised seats, transfer board, wrist rests for writing or typing, long-handled shoe horns, button hooks, Velcro closures, socks aids; voice amplification for speech; computer-assisted communication system for speech.

Interventions to Improve Speech and Swallowing

1. Use diaphragmatic breathing.
2. Use coughing techniques.

(continued)

Table 6.72 **MS Intervention Strategies** *(continued)*

3. Use upright positioning with slight forward head position and chin parallel to the patient's lap (to avoid aspiration and help with swallowing).
4. Use oral motor exercises to improve function of the mouth (for lip closure, tongue movements, and jaw control).

Interventions to Improve Cognitive Function

1. Use a memory book to log daily events and reminders.
2. Structure the environment (labeling the furniture for immediate use).
3. Give written directions for functional tasks or HEP (such as transfers, positioning, ambulation, self-stretching and strengthening).
4. Assist the caregiver/family to help the patient with directions and cueing.

Traumatic Brain Injury Interventions

Table 6.73 **TBI Intervention Strategies**[1,16]

Rancho Los Amigos (RLA) Levels 1, 2, and 3

1. Prevent contracture development. Use positioning: position the head in neutral, with rolls placed behind the neck and parallel to the head for support and to prevent lateral flexion and rotation. Position the trunk with normal alignment, with rolls behind the shoulders and hips to prevent rotation. Position the upper extremity with a cone or towel in hand to prevent finger flexion. Position the lower extremity with hips and knees in slightly flexed position and a roll between legs to prevent adduction or IR. Turn the patient every 2 hours. Position the patient correctly in a wheelchair/chair: use a reclining wheelchair or tilt-in-space wheelchair; position the head and pelvis in the wheelchair/chair. Prevent foot drop by using boots. Use gentle PROM.
2. Decrease abnormal tone. Use PROM and positioning by maintaining the head and neck in neutral position. Discourage primitive posturing that increases tone. Keep the entire body in proper alignment. Use serial casting for plantarflexion contracture.
3. Maintain skin integrity and prevent decubiti development through frequent position changes (turning every 2 hours).
4. Maintain respiratory status. Prevent respiratory complications through postural drainage, percussion, vibration, and suctioning to keep the airway clear.
5. Use sensory stimulation to improve arousal and elicit movements. Stimulate the auditory, olfactory, visual, tactile, gustatory, kinesthetic, and vestibular systems. After such stimulation, monitor the patient for changes in BP, HR, and respiration. Watch for diaphoresis. Document the patient's motor responses such as grimacing, head turning, vocalization, or changes in posture.
6. Teach the family about the recovery stages, performing ROM exercises, positioning, and sensory stimulation; work with a social worker (SW) to provide support and guidance.
7. Promote early return of functional mobility skills through upright positioning for improved arousal and proper body alignment. Support the patient's neck and head in upright posture; a tilt table may be used to allow weight bearing through the lower extremities.

RLA Level 4

1. Provide consistency through use of team-determined behavioral modification techniques. All team members should be consistent, especially when addressing inappropriate behaviors.
2. Use the same therapist for treatments.

(continued)

Table 6.73 TBI Intervention Strategies *(continued)*

3. Establish a daily routine.
4. Use calm, comforting, and focused behavior.
5. Provide structure and orientation.
6. Do not expect carry-over. The patient learns functional tasks; use charts or graphs to progress the patient with new skills.
7. Expect the patient to be self-centered and do not attempt to change the patient's attitude.
8. Provide safe and functional choices for therapy. Allow the patient to have control over the treatment, but in a safe way, such as asking whether he or she wants to walk or to play with the ball; either choice would be helpful in allowing the patient to have some control without making wrong choices.
9. Provide close supervision in a closed environment to maintain the patient's safety.
10. Teach the family about the patient's aggressive behaviors, so that they will understand and accept them as temporary and short-term behaviors. Teach the family to exhibit consistency.

RLA Levels 5 and 6

1. Continue the interventions from level 4 and focus on maximizing the patient's motor abilities. Watch for mental and physical fatigue signs, such as irritability and decreased performance.
2. Use specific and clear feedback in plain words; do not overwhelm the patient with feedback.
3. Provide verbal and physical assistance.
4. Allow rest periods.
5. Teach compensatory techniques such as dressing with one hand if hemiparesis is present in one upper extremity.
6. Involve the patient in task-specific training.
7. Break down complex tasks into component parts.
8. Provide structure and prevent overstimulation: Provide a daily schedule; use memory logs; work with the patient in a closed, reduced-stimulus environment.
9. Restore movement and functional mobility by using developmental sequence postures.
10. Use relaxation techniques.
11. Teach and emphasize safety with the patient and the patient's family.
12. Teach the family how to assist the patient with functional mobility (such as bed mobility, transfers, gait training, wheelchair mobility), PROM, and strengthening exercises.

RLA Levels 7 and 8

1. Physical therapy general goals are geared toward increasing the patient's independence through weaning from structure and using open environments (instead of closed).
2. The patient should be involved in decision making.
3. The patient needs assistance with behavioral, cognitive, and emotional reintegration (through honest feedback and preparation for community reentry).
4. Promote independence in functional tasks through mobility skills, and ADLs (using real-life environments).
5. Promote improvement of postural control, symmetry, and balance.
6. Encourage the patient to have an active lifestyle and show him or her how to increase cardiovascular endurance.
7. Provide emotional support, and encourage socialization, behavioral control, and motivation.
8. Provide patient and family education about patient compensation for impairments or disabilities; ensure that the family is acquainted with the community resources for TBI.

Spinal Cord Injury Interventions

Table 6.74 SCI Intervention Strategies[1,16]

Improve Respiratory Capacity

1. Teach deep breathing exercises, glossopharyngeal breathing, and strengthening exercises to respiratory muscles (especially diaphragm breathing by using manual contacts below the xiphoid process or weights).
2. Assist coughing: manual contacts over epigastric region by pushing quickly inward and upward while the patient is trying to cough.
3. Use respiratory hygiene with postural drainage, percussion, vibration, and suctioning.
4. Use abdominal support. Use an abdominal corset to support the abdominal contents and assist the diaphragm to rest; it decreases the possibility of orthostatic hypotension.
5. Stretch the pectoral muscles.

Maintain ROM and Prevent Contracture

1. Use PROM daily; watch for contraindicated trunk and hip motion in paraplegia such as SLR more than 60° and hip flexion more than 90° and head/neck motion in tetraplegia.
2. Use positioning. Increase the patient's tolerance to prone positioning; position the ankles at a 90° angle.
3. Use splinting—mostly for wrists, hands, and fingers in the early interventions and for ankles and hips later.
4. Use selective stretching to preserve function (e.g., keeping tight long finger flexors for tenodesis grasp or tight lower trunk for stability).

Maintain Skin Integrity, Free of Decubiti and Other Injury

1. Use a positioning program: prone positioning; gradual upright positioning when the patient is medically stabilized using an abdominal corset and elastic stockings and monitoring vital signs.
2. Use pressure-relieving devices (e.g., cushions, gel cushion, ankle boots).
3. Perform patient education for pressure relief, and pressure relief activities (push-ups) and daily skin inspection (using a long-handled or adapted mirror).
4. Provide prompt treatment of pressure sores.

Improve Strength of All Remaining Innervated Muscles

1. Use selective strengthening during the acute phase of treatment to reduce stress on the spinal segments.
2. Use resistive exercises: manually, or with cuff weights in straight planes or PNF patterns.
3. Strengthen the anterior deltoid, shoulder extensors, biceps, and lower trapezius with tetraplegia and all upper-extremity muscles with paraplegia; emphasize shoulder depressors, triceps, and latissimus dorsi for transfers and gait training.

Reorient the Patient to the Vertical Position

1. Use a tilt table and wheelchair.
2. Use an abdominal binder and elastic lower-extremity wraps to decrease venous pooling.
3. Check for signs and symptoms of orthostatic hypotension (e.g., lightheadedness, syncope, mental or visual blurring, sense of weakness).

(continued)

Table 6.74 SCI Intervention Strategies *(continued)*

Promote Early Return of Functional Mobility Skills and ADLs

1. Emphasize independent rolling using the head, neck, upper extremity, and momentum. Avoid use of adaptive devices such as bed rails or trapezes. When moving the patient from supine to prone, use flexion of the head and neck with rotation; when moving the patient from prone to supine, use extension of the head and neck with rotation. Use bilateral upper-extremities rocking when moving the patient from supine to prone. Cross the patient's ankles with the upper limb in the direction of the roll; use PNF D1 flexion and D2 extension patterns in early rolling.
2. Use bed mobility activities, such as the patient being prone on the elbows for head and neck control, prone on the hands for paraplegia, and supine on the elbows and pull-ups for tetraplegia. Strengthen the biceps and shoulder flexors for wheelchair training.
3. Train the patient to assume sitting for ADLs, transfers, self-ROM, and wheelchair training. For patients with tetraplegia, 100° SLR is required to assume a long sitting position and avoid posterior tilt and sacral sitting. Teach the patient to sit from supine on the elbows or prone on the elbows' positions.
4. Train the patient in quadruped positioning—a lead-up activity for ambulation. The patient can assume a quadruped position from being prone on the elbows by first moving backward on the elbows and then, when the hips are positioned over the knees, putting weight on each hand by extending the elbows. He or she can assume a quadruped position from a long sitting position by rotating the trunk, putting weight on each hand by extending the elbows, and using momentum and strength in the upper extremities and trunk to move in the quadruped position.
5. Train the patient in kneeling position to increase functionality in the trunk and pelvis and to promote upright control. This training is important for ambulation with crutches and KAFOs. The patient can assume a kneeling position from the quadruped position by moving the hands backward until the pelvis drops toward the heels while the therapist gives the patient mat crutches to start practicing.
6. Train the patient in transfers when the patient has good sitting balance. Start with mat transfers first using a sliding board and then without a sliding board; later, advance to other surface transfers. The patient needs to use momentum and muscle substitution depending on his or her functional levels for successful transfer. The patient should train for and practice components of transfers initially, before performing the entire transfer.
7. Teach wheelchair mobility in a customized wheelchair; the wheelchair prescription will be different for each patient depending on the level of injury. Special wheelchair considerations are needed: seat depth 1–2 inches back from the popliteal space, floor-to-seat height measurement considering the seat cushion, back height to allow functionality, fitted seat width and depth, heel loops on footrest, and removable armrests and detachable swing way leg rests.
8. Train the patient to use orthotic devices in ambulation, such as KAFOs, reciprocal gait orthosis (RGO), and AFOs.
9. Train the patient in ambulation using forearm crutches for patients with paraplegia. Use point, two-point, swing-to, or swing-through gait patterns as required.
10. Train the patient in locomotor techniques (where equipment is available).

Guillain-Barré Syndrome Interventions

Table 6.75 Guillain-Barré Syndrome Intervention Strategies[12,16]

Acute-Phase Interventions: Ascending Phase

1. Monitor the respiratory system. Use pulse oximetry to measure the oxygen saturation level in the arterial blood—it should normally be higher than 96%. Use pulmonary physical therapy as necessary to facilitate coughing and airway clearance.

(continued)

Table 6.75 Guillain-Barré Syndrome Intervention Strategies *(continued)*

2. Prevent indirect impairments. Use PROM exercises, positioning, specialty bed, gentle passive stretching, and skin care.
3. Prevent injury to denervated muscles. Use positioning and splinting and do not overuse the denervated muscles; do not overstretch. Provide light exercises using the water buoyancy in the Hubbard tank.

Subacute-Phase Interventions: Descending Phase

1. Provide muscle reeducation. Start with active assistive and active ROM exercises in straight planes and PNF patterns; continue with low- to moderate-intensity resistive exercises. Avoid overuse and fatigue with exercises; allow necessary resting periods between repetitions.
2. Provide functional training, including a gradual return to ADLs and locomotion. Teach energy conservation and activity pacing; avoid overuse and fatigue with activities.
3. Provide cardiovascular fitness and general aerobic conditioning.
4. Provide patient and family education and support.

Amyotrophic Lateral Sclerosis Interventions

Table 6.76 ALS Intervention Strategies[12]

Early-Stage Interventions

1. Patient education should focus on continuing with normal activities as long as possible. Promote the patient's health and wellness. Teach alternative means to accomplish functional activities as the disease progresses. Teach the patient to avoid overworking weakened denervated muscles through energy conservation and activity pacing; teach the patient to monitor fatigue. Teach the patient and family to use equipment and community resources as the disease progresses.
2. Use preventive treatments: AROM, AAROM, stretching, strengthening, and endurance exercises.

Middle-Stage Interventions

1. Continue interventions from the early stage.
2. Maintain the patient's respiratory status; use postural drainage and pectoral muscle stretching.
3. Maintain the patient's functional activities. Avoid overuse of denervated muscles, modify tasks and activities, and monitor the patient's fatigue. Teach wheelchair mobility. Make environmental modifications in the patient's home or work, such as installing grab bars in the bathroom or wheelchair ramps.
4. Consider the rate of disease progression, the area involved, the extent of the disease, the patient's acceptance and motivation, and available psychosocial resources.

Late-Stage Interventions

1. Prevent indirect impairments. Use PROM exercises, positioning, pressure-relieving devices such as a pressure-distributing mattress and gel cushions, a hospital specialty bed, skin care, and pulmonary physical therapy if needed.
2. Relieve pain, muscular spasms, and/or spasticity with modalities such as massage, stretching and PROM, and positioning. Provide family or caregiver education about using a daily PROM program to prevent adhesions, especially for the shoulder; transfer training; positioning; turning in bed; and skin care. Use a mechanical lift if necessary.

(continued)

Table 6.76 ALS Intervention Strategies *(continued)*

3. Address the patient's cervical muscular weakness and pain. Use an orthotic cervical collar—can be soft for mild to moderate weakness or rigid for moderate to severe weakness. Use a recliner chair; use a tilt-in-space or reclining wheelchair.
4. Address the patient's respiratory muscle weakness. Provide patient and caregiver education about energy conservation and activity pacing techniques, signs of aspiration, ways to avoid choking, and manual assisted coughing techniques. Use breathing exercises and positioning.
5. Address the patient's functional activities. Use adaptive equipment to help the patient with ADLs, including eating or feeding utensils. Use orthotic devices—especially for the ankles and knees—to assist with ambulation. Use a wheeled walker or forearm crutches to assist with ambulation.

Recent Advances in Neurological Physical Therapy: Virtual Reality

Table 6.77 Physical Therapy Using Virtual Reality

VR is a new form of physical therapy that offers the following benefits:

- Can improve the following aspects of the patient/client's functionality:
- Executive functioning
- Cortical reorganization
- Balance and trunk control
- Mobility
- Can enhance the patient/client's socialization
- Can increase the following aspects of the patient/client's psychological state:
- Sense of control
- Achievement
- Independence
- Can increase the patient/client's compliance and adherence to physical therapy
- Can be considered a form of pain diversion
- Can help the patient/client to enjoy physical therapy and engage in rehabilitation activities
- Creates a computer-generated interactive environment
- Presents true-life situations
- Is a form of "real-life" training
- Can be individualized to each patient/client
- Can be applied to individuals of all ages
- Can motivate the patient/client to learn different tasks
- Creates an objective measurement of physical therapy results (e.g., measuring the range of motion, the frequency of exercises, and the number of repetitions)
- Has a long-term impact on the patient/client's outcome
- Can be applied to remote locations as long as the patient/client has a computer

(continued)

Table 6.77 Physical Therapy Using Virtual Reality

(continued)

- Provides for continuity of care
- Can lower the cost of physical therapy
- Affects the sensory system such as vision, hearing, proprioception, touch, balance, and coordination
- Affects the motor systems for training and retraining

Table 6.78 Research-Documented Physical Therapy Using VR

1. Stroke rehabilitation: used for physical therapy for hand, thumb, fingers, balance, and gait training and retraining.
2. Multiple sclerosis and Parkinson's disease: to increase patients' walking speed and stride length.
3. Traumatic brain injury: helping patients/clients to relearn and practice planning skills, activities of daily living, and driving skills.
4. Nonpharmacologic pain control and pain reduction. Pain levels decreased from severe to mild/moderate during physical therapy ROM exercises for patients with multiple blunt-force trauma injuries (e.g., multiple fractures and internal injuries) and for patients with burn injuries. Patients' range of motion increased by 1° after just 1 day of VR therapy and by 15° during the second day of VR therapy.
5. Children with cerebral palsy, attention-deficit/hyperactivity disorder (ADHD), and autism: to improve attention, social and communication behaviors, cognitive skills, postural control, safety, and motor skills.[16,17]
6. Trunk control, limb use, balance, mobility, and gross and fine motor movements.

NEUROLOGIC SYSTEM: DATA COLLECTION AND INTERVENTIONS

Physical Therapy Interventions for the Neurological Patient in Acute Care

Table 6.79 Types of General Neurological Impairments and Physical Therapy Interventions in Acute Care[1,3]

- Increased/decreased sensation: tactile input; positioning; splinting; prevention of injury; patient/family education regarding awareness of the involved area and use of compensatory strategies (such as visual)
- Fatigue: strengthening of large muscle groups to compensate for getting fatigue early in the task; patient/family education not to overexert (may cause exacerbation of condition)
- Pain management: limiting sensory input; positioning and turning the patient; maintaining ROM; use of various modalities; use of alternative medicine if necessary
- Decreased endurance: use of a decreased number of repetitions/sets while applying therapeutic exercises; monitoring the patient for fatigue; utilization of assistive devices to conserve energy; prioritization of tasks; breathing exercises for cardiovascular conditioning
- Decreased ROM: stretching exercises (gentle); use of bracing and casting as necessary; if the patient has pain with mobility training, use of pain management (modalities, soft-tissue therapy); preserving biomechanical alignment to increase functional outcomes
- Gait deficits: increasing gait distance gradually, with rest periods between ambulation; using assistive devices and stand-by assistance; using orthotic devices; using a wheelchair while gait training; using encouragement and maintaining ambulation for functional tasks
- Decreased balance: apply interventions for proprioception to improve balance; provision of patient/family education on preventing falls; promotion of functional independence; promotion of a safe environment
- Visual impairment: using an eye patch for diplopia; checking for additional visual impairments such as nystagmus and vestibulo-ocular reflex; application of physical therapy interventions while being aware not to cause nausea or impair patient's safety
- Altered levels of consciousness and potential for cognitive and behavioral problems: work closely with other disciplines to maintain overall care of patient; work closely with the PT as patient emerges from coma; use simple commands, maintain clear communication with patient; treat patient in quiet areas with minimal distraction; provide time for processing instructions.
- Impaired respiratory function: patient may use a ventilator or have weakened muscles of respiration and impaired cough function; may need strengthening of muscles of respiration, assisted cough technique, abdominal binder to improve diaphragm function, postural drainage.

Transient Ischemic Attack

Table 6.80 Characteristics of TIA

- Temporary interruption of blood supply to the brain
- Precursor to cerebral vascular accident (CVA): approximately 10–20% of patients having TIA will have a CVA within 90 days
- Can last less than 24 hours
- Causes: emboli, reduced cerebral perfusion (arrhythmias), decreased cardiac output, hypotension, excessive use of antihypertensive medications, cerebrovascular spasm (subclavian steal syndrome—shunting blood from the left vertebrobasilar artery toward an occluded left subclavian artery and into the left arm)

Cerebral Vascular Accident

Table 6.81 Types of CVA and Their Clinical Characteristics[1]

Anterior Cerebral Artery (ACA) Syndrome

- Contralateral hemiparesis (mainly the lower extremities)
- Contralateral hemisensory loss (mainly the lower extremities)
- Urinary incontinence
- Apraxia: inability to perform purposeful movements, although there is no sensory or motor impairments
- Abulia (akinetic mutism), slowness, delay, and lack of spontaneity
- Contralateral grasp reflex and sucking reflex

Middle Cerebral Artery (MCA) Syndrome

- Contralateral hemiparesis (involving mainly the upper extremities and face)
- Contralateral hemisensory loss (involving mainly the upper extremities and face)
- Broca's (nonfluent) aphasia: limited vocabulary and slow and hesitant speech
- Wernicke's (fluent) aphasia: impaired auditory comprehension and fluent speech (with normal rate and melody)
- Global aphasia: nonfluent speech with poor comprehension
- Perceptual deficits with unilateral neglect, depth perception, spatial relations, and agnosia (inability to recognize or comprehend sights, sounds, words or other sensory information)
- Limb-kinetic apraxia: inability to perform purposive movements, although there are no sensory or motor impairments
- Contralateral homonymous hemianopsia: blindness in one-half of the visual field
- Loss of conjugate gaze to the opposite side (the paired movements of the eyes as they track moving objects)
- Sensory ataxia (impairment of muscular coordination resulting from problems in conduction of sensory responses from muscles) of the contralateral limb
- Pure motor hemiplegia

Internal Carotid Artery (ICA) Syndrome

- Occlusion of the internal carotid artery with a massive infarction in the region of middle cerebral artery that supplies blood to the brain
- Effects ranging from edema to uncal herniation, coma, and death

Posterior Cerebral Artery (PCA) Syndrome

- Contralateral homonymous hemianopsia (visual cortex involved)
- Bilateral homonymous hemianopsia
- Visual agnosia
- Prosopagnosia (difficulty naming people)
- Dyslexia (difficulty reading) without agraphia (difficulty writing)
- Anomia (color naming) and color discrimination
- Memory defect
- Topographic disorientation

NEUROLOGIC SYSTEM: DATA COLLECTION AND INTERVENTIONS

(continued)

Table 6.81 Types of CVA and Their Clinical Characteristics   *(continued)*

Vertebrobasilar Artery Syndrome

Can produce a wide variety of symptoms with ipsilateral and contralateral signs such as locked-in syndrome (with quadriplegia and coma, but good cognition) or other syndromes.

Cerebellar Hemorrhage

- Ataxia and motor weakness
- Nystagmus
- Dizziness
- Nausea and vomiting
- Impairment in postural control

Table 6.82 Medical Interventions for CVA[1,12]

- Past medical history
- Physical examination
- Diagnostic testing: Lab values; Electrocardiogram (ECG); Scanning imaging (CT scan, MRI); Transcranial Doppler (TCD); Ultrasound for blood velocity test; MRA (magnetic resonance angiography for blood flow); Positron Emission Tomography (PET)
- Manage elevated BP, raise lowered BP.
- Manage cerebral edema, control intracranial pressure.
- Oxygen by mask or canula to maintain oxygenation.
- Thrombolytic and antithrombotic agents for management of ischemic stroke.
- Anticoagulation therapy (heparin, warfarin)
- Antiplatelet therapy (aspirin, ticlopidine)
- Surgery: endarterectomy; aneurysm repair.

Table 6.83 Physical Therapy Interventions for CVA

- Physical therapy starts when the patient is medically stabilized (approximately within 72 hours). The PT or PTA should continuously monitor the patient for risk of medical emergencies (such as hypertension, arrhythmia, DVT, or another stroke).
- Focus on positioning in bed, chair, and wheelchair to reduce risk of contractures.
- Provide early stimulation of the hemiparetic side to avoid learned non-use.
- Ensure early mobilization (gait training); consider strengthening of the involved lower extremity; consider the patient's previous deconditioning.
- Promote stability of the involved upper extremity; improve motor control of the affected region; prevent injury to the affected shoulder; watch for painful shoulder syndrome; use the FES protocol for shoulder subluxation.
- Promote skill acquisition to enable ADL and functional recovery
- Facilitate lifestyle changes, to include daily exercise.
- Consider the patient's individual goals.
- Provide patient and family education from an early stage.

Post Spinal Cord Injury: Interventions

- During the acute and subacute stage of rehabilitation the PT and PTA should consider the patient's need for assistive devices, mobility devices and orthotics.
- Prevent secondary complications i.e., pressure sores, contractures, respiratory dysfunction.
- Recognize that patients with SCI will require fracture stabilization and may have undergone closed or open reduction. Effectively manage the patient with stabilization orthotics including patients with a thoracolumbosacral orthosis (TLSO) or Halo vest.

Table 6.84 Post Spinal Cord Injury: Physical Therapy Interventions[1,3]

High Cervical Levels (C2–C3 and C4)

- Breathing exercises
- Inspiratory muscle training
- PROM and positioning
- Strengthening exercises
- Patient/family/caregiver education
- Monitoring for autonomic dysreflexia (see **Table 6.55**)

Lower Cervical Levels (C5 to T1)

- Positioning
- Weight shifting
- Functional mobility training
- Strengthening exercises that include the respiratory muscles
- Patient/family/caregiver education
- Monitoring for autonomic dysreflexia

High Thoracic Levels (T2–T6)

- Positioning
- Weight shifting
- Functional mobility training that includes a standing program
- Respiratory exercises
- Patient/family/caregiver education
- Monitoring for autonomic dysreflexia

Low Thoracic Levels (T7–T12)

- Functional mobility training that includes a standing program
- Respiratory exercises
- Weight-shifting training
- Patient/family/caregiver education

Lumbar Injury Levels (L1–L5)

- Functional mobility training that includes gait training
- Weight-shifting training
- Patient/family/caregiver education

NEUROLOGIC SYSTEM: DATA COLLECTION AND INTERVENTIONS

(continued)

Table 6.84 Post Spinal Cord Injury: Physical Therapy Interventions   *(continued)*

Lumbar and Sacral Levels

- Functional mobility training that includes gait training
- Weight-shifting training
- Patient/family/caregiver education

Parkinson's Disease and Parkinsonism: Physical Therapy Interventions

Table 6.85 Parkinson's Disease and Parkinsonism: Physical Therapy Interventions

- Transfer training and bed mobility training (turning and reaching activities) facilitate patients' functional mobility and prevent falls.
- Gait reeducation with focus on step length and height, reciprocal arm swing.
- Flexibility and ROM exercises, i.e., Tai-Chi and yoga, can decrease ROM deficits, and preserve motion and ability to perform functional tasks. Examples of ROM exercises using PNF include PNF patterns (bilateral D2 flexion for the upper extremities to promote upper trunk extension and prevent kyphosis; D1 extension—hip extension, abduction, and IR) for the lower extremities to counteract flexion and adduction.
- Posture reeducation to minimize stooped and kyphotic posture.
- Therapeutic strengthening exercises can strengthen specific muscle groups and prevent deconditioning.
- Cardiopulmonary conditioning using bicycle or/and treadmill.
- Treadmill training for gait dysfunction can promote mobility for aerobic conditioning.
- Patient education to focus attention to the task can decrease the slowness of movement.
- Observe the patient for symptoms of depression; encourage, educate, and praise the patient regarding his or her efforts and ability to perform tasks.
- Physical therapy goals must be patient centered.
- Utilize cueing to assist and improve the patient's motor performance (by correcting deficits). Auditory cues are beneficial for akinesia; cues for the patient to take longer steps can assist with gait deficits.
- Teach balance exercises; can prevent falls and promote the patient's functional independence.

Traumatic Brain Injury: Medical and Physical Therapy Management

Table 6.86 Medical Management of Traumatic Brain Injury[12]

- Glasgow Coma Scale: used to determine level of consciousness. Tests the function of the brain stem and the cerebrum using the patient's eye, motor, and verbal responses. Scores from 13 to 15 indicate mild brain injury; 9 to 12 indicate moderate brain injury; and 8 and lower indicate severe brain injury.

(continued)

Table 6.86 **Medical Management of Traumatic Brain Injury**   *(continued)*

- Diagnostic Testing: computed tomography (CT); magnetic resonance imaging (MRI); functional magnetic resonance imaging (fMRI); positron emission tomography (PET); neuropsychologic testing; assessment and monitoring of intracranial pressure (ICP); Visual/auditory/somatosensory evoked potential examinations.[1]

- Medical care interventions post TBI: resuscitation; management of respiratory dysfunction including intubation and ventilation as indicated; cardiovascular monitoring—management of BP; treatment of increased intracranial pressure (using pharmacological, mechanical, or surgical procedures); maintenance of fluid and electrolyte balance; maintenance of nutrition, and eye and skin care; prevention of contractures; postural drainage; patient's safety.

Table 6.87 **Physical Therapy Management of Traumatic Brain Injury**[1,12]

- The PT and PTA are part of the interdisciplinary team that is characterized by open communication between all members of the team and open mindedness.

- Recognize importance of positioning for patients with TBI to prevent untoward events. Patients with increased ICP should be positioned with head elevated to about 30 deg. Patients with a nasogastric feeding tube should not be allowed to lie flat and an elevated head position of 30 deg is also indicated.

- General physical therapy goals may include the following: increase the patient's physical function and alertness level; reduce the risk of secondary impairments; improve motor control; decrease the effects of abnormal tone; improve postural control; increase the patient's tolerance to activities and positions; emphasize mobility, joint integrity, and function.

- Interventional goals in acute care may include the following (depending on the Ranchos Los Amigos [RLA] level): decrease abnormal posturing and primitive reflexes; improve the patient's arousal level (using sensory stimulation); manage the effects of abnormal tone and spasticity; maintain joint integrity.

- Examples of interventions in acute care may include the following (depending on the RLA level): sensory stimulation; flexibility exercises (PROM and/or AROM); bed and wheelchair positioning; patient and family education; transition to sitting when medically stable; progress to tilt table and functional tasks in sitting and supported standing; developmental sequence postures.

NEUROLOGIC SYSTEM: DATA COLLECTION AND INTERVENTIONS

Pharmacology for Neurological Pathologies

Table 6.88 Common Medications for Neurologic Conditions[18]

*Classes of Drugs	Purpose of Medication	*Common Side Effects	PTA Implications
Sedative hypnotics			
Benzodiazepines ■ Temazepam (Restoril) ■ Triazolam (Halcion) ■ Flurazepam (Dalmane)	■ Calm the patient ■ Facilitate normal sedation and sleep	■ Next day effects of drowsiness and ↓ motor performance ■ Hangover feeling the next day ■ Anterograde amnesia	■ ↑ fall risk ■ Poor memory recall of: WB status/precautions/contra-indications ■ ↑ full cooperation of patient (less anxious) ■ Potential drug tolerance ■ Potential addiction
Barbiturates ■ Amobarbital (Amytal) ■ Pentobarbital (Nembutal) ■ Phenobarbital (Solfoton)	■ CNS depressants ■ Sleep aids	■ Same as above	■ Same as above
Anti-Anxiety			
■ **Benzodiazepines** ■ Valium (diazepam) ■ Alprazolam (Xanax) ■ Clonazepam (Klonopin) ■ Lorazepam (Ativan)	■ Anti-anxiety	■ Same as above ■ Skeletal muscle relaxation ■ Rebound anxiety if stopped abruptly	■ Dizziness, drowsiness, lethargy, hypotension, drug dependence, drug tolerance, blurred vision, respiratory depression
■ **Other Anti-anxiety medications** ■ Buspirone (Buspar)	■ General anxiety disorders	■ Drowsiness ■ Personality changes ■ Nausea ■ Rashes ■ Sweating	■ Dizziness, drowsiness, fatigue, headache, blurred vision, tachycardia, myalgia, ataxia, paresthesia
Anti-Depressant			
Tricyclics ■ Amitriptyline (Elavil) ■ Doxepin (Sinequan) ■ Nortriptyline (Aventyl)	■ Treatment of depression	■ Sedation, ■ Orthostatic hypotension ■ Cardiac arrhythmias ■ Seizures	■ Drowsiness, confusion, tachycardia, orthostatic hypotension, hypotension, risk of seizures, increased fall risk,

(continued)

Table 6.88 Common Medications for Neurologic Conditions   *(continued)*

*Classes of Drugs	Purpose of Medication	*Common Side Effects	PTA Implications
MAO inhibitors ■ Phenelzine (Nardil) ■ Tranylcypromine (Parnate)	■ Treatment of depression	■ CNS excitation ■ Agitation ■ Tremor ■ Confusion ■ Hypertension ■ edema	■ Risk for hypertensive crisis, dizziness, fatigue, drowsiness, orthostatic hypotension, weakness, anxiety, paresthesia, fall risk
Second Generation Drugs ■ Fluoxetine (Prozac) ■ Paroxetine (Paxil) ■ Sertraline (Zoloft)	■ Treatment of depression	■ Risk of seizures ■ Sedation ■ Anxiety ■ Insomnia ■ Nausea	■ Anxiety, tremor, myalgia, dizziness, palpitations
Antipsychotics			
■ Aripiprazole (Abilify) ■ Chlorpromazine (Thorazine) ■ Haloperidol (Haldol) ■ Thioridazine (Mellaril)	■ Severe forms of mental illness—e.g., schizophrenia, psychosis ■ Alzheimer's agitation and confusion	■ Dysphagia ■ Tardive Dyskinesia ■ Sedation ■ Parkinsonian-like symptoms ■ Restlessness ■ Dystonia/dyskinesia ■ Neuroleptic Malignant Syndrome (NMS): Catatonia, stupor, rigidity, tremors, fever ■ Blurred vision ■ Dry mouth ■ Constipation ■ Urinary retention ■ Orthostatic hypotension	■ ↑ fall risk, orthostatic hypotension, sedation, blurred vision ■ Enhanced participation ■ Monitor for dyskinesia or other motor changes and notify medical staff immediately
Antiepileptic			
First-Generation Medications ■ Phenobarbital (Solfoton) ■ Amobarbital (Amytal)	■ Controls seizure activity in the brain for either partial seizures or general seizures ■ Same as above	■ Sedation ■ Nystagmus ■ Ataxia ■ Behavioral changes ■ GI irritation	■ Be aware of the patient's seizure plan if one is in place ■ Monitor for any changes in mm weakness, GI issues, behavioral changes

NEUROLOGIC SYSTEM: DATA COLLECTION AND INTERVENTIONS

(continued)

Table 6.88 Common Medications for Neurologic Conditions   *(continued)*

*Classes of Drugs	Purpose of Medication	*Common Side Effects	PTA Implications
■ Secobarbital (Seconal) ■ Clonazepam (Klonopin) ■ Diazepam (Valium) ■ Lorazepam (Ativan) ■ Phenytoin (Dilantin) ■ Carbamazepine (Tegretol) ■ Valproic acid (Depakote) **Second-Generation Medications** ■ Gabapentin (Neurontin) ■ Levetiracetam (Keppa) ■ Topiramate (Topomax) ■ Zonisamide (Zonegran)	■ Gabapentin is sometimes used for neuropathic pain syndromes	■ Dizziness ■ Headaches ■ Hirsutism ■ Dyskinesia ■ Akinesias ■ Temporary hair loss ■ Weight gain or loss ■ Impaired platelet function ■ Sedation ■ Fatigue ■ Dizziness ■ Ataxia ■ Generalized weakness ■ Loss of appetite	■ Beware of extra-pyramidal symptoms ■ Clinical environment triggers: lights, sounds, smells ■ Consider medication dosing and appointment scheduling if possible ■ Monitor for medication toxicity and report this immediately to a medical professional
Parkinson Disease			
■ Levodopa (Sinemet CR) ■ Bromocriptine (Parlodel) ■ Pergolide (Permax) ■ Amantadine (Symmetrel) ■ Benztropine (Cogentin) ■ Pramiperoxole (Mirapex)	■ Dopaminergic replacement therapy ■ Levodopa crosses the blood-brain barrier to transform into dopamine ■ Dopamine agonist medications (Pergolide, Bromcriptine) to decrease on-off effects (can be used alone or in combination with L-Dopa)	■ GI issues (carbidopa given with levodopa to ↓ GI issues) ■ Cardiac arrhythmias ■ Postural hypotension ■ Dyskinesia ■ ↓ effectiveness of L-dopa with prolonged use ■ On-off phenomenon Off= spontaneous reduction of L-dopa = worsening of symptoms; On = restored movement after taking L-dopa ■ Constipation and motility issues ■ Dyskinesia, dystonia ■ Decreased long term effectiveness with Levodopa	■ Coordinate PT 1 hour after taking Levodopa ■ Elderly schedule within an hour of their breakfast dose = < fatigue ■ If on drug holiday (3 days up to 3 weeks) treatment focus = maintain patient mobility Also = ↑ ↑ fall risk BP monitoring due to postural hypotension, dizziness, syncope, increased fall risk

(continued)

Table 6.88 Common Medications for Neurologic Conditions *(continued)*

*Classes of Drugs	Purpose of Medication	*Common Side Effects	PTA Implications
Skeletal Muscle Relaxants			
■ Baclofen (Lioresal)† ■ Dantrolene sodium (Dantrium)† ■ Diazepam (Valium)† ■ Gabapentin (Neurontin)† ■ Tizanidine (Zanaflex)† ■ Botulinum Toxin (Botox)†	■ †Indicated for CNS-related spasticity associated with SCI, MS ■ ††Used for skeletal muscle spasms related to PNS injury ■ †††Anticonvulsant medication used as an adjunct to other drugs for CNS dysfunctions related to SCI and MS	■ Long-term use of anti-spasmodic medications can result in sedation, physical dependence, or addiction ■ Anti-spasticity medications used to treat CNS dysfunctions may affect tone-reducing effects which may impede the reliance on muscle tone to assist in functional tasking (i.e., extensor tone in lower extremity would be reduced, thereby predisposing the patient to falls)	■ Sedation ■ Generalized muscle weakness ■ Liver toxicity - jaundice ■ Improved ability to participate in PT if well controlled with medications ■ PTA may need to schedule PT around dosing schedules to allow for optimal alertness during treatment
Medications to Manage Alzheimer's Dementia			
■ Donepezil (Aricept) ■ Memantine (Namenda)	■ Dementia management	■ Nausea/vomiting ■ Diarrhea ■ Insomnia ■ Dizziness ■ Weight loss ■ Muscle cramps ■ Drowsiness ■ Fatigue	■ ↑ fall risk ■ Hypertension

* Brand names associated with classes of medications and side effects found within this table are not representative of an all-inclusive list. It is incumbent on the clinician to research an appropriate drug information resource to obtain complete information about medications that patients may use while attending rehabilitation.
† The drugs have multi-purposes even though they are listed as skeletal muscle relaxants.

NEUROLOGIC SYSTEM: DATA COLLECTION AND INTERVENTIONS

References

1. O'Sullivan SB, Schmitz TJ. *Physical Rehabilitation.* 5th ed. Philadelphia, PA: F.A. Davis Company; 2007.
2. Rothstein JM, Roy SH, Wolf SH, Scalzitti DA. *The Rehabilitation Specialist's Handbook.* 3rd ed. Philadelphia, PA: F.A. Davis Company; 2005.
3. Umphred D, Lazaro RT. *Neurorehabilitation for the Physical Therapist Assistant.* 2nd ed. Thorofare, NJ: SLACK Incorporated; 2014.
4. Fruth SJ, Fawcett C. *Fundamentals of Tests and Measures for The Physical Therapist Assistant.* Burlington, MA: Jones and Bartlett Learning; 2020.
5. Standard neurological classification of spinal cord injury. asia-spinalinjury.org. http://asia-spinalinjury.org. Updated 2016. Accessed March 2016.
6. Stroke Engine. Constraint induced movement therapy—Upper extremity. https://strokengine.ca/en/interventions/constraint-induced-movement-therapy-upper-extremity/. Accessed August 2, 2021.
7. Taub E, Uswatte G, Morris DM.Improved motor recovery after stroke and massive cortical reorganization following constraint induced movement therapy. *Phys Med Rehabil Clin North Am.* 2003;*14*(1 suppl):S77–S91.
8. Kim YH, Park JW, Ko MH, Jang SH, Lee PK.Plastic changes of motor network after constraint induced movement therapy. *Yonsei Med J.* 2004;*45*:241–246.
9. Taub E, Uswatte G, Pidikiti R.Constraint induced movement therapy: A new approach to treatment in physical rehabilitation. *Rehabil Psychol.* 1998;*43*:152–170.
10. Reiss AP, Wolf SL, Hammel EA, McLeod EL, Williams EA.Constraint-induced movement therapy (CIMT): Current perspectives and future directions. *Stroke Research and Treatment.* 2012; *2012*:159391. doi:10.1155/2012/159391.
11. Centers for Disease Control. Mild TBI and concussion. https://www.cdc.gov/traumaticbraininjury/concussion/index.html. Accessed May 20, 2021.
12. Goodman CC, Fuller KS. *Pathology for the Physical Therapist Assistant.* 2nd ed. St. Louis, MO. Elsevier; 2017.
13. American Physical Therapy Association. Guide to physical therapist practice. Interventions. https://guide.apta.org/interventions. Updated August 1, 2014. Accessed February 3, 2021.
14. APTA. Clinical practice guidelines. https://www.apta.org/patient-care/evidence-based-practice-resources/cpgs. Accessed February 3, 2021.
15. Academy of Neurologic Physical Therapy. Practice resources—Clinical practice guidelines. https://www.neuropt.org/practice-resources/anpt-clinical-practice-guidelines. Accessed May 20, 2021.
16. *American Physical Therapy Association. Guide to Physical Therapist Practice.* 2nd ed. Alexandria, VA: APTA: 2001; revised 2003; revised 2014 for educational purposes.
17. Wang M, Reid D.Virtual reality in pediatric neurorehabilitation: Attention deficit hyperactivity disorder, autism and cerebral palsy. *Neuroepidemiology.* 2011;*36*:2–18.
18. Ciccone CD. *Pharmacology in Rehabilitation.* 4th ed. Philadelphia, PA: F.A. Davis; 2007.

Cardiopulmonary Interventions

CARDIOPULMONARY INTERVENTIONS

Review of Cardiopulmonary System and Anatomy

Overview of the Heart

See **Figures 7.1** and **7.2**.

Figure 7.1 Anatomy of the heart
Anatomy and Physiology: Understanding the Human Body by Robert K. Clark, page 293, Figure 16.4 "Anatomy of the Heart"

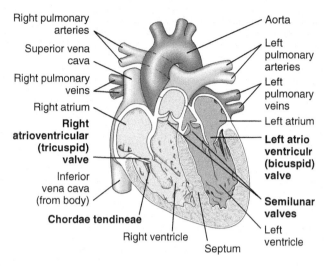

Right pulmonary arteries

Superior vena cava

Right pulmonary veins

Right atrium

Right atrioventricular (tricuspid) valve

Inferior vena cava (from body)

Chordae tendineae

Right ventricle

Septum

Aorta

Left pulmonary arteries

Left pulmonary veins

Left atrium

Left atrio ventriculr (bicuspid) valve

Semilunar valves

Left ventricle

Figure 7.2 Heart valves
Human Biology: Fifth edition by Daniel D. Chiras, page 111, Figure 6.4(a) "Heart Valves"

Table 7.1 Heart Tissue, Chambers, and Valves and Their Functions

Heart Tissue	Heart Chambers: Pumps Working in Sequence	Heart Valves: One-Way Flow of Blood
Pericardium: protective tissue that surrounds the heart	Right atrium: receives deoxygenated blood from the body through superior and inferior vena cava; occurs in the systolic phase. Blood is sent to the right ventricle. The right atrium is separated from the left atrium by the interatrial septum (wall).	Atrioventricular valves: prevent backflow of blood into the atria during ventricular systole (close when ventricular walls contract) Atrioventricular valves: tricuspid valve (right heart valve); bicuspid or mitral valve (left heart valve)
Epicardium: inside layer of pericardium	Right ventricle: pumps blood to the lungs for oxygenation via the pulmonary artery. The right ventricle is separated from the left ventricle by an interventricular septum (wall) that is thicker than the interatrial septum.	Semilunar valves: prevent backflow of blood from the aorta and pulmonary arteries into ventricles during diastolic phase Semilunar valves: pulmonary valve (prevents right backflow) and aortic valve (prevents left backflow)
Myocardium: heart muscle (major portion of heart)	Left atrium: receives oxygenated blood from the lungs (during the systolic phase); blood is sent to the left ventricle.	
Endocardium: smooth lining of the inner surface and the heart cavities	Left ventricle: pumps blood throughout entire systemic circulation via the aorta. The left ventricle is stronger than the right ventricle; it has thicker walls than the right ventricle so that it can pump the blood throughout the entire body.	

Arteries and Veins of the Body

See **Figures 7.3** and **7.4**.

Figure 7.3 Arteries of the body

Anatomy and Physiology: Understanding the Human Body by Robert K. Clark, page 304, Figure 16.17 "Overview of the arteries"

Figure 7.4 Veins of the body
Anatomy and Physiology: Understanding the Human Body by Robert K. Clark, page 306, Figure 16.19 "Overview of the veins"

Overview of the Coronary Circulation (Hemodynamics)

See **Figure 7.5**.

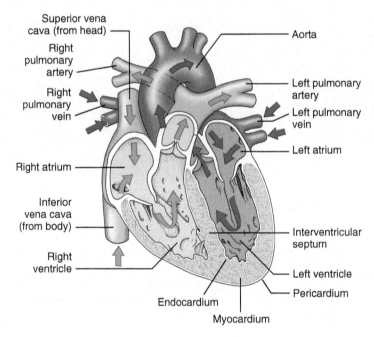

Figure 7.5 Pulmonary and systemic circulation
Human Biology: Fifth edition by Daniel D. Chiras, page 109, Figure 6.2 "Blood Flow Through the Heart"

Table 7.2 Coronary Circulation

1. Deoxygenated blood from the superior and inferior vena cava enters the heart by moving into the right atrium.
2. Blood passes down through the tricuspid valve from the right atrium to the right ventricle.
3. Blood passes through the pulmonary valve from the right ventricle into the pulmonary artery and pulmonary capillaries.
4. Gas exchange takes place in the pulmonary alveoli.
5. Oxygenated blood from the pulmonary veins passes to the left atrium.
6. Oxygenated blood passes down through the bicuspid (mitral) valve into the left ventricle.
7. Oxygenated blood goes down to the apex of the heart; during the heart's systole, it is moved from the apex of the heart to the left ventricle outflow tract and through the aortic valve into the aorta.

Blood Supply to the Heart

Table 7.3 Right Coronary Artery and Left Coronary Artery (Has Left Anterior Descending Artery and the Circumflex Artery

- Right coronary artery (RCA) supplies: right atrium; right ventricle; inferior wall of the left ventricle; atrioventricular (AV) node; Bundle of His; sinoatrial (SA) node (60% of the time)
- Left coronary artery (LCA) supplies: most of the left ventricle
- Left anterior descending (LAD) artery supplies: left ventricle; right ventricle; interventricular septum; inferior area of the apex of the heart; inferior areas of the right and left ventricles
- Circumflex artery supplies: lateral and inferior walls of the left ventricle; portion of the left atrium; SA node (40% of the time)

Overview of the Electrical Conduction of the Heart

See **Figure 7.6**.

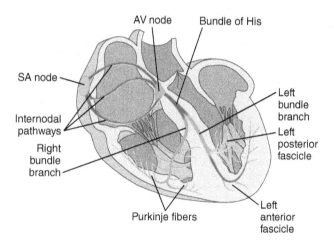

Figure 7.6 The electrical conduction system within the myocardium

Table 7.4 Conduction of the Heartbeat

- The heart has specialized conduction tissue that allows rapid transmission of electrical impulses in the myocardium (called normal sinus rhythm [NSR]). The specialized conduction tissue includes Purkinje fibers (specialized conduction tissue in both ventricles) and nodal tissue.

- The SA node initiates the electrical impulse; it is the main pacemaker of the heart. The SA node is located at the junction of the superior vena cava and the right atrium. It has both sympathetic and parasympathetic innervations, which affect the heart rate and the strength of the contraction.

- The AV node merges with the Bundle of His. The AV node is located at the junction of the right atrium and right ventricle. It has sympathetic and parasympathetic innervations.

- Contraction of the heart tissue is called systole.

- Relaxation of the heart tissue is called diastole.

- The conduction of the heartbeat starts in the SA node. The electrical impulse spreads throughout both atria (which contract together). The impulse stimulates the AV node. The impulse is transmitted down the Bundle of His to the Purkinje fibers. The impulse spreads throughout both ventricles (which contract together).

Table 7.5 Myocardial Fibers and Metabolism

- Myocardial fibers are muscle tissue made of striated muscle fibers with many mitochondria. The myocardial fibers contract as a functioning unit.

- Myocardial metabolism is essentially aerobic; it is sustained by continuous oxygen delivery from the coronary arteries. Coronary arteries have smooth muscle tissue inside their walls.

Autonomic Nervous System Influences on the Heart

Table 7.6 Parasympathetic and Sympathetic Stimulation

- Parasympathetic stimulation via the Vagus nerve: slows the heart rate and the force of myocardial contraction and decreases myocardial metabolism. It also causes vasoconstriction of the coronary arteries.

- Sympathetic stimulation (located on the sinus node and within the myocardium): increases the heart rate and the force of myocardial contraction and increases myocardial metabolism. It also causes vasodilation of the coronary arteries.

Overview of the Pulmonary Anatomy, Including the Respiratory Muscles

See **Figures 7.7** and **7.8**.

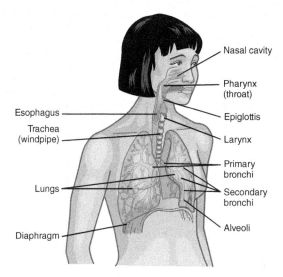

Figure 7.7 Respiratory system
Anatomy and Physiology: Understanding the Human Body by Robert K. Clark, page 326, Figure 17.6 "The lungs receive the entire output of the right ventricle"

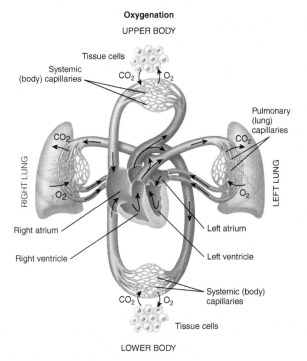

Figure 7.8 Oxygenation
Anatomy and Physiology: Understanding the Human Body by Robert K. Clark, page 326, Figure 17.6 called "The lungs receive the entire output of the right ventricle"

Table 7.7 Pulmonary Anatomy

- Nose: organ of smell; entrance to the nasal cavities; starting point of the respiratory system. Nose function is to filter, humidify, and warm the air.
- Pharynx: musculomembranous tube extending from the base of the skull to the level of C6 vertebrae, where it becomes continuous with the esophagus. It contains the nasopharynx, oropharynx, and laryngopharynx; it is innervated by the Vagus and glossopharyngeal nerves. The pharynx is a passageway for air from the nasal cavity to the larynx; it is also a passageway for food from the mouth to the esophagus. These functions are used by respiratory and digestive systems. The pharynx also participates in speech as a resonating cavity.
- Larynx: musculocartilaginous organ situated at the upper end of the trachea; contains extrinsic and intrinsic muscles; is lined with ciliated mucous membrane (part of the airway). The larynx connects the pharynx with the trachea.
- Trachea: cylindrical cartilaginous tube that goes from the larynx to the primary bronchi; extends from the C6 vertebrae to the T5 vertebrae, where (at carina) it divides into two bronchi; one bronchus goes to the right and the other to the left lung. The trachea is a conducting airway; its function is to transport air (not for gas exchange).
- Respiratory unit made of bronchi, bronchioles, alveolar ducts, alveolar sacs, and alveoli.
  - Bronchi: two main branches from trachea to lungs; provide a passageway for air
  - Bronchioles: smaller subdivisions of the bronchial tubes
  - Alveolar ducts: branch of a respiratory bronchiole that leads to the alveolar sacs of the lungs
  - Alveolar sacs: terminal portion of an air passage within the lung; the site of gas exchange
  - Alveoli: air sacs of the lungs; perform gas exchange; blood and inspired air are separated by the cell of the alveolus and that of the pulmonary capillary
- Right lung: has three lobes. Each lobe has ten bronchopulmonary segments (upper lobe: apical, anterior, and posterior segments; middle lobe: lateral and medial segments; lower lobe: superior, anterior basal, lateral basal, posterior basal, and medial basal segments) and fifty to eighty terminal bronchioles.
- Left lung: has two lobes. Each lobe has eight bronchopulmonary segments (upper lobe: apical-posterior, anterior, superior lingula, and inferior lingual segments; lower lobe: superior, anterior medial basal, lateral basal, and posterior basal segments) and fifty to eighty terminal bronchioles.

Table 7.8 Respiratory Muscles

- Muscles of inspiration: diaphragm (main muscle); accessory muscles (assist with inspiration during deeper inhalation and in the course of diseases): scalenes, sternocleidomastoid, serratus muscles, trapezius, and pectoral muscles
- Muscles of expiration: exhalation is passive when the inspiratory muscles relax; muscles that assist with forced expiration are quadratus lumborum, intercostals, abdominal muscles, and triangularis sternus

Cardiopulmonary Data Collection

Vital Signs and Normative Values

Table 7.9 Procedure for Taking Blood Pressure at the Brachial Artery[1]

1. Cuff width and length need to be appropriate for the size of the patient; cuff width needs to be 20% wider than the diameter of the arm.
2. Cuff is placed 1–2 inches above the antecubital fossa and inflated until no radial pulse can be palpated.
3. During cuff deflation, the brachial artery is auscultated over the antecubital fossa with a stethoscope.
4. Korotkoff's sounds begin: systolic blood pressure (SBP) is the first clear tapping sound that is heard; tapping sounds increase in intensity.
5. The tapping sounds are replaced by a muffled, soft blowing sound.
6. Diastolic blood pressure (DBP) is the disappearance of the muffled, soft blowing sound.

Table 7.10 Blood Pressure Normative Values: Adult[2]

Category	Systolic Blood Pressure	Diastolic Blood Pressure
Normal blood pressure (BP)	120 mm Hg or less	And 80 mm Hg or less
Elevated	120–129 mm Hg	And 80mm Hg or less
Stage I hypertension (HTN)	130–139 mm Hg	Or 80–89 mm Hg
Stage II hypertension	≥ 140mm Hg	Or ≥ 90 mm Hg
Hypertensive Crises	More than 180 mm Hg	And/or more than 120 mm Hg

Table 7.11 Blood Pressure Normative Values: Infant, Child, and Adolescent[3]

Normal BP: infant = 87–105/ 53–56 mm Hg

Normal BP: child = 97–112/57–71 mmHg

Normal BP: adolescent = 112–128/ 66–80 mm Hg

Table 7.12 Location of Pulses for Monitoring Heart Rate

- Brachial: over the medial portion of the antecubital fossa for an adult; inside of the upper arm for an infant. The inside of the upper arm is the area most commonly used to check for a pulse on an infant when performing cardiopulmonary resuscitation (CPR).
- Carotid: on either side (only on one side) of the neck between the trachea and the sternocleidomastoid muscle. It is the area most commonly checked for a pulse on an adult or a child when performing CPR.
- Femoral: in the inguinal area (inguinal triangle) at the crease between the abdomen and the thigh.
- Pedal: area over the dorsal, medial aspect of the foot.
- Popliteal: in the back of the knee at the popliteal space. The patient needs to bend the knee slightly.
- Temporal: in the area superior and lateral to the eye.

Table 7.13 **Heart Rate Normative Values**

Normal heart rate (HR): adult = 70 bpm (range = 60–100)

Abnormal HR: adult with bradycardia = less than 60 bpm; adult with tachycardia = more than 100 bpm

Normal HR: infant = 120 bpm (range = 70–170)

Normal HR: child = 125 bpm (range = 75–140)

Normal HR: adolescent = 85 bpm (range = 50–100)

Table 7.14 **Temperature and Respiratory Rate Normative Values**

	Temperature	Respiratory Rate (RR)
Adult	98.6°F (37°C)	12–18 breaths/min
Infant	95.9–99.5°F (35.5–37.5 °C)	30–50 breaths/min
Child	95.9–99.5°F (35.5–37.5 °C)	20–40 breaths/min
Adolescent	98.6°F (37°C)	15–22 breaths/min

Abnormal Breathing Patterns

Table 7.15 **Abnormal Breathing Patterns**[4]

- **Tachypnea** (rapid shallow breathing) may be observed in restrictive lung disease, pleuritic chest pain, or elevated diaphragm (because of atelectasis, pleurisy, or rib fracture).
- **Bradypnea** (slow breathing) may be observed secondary to increased intracranial pressure, diabetic coma, or drug-induced respiratory depression.
- **Hyperpnea** (rapid deep breathing) may be observed after exercise (a certain degree is normal) and in anxiety (may get hyperventilation), metabolic acidosis, comatose patients, myocardial infarction, hypoxia, or hypoglycemia. Kussmaul's breathing is deep, gasping breathing associated with severe diabetic ketoacidosis. In general, Kussmaul's breathing is also a sign of impending death.
- **Cheyne-Stokes breathing** (hyperpnea for 10–60 seconds, followed by apnea or no breathing) may be observed in congestive heart failure, drug-induced respiratory depression, uremia, or brain damage (both sides of cerebral hemispheres or diencephalon). It also may be observed in coma or basal ganglia disease. It indicates a grave prognosis in adults but may be a normal finding in children.
- **Obstructive breathing** (prolonged expiration and air trapping in the chest; breathing becomes shallow) may be observed in obstructive lung diseases.
- **Ataxic breathing** or **Biot's breathing** (several short breaths followed by long, irregular periods of apnea) may be observed in increased intracranial pressure (as in brain injury).
- **Sighing breathing** (a deep inspiration followed by a slow audible expiration)—sighs in large number may be observed in dyspnea and dizziness. Occasional sighs are normal.

Dyspnea Grades

Table 7.16 Dyspnea Grades[4]

Grade 0: The patient/client becomes short of breath at rest (while sitting or lying down). In regard to activity tolerance, grade 0 does not have an available magnitude of task. The patient/client's exertional capability cannot be precisely measured and categorized. Grade 0 is a very severe impairment. The patient/client cannot work and must give up all regular activities due to shortness of breath.

Grade 1: The patient/client becomes short of breath with light activities such as walking on a level surface, washing, standing, or shopping. Grade 1 is a severe impairment. The patient/client cannot work and must give up all regular activities due to shortness of breath.

Grade 2: The patient/client becomes short of breath with moderate or average activities such as walking up a gradual hill, climbing fewer than three flights of stairs, or carrying a light load on a level surface. Grade 2 is a moderate impairment. The patient/client will have to change his or her job and/or give up at least one regular activity due to shortness of breath.

Grade 3: The patient/client becomes short of breath with major activities such as walking up a steep hill, climbing more than three flights of stairs, or carrying a moderate load on a level surface. Grade 3 is a slight impairment. The patient/client will have to reduce at least one regular activity at work or at home. However, this impairment may not necessarily be caused by shortness of breath.

Grade 4: The patient/client becomes short of breath only with high-level activities such as carrying very heavy loads on a level surface, carrying lighter loads up the hill, or running. Typically, the patient/client in this category has no shortness of breath while performing ordinary tasks. There is no impairment; the patient/client can carry out all activities at home or at work.

Laboratory Values: Electrolytes, Blood, and Blood Gasses

Table 7.17 Lab Values: Electrolytes, Blood, and Blood Gases[4,5,6]

Test	Normal Values	Critical Values	Information for the PTA
Calcium	Infant: 10–12 mg/dL Child: 9–11.5 mg/dL Adult: 9–11 mg/dL	< 7 = tetany >12 = coma	Blood calcium levels regulated by the parathyroid hormone. Refer to Part 2, Tables 2-38 to 2-41 for management of calcium imbalance.
Potassium	Infant: 3.6–5.8 mEq/L Child: 3.5–5.5 mEq/L Adult: 3.5–5.0 mEq/L	Adult: <2.5 >6.6 Values below 3.2 mEq/L or above 5.1 mEq/L may indicate contraindication for PT.	Refer to Part 2, Tables 2-30 to 2-33 for management of potassium imbalance.

(continued)

Table 7.17 **Lab Values: Electrolytes, Blood, and Blood Gases**[4,5,6]   *(continued)*

Test	Normal Values	Critical Values	Information for the PTA
Sodium	Infant: 134–150 mEq/L Child: 135–145 mEq/L Adult: 135–145 mEq/L	≤ 110 mEq/L	Signs of hyponatremia evident when blood levels at or below 130 mEq/L. Refer to Part 2, Tables 2-34 to 2-37 for management of sodium imbalance.
Serum Creatinine	Infant: 0.2–0.4 mg/dL Child: 0.3–0.7 mg/dL Adult female: 0.5–1.1 mg/dL Adult male: 0.6–1.2 mg/dL		Evaluates kidney function. Increased levels may indicate rhabdomyolysis, dehydration, or renal disease. Decreased levels may be present with older age, pregnancy, or liver disease.
Blood Urea Nitrogen (BUN)	Infant: 5–18 mg/dL Child: 5–18mg/dL Adult: 10–20 mg/dL		Evaluates kidney function. BUN may be elevated in patients with burns, renal failure, and congestive heart failure (CHF).
Glucose (Fasting)	Child: 60–100 mg/dL Adult: 70–100 mg/dL Adult >60 years: 80–110mg/dL	> 126 mg/dL fasting = diabetes >200 mg/dL 2 hour post prandial = diabetes Hypoglycemia < 70 mg/dL—do not exercise, provide carbohydrates. Hyperglycemia > 200 mg/dL. Do not exercise if above 300 mg/dL	Refer to Part 2, Tables 2-27 to 2-28 for management of blood glucose imbalance.
Hgb A1C	Adult Normal: < 5.7% Pre-diabetes: 5.7–6.4% Poor glucose control: > 6.5%		Measures average level of blood glucose over prior 2–3 months.
Hematocrit	Child: 30–49% Adult female: 36–46% Adult male: 39–52%	< 25% no exercise 26–29% light exercise 30–32% add resistance as tolerated.	Determines relative volume of red blood cells as a percentage of blood volume.
Hemoglobin	Child: 14-17 g/dL Adult female: 12–16 g/dL Adult male: 13–18 g/dL	Low critical < 5–7g/dL High critical > 20 g/dL < 8g/dL no exercise 8–10 g/dL light exercise	Measure of hemoglobin levels in blood. Assess anemia, blood loss.

(continued)

Table 7.17 Lab Values: Electrolytes, Blood, and Blood Gases[4,5,6]   *(continued)*

Test	Normal Values	Critical Values	Information for the PTA
Lipids	HDL: Males ≥ 40 mg/dL Females ≥ 50 mg/dL LDL: < 130 mg/dL Triglycerides: < 150 mg/dL Total Cholesterol: < 200 mg/dL	LDL: high >160 mg/dL Triglycerides: high >200 mg/dL Total Cholesterol: high ≥ 240 mg/dL	Lipid levels are key factors to evaluate risk for cardiovascular disease.
Oxygen Saturation	95% or higher	Terminate activity if O_2 Sat drops below 90%. Supplemental oxygen may be indicated and prescribed by the physician.	Measures arterial blood oxygen.
PCO_2 (partial pressure of carbon dioxide)	Infant: 35–55 mm Hg Adult: 35–45 mm Hg		Measure of carbon dioxide within the blood. Used to monitor patients on ventilators and with respiratory disease and acid base imbalance.
PaO_2 (partial pressure of oxygen)	Infant: 75–80 mm Hg Adult: 75–100 mm Hg		Measures oxygen concentration in arterial blood.
Blood PH	Child: 7.39–7.41 Adults: 7.35–7.45	≥ 7.45 = Respiratory or Metabolic Alkalosis ≤ 7.35 Respiratory or Metabolic Acidosis	Refer to Part 2, Tables 2-42 to 2-45 for management of acid-base disorders.

Heart and Lung Sounds

Table 7.18 Heart Sounds[4]

- S_1—the normal heart sound (called also "lub") that occurs when the bicuspid (mitral) and tricuspid valves close, the beginning of systole. S_1 can be auscultated over the left lower sternal border (called the apex of the heart).

- S_2 —the normal heart sound (called also "dub") that occurs when the aortic and pulmonary valves close; the end of systole (the period between S_1 and S_2) and beginning of diastole (the period between S_2 and the next S_1). S_2 can be auscultated over the left upper sternal border (called the base of the heart).

- S_3—the abnormal heart sound that can be heard only with a stethoscope. Called a ventricular gallop, it occurs after S_2 and is associated with left ventricular failure. S_3 can be found in CHF.

(continued)

Table 7.18 **Heart Sounds**[4] (continued)

- S_4—the abnormal heart sound that can be heard only with a stethoscope; it is called an atrial gallop. S_4 occurs before S_1 and is associated with hypertension, myocardial infarction, coronary artery disease (CAD), and aortic stenosis.

- Pericardial friction rub—the abnormal heart sound that can be heard only with a stethoscope; it is heard as a high-pitched, rough, and creaking or squeaking sound. Pericardial friction rub is associated with inflammation of the pericardial sac with or without excessive fluid (called pericardial disease). Pericardial disease or pericarditis can result from myocardial infarction, trauma, or infection (bacterial, viral, or fungal).

- Murmur—the abnormal heart sound that can be heard without the stethoscope for murmur grades of 1, 2, 3, and 4; it can be heard only with a stethoscope for murmur grades of 5 and 6. Heart murmurs can be rumbling, soft, blowing, loud, or booming and can be heard during systole, diastole, or both. Diastolic murmur is a turbulence between S_2 and S_1; systolic murmur is a turbulence between S_1 and S_2. Murmurs do not necessarily indicate heart disease, and many heart diseases do not necessarily produce murmurs. Murmurs can be heard in a stenotic valve (a valve that has an impaired opening) or in a regurgitant valve (a valve that has an impaired closing).

Table 7.19 **Lung Sounds**[4]

- Vesicular breath sounds—the normal, low-pitched breath sounds heard over the lungs. Vesicular breath sounds are produced by air passing in and out of the airways. Bronchial and tracheal breath sounds—the normal breath sounds heard over the bronchi and trachea—are higher pitched and louder than vesicular sounds; they are produced by air passing over the walls of bronchi and trachea.

- Wheezes—the abnormal lung sounds that can be heard with a stethoscope during expiration; these whistling, musical sounds are caused by narrowing of the lumen of the airways. Wheezes are the result of asthma, bronchitis, mitral stenosis, emphysema, airway obstruction (caused by foreign bodies), pulmonary infections, pulmonary edema, or other chronic obstructive pulmonary disease (COPD).

- Crackles—the abnormal lung sounds that can be heard with a stethoscope; these rustling or bubbling sounds are also called rales. Crackles are the result of atelectasis (collapsed lung). They can also be caused by air passing over airway secretions or opening of collapsed airways.

- Friction—the abnormal lung sounds that can be heard with a stethoscope. Friction is produced by rubbing together of roughened pleural surfaces; it is similar to crackles but more superficial.

- Stridor—the abnormal, high-pitched (harsh) sound occurring during inspiration that can be heard without a stethoscope. It is a sign of upper airway obstruction indicating a life-threatening condition (such as epiglottitis). However, difficulty breathing without stridor can still be interpreted as an obstructed upper airway.

CARDIOPULMONARY INTERVENTIONS

Sputum Analysis

Table 7.20 Sputum Analysis[6]

Sputum should be analyzed and documented for quantity, viscosity, color, odor, frequency, time of day, and ease of expectoration.

Types of Sputum

- Fetid: foul smelling; signifies anaerobic infection; occurs with bronchiectasis, lung abscess, or cystic fibrosis
- Mucoid: white or clear; present with chronic cough due to acute or chronic bronchitis and cystic fibrosis; not necessarily associated with bronchopulmonary infection
- Frothy: white or white with a shade of pink; foamy; thin frothy sputum can be associated with pulmonary edema
- Hemoptysis: blood or bloody sputum expectoration; can be a small amount or massive hemorrhage; present in a variety of pathologies
- Purulent: pus; yellow or greenish sputum; sometimes thick and copious sputum; common in acute and chronic infection
- Mucopurulent: mix of mucoid sputum and pus; yellow to green color; common in infection
- Tenacious: thick and very sticky sputum
- Rusty: rusty-colored sputum; common in pneumococcal pneumonia

Cardiopulmonary Signs and Symptoms

Table 7.21 Cardiopulmonary Signs and Symptoms

Cyanosis

- Blue, gray, or dark purple discoloration of the skin, lips, nails, and tongue caused by deoxygenated or reduced hemoglobin in the blood; oximetry of the arterial blood saturation may be 85% or less.
- Cyanosis of the mucous membranes such as in the mouth indicates hypoxemia and respiratory failure.
- Cyanosis of retinae indicates congenital heart disease or cardiac failure.
- Peripheral cyanosis of the digits (of fingers and toes) indicates chronic hypoxia; it may indicate respiratory obstruction, reduced pulmonary function, or inadequate ventilation.
- For African American patients/clients, cyanosis can be seen by close inspection of lips, tongue, conjunctiva (of the eyelids), palms of the hands, and the soles of the feet.
- One method of testing is pressing the palms; slow blood return indicates cyanosis. Another sign is ashen gray lips and tongue.

(continued)

Table 7.21 Cardiopulmonary Signs and Symptoms   *(continued)*

Clubbing

- Enlarged terminal phalanx of the finger; excessive growth of the soft tissues of the ends of the fingers (giving a beak appearance from the side and a sausage appearance from above).
- Clubbing indicates COPD, lung fibrosis, lung carcinoma, and other pulmonary illnesses.

Diaphoresis

- Sweating is profuse, and skin is cold and clammy.
- Diaphoresis indicates inadequate cardiovascular response or excessive effort.

Pulse Palpation

- *Normal* or regular pulse—a pulse when the force and frequency are the same. It is documented as 3+.
- *Bounding* pulse—an abnormal pulse that reaches a high intensity and then disappears quickly. Also called a collapsing pulse, it is documented as 4+.
- *Thready* pulse—an abnormal pulse characterized as fine, scarcely perceptible. It is documented as 1+.
- *Weak* or slow pulse—an abnormal pulse characterized by a rate of less than 60 beats per minute. It is documented as 2+.

Pitting Edema

- Edema of the extremities characterized by maintenance of the skin depression after moderate pressure was applied.
- Bilaterally, it may indicate CHF.

Electrocardiogram (EKG or ECG)

Table 7.22 Electrocardiogram (EKG or ECG)

- Electrocardiogram (EKG or ECG): records the electrical activity of the heart; determines different waves patterns in cardiac rhythm; evaluates the abnormal heart rhythms, identifies if patient had prior heart attack.
- EKG/ECG is used with the exercise tolerance test (ETT), also called the graded exercise test, to record the patient's/client's electrical activity of the heart during graded increases in the rate of exercise.

See **Figure 7.9**.

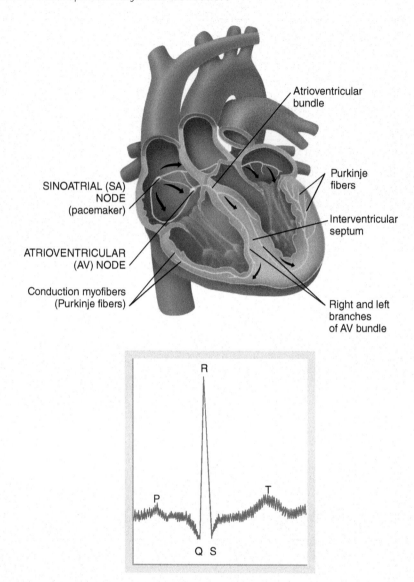

Figure 7.9 Conduction system of the heart and normal EKG

Anatomy and Physiology: Understanding the Human Body by Robert K. Clark, page 296, Figure 16.9 "The impulse generation and conduction system of your heart"

Table 7.23 Electrocardiogram Waves[4,7]

- **P wave:** first wave caused by atrial depolarization. A normal P wave is upright, rounded, and 1–3 mm tall. Abnormally shaped P waves include flutter (F) waves, fibrillation (f) waves (small with irregular deflections on the baseline), and premature (P) waves (have a different PR interval in a rhythm group and look different than regular P waves).
- **PR Interval:** measures conduction time from atrium to ventricle.
- **QRS complex:** ventricular depolarization. Irregularities in the ventricular conduction include flutter and fibrillation (develop with ventricular tachycardia). Premature ventricular contractions (PVCs) are wide, bizarre QRS complexes.
- **ST segment:** beginning of ventricular repolarization; it can be used to identify ischemia, injury, or infarction. Abnormal "ST Segment" includes the following:
  - Depressed ST segment—indicates ischemia or a nontransmural myocardial injury (part of the tissue of a portion of the cardiac wall is injured)
  - Elevated ST segment—indicates transmural myocardial injury (such as an infarction, in which the tissue in the entire thickness of a portion of the cardiac wall dies)
- **T wave:** completion of ventricular repolarization.
- **Regular sinus rhythm:** each QRS complex is preceded by a P wave; QRS complexes are equally spaced.

Cardiac Cycle

Table 7.24 Cardiac Cycle

Atrial Systole

- Contraction of the heart muscles (myocardium) involving the right and left atria (that contract at the same time).
- Includes an electrical systole (which stimulates the myocardium of the chambers of the heart to contract) and a mechanical systole (contraction of the heart).
- As the atria contract, the blood pressure in each atrium increases, forcing additional blood into the ventricles (called atrial kick). If normal electrical conduction of the heart is absent (e.g., in atrial fibrillation, atrial flutter, or complete heart block), the atrial kick is absent.
- Electrical systole of the atria begins with the onset of the P wave on the EKG.

Ventricular Systole

- Contraction of the myocardium involving the right and left ventricles.
- At the beginning of ventricular systole, both the bicuspid (mitral) and tricuspid valves (known together as the atrioventricular valves) close. When these valves close, S_1 takes place.
- At the end of the ventricular systole, the aortic and pulmonic valves close. When these valves close, S_2 takes place.
- As the left ventricle empties, its pressure falls below the pressure in the aorta, and the aortic valve closes.
- As the pressure in the right ventricle falls below the pressure in the pulmonary artery, the pulmonic valve closes.
- Ventricular systole occurs between S_1 and S_2.
- In an EKG, the electrical systole of the ventricles begins at the beginning of the QRS complex.

(continued)

Table 7.24 Cardiac Cycle *(continued)*

Cardiac Diastole (Complete Cardiac Diastole)

- Period of time when the heart relaxes after the contraction in preparation for refilling with blood; the filling stage of the heart.
- Diastole has two phases: ventricular diastole (when the ventricles are relaxing), and atrial diastole (when the atria are relaxing).
- During ventricular diastole, the pressure in the ventricles (right and left) drops from the peak that it reached in the systole.
- When the pressure drops in the left ventricle (below the pressure in the left atrium), the bicuspid (mitral) valve opens, and the left ventricle fills with blood (which was accumulating in the left atrium).
- When the pressure drops in the right ventricle (below the pressure in the right atrium), the tricuspid valve opens, and the right ventricle fills with blood (which was accumulating in the right atrium).
- Diastole occurs between S_2 and S_1.

Coordination of the Cardiac Cycle

- During the cardiac cycle, the rhythmic sequence of contractions is coordinated by the SA and AV nodes.
- The SA node is the "cardiac pacemaker" of the heart and is located in the upper wall of the right atrium. SA node is responsible for the electrical stimulation (action potential) that initiates atrial contraction.
- The electrical wave then reaches the AV node (situated in the lower right atrium) and through the Bundles of His and Purkinje fibers leads to contraction of the ventricles.

Cardiac Terminology and Normative Values

Table 7.25 Cardiac Terminology and Normative Values

- **Cardiac output (CO):** amount of blood/minute that leaves the right or left ventricles. It is expressed in L/min. Normal CO = 4–6 L/min. CO is influenced by the heart rate and the stroke volume; it is calculated by multiplying the stroke volume by the heart rate (CO = HR x SV).
- **Stroke volume (SV):** amount of blood that is ejected by the left ventricle with each heartbeat (myocardial contraction). SV is influenced by contractility (ability of the ventricle to contract), preload (amount of blood in the ventricle at the end of diastole), and afterload (the left ventricle force needed to overcome aortic pressure and open the aortic valve during systole). SV is also influenced by the patient's age and gender and the amount of exercise performed by the patient. SV average values = 60–80 mL.
- **Ejection fraction (EF):** percentage of blood emptied from the ventricle during systole. The EF of the left ventricle averages (in healthy hearts) is 55–70%. After myocardial infarction, EF can be reduced. EF is used as an index of contractility.
- **Cardiac index (CI):** similar to but more accurate than CO; takes into consideration the relationship between CO and the body surface area (BSA). It can be expressed as CI = CO/BSA normal values for average adult at rest = 3.0 L/min/m^2.

Pulmonary Terminology and Normative Values

Table 7.26 Pulmonary Terminology[4]

- **Ventilation:** movement of air into and out of the lungs. It can be estimated by spirometry.

- **Respiration:** the exchange of gas, supplying oxygen to the tissues and removal of carbon dioxide. External respiration is diffusion of gas across the alveolar and capillary membranes; internal respiration is exchange of gas between capillaries and tissues of the body.

- **Arterial oxygenation:** ability of arterial blood to carry oxygen. Normal adult and child arterial blood oxygen saturation is between 95% and 98%.

- **Alveolar ventilation:** ability of lungs to take in oxygen and to remove carbon dioxide from the pulmonary circulation and maintain the normal potential of hydrogen = pH. (pH measures the concentration of free-floating hydrogen ions within the body.) Blood is a solution that is neither acid nor alkaline; the body's normal blood plasma pH is between 7.35 and 7.45.

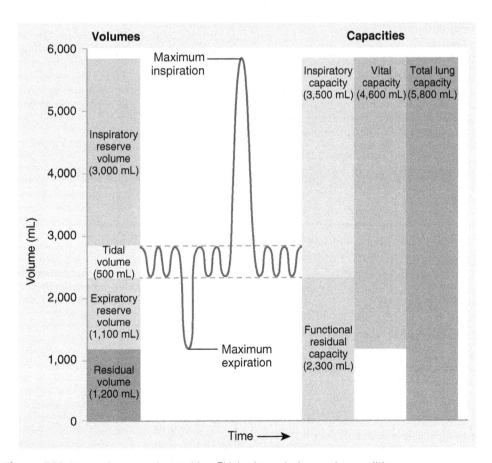

Figure 7.10 Lung volumes and capacities. Tidal volume during resting conditions

See **Figure 7.10**.

Table 7.27 Lung Volumes[4]

- **Tidal volume (TV):** volume of air inhaled (inspired) and exhaled (expired) in a normal, quiet breath. It can be 500 mL for a child and an adult, and 20 mL for an infant.
- **Inspiratory reserve volume (IRV):** maximal amount of air that can be forcefully inhaled after a normal inspiration.
- **Expiratory reserve volume (ERV):** maximal amount of air that can be forcefully expelled from the lungs after a normal expiration.
- **Residual volume (RV):** volume of air remaining in the lungs after a maximal, full expiration. RV is necessary for continuous gas exchange.
- **Inspiratory capacity (IC):** volume of air that can be inspired after a resting exhalation (expiration); IC = IRV + TV.
- **Vital capacity (VC):** volume of air that can be exhaled from the lungs after a maximal inspiration; VC = IRV + TV + ERV. VC is important to evaluate the ability of the lung to exchange O_2 and CO_2. Normal VC is more than 80% of the predicted value; mild VC is between 66% and 80% of the predicted value; moderate VC is between 50% and 65% of the predicted value; severe VC is less than 50% of the predicted value.
- **Functional residual capacity (FRC):** amount of air remaining in the lungs after a normal expiration (exhalation); FRC = ERV + RV.
- **Total lung capacity (TLC):** volume of air in the lungs after a maximal inspiration (inhalation); TLC = IRV + TV + ERV + RV. Normal TLC is more than 80% of the predicted value; mild TLC is between 66% and 80% of the predicted value; moderate TLC is between 50% and 65% of the predicted value; severe TLC is less than 50% of the predicted value.
- **Forced expiratory volume (FEV):** amount of air forcefully exhaled after a full inspiration (inhalation). When testing FEV, the expiration is performed quickly as possible and the volume is measured at 0.5 second, at 1 second, at 2 seconds, and at 3 seconds. Normal FEV is more than 80% of the predicted value; mild FEV is between 66% and 80% of the predicted value; moderate FEV is between 50% and 65% of the predicted value; severe FEV is less than 50% of the predicted value.

Contraindications to Exercise Tolerance Tests

See also Section 2-3.

Table 7.28 Contraindications to Exercise Tolerance Tests (ETT)

Absolute Contraindications	Relative Contraindications
Recent complicated myocardial infarction (MI); any acute cardiac event or injury	More than 200 mm Hg resting SBP or more than 110 mm Hg resting DBP or hypertensive response (SBP more than 250 mmHg and/or DBP more than 115 mmHg)
Unstable angina; uncontrolled ventricular arrhythmia	Electrolyte imbalances (such as hypokalemia or hypomagnesemia)
Uncontrolled atrial arrhythmia; third degree AV heart block (without pacemaker)	Frequent and complex ventricular ectopy; ventricular aneurysm
Aortic aneurysm (known or suspected); myocarditis (or pericarditis)	Uncontrolled diabetes or other metabolic disease
Thrombophlebitis; pulmonary embolus	Moderate valvular disease
Acute infections; psychosis	Neuromuscular, musculoskeletal, or rheumatoid disorders that can be exacerbated by exercise
Acute CHF; severe aortic stenosis	Advanced or complicated pregnancy

Termination Criteria for Exercise Tolerance Test

Table 7.29 ETT Termination Criteria

- Onset of angina
- Fall in arterial blood gas for oxygen (PaO_2) of more than 20 mm Hg or PaO_2 being less than 55 mm Hg
- Rise in partial pressure of carbon dioxide ($PaCO_2$) of more than 10 mm Hg or an increase in $PaCO_2$ more than 65 mm Hg
- Maximal shortness of breath (dyspnea); symptoms of fatigue; total fatigue
- Cardiac ischemia or cardiac arrhythmia
- Failure of heart rate to increase with increased intensity
- Increase in diastolic BP of more than 115 mm Hg; increase in systolic BP of more than 250 mm Hg; decrease in BP with increased exercise – drop in DBP of > 10 mm Hg from baseline.
- Leg cramps or claudication; pallor; cyanosis; cold sweat (diaphoresis); ataxia
- Patient/client delayed (several hours) responses to ETT: insomnia; prolonged fatigue; sudden weight gain caused by fluid retention
- Patient's request to stop

Body Structure and Function Impairments Related to the Cardiopulmonary System

Coronary Artery Disease (CAD): Impairments

Table 7.30 CAD Impairments[6]

CAD

- Narrowing of the coronary arteries due to atherosclerosis; more common in men than in women.
- In CAD, blockages within the coronary arteries limit the flow of oxygenated blood to the myocardium, causing infarction or ischemia of the heart muscle.

Angina Pectoris

- Classic CAD symptom: pain, burning, or pressure in the chest. Chest pain or discomfort is caused by ischemia, which is a temporary condition (secondary to an imbalance of myocardial oxygen supply and demand).
- Angina can start with exertion, emotion, exposure to cold air, or consumption of a large meal. It can also be precipitated by exertion and can progress to full MI if symptoms are not treated.
- Levels of angina: light pain (1+) to most severe (4+). On a 1 to 10 pain scale, patients may rate the pain as 10.
- Classical presentation of angina includes the Levine sign, when the patient is clenching his or her fist over the sternum; angina symptoms can also present with radiating pain down the left arm, pain going up into the chin or the jaw, and pain between the shoulder blades. Females often present with atypical symptoms i.e., pain between shoulder blades, in right upper arm, anxiety, and weakness.
- Angina can be confirmed by a 12-lead EKG showing ischemia with a depressed ST segment and an inverted (flipped) T wave.
- Angina is classified as stable or unstable:
  - Stable angina has less intensity (pain 5/10 that improves to 0/10 with rest and administration of oxygen and nitroglycerin).
  - Unstable angina (also called pre-infarction angina) does not improve (as the stable angina) and requires immediate (emergency) medical intervention.
- In general, any angina symptoms require medical interventions.

Other CAD Impairments

- Cough
- Dyspnea
- Orthopnea: labored breathing while lying flat that is relieved by sitting up; the classic symptom of left ventricular heart failure
- Weakness
- Weight gain and venous stasis (due to peripheral edema)
- Anorexia
- Nausea
- Increased pulmonary arterial pressure
- Hypertension
- Sweating
- Lightheadedness
- Possibly hypotension (depending on the cardiac disease)

(continued)

Table 7.30 CAD Impairments[6]   *(continued)*

Myocardial Infarction

- Loss of living heart muscle as a result of coronary occlusion; occurs when the atherosclerotic plaque in a coronary artery ruptures, forming a thrombus that obstructs the injured blood vessel.
- Most MIs heal initially without incident, but complications can occur.
- EKG identifies MI with a (pathologic) Q wave (transmural MI with full thickness of the ventricular wall) or a non-Q wave (nontransmural MI involving the endocardium). Newer MI classification indicates that a non-Q wave EKG (absent Q wave) may also be a transmural MI.
- Typically, after an hour from the transmural MI, the EKG will show an elevated ST segment. After a few hours from the transmural MI, the EKG will show a pathologic Q wave. A nontransmural MI will appear on the EKG as an ST depression (without a Q wave).

Congestive Heart Failure (CHF): Impairments

Table 7.31 CHF Impairments

CHF, a frequent complication of ischemic and hypertensive heart disease, is the inability of the heart to circulate blood effectively to meet the body's metabolic demands; can affect the left ventricle, right ventricle, or both. It is associated with the following impairments:

- Dyspnea
- Orthopnea
- Dyspnea with exertion
- Muscular fatigue
- Tachycardia
- Cyanosis
- Productive cough
- Pulmonary edema (increased hydrostatic pressure in the pulmonary veins and interstitial space of the lung)
- Peripheral edema (with bilateral pitting edema)
- Fluid weight gain
- Presence of an abnormal S_3 heart sound
- Renal dysfunction
- Heart murmurs (from mitral regurgitation of enlarged left ventricle)
- Obstructive sleep apnea
- Failure of the left ventricle can result in inadequate CO with resultant fatigue, weakness, and reduced tolerance to exercise and can cause pulmonary edema along with dyspnea and orthopnea.
- Failure of the right ventricle results in peripheral edema, venous congestion, weight gain and cyanosis.

Chronic Obstructive Pulmonary Disease (COPD): Impairments

Table 7.32 COPD Impairments

Definition

- COPD includes the most common chronic respiratory disorders affecting normal expiratory volumes; they cause narrowing obstruction or destruction of the bronchi/bronchioles and alveolar (bronchial) tissue.
- The main form of COPD is emphysema (characterized by air flow limitation that is not fully reversible).
- COPD causes: tobacco smoking (most common); exposure to environmental dust, smoke, or particular pollution; deficiency of alpha-1 antitrypsin (inadequate protection against destructive enzyme activity in the lungs).

Classification of COPD

- 0 = at risk for COPD (may have chronic impairments such as cough and sputum production)
- I = mild COPD (FEV in 1 second is equal or more than 80% of the predicted value; may have or not have chronic impairments such as cough and sputum production)
- II = moderate COPD (FEV in 1 second is less than 80% of the predicted value; may have or not have chronic impairments such as cough and sputum production)
- III = severe COPD (FEV in 1 second is less than 50% of the predicted value; may have or not have chronic impairments such as cough and sputum production)
- IV = very severe COPD (FEV in 1 second is less than 30% of the predicted value; has chronic respiratory failure)

Emphysema Impairments

- Chronic cough
- Expectoration (of pink thin sputum)
- Exertional dyspnea
- Enlarged thorax (due to loss of elastic recoil of the lungs)
- Increase in the anterior–posterior diameter of the chest
- Dorsal kyphosis
- Barrel chest appearance
- Distant breath and heart sounds
- Expiratory wheezing
- Crackles
- Mild to moderate weight loss
- Decreased exercise tolerance
- Repeated respiratory infections

Advanced stages

- Hypertrophy of accessory muscles
- Cyanosis
- Digital clubbing
- Breathing using only pursed-lip breathing

(continued)

Table 7.32 COPD Impairments *(continued)*

Other Specific Pulmonary Impairments of Emphysema

- Decreased vital capacity
- Increased residual volume and functional residual capacity
- Decreased FEV_1
- Hypoxemia (decreased oxygen concentration in the arterial blood—PaO_2)
- Hypercapnia (increased partial pressure of carbon dioxide in the blood—$PaCO_2$—to levels of 45 or 50 mm Hg)

Asthma

- A type of COPD characterized by increased sensitivity to irritants such as cold air, chemicals, exercise, infection, or stress.
- Manifests as spasms in the bronchi, resulting in narrowing of the airways and production of mucus and secretions in the affected bronchial area.
- Asthma impairments include (1) cough, (2) dyspnea, (3) wheezing during expiration, (4) crackles, (5) anxiety, (6) tachycardia, (7) tachypnea, (8) cyanosis, and (9) increased use of accessory muscles.

Chronic Bronchitis

- A type of COPD characterized by chronic cough and sputum production, mostly as a result of cigarette smoking.
- Chronic bronchitis impairments include (1) crackles, (2) wheezing, (3) increased respiratory infections, (4) hypoxemia, (5) variable $PaCO_2$ to levels, (6) edema from right sided heart failure, and (7) decreased expiratory rates.

Cystic Fibrosis

- A genetic pulmonary disease transmitted by an autosomal recessive trait that causes a malfunction of the exocrine glands, resulting in increased secretions in the lung. Cystic fibrosis affects other organs as well.
- Cystic fibrosis impairments include (1) thick secretions (leading to obstruction), (2) frequent respiratory infections, (3) weight loss (despite caloric intake), (4) salty taste to the skin, (5) chronic cough, (6) viscous secretions, (7) cyanosis, (8) dyspnea, (9) tachypnea, (10) decreased expiratory flow (decreased FEV in 1 second), (11) increased residual volume, (12) hyperinflation of lungs, (13) poor endurance, and (14) gastrointestinal dysfunction (or diabetes).

Bronchiectasis

- A type of COPD characterized by chronic dilation of a bronchus or bronchi, caused by the damaging effects of a longstanding infection, usually experienced in the patient's childhood.
- Bronchiectasis impairments include (1) dyspnea, (2) copious thick secretions, (3) productive cough, (4) crackles, (5) digital clubbing, (6) hemoptysis (expectoration of blood), (7) recurrent secondary infections, and (8) decreased breath sounds.

CARDIOPULMONARY INTERVENTIONS

Chronic Restrictive Lung Disease (CRLD): Impairments

Table 7.33 CRLD Impairments[6]

Definition

- A group of disorders with different etiologies resulting in difficulty expanding the lungs and reduced lung volume
- Causes: pleural disease, trauma, surgery, infection, radiation therapy, inorganic dust, oxygen toxicity, asbestos exposure, inhalation of noxious gases, pulmonary edema (effusion of serous fluid into the alveoli and interstitial tissue of the lungs), pulmonary embolism, pulmonary fibrosis, hyaline membrane disease, normal aging
- Extrapulmonary causes: neurologic disorders i.e., SCI, ALS, Guillain Barre syndrome; musculoskeletal disorders i.e., kyphosis, scoliosis, chest wall deformity; post-surgical conditions involving abdomen or chest wall

Types of CRLDs

- Idiopathic pulmonary fibrosis: the most common CRLD, characterized by formation of scar tissue in the parenchyma of the lungs following inflammation of the alveoli
- Pneumoconiosis: Asbestosis, black lung disease, silicosis

CRLD General Impairments

- Dyspnea
- Nonproductive cough
- Early fatigue
- Rapid shallow breathing
- Limited chest expansion
- Decreased ability to take a deep breath
- Use of accessory muscles for ventilation
- Cyanosis
- Crackles
- Weight loss
- Postural deviations (kyphosis) for breathing difficulties
- Decreased chest mobility
- Hypoxemia
- Hypocapnia
- Reductions in vital capacity (VC), forced residual capacity (FRC), and total lung capacity (TLC). Hypercapnia is the terminal stage of the idiopathic pulmonary fibrosis

(continued)

Table 7.33 CRLD Impairments[6]   *(continued)*

Other Causes of CRLD

- CRLD can be caused by alterations in the neuromuscular apparatus characterized by decreased muscular strength and inability to expand the rib cage, such as may occur with multiple sclerosis, muscular dystrophy, Parkinson's disease, spinal cord injury, or cerebral vascular accident.

- CRLD impairments with the above conditions include (1) dyspnea; (2) hypoxemia; (3) crackles; (4) digital clubbing; (5) cyanosis; (6) decreased breath sounds; (7) reduced cough effectiveness; (8) reduced lung volume; and (9) atelectasis (collapsed lungs).

- CRLD can be caused by pulmonary restrictions as a result of pulmonary or cardiac surgery (secondary to lung abscesses, lung abnormalities, tuberculosis, tumors, CAD, arrhythmias, aneurysm, congenital heart abnormalities, or cardiac valve disorders).

- CRLD can be caused by trauma to the chest area resulting in rib fractures and puncture of the lungs, causing pneumothorax—air in the pleural space—or hemothorax—blood in the pleural space or lung contusions. Impairments may include shallow breathing, pain with deep inspiration or cough, crepitation, dyspnea, absent or decreased breath sounds, cyanosis, and cough with hemoptysis.

Patient Safety During Cardiopulmonary Interventions

Basic Cardiac Life Support for Adults

Table 7.34 **Adult Basic Life Support—Healthcare Provider**[8]

- Verify safety of scene.
- Check for responsiveness.
- Activate emergency response system (via mobile device if appropriate).
- Get automated external defibrillator (AED) or send someone to get a device.
- Look for breathing and check pulse.
- If not breathing and no pulse felt after 10 seconds, begin CPR.
- Perform cycles of 30 compressions and 2 breaths at rate of 100 to 120 compressions per minute.
- Use head tilt and chin tilt to open the airway.
- Use AED as soon as available.
- Assess rhythm and follow prompts on AED.

Table 7.35 **Choking**

The finger sweep and tongue-jaw lift should be used only in an unresponsive/unconscious patient/client, and only if the foreign object is visible. Attempt other methods before attempting a finger sweep. Never do a blind finger sweep.

Adults: For a mild obstruction stay with the person and encourage them to cough. For a severe obstruction perform abdominal thrusts (Heimlich maneuver), call the EMS, and prepare to provide basic life support if person loses consciousness.

Infants: for a mild obstruction, stay with the child but be prepared to activate EMS if infant unable to dislodge the foreign object. Do not do a blind finger sweep. For severe obstruction use back blows and chest thrusts, call EMS and be prepared to provide CPR if infant becomes unresponsive.

Finger Sweep and Tongue-Jaw Lift

1. With the patient/client face up, open the patient/client's mouth by grasping both the tongue and lower jaw between the thumb and fingers and lifting the mandible (tongue-jaw lift). This maneuver alone may be sufficient to relieve an obstruction.
2. Insert the index finger of the other hand deeply into the patient/client's throat to the base of the tongue.
3. Use a hooking action to dislodge the foreign body and maneuver it into the mouth.
4. It is sometimes necessary to use the index finger to push the foreign body against the opposite side of the throat to dislodge and remove it.

Table 7.36 **Heimlich Maneuver: Removal of a Foreign Body Blocking the Air Passage**[7]

Maneuver for a Standing Victim

Place the clasped hands just below the middle of the rib cage. The rescuer forms a fist with one hand and places it below the sternum. The rescuer then grasps the wrist of the hand, forming the fist. The hands are then rapidly brought inward and upward.

Maneuver for a Supine Victim

Place the hands just below the rib cage at the distal end of the sternum. As in the standing position, the rescuer then grasps the wrist of the hand, forming the fist. The hands are then rapidly brought distal to proximal.

Signs and Symptoms That Warrant Discontinuing Cardiac Interventions

Table 7.37 **Signs and Symptoms That Warrant Discontinuing Cardiac Interventions**[6]

- Temperature of more than 100°F
- Systolic BP of more than 250 mm Hg
- Diastolic BP of more than 110 mm Hg
- Fall in systolic BP of more than 10 mm Hg
- Rise in HR of more than 20 bpm or as prescribed by physician
- Resting HR of more than 130 bpm and/or less than 40 bpm
- Chest pain, palpitations, and/or irregular pulse
- Oxygen saturation of less than 90%
- Blood glucose of more than 250 mg/dL
- Cyanotic and/or diaphoretic
- Dizziness and/or syncope
- Bilateral leg/foot edema

Signs and Symptoms That Warrant Changing or Discontinuing Interventions in Pulmonary Rehabilitation

Table 7.38 **Signs and Symptoms That Warrant Changing or Discontinuing Interventions in Pulmonary Rehabilitation**

- Increased cyanosis
- Severe dyspnea
- Decreased oxygen saturation levels
- Moderate to severe blood-streaked sputum
- Severe fatigue
- Severe pain
- Deep vein thrombosis (DVT)
- Pneumothorax
- Pulmonary embolism
- Severe pulmonary edema
- Cardiac arrhythmia
- Congestive heart failure
- Severe hypertension
- Severe pleural effusion
- Intervention over an area of fracture or tumor

CARDIOPULMONARY INTERVENTIONS

(continued)

Table 7.38 Signs and Symptoms That Warrant Changing or Discontinuing Interventions in Pulmonary Rehabilitation *(continued)*

- Unstable angina or recent myocardial infarction
- Intervention involving direct pressure on the xiphoid process
- Uncontrolled coughing
- Forced expiration should not be used during pursed lip breathing
- Avoid prolonged expiration and hyperventilation

The physical therapist assistant (PTA) needs to immediately report to the physical therapist (PT) any change in the patient's condition during interventions or any new contraindication and precaution related to the intervention. When any patient experiences a life-threatening condition, the PTA needs to provide CPR, call EMS, reposition the patient, and report the incident to the PT or nursing personnel.

Postural Drainage: Possible Complications and Safety Interventions During Pulmonary Rehabilitation

Table 7.39 Postural Drainage: Complications and Safety Interventions

Hypoxemia

- Definition: decreased oxygen concentration of the arterial blood.
- Safety interventions for hypoxemia: Call the PT and the nursing staff (if in a hospital or skilled nursing facility); call the PT and EMS (for home health care). The patient needs higher oxygen concentrations during the procedure if the potential for or observed hypoxemia exists. If the patient becomes hypoxemic during treatment, stop pulmonary therapy immediately, return the patient to the original resting position, and consult the PT (or nursing staff/EMS), depending on where the interventions were rendered. Ensure adequate ventilation until help arrives.
- Hypoxemia during postural drainage may be avoided in unilateral lung disease by placing the involved lung in the uppermost position with the patient on his or her side.

Increased Intracranial Pressure

- Definition: increased pressure of the cerebrospinal fluid in the head.
- Normal intracranial pressure is between 4 and 15 mm Hg. Pressure higher than 20 mm Hg can cause risk of compression or herniation of the brain or brain stem[6].
- Safety interventions for increased intracranial pressure: Stop pulmonary therapy, return the patient to the original resting position, and consult the PT (or nursing staff/EMS), depending on where the interventions were rendered.

(continued)

Table 7.39 **Postural Drainage: Complications and Safety Interventions** *(continued)*

Acute Hypotension

- Definition: blood pressure decreased below the normal level.
- Safety interventions for acute hypotension: Stop pulmonary therapy, return the patient to the original resting position, monitor the patient, and consult the PT.

Pulmonary Hemorrhage

- Definition: hemorrhage from the lung, with bright red and frothy blood that is typically coughed up.
- Safety interventions for pulmonary hemorrhage: Stop pulmonary therapy, return the patient to the original resting position, and call the PT (or nursing staff/EMS), depending on where the interventions were rendered. Administer oxygen and maintain the airway until nursing or EMS personnel respond.

Pain or Injury to Muscles, Ribs, or Spine

- Safety interventions for pain or injury: Stop pulmonary therapy that appears directly associated with pain or injury, be careful in moving the patient, and consult the PT.

Vomiting and Aspiration

- Vomitus may be aspirated into the nose, throat, or lungs.
- Safety interventions for vomiting and aspiration: Stop pulmonary therapy, administer oxygen, maintain the airway, return the patient to the previous resting position, and contact the PT (or nursing staff/EMS) immediately, depending on where the interventions were rendered. The patient needs to have the airway cleared using suctioning.

Bronchospasm

- Definition: abnormal narrowing and partial obstruction of the lumen of the bronchi (caused by spasm of the peribronchial smooth muscle). The patient experiences coughing and wheezing.
- Safety interventions for bronchospasm: Stop pulmonary therapy, return the patient to the previous resting position; administer or increase oxygen delivery while contacting the PT. The patient may need physician-ordered bronchodilators.

Dysrhythmia

- Definition: irregular heart rate (disordered or disrupt heart rhythm).
- Safety interventions for dysrhythmia: Stop pulmonary therapy, return the patient to the previous resting position, contact the PT (or nursing staff/EMS) immediately, depending on where the interventions were rendered.

Oxygen Safety

Table 7.40 Oxygen Safety in Home Health Pulmonary Rehabilitation

- Oxygen is a drug and dosage, and usage will be prescribed by the physician.

- Long-term home oxygen is available from three different delivery systems: electrically driven oxygen concentrators, liquid systems, and compressed gas. Inside the home, liquid and compressed gas systems use large tanks to store oxygen. Small, portable tanks of compressed oxygen also may be needed for brief periods (such as a few hours) outside the home. Each system has advantages and disadvantages.

- Oxygen is typically administered with continuous flow through a two-pronged nasal tube (cannula), even though this system is highly wasteful of oxygen (delivering maximum oxygen concentrations of only 40%). To improve efficiency and increase the patient's (client's) mobility, several devices, including reservoir cannulas, Ambu bags, demand-type systems, and transtracheal catheters (cannula placed directly into the trachea), can be used. Usually, a respiratory therapist or a physician instructs the patient about the proper oxygen use.

- When the patient (client) is using oxygen therapy at home, it is important to stabilize the tank (possibly using a stand) and store it in an area that is out of the way so the tank will not fall. The tank should be closed tightly when not in use.

- Because oxygen can cause an explosion, it is essential to keep the tank away from any flammable source, such as matches, heaters, or hair dryers. No one in the house should smoke when oxygen is in use.

Medical Cardiac Tests and Procedures: Left Heart Cardiac Catheterization, Echocardiogram, Coronary Artery Bypass Graft Surgery, and Percutaneous Transluminal Coronary Angioplasty

Table 7.41 Medical Cardiac Tests and Procedures[4,6]

Left Heart Cardiac Catheterization

- Percutaneous intravascular insertion of a catheter into any chamber of the heart or great vessels for diagnosis, assessment of abnormalities, interventions, and evaluation of the effects of pathology on the heart and great vessels.

- During left heart cardiac catheterization, the following diagnostic cardiac tests can be performed: assessment of coronary artery anatomy and its normality, estimation of the cardiac ejection fraction (of left ventricle function), assessment of the cardiac valves, measurements of the intracardiac pressures, and biopsies of the endocardium.

- The normal cardiac ejection fraction is 55–70% of the volume of blood left in the left ventricle at the end of the diastole that has been ejected into the aorta during the systole. A lower cardiac ejection fraction indicates an impaired left ventricle.

- During cardiac catheterization, the patient may also receive a coronary angiogram to record the size, shape, and location of the heart and blood vessels. The angiogram can be of the aorta (to diagnose aneurysm or tumors) and/or of the heart (to determine the size and shape of the chambers and the valves).

(continued)

Table 7.41 **Medical Cardiac Tests and Procedures**[4,6]   *(continued)*

Echocardiogram

- Noninvasive procedure using ultrasound waves to evaluate cardiac structures (such as the heart's valves, chambers, walls, and abnormal intracardiac masses or blood clots).

- Dobutamine stress echocardiogram: dobutamine is given to the patient to increase the heart's workload and evaluate the adequacy of blood flow.

- Prior myocardial infarction can be diagnosed.

- Multidimensional visualization echocardiogram: uses computer technology to visualize three-dimensional cardiac structures.

- Stress echocardiogram: identifies segments of the heart when the patient is performing a treadmill test or is taking a vasodilator medication.

- Transesophageal echocardiogram: invasive echocardiogram into the esophagus; detects cardiac sources of emboli, valves' malfunctions, endocarditis, or congenital heart disease.

Coronary Artery Bypass Graft Surgery (CABG)

- Surgical procedure to treat severe coronary artery disease by using a shunt (or a graft from a donor artery or vein) to install an alternative route for the blood flow and to bypass an obstruction (blockage) in one or more of the coronary arteries.

- The graft can be taken from the radial artery of the nondominant hand or from the saphenous vein.

- In the CABG surgery, the graft is attached and sutured above (into the aorta) and below into the obstructed artery (beyond the occlusion) so that blood flows around it and to the area of the heart below the obstruction. The graft improves the blood flow and the heart's function, relieves angina pectoris symptoms, and prevents MI.

- CABG surgery techniques are continually improving, with less sternal cutting or no sternal cutting at all.

- After CABG surgery, the patient is monitored postoperatively in the intensive care coronary unit (ICCU) with breathing/suctioning tube (and ventilator), vascular catheters (including a pulmonary artery pressure monitor, an arterial catheter for BP monitoring, and IV tubes), heart monitor, chest drainage tubes, bladder catheter, and nasogastric tube.

Percutaneous Transluminal Coronary Angioplasty (PTCA)

- Also called balloon angioplasty or angioplasty; a nonsurgical method of treating localized coronary artery narrowing.

- During PTCA, under X-ray guidance, a double-lumen catheter with a deflated balloon on the tip is inserted transcutaneously in an artery (in the femoral or radial artery). X-ray guides the catheter up into the involved (narrowed by plaque) coronary artery of the heart. The balloon is then inflated and deflated several times to open the narrow artery by compressing the plaque deposits against the wall of the artery.

- During PTCA, stents may be placed permanently inside the opened artery to hold it open. Stents are tiny mesh-like tubes of stainless steel that are inserted in the involved artery (that was just opened) using the catheter with a deflated balloon on the tip. The balloon is inflated, expanding the stent and pressing it against the artery wall.

- Stents are coated with a special medication to prevent endothelial cell proliferation (as a result of endothelial cell trauma and having a foreign object placed into the artery).

- At the end of the PTCA, the balloon is deflated, and the catheter and balloon removed. The stent remains permanently expanded and in place to help keep the narrowed portion of the artery open.

(continued)

CARDIOPULMONARY INTERVENTIONS

Table 7.41 Medical Cardiac Tests and Procedures[4,6]   (continued)

Left Ventricular Assistive Device (LVAD)

- A pump, which may be temporary or permanent, assists with the function of the left ventricle. A temporary pump is used with patients who are waiting for transplant surgery. A permanent device is used if the patient is not a surgical candidate.
- Surgery to implant the device requires opening through the sternum to allow access to the heart.
- The pump involves a tube carrying blood from the left ventricle and another delivering the blood to the aorta. The pump is connected to an external battery pack.
- During surgery the patient may be placed on a heart lung bypass machine.
- Some pumps are placed externally and are mainly for temporary use while the patient awaits a heart transplant.
- Post-surgery the patient will remain in ICU and may be on a ventilator during this time.

Artificial Cardiac Pacemaker

- Device is used to trigger mechanical contractions of the heart by emitting periodic electrical discharges.
- Pacemakers are used for bradycardia, A-V conduction block (may be post MI), other types of A-V block (bifascicular or trifascicular second degree), recurrent syncope (due to carotid sinus abnormalities), sinus node dysfunction, certain arrhythmias, and certain types of CHF (class III CHF).

Automatic Implantable Cardioverter Defibrillator (AICD)

- Surgically implanted defibrillator for patients at high risk for sudden cardiac arrhythmia (which can be life threatening).

Cardiac Safety Rehabilitation Guidelines After Medical Cardiac Procedures

Table 7.42 Safety Guidelines After Medical Cardiac Procedures

Guidelines After CABG Surgery

Physical therapy interventions immediately after CABG surgery may consist of the following treatments: (1) transfers and early ambulation; (2) upper-extremity flexibility exercises (as per the surgeon's choice; some doctors limit upper extremity flexibility exercises in first 4 or 6 weeks postoperatively); (3) postural training; (4) functional training; (5) pain management for areas of incision (using PNF UE diagonal patterns, and ROM exercises with ten repetitions for one to two times per day); and (6) patient education after CABG surgery to avoid lifting, pushing, and pulling objects until sternum is healed. After CABG surgery, patients may have postoperative fatigue and need to increase ambulation gradually. At 6 weeks after CABG surgery, cardiac rehabilitation can begin with aerobic training after a maximal ETT.

Guidelines After PTCA

Physical therapy interventions immediately after PTCA may consist of transfers, ambulation, and activities of daily living (ADLs) at comfortable low intensity. Aerobic training may start 2 to 3 weeks after PTCA (to allow a decrease in the inflammatory response). The exercise prescription for aerobic training should be based on the post-PTCA ETT (not pre-PTCA ETT).

(continued)

Table 7.42 Safety Guidelines After Medical Cardiac Procedures *(continued)*

Guidelines After LVAD Surgery[9]

Physical therapy interventions immediately post LVAD surgery may consist of transfers, ambulation, and light ADLs. Low intensity exercise with a Borg RPE no greater than 13/20. LVAD flow rates to remain between 3 and 4 L/min during exercise. Patients may begin cardiac rehab two weeks after surgery. Sternal precautions should be followed for up to 6 weeks post-surgery median sternotomy to allow for tissue healing.

Guidelines After AICD or Pacemaker Implant

Check with the doctor when to start upper-extremity aerobic exercises. Also, consider the patient's heart rate settings and limit activities (such as functional training or ambulation) at the programmed heart rate. Interventions should avoid intensities that might accidentally activate the device. Initially, upper-extremity aerobic exercises should be avoided so as not to accidentally dislodge the device. In addition, patients with an AICD or pacemaker should receive education about keeping away from electromagnetic signals (such as antitheft devices) that may cause a discharge of the AICD or cause the pacemaker to slow down or speed up.

Orthostatic Hypotension in Cardiopulmonary Rehabilitation

Table 7.43 Orthostatic Hypotension[6]

- Orthostatic hypotension occurs when a person assumes an upright position when getting up from bed (or chair).
- During orthostatic hypotension, the patient's blood pressure suddenly drops ≥20 mm Hg in systolic BP or a drop of ≥ 10 mm Hg in both systolic and diastolic BP with a pulse increase of ≥ 15 BPM when changing positions from lying to sitting or standing. At the same time, a patient with orthostatic hypotension may have a blood pressure of 100 mm Hg (or less) while standing. During orthostatic hypotension, symptoms include lightheadedness, dizziness, and loss of balance. Guard the patient closely due to increased risk of falling on first coming to stand.
- Patients at risk for orthostatic hypotension:
  - Patients who were in bed rest for long periods of time
  - Patients who took vasodilators or antihypertensive medications
  - Patients who became dehydrated
  - Patients who have peripheral vascular disease or muscular atrophy
- Suggested interventions:
  - Use a slow, stepwise progression from supine to sit.
  - Elevate the head of the bed gradually.
  - Provide patient education for deep breathing and ankle pumps prior to moving into sitting and while the patient is sitting at the edge of the bed.
  - Support the patient's feet while the patient is sitting at the edge of the bed.
  - Use a support stocking, and in extreme cases an abdominal binder may be indicated.
  - Use a tilt table.

Types of Cardiopulmonary Interventions

Methods for Monitoring Patients During Cardiopulmonary Rehabilitation/Interventions

Table 7.44 Target Heart Rate

- Target heart rate (THR) needs to be determined by the PT. In cardiopulmonary rehabilitation, it can also be determined during an ETT (also called a graded exercise test).

- During exercises, the patient must be monitored not to exceed the determined THR.

- Formula for calculating THR:

  1. Calculate the patient's maximal heart rate (HR_{max}). The HR_{max} is calculated by subtracting the patient's age from 220 (220 – patient's age). For example, for a patient who is 60 years old, the HR_{max} is 220 – 60 = 160.

  2. Calculate the patient's THR. A patient having a cardiac pathology needs to exercise starting between 50% and 75% of the HR_{max}. Continuing the previous example, the THR for a patient who is 60 years old and has cardiac disease would be 160 (50% – 75%) = 80 bpm – 120 bpm. This patient should start exercises that do not exceed a THR of 80 bpm (50% of the HR_{max}). The patient can then gradually build up his or her exercise program to a THR of 120 bpm (75% of the HR_{max}).

- When using the THR formula, the therapist must take into consideration the patient's medications (such as beta blockers that may decrease the HR_{max}).

Rating of Perceived Exertion (RPE)

Table 7.45 Patient Education Related to RPE Scales Assessment Tools

Assessment Tools

Physical activity for patients who have cardiopulmonary dysfunctions needs to be monitored carefully. A rapid assessment done by the patient (client) himself or herself is very important, especially for patients (clients) who experience dyspnea. Two assessment tools are commonly used to teach the patient (client) to monitor physical activity intensity:

- Borg Rating of Perceived Exertion (RPE) scale:[10] a 15-point scale that starts at 6 as "very light" and ends up at 20 with 19 being very, very hard.

- Modified Borg scale: a 10-point scale scientifically tested in a research study in California.[11]

Research studies [11,12] evaluating these RPE scales showed that the Borg scale had a high correlation with a person's actual heart rate during physical activity and provided a fairly good estimate of the actual heart rate during activity. Other studies[10] found that the Borg RPE scale correlated with many physiological variables such as heart rate, lactate concentration, percentage of VO_{2max2}, VO_2, ventilation, and respiratory rates; however, inconsistencies existed such that some variables affected the validity of the RPE score as a measure of exercise intensity. For example, although the RPE correlated with the heart rate in some studies, research [11,12] that used sedentary patients as subjects found weaker correlations (between RPE and the heart rate) compared to studies that used trained subjects. Studies [11,12] also indicated that there were variations between the scale depending on the exercise protocols used and the subjects' gender. Male RPE scores showed weaker correlations than female RPE scores.

(continued)

Table 7.45 **Patient Education Related to RPE Scales Assessment Tools** *(continued)*

Patient Education Program

The patient should be introduced to the Borg RPE scale before starting the exercise or activity. The following is an example of patient education information about the 15-point RPE Borg scale:

1. While doing exercises or physical activity, we want you to rate your perception of exertion. This feeling should reflect how heavy and strenuous the exercise feels to you, combining all sensations and feelings of physical stress, effort, and fatigue.
2. Try to appraise your feeling of exertion as honestly as possible without thinking about what the actual physical load is. Your own feeling of effort and exertion is important, not how it compares to other people's feelings.
3. The number 6 on the RPE scale corresponds to "no exertion at all," such as lying in bed or sitting in a chair relaxed.
4. The number 9 on the RPE scale corresponds to "very light" exercises. For a healthy person, it is like walking slowly at his or her own pace for a few minutes.
5. The number 13 on the RPE scale is "somewhat hard" exercise, but at which it still feels okay to continue.
6. The number 17 on the RPE scale is "very hard." It means that the exercise is very strenuous. A healthy person can still go on, but the person needs to push himself or herself. The exercise or activity feels very heavy, and the person is very tired.
7. The number 19 on the RPE scale is an extremely strenuous exercise level. For most people, this is the most strenuous exercise they have ever experienced.

Metabolic Equivalents and Activities

Table 7.46 **Overview of Metabolic Equivalents**

- Metabolic equivalents (METs) estimate the metabolic cost of physical activity by evaluating the basic oxygen requirements at rest.
- 1 MET = approximately 3.5 mL of O_2/kg/min.
- Clinically, every activity can be expressed in METs, and the activity METs are compared with the METs at rest.

Table 7.47 **METs and Activities[4]**

- 1–2 METs: walking at 1 mph (on a level surface); active exercises to the upper or lower extremities (can be supine or standing); driving a car; desk work; light housework; electric calculating machine operation; washing clothes; polishing furniture; feeding self; needlework; sewing; standing; motorcycling; playing cards
- 2–3 METs: walking at 2 mph (on a level surface); biking at 5 mph (on a level surface); active exercises while standing; light exercises on a mat; playing billiards; bowling; shuffleboard; driving a powerboat; golfing with power cart; canoeing; horseback riding at a walk; light wood working; riding lawn mower; auto repair; radio and television repair; bartending; janitorial work
- 3–4 METs: biking at 6 mph; walking at 3 mph; walking stairs slowly; playing volleyball with another five people (noncompetitive); golfing and pulling the bag cart; sailing in a small boat; horseback riding (trotting); playing badminton (socially, doubles); vacuuming; pushing light power mower; cleaning windows; mopping floors; laying bricks; plastering; using a wheelbarrow (with 100-pound load); welding (with moderate load); machine assembly

(continued)

Table 7.47 METs and Activities[4] *(continued)*

- 4–5 METs: biking at 8 mph; walking at 3.5 mph (on a level surface); active exercises to the upper or lower extremities (can be supine or standing); playing table tennis; golfing and carrying the golf clubs; dancing the foxtrot; playing badminton (single); playing tennis (doubles); ballet; raking leaves; scrubbing floors; washing the car; painting; performing masonry work; performing paperhanging work; performing light carpentry work

- 5–6 METs: biking at 10 mph; walking at 4 mph; performing step aerobics to tolerance; canoeing at 4 mph; horseback riding (posting to trotting); stream fishing; ice or roller skating at 9 mph; digging a garden; shoveling light earth

- 6–7 METs: walking at 5 mph; biking at 11 mph; playing tennis (singles); swimming (20 yards/min); playing competitive badminton; skiing (light) down the hill; water skiing; folk and square dancing; shoveling light snow; shoveling 10 times/min (4.5 kg or 10 pounds); splitting wood; hand lawn mowing

- 7–8 METs: jogging at 5 mph; biking at 12 mph; playing basketball; skiing (vigorous) downhill; mountain climbing; canoeing at 5 mph; playing ice hockey; playing touch football; playing paddle ball; sawing hardwood; carrying 36 kg or 80 pounds; digging ditches

- 8–9 METs: running at 5.5 mph; bicycling at 13 mph; swimming (at 30 yards/min); skipping rope; playing squash (socially); playing handball (socially); playing basketball (vigorous); ski touring at 4 mph; shoveling 10 times/minute (5.5 kg or 14 pounds)

- 10 METs and more: running at 6 mph (10 METs); running at 9 mph (15 METs); running at 10 mph (17 METs); playing competitive handball; playing competitive squash; swimming (greater than 40 yards/min); ski touring of more than 5 mph; shoveling 10 times/min (7.5 kg, or 16 pounds)

Patient Education Topics for Cardiac Disease

Table 7.48 Patient Education Topics Offered by the Entire Medical Team

- Medications: action of medications; effects of medications considering quality of life and survival; general side effects and what to do about it; dosage; availability of lower-cost medications and financial assistance; patient's disclosure of herbal remedies and supplements.

- Dietary recommendations: patient's regular dietary habits; instructions how to reduce fat intake (for most of the heart diseases); instructions how to monitor salt and fluid intake (for CHF); restrictions on alcohol consumption.

- Activity guidelines: education about the planned exercises, activities at home (including sex, sexual difficulties, and coping strategies), leisure activities, and work activities.

- Patient self-monitoring during activities: education about monitoring HR if the patient is able to feel the pulse; monitoring activities or exercises using the Borg RPE scale; awareness of signs and symptoms suggesting exercise intolerance (e.g., lightheadedness, dyspnea, mental confusion, inability to carry a brief conversation while performing activities or exercises). Patients having CHF may use the Borg dyspnea scale (whose values correspond to the patient's current perceived respiratory effort, such as 10 = completely out of breath; 5 = somewhat breathless; 1 = breathing easily) or the Borg RPE scale.

(continued)

Table 7.48 **Patient Education Topics Offered by the Entire Medical Team** *(continued)*

- Patient's recognition of symptoms and patient's response: written information about the patient's action when symptoms occur (such as calling the physician or going to hospital); recognizing weight gain (2 pounds or more in 1–2 days for CHF); expected symptoms; explanation of the medical treatment plan by the physician; clarification of the patient's responsibilities; importance of smoking cessation; roles of the family members (or other caregivers) in the medical treatment plan.

- Lifestyle topics: resumption of sexual activity (depends on the patient being comfortable enough to discuss the issue; the patient and patient's partner need to be encouraged to bring up the issue). In general, when patients are able and comfortable to climb stairs or walk outdoors, they may be ready for sexual activity. The patient needs to know that in terms of the amount of energy used, sexual activity is different than other physical activities, and needs planning, pacing, and warm-up.

- Psychosocial and social topics: emotional depression. Studies show that emotional depression is common post-CABG surgery (especially for women as compared with men). The patient needs encouragement to seek guidance and counseling.

Phases of Cardiac Rehabilitation After Myocardial Infarction

Table 7.49 **Interventions for Cardiac Rehabilitation Phases**[4]

Cardiac Rehabilitation Post-MI: Team Approach

The multidisciplinary team includes the MD/DO, nurse, PT, PTA, OT, COTA, exercise physiologist, nutritionist, and social worker. Cardiac rehabilitation includes three phases: phase I—inpatient phase; phase II—outpatient phase; and phase III—community-based phase.

Phase I: Inpatient Phase

Inpatient cardiac rehabilitation programs differ based on the pace of increasing MET levels. General interventions in phase I include the following:

- Patient and patient family education for life changes, risk factor modifications, family support, self-monitoring of vital signs (precautions: HR should not rise with activity more than 20 bpm above the resting HR), recognizing adverse symptoms with activity (teaching the Borg RPE scale), and HEP (walking on a level surface at 1 mph).

- Bed mobility skills: ankle pumps to decrease possibility of DVT; transfers with assistance to decrease possibility of pneumonia.

- Activities starting at 1 MET and continuing gradually to 2 METs; some hospitals may progress the patient's activities to 4–5 METs depending on the patient's individual response and medical history.

Phase II: Outpatient Phase

Phase II is based on the results of ETT (at 4–6 weeks post-MI); it uses an exercise prescription of 70–85% of maximum heart rate, with a more conservative exercise prescription reserved for patients with a negative ETT (positive for ischemia). General interventions include the following measures:

(continued)

Table 7.49 **Interventions for Cardiac Rehabilitation Phases**[4] *(continued)*

- Patient education (continuing from phase I) for self-monitoring of vital signs, lifestyle changes, regulation of diet, performing independent ADLs, and an HEP (to include up to 5 METs)
- Activities at 5 METs: treadmill walking at 3.5 mph on a level surface; active exercises to the upper or lower extremities while supine or standing; stationary bicycling; golfing using a power cart; vacuuming; mild resistance exercises
- Resistance exercises (starting at approximately 5 weeks post-MI): Teach the patient to exercise large muscle groups first before exercising small muscle groups; exercise at levels 11–13 on the Borg RPE scale (light to somewhat hard); use slow, controlled movements; stop exercises if become uncomfortable

Phase III: Community-Based or Voluntary Program

Phase III focuses on long-term physical fitness and cardiopulmonary function. The patient self-monitors vital signs during exercise and is aware of his or her target rate. The target MET activity is set based on the patient's individual activities at work and play.

Prevention Interventions for Coronary Artery Disease

Table 7.50 **Prevention Interventions for CAD**[4]

Dietary Guidelines

To be provided by a nutritionist or dietician:

- Patient needs to adopt a low-fat diet (decrease saturated fats and avoid trans fatty acids), decrease salt intake, and have adequate fiber, minerals, and vitamins in the diet.
- Patient may require a sensible diet plan designed by a nutritionist to lose weight.

Exercise Guidelines

To be provided by the PT/PTA:

- Patient needs to gradually increase the endurance activity (such as increasing walking as the aerobic exercise to 40–45 minutes per session).
- Patients older than age 40 with two or more risk factors for heart disease need an ETT before starting an aerobic program or a strengthening exercise program.
- The ETT can identify latent ischemia.
- Exercise programs (prescriptions) for patients older than age 40 with two or more risk factors and a normal ETT can start at 70–80% of the HR_{max} for 30–40 minutes, three to four times per week, with 5–10 minutes of warm-up and cool down.

Community-Based Smoking Cessation Programs (or Medically Supervised Smoking Cessation Programs)

- Program can be recommended for patients who smoke to assist them to stop smoking.

(continued)

Table 7.50 **Prevention Interventions for CAD**[4] *(continued)*

Stress Management

- Programs of different type can be recommended and adapted to the patient's individual needs.

Medications

- Medications may be prescribed to control risk factors such as hypertension, diabetes mellitus, hypercholesterolemia, anxiety, or depression.
- All medications should be used in a proper and consistent mode.

Manage Diabetes or Impaired Glucose Tolerance

- Impaired glucose metabolism is a significant risk factor for coronary artery disease.
- Educate on importance of maintaining blood glucose levels within acceptable limits. Patients who struggle may benefit from referral to a dietician.

Control of Hypertension

- A multifactorial approach that involves, in addition to medications, lifestyle modifications (including weight reduction), dietary reduction of sodium intake, and increased physical activity.

Pulmonary Interventions: Terms Related to Postural Drainage

Table 7.51 **Postural Drainage Terms**

Turning

Turning is the rotation of the body around the longitudinal axis to promote unilateral or bilateral lung expansion and improve arterial oxygenation. Regular turning can be to either side or to the prone position (proning), with the bed at any degree of inclination (as indicated and tolerated). Patients may turn themselves, or they may be turned by the caregiver or by a special bed or device.

Postural Drainage

Postural drainage is the drainage of secretions, by the effect of gravity, from one or more lung segments to the central airways (where they can be removed by cough or mechanical aspiration). Each position consists of placing the target lung segment(s) superior to the carina tracheae (the ridge at the lower end of the trachea separating the openings of the two primary bronchi). Positions should generally be held for 3–15 minutes (longer in special situations). Standard positions are modified as the patient's condition and tolerance warrant.

(continued)

Table 7.51 **Postural Drainage Terms**   *(continued)*

Percussion

Percussion is a manual technique for mobilizing secretions from the lungs by striking the chest wall. It is also referred to as cupping, clapping, and tapotement. The purpose of percussion is to intermittently apply kinetic energy to the chest wall and lung. This goal is accomplished by rhythmically striking the thorax with a cupped hand or mechanical device directly over the lung segment(s) being drained. No convincing evidence demonstrates the superiority of one method over the other.

Vibration

Vibration is another manual technique that involves the application of a fine tremulous action (manually performed) by pressing in the direction that the ribs and soft tissue of the chest move during expiration (over the draining area).

Postural Drainage Positions: Indications, Contraindications, and Precautions

Table 7.52 **Postural Drainage: Indications, Contraindications, and Precautions**

Postural drainage uses gravity to assist the removal of secretions from specific lobes of the lung, bronchi, or lung cavities. Postural drainage positions increase anteroposterior lung expansion and height, allowing for effective breathing. To perform postural drainage, the patient should be positioned so that the involved segmental bronchus is uppermost.

Indications for Postural Drainage Positions

- Aspiration
- Increased pulmonary secretions
- Atelectasis (lung collapse) due to excess mucus

Contraindications for All Postural Drainage Positions (see also Table 7.39)

- Intracranial pressure > 20 mm Hg
- Head and neck injury (until stabilized)
- Active hemorrhage with hemodynamic (circulating blood forces) instability
- Recent spinal surgery (such as laminectomy)
- Acute spinal injury or active hemoptysis (expectoration of blood from larynx, trachea, bronchi, or lungs)
- Emphysema (COPD)
- Bronchopleural fistula (an abnormal opening between the pleural space and an airway in the lung)
- Pulmonary edema associated with congestive heart failure
- Large pleural effusions (fluid in the pleural cavity)
- Pulmonary embolism (obstruction of pulmonary artery or one of its branches)

(continued)

Table 7.52 **Postural Drainage: Indications, Contraindications, and Precautions** *(continued)*

- Aged, confused, or anxious patients who do not tolerate position changes
- Rib fracture, with or without flail chest (in flail chest, the affected rib segment is not attached on either end, and moves in and out during breathing)
- Surgical wound or healing tissue

Contraindications for Trendelenburg Position*

- Intracranial pressure > 20 mm Hg
- Patients in whom increased intracranial pressure is to be avoided (such as after neurosurgery, aneurysms, or eye surgery)
- Uncontrolled hypertension
- Distended abdomen
- Esophageal surgery
- Recent gross hemoptysis related to recent lung carcinoma treated surgically or with radiation therapy
- Uncontrolled airway at risk for aspiration (tube feeding or recent meal)

Precautions for Trendelenburg Position*

- Pulmonary edema
- Shortness of breath
- Congestive heart failure
- Medication-controlled hypertension
- Hiatal hernia
- Obesity
- Nausea

Contraindications for Reverse Trendelenburg Position†

- Hypotension
- Vasodilator medications

Precautions for Side-Lying Positions

- Arthritis
- Recent rib fracture
- Shoulder tendonitis/bursitis
- Patient's discomfort
- Axillofemoral bypass graft

* In Trendelenburg position, the patient's head is low, and the body and legs are on an elevated and inclined plane.
† In reverse Trendelenburg position, the patient's head is elevated and the body and legs are low.

CARDIOPULMONARY INTERVENTIONS

Table 7.53 **Bronchial Drainage Positions and Percussion**[4]

Upper Lobes—Apical Segments

The patient can be positioned on a bed or a drainage table (that is flat). The patient leans back on a pillow at a 30° angle against the therapist. The therapist claps with markedly cupped hand over area between the clavicle and the top of scapula on each side.

Upper Lobes—Posterior Segments

The patient can be positioned on a bed or a drainage table (that is flat). The patient leans over a folder pillow at a 30° angle. The therapist stands behind and claps over the upper back on both sides.

Right Middle Lobe

With the foot of the table or bed elevated 16 inches, the patient lies head down on the left side and rotates one-fourth turn backward. A pillow may be placed behind, from shoulder to hip. The patient's knees should be flexed. The therapist claps over the right nipple area. In females with breast development or tenderness, use cupped hand with heel of the hand under the armpit and fingers extending forward beneath the breast.

Left Upper Lobe—Lingular Segments

With the foot of the table or bed elevated 16 inches, the patient lies head down on the right side and rotates one-fourth turn backward. A pillow may be placed behind, from shoulder to hip. The patient's knees should be flexed. The therapist claps with moderately cupped hand over the left nipple area. In females with breast development or tenderness, use cupped hand with heel of the hand under the armpit and fingers extending forward beneath the breast.

Lower Lobes—Lateral Basal Segments

With the foot of table or the bed elevated 20 inches, the patient lies on the abdomen, head down, and then rotates one-fourth turn upward. The patient's upper leg is flexed over a pillow for support. The therapist claps over the uppermost portion of the lower ribs. For left lateral basal segment, the patient should lie slightly on his or her right side in the same position, whereas for the right lateral basal segment, the patient should lie slightly on his or her left side in the same position.

Lower Lobes—Posterior Basal Segments

With the foot of the table or bed elevated 20 inches, the patient lies on the abdomen. The patient's head is down, and a pillow is under the hips. The therapist claps over the lower ribs close to the spine on each side.

Upper Lobes—Anterior Segments

On a bed or drainage table that is flat, the patient lies on back with a pillow under the knees. The therapist claps between the clavicle and the nipple on each side.

Lower Lobes—Anterior Basal Segments

With the foot of the table or bed elevated 20 inches, the patient lies on his or her side, with head down, and a pillow under the knees. The therapist claps with slightly cupped hand over the lower ribs. To drain the right anterior basal segment, the patient should lie on his or her left side in the same position, whereas for the left anterior basal segment, the patient should lie on his or her right side on the same position.

Lower Lobes—Superior Segments

On a bed or table that is flat, the patient lies on the abdomen with two pillows under the hips. The therapist claps over the middle back at the tip of the scapula on either side of the spine.

Percussion and Shaking Techniques: Indications, Contraindications, and Precautions

Table 7.54 Percussion and Shaking Techniques: Indications, Contraindications, and Precautions

Percussion

Percussion is a tapotement technique used in pulmonary physical therapy to strike the chest wall with cupped hands to mobilize lung secretions. It can be applied in combination with postural drainage positions for specific lung segments.

Indications for Percussion

- Aspiration
- Increased pulmonary secretions
- Atelectasis (lung collapse) caused by excess mucus

Contraindications for Percussion (in Addition to Postural Drainage Contraindications)

- Subcutaneous emphysema
- Recent epidural spinal infusion or spinal anesthesia
- Recent skin grafts, or flaps, on the thorax
- Burns, open wounds, and skin infections of the thorax
- Recently placed transvenous pacemaker (temporary pacemaker inserted transvenously into right ventricular apex) or subcutaneous pacemaker (particularly if mechanical devices are to be used)
- Suspected pulmonary tuberculosis
- Lung contusion
- Bronchospasm
- Osteomyelitis (inflammation of bone and marrow) of the ribs; osteoporosis
- Coagulopathy (blood clotting defect)
- Complaint of chest-wall pain

Shaking

Shaking is a vibration technique used in pulmonary physical therapy to mobilize lung secretions. PTA may use five to seven shaking techniques for a specific lung segment in combination with postural drainage positions. Use of fewer than five techniques is ineffective and use of more than ten techniques (with inhalations) can cause hyperventilation.

Indications for Shaking

- Aspiration
- Increased pulmonary secretions
- Atelectasis (lung collapse) caused by excess mucus

(continued)

Table 7.54 **Percussion and Shaking Techniques: Indications, Contraindications, and Precautions** *(continued)*

Precautions When Applying Percussion or Shaking

- Fractured ribs
- Degenerative bone disease
- Hemoptysis (expectoration of blood)
- Coagulation disorders
- Increased partial thromboplastin time (PTT—blood coagulation) to more than 38 seconds (normal = 25–38 seconds)
- Platelet count less than 50,000

Other Interventions for Pulmonary Rehabilitation

Table 7.55 **Breathing Techniques, Activity Pacing, Coughing, and Aerobic Training**

For relaxation exercises, see Part 4.

Breathing Exercises

Breathing exercises are taught in a quiet environment, with the patient in a relaxed and comfortable position (free of restrictive clothing). At the beginning of the exercises, the patient should be sitting in a semi-reclined position with the head and the trunk elevated at approximately 45°, allowing the abdominal musculature to relax. The patient's knees and hips are flexed and supported with a pillow.

Precautions During Breathing Exercises

- Do not allow the patient to perform forced expiration (because it can cause bronchospasm); expiration should be passive, relaxed, or controlled.
- Do not allow the patient to start inspiration using the accessory muscles and the upper chest; the upper chest should be quiet during breathing.
- Do not allow the patient to take a very prolonged expiration (because it causes the patient to gasp with the next inspiration and becomes an irregular breathing pattern).
- Allow the patient to perform deep breathing for only three or four inspirations and expirations at a time (to avoid possibility of hyperventilation).

Glossopharyngeal Breathing

Glossopharyngeal breathing is a breathing technique for patients who have weakness in the muscles of inspiration (diaphragm and accessory muscles). The patient takes several "gulps" of air and then closes his or her mouth, forcing the air into the lungs.

Pursed-Lip Breathing

Pursed-lip breathing is an expiratory breathing technique for patients who have dyspnea caused by (most often) COPD. It may prevent premature closing of intrapulmonary airways. First the patient inhales through the nose for several seconds with the mouth closed. Then the patient exhales through puckered lips (such as whistling or kissing) to slow the expiratory flow. This creates slight back-pressure, allowing for better gas exchange. During pursed-lip breathing, there should not be expiratory flow through the nose.

(continued)

Table 7.55 Breathing Techniques, Activity Pacing, Coughing, and Aerobic Training *(continued)*

Diaphragmatic Breathing

Diaphragmatic breathing is a breathing technique that retrains the patient to use the diaphragm while relaxing the abdominal muscles during inspiration (such as having the abdomen rising while the chest wall remains stationary). The patient inhales slowly so that the abdomen swells out and the lower part and the upper part of the chest expand and slightly lift. Then the patient holds the breath momentarily and releases the expiratory flow slowly (exhaling) as the abdomen is drawn in, the diaphragm is lifted, and the chest relaxes. Diaphragmatic breathing is used for COPD and CRLD. It is also a relaxation technique. The therapist may use a biofeedback machine to help use of diaphragm and inhibit use of accessory muscles.

Diaphragmatic breathing is performed as follows:
1. The patient is relaxed in a semi-reclined position, and the procedure is explained to the patient.
2. The therapist places his or her hand gently over the subcostal angle of the patient's thorax.
3. The therapist applies gentle pressure throughout the exhalation phase of breathing. Toward the end of the exhalation, the therapist increases to firm pressure. The patient is asked to inhale against the resistance of the therapist's hand.
4. As the therapist feels the diaphragm moving, the hand resistance is released, allowing the patient a full inhalation.
5. The patient is taught the technique first in a semi-reclined sitting position (also called semi-Fowler position) and then in sitting, standing, walking, and stair climbing positions.

Segmental Breathing

Segmental breathing is a breathing technique to help the hypoventilated segments of the lungs in patients with pleuritic pain, splinting (from surgery or trauma), and segmental atelectasis. Before segmental breathing, the patient needs to clear the airways (of mucus) by using secretion removal techniques. The patient inhales against the resistance of the therapist's hand (placed at the thorax over the area of hypoventilation). As the therapist feels the local expansion of the thorax, the hand resistance is slowly released to allow for full inhalation.

Active Cycle of Breathing Techniques (ACBT)

ACBT are used to help clear secretions from airways. ACBT is performed as follows:
■ The breathing control phase: ACBT begins with patient performing a few minutes of relaxed diaphragmatic breathing.

■ Deep breathing or thoracic expansion exercises: The patient performs three to five deep inhalations with a 3-second hold followed by a passive exhalation. If the patient gets lightheaded return to the breathing control phase.

■ Huffing or forced expiration techniques: The patient performs a deep breath in followed by one or two huffs out. This forced expiration helps to mobilize secretions.

■ Coughing: may be added to clear secretions.

■ Repeat the cycle for up to 10 minutes to clear secretions from the lungs.

Activity Pacing

Activity pacing teaches the patient how to perform an activity (such as ADLS, ambulation, stair climbing, and other tasks) within his or her breathing capacity limits. The patient needs to break an activity into several small components. The patient then performs each component with rest periods between them, eliminating dyspnea and fatigue. While performing each small component of the activity, the patient may use the pursed-lip breathing technique. For example, to climb one flight of stairs, the patient inhales at rest and then, on exhalation while using pursed-lip breathing, ascends one or two steps. Then the patient stops to rest until full recovery. The patient repeats the process until the whole flight is ascended without dyspnea and fatigue.

(continued)

Table 7.55 Breathing Techniques, Activity Pacing, Coughing, and Aerobic Training

Coughing

Coughing is the easiest way to clear the airway. Assisted cough takes place with the patient in a sitting position (against a wall), and the PTA placing both hands below the patient's subcostal angle (against the patient's abdomen between the navel and the rib cage). As the patient inhales deeply and attempts to cough, the PTA's hands push inward and upward assisting the exhalation of air.

Huffing

Huffing is similar to coughing. The patient must take a deep breath and immediately try to forcibly expel the air by saying, "Ha, ha, ha."

Mucus Expulsion

Mucus (phlegm) expelled through coughing may need to be sent to the laboratory for analysis. In pneumonia, the mucus is viscid, tenacious, and sticky. Its appearance is rusty and containing blood. In bronchitis, the mucus is mucoid, streaked with blood, and greenish yellow (from pus).

Suctioning

Suctioning is removal of secretions from the larger airways. It is performed as follows:
1. Use aseptic technique.
2. Provide supplemental oxygen.
3. Insert the suction catheter without applying suction, as fully as possible (be gentle).
4. Apply suction while withdrawing the catheter.
5. Re-expand the lung with a mechanical ventilator or manual inflation by use of a resuscitator bag attached to the tracheal tube.

Warning: The suctioning procedure should be done by an experienced PT (check your state practice act). Tracheal suctioning can be used only with patients who have an artificial airway in place. Suctioning must be avoided in patients with hypoxemia, cardiac dysrhythmias, mechanical trauma, bacterial contamination of the tracheobronchial tree, or increased intracranial pressure.

Bagging

Bagging provides artificial ventilation, restores oxygen, and re-expands the lungs after suctioning. It is performed as follows:
1. Attach the manual resuscitator bag to an oxygen source.
2. Connect the manual resuscitator bag to the tracheal tube.
3. Squeeze the bag rhythmically to deliver the desired volume of air to the patient.
4. The patient exhales passively.

Bagging is used before and after suctioning for patients who are not mechanically ventilated.

Turning, Positioning, and Movement Techniques

Turning, passive positioning, using splints, PROM, AROM, sitting, standing, and ambulation are used with every patient in a cardiopulmonary acute care unit (ICU/CCU); the selection of a technique depends on the patient's diagnosis and tolerance. The therapist should be careful with intravascular lines and tubes. In addition, the therapist should watch the patient for orthostatic hypotension, dyspnea, and changes in vital signs.

(continued)

Table 7.55 **Breathing Techniques, Activity Pacing, Coughing, and Aerobic Training** *(continued)*

Aerobic Training

Aerobic training is part of cardiopulmonary rehabilitation in post-acute care. It includes warm-up, aerobic exercise, and cool-down. Stretching exercises during exhalation (to prevent a Valsalva maneuver) are recommended before aerobic training. The warm-up period (5–15 minutes) consists of the same exercise as the aerobic exercise but is performed at a lower intensity while using controlled breathing. The aerobic exercise (20–60 minutes) should maintain the calculated THR of the exercise prescription. The patient can be monitored using a rating of perceived shortness of breath, heart rate values, respiratory rate, and oximetry (oxygen saturation measurement). The cool-down (5–15 minutes) consists of low-level aerobic activities that slowly return the cardiopulmonary system to pre-exercise levels.

Examples of Pulmonary Exercises

Table 7.56 **Examples of Pulmonary Exercises**

Lateral Chest Mobilization Exercises

These exercises are performed during inspiration and expiration and mobilize the lateral rib cage. To perform mobilization to the lateral side of the chest:
1. During inspiration, the patient (sitting) bends away from the tight side of the chest (to lengthen hypomobile structures and expand the chest).
2. During expiration, the patient (sitting) pushes a fisted hand onto the lateral aspect of the chest while bending toward the tight side.
3. To progress these exercises, ask the patient to raise his or her arm on the tight side over the head and side-bend away from the tight side (increasing the stretch on the hypomobile structures).

Upper Chest Mobilization Exercises

These exercises are performed to stretch the pectoralis muscles. Do the following to perform upper chest mobilization for pectoralis stretch:
1. During the exercise, the patient sits in a chair with hands clasped behind the head.
2. During inspiration, the patient abducts the arms horizontally.
3. During expiration, the patient brings the elbows together while bending forward.

Upper Chest Mobilization Exercises

These exercises provide for upper chest expansion and stretching the shoulders. Do the following to perform upper chest mobilization for chest expansion and shoulders stretch:
1. During the exercise, the patient sits in a chair.
2. During inspiration, the patient reaches with both arms overhead (at 180° in bilateral shoulder flexion and slight abduction).
3. During expiration, the patient bends forward at the hips while reaching forward with both arms toward the floor.

Cardiopulmonary Intervention Patterns

CARDIOPULMONARY INTERVENTIONS

American Physical Therapy Association (APTA) Guide to Physical Therapist Practice: APTA's Cardiopulmonary Intervention Patterns

Table 7.57 Therapeutic Exercises[13]

1. Strength, power, and endurance training for the head, neck, limb, pelvic floor, trunk, and ventilatory muscles: active assistive, active, and resistive exercises, including concentric, dynamic, isotonic, isometric, and plyometric; aquatic programs; standardized, programmatic, complementary exercise approaches task-specific performance training
2. Flexibility exercises: muscle lengthening, range of motion, stretching
3. Relaxation exercises: breathing strategies; movement strategies; relaxation techniques; standardized, programmatic, complementary exercise approaches
4. Aerobic capacity and endurance conditioning and reconditioning: aquatic programs, gait and locomotor training, increased workload over time, task-specific performance training, walking and wheelchair propulsion programs
5. Body mechanics and postural stabilization: body mechanics training, posture awareness training, postural control training, postural stabilization activities
6. Gait and locomotion training: developmental activities training; gait training; implement and device training; perceptual training; standardized, programmatic, complementary exercise approaches wheelchair training
7. Neuromotor development training: developmental activities training, motor training, movement pattern training, neuromuscular education or re-education
8. Balance, coordination, and agility training: developmental activities training; motor function such as motor control and motor learning training and retraining; neuromuscular education and re-education; standardized, programmatic, complementary exercise approaches

Table 7.58 Functional Training in Self-Care and in Domestic Education, Work Community, and Social and Civic Life [13,14]

1. ADL training: bathing, bed mobility and transfer training, developmental activities, dressing, eating, grooming, toileting
2. Devices and equipment use and training: assistive and adaptive device and equipment training during ADLs and instrumental activities of daily living (IADLs); orthotic, protective, or supportive device or equipment training during ADLs and IADLs; prosthetic device or equipment training during ADLs and IADLs
3. Functional training programs: simulated environments and tasks
4. IADL training: caring for dependents, home maintenance, household chores, shopping, structured play for infants and children, yard work
5. Injury prevention or reduction: safety awareness training during self-care and home management, injury prevention or reduction with use of assistive devices and equipment
6. Devices and equipment use and training: assistive and adaptive device and equipment training during IADLs; orthotic, protective, or supportive device or equipment training during IADLs; prosthetic device or equipment training during IADLs
7. Functional training programs: simulated environments and tasks, task adaptation, task training, work conditioning, work hardening
8. IADL training: community service training involving instruments, school and play activities training including tools and instruments, work training with tools
9. Injury prevention or reduction: injury prevention education during work at job, school, or play, community, and leisure integration or reintegration; injury prevention or reduction with use of devices and equipment; safety awareness training during work at job, school, or play, community, and leisure integration and reintegration
10. Leisure and play activities and training

Table 7.59 **Prescription, Application, and (as Appropriate) Fabrication or Modification of Locomotive Aids, Orthotic and Prosthetic Devices**[14]

---

1. Adaptive devices: seating systems
2. Assistive devices: canes, crutches, long-handled reachers, walkers, power devices, static and dynamic splints, wheelchairs
3. Orthotic devices: braces, casts, splints, shoe inserts
4. Protective devices: braces, cushions
5. Supportive devices: compression garments, corsets, elastic wraps, neck collars, supplemental oxygen, mechanical ventilators

---

Table 7.60 **Manual Therapy Techniques (Excludes Joint Mobilization)**[13]

---

1. Manual lymphatic drainage
2. Passive range of motion (PROM)
3. Massage (such as connective tissue massage, therapeutic massage)
4. Soft-tissue mobilization

Table 7.61 **Electrotherapeutic Modalities** [13]

Electrical muscle stimulation, such as EMS and TENS

- Electrical modalities may be contraindicated in certain cardiac conditions (see Tables 2-60 and 4-5).

Table 7.62 **Patient/Client-Related Instruction**[13]

Instruction, education, and training of patients/clients and caregivers regarding the following topics:
- Risk factors for pathology and pathophysiology (disease, disorder, or condition) impairments
- Functional limitations or disabilities
- Enhancement of performance
- Health, wellness, and fitness programs
- Plan for intervention
- Current condition—pathology and pathophysiology (diseases, disorder, or condition), impairments, functional limitations, and disabilities
- Plan of care
- Transitions across settings
- Transitions to new roles

CARDIOPULMONARY INTERVENTIONS

Table 7.63 Airway Clearance Techniques[13]

- Breathing strategies: active cycle of breathing or forced expiratory techniques; assisted cough/huff techniques; autogenic drainage; paced breathing; pursed-lip breathing; techniques to maximize ventilation: maximum inspiratory hold, staircase breathing, manual hyperinflation
- Positioning: positioning to alter the work of breathing, positioning to maximize ventilation and perfusion, pulmonary postural drainage
- Manual and mechanical techniques: assistive devices; chest percussion, vibration, and shaking; chest wall manipulation; suctioning; ventilatory aids

Clinical Practice Guidelines

Clinical Practice Guidelines (CPGs), developed by APTA sections, other organizations, societies, and health care organizations, are based on a systematic review of the evidence and provide therapists with resources to help guide clinical decision making. The Academy of Cardiovascular and Pulmonary Physical Therapy, a Section of the APTA, provides access to CPGs relevant to the management of patients with cardiovascular and pulmonary diagnoses. Examples of topics addressed by the Academy of Cardiovascular and Pulmonary Physical Therapy include the following:[15] Role of Physical Therapists in the Management of Individuals at Risk for or Diagnosed with Venous Thromboembolism: Evidence-Based Clinical Practice Guideline; Supplemental Oxygen Utilization During Physical Therapy Interventions; Physical Therapist Clinical Practice Guideline for the Management of Individuals with Heart Failure. A full listing and links to the published CPGs can be found at https://www.aptacvp.org/clinical-practice-guidelines.

Coronary Artery Disease: Intervention Patterns

Table 7.64 Basic Physical Therapy Goals for CAD Interventions (Included in the APTA's Guide to Physical Therapist Practice)[13,14]

- To improve physiological response to increased oxygen requirements; to decrease symptoms associated with increased oxygen requirements
- To increase power, strength, endurance, and aerobic capacity
- To increase capability of performing ADLs, IADLs, home management, and community and work integration/reintegration
- To improve ability to recognize a recurrence and seek immediate interventions; to decrease the risk of recurrence
- To acquire behaviors that promote wellness, healthy habits, and prevention
- To increase patient/client, family, and caregiver decision-making ability in regard to patient (client) health and use of healthcare resources

Table 7.65 Exercise Guidelines for CAD

- The aerobic exercise prescriptions should be based on the FITT equation: F = frequency, I = intensity, T = time (duration), T = type (mode).

- Aerobic exercise training is recommended three to five times per week for 12 or more weeks.

- Each aerobic exercise training session consists of 20–40 minutes of aerobic exercise, 5–10 minutes of warm-up, and 5–10 minutes of cool down. Patients (clients) who are deconditioned may need rest periods of 5 minutes between exercises.

- The aerobic exercise intensity may start at approximately 70–85% of the HR_{max}. Patients (clients) who are deconditioned may need to start at a lower intensity of 50–60% of the HR_{max}. However, the safest method of calculating the exercise intensity for patients/clients having CAD is through use of the medically supervised ETT. During the ETT, EKG monitoring can detect exercise-induced ischemia.

- Exercise intensity can be based on either exercise prescription or patient (client) report of rating of perceived exertion (Borg RPE scale). When using the Borg RPE scale, patients (clients) need to limit their exertion to the range between "fairly light" [11] and "somewhat hard" [13].

- During exercises, the patient (client) should not experience fatigue as a result of exercises. If fatigue occurs, the exercise intensity or frequency should be decreased. Patients (clients) should be aware that symptoms of fatigue and overexertion may occur during the exercises (activities), or may occur later in the day or the following day.

- The type (mode) of exercise or activity can be treadmill, bicycle, stair climber, rower, reclining bicycle, stepper, cross-country ski stimulator, and arm ergometer. Patients (clients) have a large variety of equipment from which to choose. It is important to allow patients (clients) to choose the equipment that they enjoy the most.

- The exercise or activity should progressively increase in a logical fashion, with increasing energy costs (such as METs) being matched with appropriate BP and HR monitoring.

- Contraindications to aerobic exercise training include the following: [1] unstable angina, [2] symptomatic heart failure, [3] uncontrolled arrhythmia, [4] moderate to severe aortic stenosis, [5] uncontrolled diabetes, [6] acute systemic illness or fever, [7] uncontrolled tachycardia, [8] resting systolic BP of equal or more than 200 mm Hg, [9] resting diastolic BP of equal or more than 110 mm Hg, and [10] thrombophlebitis.

- As a safety precaution, patients (clients) need to know to stop the exercise (activity) immediately with any ischemia symptom i.e., angina.

- If the patient (client) experiences angina pain in the outpatient facility, the PTA should stop the activity, have the patient (client) lie down, take the patient's BP and HR, and call the PT. From the results of the BP and HR, the PT will determine patient's ischemic threshold (maximum volume of oxygen when the patient experienced ischemia). In an outpatient facility, patients (clients) may use nitroglycerin (NTG) medication to reduce ischemia; NTG is taken sublingually or using a spray. The patient (client) waits 5 minutes and repeats administration of NTG. Patients (clients) know that if the symptoms do not resolve after three administrations of NTG (at 5-minute intervals), they need to go to the emergency room.

- When the patient's symptoms of ischemia amplify (instead of abating) after the exercise or activity stopped, the patient needs to be assisted to a position of comfort and emergency medical services needs to be alerted.

- If the patient (client) is alone while ascending stairs and the symptoms of ischemia appear, he or she must stop, take a few easy deep breaths, and wait for the symptoms to abate. Then the patient (client) can descend stairs slowly to the first available help.

- As a safety precaution in cases of ischemia in an inpatient facility, the PTA should follow the facility's guidelines by seeking immediate nursing personnel help. The facility may administer to the patient oxygen, EKG, and/or NTG or other anti-ischemic medication.

Table 7.66 **Strength Training in Cardiac Rehabilitation After MI**

- Strength training is a recent exercise addition in cardiac rehabilitation. According to research studies, it is considered safe and effective.
- Strength training can start with light resistance using light elastic bands or weights (1–3 pounds) for 12–15 repetitions. The resistance can be gradually increased to the patient's comfort level.
- Strength training should begin at approximately 5 weeks after MI or 8 weeks after CABG surgery, although this may vary by facility.
- Strength training guidelines include the following: (1) use the patient's large muscle groups before exercising the small muscle groups; (2) stress exhalation with exertion; (3) avoid sustained tight grip; (4) use slow controlled movements; (5) focus on the Borg RPE scale range of 11 to 13; and (6) stop exercises with any warning that the patient is experiencing uncomfortable signs and symptoms.
- When starting and during cardiac strength training, the PTA should have the immediate availability of the PT (in the event of an emergency).

Congestive Heart Failure: Interventions

Table 7.67 **Basic Physical Therapy Goals for CHF Interventions (Included in the APTA's Guide to Physical Therapist Practice)[13]**

- To improve physiological response to increased oxygen requirements
- To improve the patient's self-management of symptoms; to increase the patient's awareness of relevant community resources
- To increase the capability of performing independent ADLs and physical tasks
- To acquire behaviors that promote wellness, healthy habits, and prevention
- To reduce disability associated with acute or chronic illness
- To reduce the risk of secondary impairments

Table 7.68 **Exercise Guidelines for CHF**

- Low-level exercises can start when the functional status of the cardiac system (hemodynamic system) is stable. Exercises should consider the patient's systemic conditioning, peripheral endurance training, low-level resistance training, and respiratory muscle training.
- During exercises, the patient needs to be monitored through oxygen saturation (using pulse oximetry with finger probe), vital signs (BP, HR, RR), observation, auscultation, and recording the RPE (Borg RPE scale). Also, the patient needs to be observed for orthostatic hypotension caused by exertion, angina, and significant dysrhythmias.
- The exercise intensity should be low (40-60% VO_{2max}); the duration of exercise can be gradually increased as per the patient's tolerance. Initially duration could be as little as 2–6 minutes, followed by a 2 minute rest, increasing duration as tolerated. The exercise HR should be less than 115 bpm. The PTA needs to recognize that some cardiac medications blunt the HR response to exercise, finding patient's HR only increases by 10–20 BPM above resting during exercise. Use of Borg's RPE scale is indicated with this population as a better reflection of intensity during exercise.
- For patients who are deconditioned, light calisthenics in sitting position are recommended to begin the exercise program. Also, the exercises need to start with a prolonged warm-up and end with a prolonged cool down. Isometrics are contraindicated.
- Resistance training can start with elastic bands (yellow) or light weights for the upper and lower extremities.

Chronic Obstructive Pulmonary Disease: Interventions

Table 7.69 Basic Physical Therapy Expected Outcomes for Pulmonary Interventions (Included in the APTA's Guide to Physical Therapist Practice)[13,14]

- To improve the patient's (and family's) understanding of the disease process, expectations, goals, and outcomes
- To increase the strength, power, and endurance of the peripheral and ventilatory muscles; to increase cardiovascular endurance; to improve independence in airway clearance; to decrease the work of breathing
- To increase the capability of performing physical tasks and ADLs/IADLs
- To improve decision-making capability in regard to the use of healthcare resources
- To enhance the patient's self-management of the symptoms and of the pulmonary disease

Table 7.70 General Interventions for COPD

- Patient education
  - Topics such as smoking cessation (if the patient continues to smoke)
  - Types of exercises and activities (including effects, contraindications, and adherence)
  - Monitoring the use of bronchodilators, before engaging in activity/exercise; bronchodilators are used to expand the bronchi by relaxing the bronchial muscles.
  - Monitoring the use of antibiotics
  - Relaxation techniques
  - Energy conservation
  - Use of home humidifier (to increase moisture content of the air)
  - For asthma, avoidance of allergens or other environmental triggers
  - For cystic fibrosis, performing chest physical therapy and postural drainage (on a regular schedule either BID, QID, or PRN)
- Secretion removal and postural drainage techniques
- Breathing techniques (diaphragmatic and pursed-lip breathing) and activity pacing; monitoring the breathing pattern with exercises and activities
- Cough techniques
- Exercises
  - During all interventions monitor HR, BP, respiratory rate, and oxygen saturation.
  - Shoulder shrugs, arm circles, chest mobility exercises, and postural exercises increase expansibility of the lungs.
  - Exercise intensity for a patient with mild to moderate COPD ranges between 50–70% of heart rate reserve. Exercise duration of 20–30 minutes is recommended although patients may require frequent rest periods in each session. A frequency of three to five sessions a week can be used with patients who tolerate 20–30 minutes of continuous exercise.
  - Exercise should include aerobic and resistance exercise in addition to flexibility already mentioned. Patients with COPD benefit from a longer warm-up period. Resistance training should include upper and lower extremities.

Table 7.71 COPD Patient Education Topics (Delivered by the Entire Rehabilitation Team)

- Anatomy and physiology of respiratory disease
- Nutritional guidelines
- Airway clearance techniques
- Stress management and relaxation techniques
- Energy-saving techniques
- Benefits of being smoke free
- Use of medications
- The effects of environmental factors on COPD
- Oxygen delivery systems
- Psychosocial aspects of COPD
- Management of COPD
- Community resources

Chronic Restrictive Lung Diseases, Atelectasis, and Pulmonary Edema: Intervention Patterns

Table 7.72 General Intervention Patterns: CRLDs, Atelectasis, and Pulmonary Edema

CRLDs from Surgical Procedures

- Preoperative physical therapy interventions to assist the patient following surgery with deep-breathing exercises
- Incentive spirometer
- Coughing techniques with proper incisional splinting
- Secretions removal
- Bed mobility training
- Patient education
- Ankle pumps to decrease DVT

CRLDs from Surgical Procedures

- Postoperative physical therapy interventions to assist the patient with monitoring vital signs
- Incentive spirometer
- Monitoring sputum production
- Patient education on deep breathing and coughing techniques
- Proper splinting techniques for the incisional line
- Ankle pumps to decrease DVT and increase blood flow
- Transfers to the edge of the bed
- Early postoperative ambulation

(continued)

Table 7.72 General Intervention Patterns: CRLDs, Atelectasis, and Pulmonary Edema   *(continued)*

Atelectasis

Pulmonary disorder due to collapse of one or more lobes of the lungs

- Postural drainage with percussion
- Segmental breathing exercises
- Incentive spirometer
- Patient education for proper splinting with coughing or movement

Pulmonary Edema

Effusion of serous fluid into the alveoli and interstitial tissue of the lungs; can be caused by failure or weakening of the left ventricle

- Deep breathing and coughing techniques
- Paced activity with pursed-lip breathing

Pharmacology for Cardiovascular and Pulmonary Conditions

CARDIOPULMONARY INTERVENTIONS

Effects of Medications in Cardiac Rehabilitation

Table 7.73 Effects of Medications in Cardiac Rehabilitation[4]

Angiotensin-Converting Enzyme (ACE) Inhibitors

- Group of drugs used to treat HTN, CHF, and other diseases; suppress the rennin–angiotensin–aldosterone system
- Examples: Capoten (Captopril), Lotensin (Benazepril), Prinivil (Lisinopril), Zestril (Lisinopril), and Univasc (Moexipril)
- Effects
  - Have no effect on HR
  - Decrease BP at rest and with exercise
  - Have no effect in exercise capacity
  - Increase or have no effect in exercise capacity in patients with CHF

Beta Blockers

- Group of drugs used to treat angina pectoris, HTN, and dysrhythmias; decreases sympathetic activity at beta receptors in the heart
- Examples: Sectral (Acebutolol), Tenormin (Atenolol), Lopressor (Metoprolol), Inderal (Propranolol), Corgard (Nadolol), Levatol (Penbutolol), Coreg (Carvedilol)
- Effects
  - Decrease HR and BP at rest and with exercise
  - Increase exercise capacity in patients with angina
  - Decrease exercise capacity or have no effect in exercise capacity in patients without angina

Calcium-Channel Blockers

- Group of drugs used to treat angina pectoris, HTN, vascular spasm, CHF, supraventricular tachycardia; slow the influx of calcium into coronary smooth muscles, dilate coronary and peripheral arteries, and decrease arterial resistance and oxygen demand
- Examples: Plendil (Felodipine), Cardene (Nicardipine), Cardizem (Diltiazem), Verelan (Verapamil)
- Effects
  - Increase HR at rest and with exercise (Felodipine, Nicardipine)
  - Decrease HR at rest and with exercise (Diltiazem, Verapamil)
  - Decrease BP at rest and with exercise (all calcium-channel blockers)
  - Increase exercise capacity in patients with angina (all calcium-channel blockers)
  - Have no effect on exercise capacity in patients without angina (all calcium-channel blockers)

Digitalis

- An antiarrhythmic and cardiotonic drug that is used to treat CHF, atrial fibrillations, atrial flutter, supraventricular tachycardia; increases the force of myocardial contraction and decreases conduction through the AV and SA nodes, slows HR
- Examples: Lanoxin (Digoxin)
- Effects

(continued)

Table 7.73 **Effects of Medications in Cardiac Rehabilitation**[4]   *(continued)*

- Decreases HR in patients with CHF and atrial fibrillations
- Has no effect on BP
- Increases exercise capacity in patients with CHF and atrial fibrillations

Diuretics

- Group of drugs used to treat HTN, CHF, and edema; increase urine secretion
- Examples: Lasix (Furosemide), Naturetin (Bendroflumethiazide), Hydrodiuril (Hydrochlorothiazide), Aldactone (Spironolactone)
- Effects
  - Have no effect on HR
  - Have no effect on BP or may decrease BP at rest or with exercise
  - Have no effect on exercise capacity except for patients with CHF

Nitrates

- Group of drugs used to treat angina pectoris, HTN, and CHF; arteriovenous dilators
- Examples: Amyl Nitrite, Novo Sorbide (Isosorbide Dinitrate), Isordil (Isosorbide Dinitrate), Nitrostat (Nitroglycerin)
- Nitroglycerin (NTG)
  - Also a type of nitrate used as an arterial and venous dilator; used to treat angina pectoris, CHF, and acute pulmonary edema
  - Forms of NTG: intravenous infusion (in critical care), ointment (applied to the chest), transdermal patches, and oral drug (either tablet dissolving under tongue or a spray of the mouth)
  - Contraindications for NTG: should not be used in men using Sildenafil for erectile dysfunction (can cause a fatal heart attack)
- Effects of nitrates
  - Increase HR at rest
  - Increase HR or have no effect with exercise
  - Decrease BP at rest
  - Decrease BP or have no effect with exercise
  - Increase exercise capacity in patients with angina
  - Have no effects on exercise capacity in patients without angina or patients with CHF

Vasodilators (Non-Nitrates)

- Group of drugs used to treat mostly severe to moderate HTN and CHF; dilate blood vessels by relaxing smooth muscles; depress heart conduction and irritability.
- Examples: Hydralazine (Apresoline), Minoxidil (Loniten), Nifedipine (Procardia)
- Effects
- Increase HR or have no effect at rest or with exercise
- Decrease BP at rest or with exercise
- Have no effect on exercise capacity
- Increase or have no effect on exercise capacity with CHF

Table 7.74   **Medications for Common Cardiovascular Conditions[16]**

*Classes of Drugs	Purpose of Medication	*Common Side Effects	PTA Implications
Antihypertensive Medications: Ace Inhibitors <ul><li>Captopril (Capoten)</li><li>Lisinopril (Zestril)*</li><li>Enalapril (Vasotec)</li><li>Banezapril (Lotensin)</li></ul>* Lisinopril also used to prevent migraines	<ul><li>BP control</li><li>Manage CHF</li><li>Chronic kidney disease</li><li>Post MI</li><li>↓BP, ↓ overt heart failure</li></ul>	<ul><li>Dizzy</li><li>Cough</li><li>Fatigue</li><li>HA</li><li>Rash</li></ul>	<ul><li>Angioedema</li><li>↑ fall risk</li></ul>
Beta Blockers <ul><li>Propanolol (Inderal)</li><li>Nadolol (Corgard)</li><li>Atenolol (Tenormin)</li><li>Metoprolol (Toprol, Lopressor)</li></ul>	<ul><li>HTN</li><li>Angina</li><li>Prevention of MI</li><li>↓ HR & BP</li></ul>	<ul><li>Orthostatic hypotension</li><li>Bradycardia</li><li>Shortness of breath (SOB)</li><li>Increased cholesterol and blood glucose levels</li><li>Impotence</li><li>Depression</li><li>Fatigue</li></ul>	<ul><li>↑ fall risk</li><li>Blunts heart rate and cardiac output responses to exercise.</li><li>Monitor for diabetic reactions</li></ul>
Diuretics <ul><li>Chlorothiazide (Diuril)</li><li>Furosemide (Lasix)</li><li>Hydrocholorothiazide (HydroDiuril)</li></ul>	<ul><li>HTN</li><li>Peripheral edema due to CHF</li><li>↑ excretion of electrolytes and H_2O working on the renal system</li></ul>	<ul><li>Hypokalemia</li><li>Hyperuricemia</li><li>Dizziness</li><li>Cramping</li><li>Hyponatremia</li><li>Blood glucose abnormalities</li><li>Dry mouth</li></ul>	<ul><li>↑ fall risks</li><li>Monitor for blood sugar reactions during exercise</li><li>Electrolyte imbalances can affect cognition</li></ul>
Anti-Angina <ul><li>Minitran (nitroglycerin)</li><li>Nitro-Dur (nitroglycerin)</li><li>Isosorbide mononitrate (Imdur)*</li></ul>	<ul><li>Angina-reducing medication</li></ul>	<ul><li>Dizziness</li><li>Drowsiness</li><li>Fatigue</li><li>Flushing</li><li>Nausea/vomiting</li><li>Headache*</li></ul>	<ul><li>↑ fall risk</li></ul>

(continued)

Table 7.74   **Medications for Common Cardiovascular Conditions**[16]   *(continued)*

*Classes of Drugs	Purpose of Medication	*Common Side Effects	PTA Implications
Lipid Lowering "Statins" ■ Atorvastatin (Lipitor) ■ Rosuvastatin (Crestor) ■ Lovastatin (Mevacor) ■ Simvastatin (Zocor) ■ Pravastatin (Pravachol) ■ Niacin (Nicobid)	■ ↓ blood lipids ■ ↓ atherosclerotic disease ■ Inhibits cholesterol synthesis	■ Abdominal discomfort ■ Constipation ■ Nausea ■ Muscle pain/ache not associated with exercise ■ ↑ liver enzymes	■ Monitor for muscle soreness as a potential sign of drug toxicity
Antiplatelet Agents ■ Clopidogrel (Plavix) ■ Dipyridamole (Persantine) ■ Ticlopidine (Ticlid) ■ Aspirin (Bayer)*	■ Stroke prevention ■ Heart attack ■ Peripheral artery disease ■ Acute coronary syndrome ■ Inhibits platelet aggregation	■ Bleeding ■ GI issues*	■ Bruising / bleeding during interventions
Anticoagulants ■ Warfarin (Coumadin)** ■ Heparin (IV) ■ Enoxaparin (Lovenox) * (injectable) * Does not need PT-INR monitoring	■ Clotting diseases ■ Atrial fibrillation ■ Thins blood	■ Dizziness ■ Bleeding ■ Anemia ■ Thrombocytopenia	■ ↑ fall risk ■ ↑ incidence of bruising/bleeds * Acute care—check with RN ■ Reference PT-INR values ■ Follow physician protocol for PT participation
Cardiac Glycosides ■ Digoxin (Digitek) ■ Lanoxin	■ Improves heart pumping efficiency ■ Anti-arrhythmia medication	■ Nausea/vomiting ■ Rash ■ Diarrhea ■ Blurred vision ■ Electrolyte imbalances may = drowsiness, fatigue, dizziness, dry mouth, low BP, fast heart rate, muscle cramps/pain	■ ↑ fall risk if electrolyte imbalances occur ■ blurred vision

General Guidelines for Therapeutic PT INR Levels

PT INR: Normal = 0.9–1.2.

Post-surgical total joint patients = 1.9–2.9; Atrial fibrillation patient = 2.3–3.3.

PE, DVT, Valvular Heart Disease = 2.0–3.0; Prosthetic valve or recurrent systemic embolism = 2.5–3.5.

** Know your PT INR guidelines for interventions with PT-INR's > 3.0. Check with RN or MD protocols before proceeding.

* Brand names associated with classes of medications and side effects found within this table are not representative of an all-inclusive list. It is incumbent on the clinician to research an appropriate drug information resource to obtain complete information about medications that patients may use while attending rehabilitation.

CARDIOPULMONARY INTERVENTIONS

Bronchodilators Commonly Used in Pulmonary Rehabilitation

Table 7.75 Commonly Used Bronchodilators and Their Side Effects[16]

Bronchodilator	Characteristics	Side Effects
B_2 agonists (e.g., Albuterol (Ventolin), Terbutaline (Breathaire), Isoproterenol (Isuprel))	Taken orally, subcutaneously or by inhalation and may be administered in metered dose inhalers (MDI) or nebulizers; used to promote bronchial smooth muscle relaxation, for intermittent attacks of wheezing and exercise-induced asthma	Palpitations, tachycardia, tremor and nervousness
Methylxanthines (e.g., Theophylline (Theo-Dur), Dyphylline (Dilor))	Taken orally or intravenously; used for asthma and COPD to improve bronchodilation	Palpitations, tachycardia, vomiting, nausea, and seizures
Anticholinergics (e.g., Ipratropium (Atrovent), Atropine (Atro-Pen))	Used for COPD and acute asthma (combined with B_2 agonist medication)	Dry mouth, nausea, and cough, tachycardia, blurred vision, confusion

Table 7.76 Medications for Common Pulmonary Conditions[16]

*Classes of Drugs	Purpose of Medication	*Common Side Effects	PTA Implications
Bronchodilators ■ Albuterol (Proventil) ■ Pirbuterol (Maxair) ■ Montelukast (Singulair)	■ COPD ■ Bronchospasms ■ Asthma	■ Anxiety ■ Tremor ■ Headaches ■ Palpitations ■ Fever ■ Sore throat ■ Diarrhea	■ Inhalers ARE NOT rescue inhalers—do not use for acute attacks
Corticosteroids ■ Budesonide (Pulmicort) ■ Fluticasone (Flovent) ■ Prednisone (Sterapred) ■ Dexamethasone (Decadron)	■ Asthma- inhibit the inflammatory response in the airways.	■ Runny nose ■ Sore throat ■ Fluid retention ■ Insomnia ■ Mood swings ■ Upset stomach ■ Immunosuppression (long term corticosteroid use) ■ ↑ blood sugar (steroid use) ■ Bone density	■ Immune system suppression = wear PPE/hand washing ■ Monitor for hypoglycemic reactions with exercise and corticosteroid use ■ Osteoporotic bone changes with prolonged corticosteroid use PPE = Personal Protective Equipment

(continued)

Table 7.76 **Medications for Common Pulmonary Conditions**[16] *(continued)*

*Classes of Drugs	Purpose of Medication	*Common Side Effects	PTA Implications
Combination ■ Advair (BD & CCS) ■ Dulera (BD & CCS) ■ Combivent* (2 BD) BD = Bronchodilator CCS = Corticosteroid	■ COPD ■ Asthma	■ Headache ■ Sore throat ■ Anxiety ■ Palpitations ■ Rapid heart rate ■ Tremor ■ Glaucoma*	■ Immune system suppression = wear PPE/hand washing ■ Osteoporotic bone changes with prolonged corticosteroid use

* Brand names associated with classes of medications and side effects found within this table are not representative of an all-inclusive list. It is incumbent on the clinician to research an appropriate drug information resource to obtain complete information about medications that patients may use while attending rehabilitation.

References

1. Dreeben-Irimia BC. *Dreeben-Irimia's Introduction to Physical Therapy for Physical Therapist Assistants.* 4th ed. Burlington, MA: Jones & Bartlett Learning; 2020.
2. American College of Cardiology. New high blood pressure guidelines. https://www.acc.org/latest-in-cardiology /articles/2017/11/08/11/47/mon-5pm-bp-guideline-aha-2017. Accessed June 1, 2021.
3. Vital Signs: Normal blood pressure. https://uichildrens.org/health-library/vital-signs-normal-blood-pressure-mmhg-picu-chart. Accessed July 29, 2020.
4. O'Sullivan SB, Schmitz TJ. *Physical Rehabilitation.* 5th ed. Philadelphia, PA: F.A. Davis Company; 2007.
5. Academy of Acute Care Physical Therapy. Laboratory values interpretation resource. https://cdn.ymaws.com/www .aptaacutecare.org/resource/resmgr/docs/2017-Lab-Values-Resource.pdf. Accessed June 2, 2021.
6. Goodman C, Fuller K, Marshall C. *Pathology for the Physical TherapistAssistant. 2nd ed. :St Louis* , MO: Elsevier; 2017.
7. Rothstein JM, Roy SH, Wolf SL, Scalzitti DA. *The Rehabilitation Specialist's Handbook. sh* Philadelphia, PA: 3rd ed. F.A. Davis Company; 2005.
8. Panchal AR, Bartos JA, Cabanas JG, et al.Circulation. Part 3: Adult basic and advanced life support: 2020 American Heart Association guidelines for cardiopulmonary resuscitation and emergency cardiovascular care. Accessed June 3, 2021. https:// www.ahajournals.org/doi/10.1161/CIR.0000000000000916.
9. Academy of Acute Care Physical Therapy. *Adult vital sign interpretation in acute care guide 2021.* https://www.aptaacutecare.org /page/ResourceGuides. Accessed May 21, 2021.
10. Physical activity for everyone: Measuring physical activity intensity: Perceived exertion (Borg rating of perceived exertion scale). cdc.gov. http://www.cdc.gov/physicalactivity/everyone/measuring/exertion.html. Reviewed September 2020. Accessed August 2, 2021.
11. Kendrick KR, Baxi SC, Smith RM.Usefulness of the modified 0-10 Borg scale in assessing the degree of dyspnea in patients with COPD and asthma. *J Emerg Nurs.* 2000 Jun;26(3):216–222. PubMed PMID: 10839848. Accessed April 2016. *DOI* : http:// dx.doi.org/10.1016/S0099-1767(00)90093-X.
12. Lavietes MH, Matta MH, Tiersky LA, Natelson BH, Bielroy L, Chernial NS. The perception of dyspnea in patients with mild asthma. *Chest.* 2002;120–122.
13. American Physical Therapy Association. *Guide to PT Practice.* 2nd ed. Alexandria, VA: APTA; 2001; revised 2003.
14. American Physical Therapy Association. Guide to physical therapist practice 3.0. apta.org. https://guide.apta.org/interventions. Updated August 1, 2014. Accessed February 3, 2021.
15. Academy of Cardiovascular and Pulmonary Physical Therapy. *Clinical practice guidelines.* https://www.aptacvp.org/clinical -practice-guidelines. Accessed June 7, 2021.
16. Ciccone CD. *Pharmacology in Rehabilitation.* 4th ed. Philadelphia, PA: F.A. Davis; 2007.

Integumentary Interventions

INTEGUMENTARY INTERVENTIONS

Review of Integumentary System Anatomy

Skin Anatomy

See **Figure 8.1**.

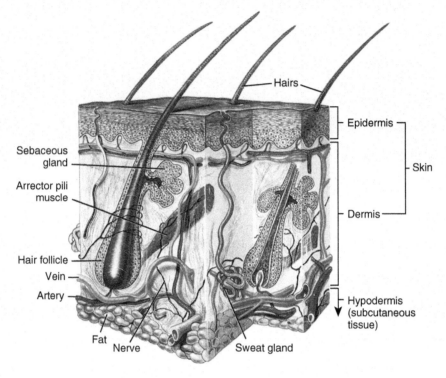

Figure 8.1 Anatomy of the skin.
Source: Chiras, D. D. (2005). Human biology. Jones & Bartlett Publishers, page 200, Figure 11-3 "General Sense Receptors"—only the illustration.

Table 8.1 Skin: The Largest Organ in the Body

- **Skin function:** shields the body against infection (bacteria and chemicals), dehydration, and temperature changes; first defense against pain; provides sensory information about the environment; manufactures vitamin D; excretes salts and small amounts of urea (through perspiration); maintains fluid balance.

- **Epidermis:** outermost skin layer made of stratified epithelium; produces melanin, which is responsible for skin color.

- **Dermis** (also called the "true skin"): inner layer of the skin made of collagen and elastin fibrous connective tissues; contains lymphatic structures, blood vessels, nerves and nerve endings, and sebaceous and sweat glands. The dermis has two layers: papillary and reticular.

- **Subcutaneous layer:** not part of the skin, beneath the dermis, made of loose connective tissue and fat tissue (that provides insulation), and supports and cushions the skin. Fasciae and muscles are below the subcutaneous layer.

- **Skin appendages:** hair and nails. Skin can also be classified as thin and hairy or thick and hairless (glabrous). Glabrous skin does not contain hair follicles and covers the surface of the palms of the hands, soles of the feet, and flexor surfaces of the digits.

Sensory Receptors Location in the Skin: Identification of Burn Depth

Table 8.2 Sensory Receptors: Location and Function

- **Epidermis:** contains free nerve endings, which function as receptors for pain and itch; Merkel's disk (also found in the epithelial root sheath of a hair) functions as touch receptor.

- **Dermis:** contains free nerve endings, which function as pain receptors.

- **Papillary dermis:** contains Meissner's corpuscles, which function as touch receptors (most numerous in palmar and plantar surfaces, lips, eyelids, nipples, and tip of the tongue); Ruffini's corpuscles (also in subcutaneous tissue) function as pressure receptors (once thought to mediate the sense of warmth); Krause's corpuscles function as cutaneous touch receptors; and Krause's end bulbs (also found in cornea) function as touch receptors.

- **Reticular dermis:** contains Pacinian corpuscles (also found in pancreas, penis, nipple, and clitoris), which function as deep and heavy pressure (and vibration) receptors. Pacinian corpuscles are also called Vater's corpuscles.

Integumentary Overview

Normal Physiology of Wound Healing

Table 8.3 Wound Healing Phases[1]

Wound healing is a continuous process, and its phases are not distinct, but rather overlap with one another. Wound healing depends on the patient's (client's) age, size of wound, trauma, nutrition, blood flow, medications, infection, and stress.

Phase I

Inflammation: a normal immune system reaction to injury. Phase I can last from the beginning of injury to approximately day 10. The phase I healing rate is affected by the blood supply, extrinsic environment, and available nutrients. Interruption or delay of phase I can cause chronic inflammation (months to years).

Events:

1. Injury occurs.
2. Temporary repair, coagulation and short-term decreased blood flow.
3. Injured cells undergo necrosis.
4. Pathogens spread slowly; debris and bacteria are attacked by a host of cells; pus may be formed.
5. Oxygen delivery through increased blood flow to keep phagocytic cells working.
6. Permanent repair facilitation begins; wound becomes clean to set the stage for re-epithelialization.

Phase II

Proliferation: new tissue fills in the wound. Phase II can last from the third day after the injury to approximately day 20. The phase II healing rate is affected by blood supply, extrinsic environment, and available nutrients. New scar tissue formed in this phase needs to be protected. Interruptions or delay of phase II can cause a chronic wound.

Events:

1. Fibroblasts secrete collagen.
2. New blood vessels grow from endothelial cells (angiogenesis).
3. Capillary buds grow into the wound bed.
4. New reddish (slightly bumpy) granulation tissue is formed.
5. Epithelial cells differentiate into type I collagen.
6. Collagen synthesis occurs and new fragile scar tissue is formed.

Phase III

Maturation/remodeling: granulation that began in the proliferative phase continues. Phase III can last from approximately day 9 after injury to approximately 2 years. The phase III healing rate is affected by blood supply, extrinsic environment, and available nutrients.

Events:

1. Epithelial cells continue to differentiate into type I collagen.
2. New skin acquires tensile strength (15% of normal strength).
3. Scar tissue is rebuilt over time (80% of original tensile strength).
4. Granulation tissue is replaced by less vascular tissue.
5. In deep wounds, dermal appendages (such as hair follicles, and sebaceous and sweat glands) are replaced by fibrous tissue.
6. Scar tissue matures and changes appearance (from red to pink to white and from raised and rigid to flat and flexible).

Burn Classification

Table 8.4 Burn Classification[1]

Superficial Burn (Epidermal Burn)

- Damage occurs only to the epidermis (such as the classic sunburn or a brief scald).
- The skin is red and erythematous (because of epidermal damage and dermal irritation). The skin has slight (minimal) edema.
- There are no blisters, and the skin is dry.
- Pain and tenderness to touch will appear later. In 2–3 days, the injured epidermis will peel off (desquamate), and the skin will heal on its own without any scarring.

Superficial Partial-Thickness Burn

- Damage occurs to the epidermis and the papillary layer of the dermis (such as scalds or flash flame burn).
- The epidermis is destroyed completely, and the dermal layer is inflamed with mild to moderate damage.
- The skin is bright pink or red (or mottled red), with blanching and capillary refill (when pressure is exerted against the tissue).
- There are intact blisters, and the skin surface is moist. When blisters are removed (evacuated to speed up the healing), the skin weeps.
- Extreme pain and skin sensitivity are present with light touch and changes in temperature or exposure to air (because of nerve endings involvement).
- If infection is present, the patient (client) will have fever. Edema is moderate.
- This burn will heal on its own in approximately 7–10 days without surgical intervention. After healing, minimal scarring is possible.

Deep Partial-Thickness Burn

- Damage occurs to the epidermis and dermis deep to the reticular layer of dermis (such as scalds or flash flame burn).
- This burn starts to resemble a full-thickness burn.
- Because most of the dermis is destroyed, the nerve endings, hair follicles, and sweat ducts are also injured.
- The skin is mixed red and waxy white, with blanching and very slow capillary refill (when pressure is exerted against the tissue). The deeper the damage, the whiter the blanching appears.
- There are broken blisters, and the skin surface is very moist (because of leakage of plasma fluid).
- There is also water loss (through evaporation) because of vascular destruction.
- The patient (client) has no pain or sensitivity to light touch or gentle pin prick.
- There is sensitivity to pressure (because of the location of Pacinian corpuscles in the deep reticular dermis). Edema is very distinct.
- The wound may need a few days to stage itself as a deep partial-thickness and clearly differentiate from a full-thickness burn.

(continued)

INTEGUMENTARY INTERVENTIONS

Table 8.4 **Burn Classification** *(continued)*

- Typically, the dead tissue will begin to slough, and preservation of hair follicles and new hair growth will indicate a deep partial-thickness and spontaneous healing.
- Healing is slow (usually in 3–5 weeks without infection), with new tissue that appears dry and scaly, easily abraded, and itchy.
- The burn needs to be kept free of infection.
- Creams need to lubricate the new surface of the skin artificially.
- After healing, scarring is excessive with a possibility of hypertrophic and keloid scars.
  - A hypertrophic scar is a firm raised scar within the boundaries of the burn wound.
  - A keloid scar spreads beyond the borders of the original burn and is made of collagen and fibroblasts. It appears shiny and rubbery.

Full-Thickness Burn

- Complete damage to all the epidermal and dermal layers (such as flame or contact with hot objects burn).
- The subcutaneous layer may also be damaged to some extent.
- This burn is white (without blood supply) and has a hard, charred, parchment-like eschar that covers the area. Eschar is dead tissue with crusty or scabbed black, deep red, or white material. White eschar indicates total ischemia (deficiency of blood) of the tissue. Red eschar indicates hemoglobin from the destroyed red blood cells.
- There is no blanching of the skin. Bodily hair will pull out because of complete damage to hair follicles. Nerve endings are destroyed, and the wound has anesthesia.
- There is also damage to the peripheral vascular system that leaks fluid into the interstitial spaces (under the eschar), constricting the deep blood circulation (and possibility of blood flow occlusion and necrosis). An escharotomy may be necessary to improve the peripheral blood flow.
- This burn heals only with surgical skin grafting because all the epithelial cells are destroyed. There will be a large amount of scarring, and plastic surgery is necessary.

Subdermal Burn

- Complete destruction of all tissue from the epidermis to the subcutaneous tissue. The burn is charred.
- The wound is anesthetic with muscle and nerve damage.
- Excessive surgical management using skin grafting is necessary.

Electrical Burn

- A different type of burn occurring from the passage of electrical current through the body after the skin made contact with an electrical source. Usually, the bone offers the most resistance to electricity, whereas muscles and nerves offer the least resistance.
- The wound of the initial contact is charred, and the skin is yellow and ischemic.
- The exit wound is dry with damaged tissue (appearing as an explosion out of the tissue). An area that may be viable becomes necrotic in a few days.
- The blood supply is altered and may have necrosis of the vascular wall.
- Other problems associated with electrical burns include cardiac arrhythmias, ventricular fibrillations, renal failure, acute spinal cord damage, and vertebral fracture.

Burn Wound Zones

Table 8.5 Burn Wound Zones[1]

- **Zone of hyperemia:** area of minimal tissue damage. The tissue can recover within several days; no long-lasting effects.
- **Zone of stasis:** area of tissue surrounding the burn that contains injured cells that may die within 24–48 hours without treatment. Infection, wound dryness, and inadequate perfusion can result in complete damage and necrosis of the tissue (that could have initially been saved). Splints and compression bandages should not be placed too tightly, so as not to compromise the tissue.
- **Zone of coagulation:** the area of maximum tissue damage exhibits irreversible cell damage and skin death; similar to a full-thickness burn. A skin graft is required for this area to heal. This area is subject to an increased risk of infection due to eschar; the patient needs care in a specialized burn center.

Rule of Nines and Lund-Browder Burn Classifications

Table 8.6 Rule of Nines and Lund-Browder Burn Classifications

Rule of Nines Burn Classification

The rule of nines is a formula for estimating percentage of body surface area, judging the portion of the skin that has been burned.

- For the adult, the head represents 9%.
- Each upper extremity is 9%.
- The anterior trunk is 18% (each half of the anterior trunk is 9%).
- The posterior trunk is 18% (each half of the posterior trunk is 9%).
- Each lower extremity is 18% (anterior lower extremity is 9%, and posterior lower extremity is 9%).
- The perineum is 1%.

Lund-Browder Burn[1] Classification

This series of burn calculations is more accurate, especially for children, because the formulas estimate the burn size based on the patient's age and changes that occur during normal growth.

Newborns

- Each surface of the head is 9.5%.
- Each surface of the thigh is 2.75%.
- Each surface of the leg is 2.5%.

Children Up to 1 Year Old

- Each surface of the head is 8.5%.
- Each surface of the thigh is 3.25%.
- Each surface of the leg is 2.5%.

(continued)

Table 8.6 Rule of Nines and Lund-Browder Burn Classifications *(continued)*

Children Up to 5 Years Old

- Each surface of the head is 6.5%.
- Each surface of the thigh is 4.0%.
- Each surface of the leg is 2.75%.

Children Between 10 and 14 Years Old

- Each surface of the head is 5.5%.
- Each surface of the thigh is 4.25%.
- Each surface of the leg is 3.0%.

Children 15 Years and Older

- Each surface of the head is 4.5%.
- Each surface of the thigh is 4.5%.
- Each surface of the leg is 3.25%.

(See **Figure 8.2**, Rule of Nines) following Table 8.6.
(See **Figure 8.3**, Lund Browder chart) following Table 8.6.

Figure 8.2 Rule of Nines.

Entire head
9%

Anterior torso 9%

Upper back 9%

Entire arm
9%

Anterior abdomen 9%

Lower back 9%

Perineum 1%

Anterior leg 9%   Posterior leg 9%

Adult skin area	
Head and neck	9%
Torso	36%
Arms	18%
Legs	36%
Perineum	1%
	100%

INTEGUMENTARY INTERVENTIONS

Age (years)	A ($\frac{1}{2}$ of head)	B ($\frac{1}{2}$ of one thigh)	C ($\frac{1}{2}$ of one leg)
0	$9\frac{1}{2}$	$2\frac{3}{4}$	$2\frac{1}{2}$
1	$8\frac{1}{2}$	$3\frac{1}{4}$	$2\frac{1}{2}$
5	$6\frac{1}{2}$	4	$2\frac{3}{4}$
10	$5\frac{1}{2}$	$4\frac{1}{4}$	3
15	$4\frac{1}{2}$	$4\frac{1}{2}$	$3\frac{1}{4}$
Adult	$3\frac{1}{2}$	$4\frac{3}{4}$	3

Figure 8.3 Lund-Browder chart.

Systemic Complications of Burn Injury

Table 8.7 Systemic Complications of Burns

- **Complications caused by infections:** very high risk of developing infection secondary to exposed tissue. Various types of bacteria may infect the wound, with the two most powerful strains being *Pseudomonas aeruginosa* and *Staphylococcus aureus.* When the burn is infected, the wound (or the drainage) is discolored. The healing is delayed, and necrosis and tissue death can take place.
- **Respiratory system complications:** respiratory system shock or inhalation injury (can be caused by exposure to smoke inhalation and fire). Inhalation injury is a life-threatening complication, especially in those persons who have suffered facial burns. Other (early or late) respiratory system complications of burns include pulmonary edema, airway obstruction, respiratory failure, restrictive lung disease, pneumonia, and dyspnea.
- **Metabolic system complications:** weight loss, decreased energy, and negative nitrogen balance (or equilibrium). Negative nitrogen balance occurs because of the decreased nitrogen amount in the body—a larger than normal amount of nitrogen is eliminated mostly through the skin sweat (also eliminated in feces and urine).
- **Cardiac and peripheral vascular systems complications:** decreased or absent pulses, fluid and plasma loss that can lead to decreased cardiac output, increased pain with active range of motion (AROM), and numbness and tingling.
- **Urinary system complications:** red (indicating blood) or dark brown (indicating infection, ketone bodies, blood, bacteria, or pus) urine.
- **Gastrointestinal system complications:** ileus (intestinal obstruction) with distended abdomen, abdominal cramps, and abdominal collapse; gastric ulcer.
- **Psychological Dysfunctions/Complications:** Depression, anxiety, confusion, post-traumatic stress disorder, inappropriate behavior, sleep disturbances.[2]

Burn Healing

Table 8.8 Burn Healing[1]

Wound Healing

Wound healing of the burn depends on the patient's age, size of the burn, type of the burn, area of the burn, trauma, nutrition, blood flow, medications, infection, and stress.

Epidermal Healing

Epidermal healing includes epithelialization of the viable cells. The intact epithelial cells grow and proliferate and then cover the wound. Such epithelialization can occur in a partial-thickness burn that has intact hair follicles and glands. When there is damage to the sebaceous glands causing dryness and itching of the wound, the therapist should teach the patient to apply moisturizing cream (to lubricate the newly healed tissue).

Dermal Healing

Dermal healing includes scar formation over the burn wound. Scar formation is divided into three phases: inflammatory, proliferative, and maturation.

- **Inflammatory phase:** begins at the time of injury and ends in about 3–5 days; characterized by redness, edema, warmth, pain, and decreased range of motion (ROM). Physiologically, when the blood vessel is ruptured, the vessel wall contracts to decrease blood flow (vasoconstriction) to the area. Platelets then clump together, and fibrin is deposited to form a clot over the area. Fibrin partially retains body fluids, provides a firm coagulated clot, protects the underlying cells from destruction, and helps the blood cells to heal the wound. After a short vasoconstriction, vasodilation (increased blood flow to the wound) occurs, and increased permeability of the blood vessels brings plasma into the interstitial space. This process of healing causes edema formation. Leukocytes clean the area of contamination, whereas macrophages clear the debris and attract fibroblasts to the wound.

- **Proliferative phase:** characterized by fibroblasts that synthesize scar tissue (made of collagen and protein polysaccharides), formation of granulation tissue (made of macrophages, fibroblasts, collagen, and blood vessels), and wound contraction (to close the wound). In this phase, skin grafting can help to decrease wound contraction and prevent scarring.

- **Maturation phase:** includes remodeling of the scar tissue and can last as long as 2 years. During this phase, the number of fibroblasts declines, and a remodeling of collagen (parallel alignment of collagen fibers) occurs. When the ratio of collagen production equals or exceeds breakdown, hypertrophic or keloid scars will result. Keloids scars form at the site of the wound. For African American patients (clients), keloids appear on a wound highly elevated and irregular, continuing to enlarge.

- **Surgical Management:** wounds are surgically excised to remove as much eschar as possible. Many times, the wound is closed with a graft when the eschar is removed. Some grafts may only be temporary i.e., xenograft. (For additional information see **Table 8.26**).

Table 8.9 Types of Grafts Used in Burn Management

- Autograft: use of patient's own skin
- Allograft: typically use of cadaver skin
- Xenograft: typically use of pigskin
- Biosynthetic grafts: combination of collagen and synthetic material

Pressure Injury Staging

According to the National Pressure Injury Advisory Panel, a pressure injury is defined as follows: "A pressure injury is localized damage to the skin and/or underlying soft tissue usually over a bony prominence or related to a medical or other device. The injury can present as intact skin or an open ulcer and may be painful. The injury occurs as a result of intense and/or prolonged pressure or pressure in combination with shear. The tolerance of soft tissue for pressure and shear may also be affected by microclimate, nutrition, perfusion, co-morbidities, and condition of the soft tissue."[3]

Table 8.10 Pressure Injury Staging Classification Developed by the National Pressure Injury Advisory Panel (NPIAP)[3]

Stage 1 Pressure Injury: Non-blanchable erythema of intact skin

Intact skin with a localized area of non-blanchable erythema, which may appear differently in darkly pigmented skin. Presence of blanchable erythema or changes in sensation, temperature, or firmness may precede visual changes. Color changes do not include purple or maroon discoloration; these may indicate deep tissue pressure injury.

Stage 2 Pressure Injury: Partial-thickness skin loss with exposed dermis

The wound bed is viable, pink or red, moist, and may also present as an intact or ruptured serum-filled blister. Adipose (fat) is not visible, and deeper tissues are not visible. Granulation tissue, slough, and eschar are not present. These injuries commonly result from adverse microclimate and shear in the skin over the pelvis and shear in the heel. This stage should not be used to describe moisture associated skin damage (MASD) including incontinence associated dermatitis (IAD), intertriginous dermatitis (ITD), medical adhesive related skin injury (MARSI), or traumatic wounds (skin tears, burns, abrasions).

Stage 3 Pressure Injury: Full-thickness skin loss

Full-thickness loss of skin, in which adipose (fat) is visible in the ulcer and granulation tissue and epibole (rolled wound edges) are often present. Slough and/or eschar may be visible. The depth of tissue damage varies by anatomical location; areas of significant adiposity can develop deep wounds. Undermining and tunneling may occur. Fascia, muscle, tendon, ligament, cartilage, and/or bone are not exposed. If slough or eschar obscures the extent of tissue loss, this is an unstageable pressure injury.

Stage 4 Pressure Injury: Full-thickness skin and tissue loss

Full-thickness skin and tissue loss with exposed or directly palpable fascia, muscle, tendon, ligament, cartilage, or bone in the ulcer. Slough and/or eschar may be visible. Epibole (rolled edges), undermining, and/or tunneling often occur. Depth varies by anatomical location. If slough or eschar obscures the extent of tissue loss this is an unstageable pressure injury.

Unstageable Pressure Injury: Obscured full-thickness skin and tissue loss

Full-thickness skin and tissue loss in which the extent of tissue damage within the ulcer cannot be confirmed because it is obscured by slough or eschar. If slough or eschar is removed, a stage 3 or stage 4 pressure injury will be revealed. Stable eschar (i.e., dry, adherent, intact without erythema or fluctuance) on the heel or ischemic limb should not be softened or removed.

(continued)

Table 8.10 Pressure Injury Staging Classification Developed by the National Pressure Injury Advisory Panel (NPIAP)   *(continued)*

Deep Tissue Pressure Injury: Persistent non-blanchable deep red, maroon, or purple discoloration

Intact or nonintact skin with localized area of persistent non-blanchable deep red, maroon, purple discoloration or epidermal separation revealing a dark wound bed or blood-filled blister. Pain and temperature change often precede skin color changes. Discoloration may appear differently in darkly pigmented skin. This injury results from intense and/or prolonged pressure and shear forces at the bone–muscle interface. The wound may evolve rapidly to reveal the actual extent of tissue injury, or it may resolve without tissue loss. If necrotic tissue, subcutaneous tissue, granulation tissue, fascia, muscle, or other underlying structures are visible, this indicates a full thickness pressure injury (unstageable, stage 3, or stage 4). Do not use deep tissue pressure injury (DTPI) to describe vascular, traumatic, neuropathic, or dermatologic conditions.

Additional Pressure Injury Definitions

Medical Device Related Pressure Injury (describes an etiology): Medical device related pressure injuries result from the use of devices designed and applied for diagnostic or therapeutic purposes. The resultant pressure injury generally conforms to the pattern or shape of the device. The injury should be staged using the staging system.

Mucosal Membrane Pressure Injury: Mucosal membrane pressure injuries are found on mucous membranes with a history of a medical device in use at the location of the injury. Due to the anatomy of the tissue, these injuries cannot be staged.

A. Stage 1 pressure ulcer.

B. Stage 2 pressure ulcer.

C. Stage 3 pressure ulcer.

D. Stage 4 pressure ulcer.

E. Unstageable pressure ulcer.

F. Suspected deep tissue injury.

Figure 8.4 Pressure injury stages.
© Duangnapa Kanchanasakun/Shutterstock.

Wound Terminology

Table 8.11 Wound Terminology [1,4]

- Exudate: Fluid that has leaked from the blood vessels into surrounding tissues. Contains proteins and cells and may contain pus and or blood cells.
- Necrosis: Breakdown and death of cells due to injury. Is irreversible.
- Eschar: Dead tissue found in a full thickness wound. Typically burns and pressure ulcers.
- Slough: Necrotic tissue found in a wound. Frequently creamy yellow in color, soft and moist.
- Granulation Tissue: Newly formed tissue in a healing wound. Consists of endothelial cells, fibroblasts, and some macrophages.
- Epithelialization: The process of epithelial cells closing the wound.
- Hemosiderin staining: Dark pigmentation of the skin, typically associated with venous insufficiency. Often associated with vascular incompetence.

Wound Characteristics

Table 8.12 **Wound Characteristics (To Be Documented Throughout Wound Healing Phases)**

- Location: location of the wound on the patient's body
- Size: depth, width, length
- Shape: distinct or irregular
- Edges: shape of the wound edges, evidence of premature healing
- Tunneling, undermining, and sinus tracts: presence of these and their depth
- Base of the wound: characteristics of the base of the wound (compared with the sides and edges of the wound); exudate (amount of exudate, and its color and odor); granulation tissue (has or does not have granulation tissue, amount of granulation tissue, location of granulation tissue); necrosis, eschar, slough (including the amount, texture and color, and adherence to the wound bed); epithelialization (has or does not have epithelialization; is epithelialization on schedule or is premature); other structures exposed to the wound (bone, tendon, ligament)
- Wound drainage signs:
  - Serous: clear, shiny exudate; can have a slightly yellow appearance; signifies a healthy wound
  - Seropurulent: brighter yellow drainage; slightly thicker exudate than the serous drainage; slightly malodorous; signifies a contaminated or infected wound
  - Sanguineous: red or bloody drainage; signifies a healthy wound
  - Serosanguineous: pinkish, red-colored exudate; signifies a healthy wound
  - Purulent or pus: thick, cloudy or opaque exudate; malodorous; signifies an infected wound
- Clinical signs of wound infection:
  - Erythema (redness): can present as a red periwound border or as a darker border in darker skin
  - Edema: describe volume, girth, quality, fluctuance, pitting, or nonpitting
  - Induration: a raised swollen area of the periwound; commonly found in chronic infected wounds
- Periwound area: has or does not have edema, induration, and maceration
- Bacteria: are or are not present in the wound; the amount
- Pain: patient's pain level

Wound Closure

Table 8.13 **Wound Closure Terms[1]**

- **Primary intention:** healing after the wound was closed using surgery (the edges were brought together with staples, sutures, glue, and/or skin grafts or skin flaps). Primary intention wound healing goes through the stages of healing but on a smaller scale.
- **Dehiscence** (bursts open): process by which the wound healed through primary intention opens up again because of infection or maceration. Dehiscence typically happens in surgical abdominal wounds. In cases of dehiscence wound, the surgeon is immediately informed. The wound needs to be covered with sterile dressing or towel moistened with warm sterile physiological saline solution.

(continued)

INTEGUMENTARY INTERVENTIONS

Table 8.13 Wound Closure Terms   *(continued)*

- **Secondary intention:** healing when the wound is left to heal on its own. The wound closes through contraction, reepithelialization, or a combination of the two. During secondary intention wound healing, contact inhibition (inhibition of cell division caused by the close contact of similar cells) can happen. In case of contact inhibition, wound healing may need to continue for several years (although the wound is closed). Also, the clinician may have to use different interventions to allow the wound to heal. Factors affecting wound closure by secondary intention include wound depth (if the wound is shallow, the closure can be quicker), wound shape (linear wounds contract most rapidly; circular wounds contract slowly), superficial wounds (close by reepithelialization), partial-thickness wounds (close by reepithelialization with minimal contraction), full-thickness wounds (close by contraction and scar formation, although epithelial cells migrate from the wound edges to assist in wound closure if the environment is homeostatic), wound location (areas with least pressure close more rapidly than areas with most pressure), and wound etiology (a less traumatic wound such as a surgery wound closes more rapidly than a traumatic wound such as a pressure injury wound).
- **Tertiary intention** (delayed primary): wound is allowed to heal by secondary intention and then is closed by primary intention (as the final treatment).

Signs of Potential Wound Infection

Table 8.14 Potential Infection Signs

- Change in wound drainage (amount, color, and odor)
- Redness or warmth of the periwound areas (less obvious in darker skin; may need to palpate the area)
- Swelling
- Increase in pain or tenderness
- Patient has fever, nausea, fatigue, or loss of appetite
- Change in the quality of granulation tissue or failure to produce good-quality tissue—for example, granulation tissue that is soft, pale, or easy to break
- Malaise
- May have red streaks leading from the wound

Factors Contributing to Abnormal Wound Healing

1. **Intrinsic factors** (internal factors): inadequate blood flow and oxygen; decreased moisture; decrease in elasticity, and collagen, and mast cell production; decrease in vascularity; and the underlying disease (such as diabetes, cancer, circulatory insufficiency, HIV infection, and/or connective tissue diseases)
2. **Extrinsic factors** (environmental factors): chemotherapy or radiation effects; incontinence; smoking; medications; recreational drugs; alcohol intake; malnutrition; dehydration; infection (bioburden infection, when healing is slowed by pathogens, granulomas, or necrotic tissue); and patient's stress

3. **Iatrogenic factors**: injury or illness that occurs as a result of medical care (such as poor wound care because of inappropriate dressings or lack of moisture; sheer injuries such as skin tears during transfers and repositioning; inadequate or absent pressure-relieving devices causing ischemia)

Arterial/Venous Insufficiency and Ulcers

Table 8.15 Peripheral Vascular Disease and Ulcerations[4]

Arterial or Venous Insufficiency

- Causes of peripheral vascular disease (PVD). PVD includes any condition that causes partial or complete obstruction of the flow of blood to and from the arteries or veins outside the chest.
- PVD includes atherosclerosis of the carotid, aortoiliac, femoral, and axillary arteries as well as deep venous thrombosis of the limbs, pelvis, and vena cava.

Venous Insufficiency

- A failure of the valves of the veins to function, which interferes with venous return to the heart and may produce edema. Chronic venous insufficiency (CVI) is venous insufficiency that persists for a long period of time. The majority of patients who are diagnosed with PVD also have CVI.
- Eighty percent of all leg ulcers are caused by venous insufficiency disease. In addition to venous insufficiency, many patients with ulceration also have deep vein thrombosis (DVT).
- Clinical signs of venous insufficiency:
  1. Swelling of unilateral or bilateral lower extremities
  2. Itching, fatigue, aching, and heaviness in the involved limb(s)
  3. Skin changes (hemosiderin staining, involving iron-containing pigment on the skin)
  4. Fibrosis of the dermis
  5. Increase in skin temperature of the lower legs
  6. Wounds on the lower extremities (proximal to medial malleolus); wounds can be very painful; minor dull leg pain around the wound; pain eases with leg elevation; tissue is wet from excessive draining exudates; wound is shallow with irregular edges; wound base is red
  7. Lymphedema of the lower extremities

PVD from Arterial Insufficiency

- Ten percent to twenty-five percent of lower-extremity ulcers are caused by the PVD from arterial insufficiency disease.
- Factors that lead to PVD from arterial insufficiency: hypertension, cardiac disease, arteriosclerosis, diabetes, smoking, renal disease, and elevated cholesterol and triglycerides.
- Contributors to PVD from arterial insufficiency: obesity and sedentary lifestyle.
- Clinical signs of arterial insufficiency:
  1. Ulcers located on the lower extremities (at lateral malleoli, dorsum of feet, and toes); wounds are painful with legs elevated and relieved in the dangling position; wound has well-defined edges and minimal exudate; wound bed and surrounding tissue is pale.
  2. Abnormal nail growth with thick toenails.
  3. Decreased or absent leg and foot hair.
  4. Dry and shiny skin of the lower extremities.
  5. Pale skin of the lower extremities (in Caucasian people).

(continued)

Table 8.15 Peripheral Vascular Disease and Ulcerations   *(continued)*

6. Skin is cool on palpation.
7. Patients have pain in the legs or feet (due to intermittent claudication—during exercise, muscles do not receive enough blood supply for normal function).
8. Skin around the wound is black and may have gangrene (dry)
9. Lower-extremity pulses are decreased or absent.
10. Lower extremity is pale on elevation.
11. Rubor (redness) of the lower extremity is observed in a dependent position.
12. Patients with clinical signs of arterial insufficiency may also have diabetes.

See **Figure 8.5**.

A. Arterial insufficiency wound.

B. Arterial insufficiency wound.

C. Venous insufficiency wound.

D. Venous insufficiency wound.

Figure 8.5 Arterial and venous ulcers.

Neuropathic Ulcers

Table 8.16 Neuropathic Ulcers[1,4]

- Neuropathy is any disease of nerves, including peripheral and cranial nerves and/or the autonomic nervous system.
- The disease process most commonly associated with neuropathy is diabetes mellitus. Diabetic neuropathy affects mostly the lower extremities and is characterized by foot insensitivity and ulcerations.
- Diabetic neuropathy (diabetic sensory neuropathy) affects the feet, the lower extremities, and sometimes the hands (late in the course of the disease). Usually with diabetic sensory neuropathy, the patient is unable to sense pain and pressure, and there is a risk of skin breakdown without the patient being aware of it. Mechanical, repetitive stresses are the main causes of neuropathic ulcers.
- Sometimes patients with diabetic sensory neuropathy may also have foot drop, claw toe or hammer toe deformities, decreased or absent skin sweat and oil production (dry and inelastic skin), heavy callus formation, arterial disorders, and increased vulnerability to skin breakdown.
- Neuropathic ulcers are most frequently found on the plantar weight-bearing surface of the foot and at sites of bony prominences (or any other sites on the lower extremity). The wound can be deep, circular in shape, and without any pain (secondary to sensory loss); it bleeds easily (except for associated arterial insufficiency). Skin adjacent to the neuropathic ulcer wound is usually healthy but has also sensory deficits.
- Clinical signs of neuropathic ulcers:[4]
  1. Typically are found on the plantar aspect of the foot with a callous ring surrounding the perimeter of the wound; usually round (may have a crater-like appearance).
  2. Decreased pain or no pain will be reported subjectively.
  3. Drainage will be little to none.
  4. Wound base is typically non-necrotic.
  5. Dry, calloused, cracking appearance typically associated with the periwound.
  6. Pulses may be normal or of poor quality.
  7. Skin temperature is typically normal but may be increased.

Table 8.17 The Modified Wagner Scale for Classification of Neuropathic Ulcers

Depth Classification

0: The "at risk" foot: Risk factors present, prior ulcer evident; foot deformity with increased pressure points

1: Superficial, noninfected ulceration

2: Deep ulceration with tendon or joint exposed (with or without local infection)

3: Extensive ulceration with bone exposed and/or deep infection (osteomyelitis, abscess)

Ischemic Classification

A: Nonischemic

B: Ischemia (no gangrene)

C: Gangrene on part of foot (forefoot)

D: Gangrene on entire foot

Data from Brodsky J. An improved method for staging and classification of foot lesions in diabetic patients. In: Bowker J, Pfeifer MA, eds. *Levin and O'Neal's The Diabetic Foot.* 7th ed. St. Louis, MO: Mosby; 2007:222–223.

INTEGUMENTARY INTERVENTIONS

See **Figure 8.6**, neuropathic wounds.

A. Charcot foot deformity with mid-foot ulcer.

B. Ulcer over first metatarsal head.

C. Ulcer on distal aspect of limb with prior amputation.

Figure 8.6 Diabetic wounds.

Causes and Classification of Edema[1,4]

Edema is a local or generalized condition in which the body tissues contain an excessive amount of tissue fluid.

Causes of Edema

- Increased permeability of the capillary walls
- Increased capillary pressure caused by venous obstruction or heart failure
- Lymphatic obstruction
- Disturbances in renal function
- Reduction of plasma proteins
- Inflammatory conditions
- Fluid and electrolyte disturbances (caused by sodium retention)
- Malnutrition
- Starvation
- Bacterial toxins, venoms, histamine, or caustic substances

Table 8.18 Edema Classification

Types of Edema

- **Pitting:** edema of the extremities (usually). When pressed firmly with a finger for 5 seconds, the skin maintains the depression produced by the finger. (1+: indentation is barely detectable and skin rebounds quickly; 2+: slight indentation visible when skin is depressed but returns to normal in 15 seconds; 3+: deeper indentation when pressed but returns to normal within 15–30 seconds; 4+: indentation between 1.3 and 2.5 centimeters that lasts for more than 30 seconds).

- **Nonpitting:** When pressed firmly with a finger, the skin immediately rebounds to its original contour.

- **Brawny:**[5] chronic nonpitting edema that is golden brown in color due to hemosiderin.

- **Fibrosis:**[5] chronic edema containing fibrous tissue.

- **Transudate:** mild edema that is part of the inflammatory process; contains clear fluid made of water and dissolved electrolytes.

- **Inflammatory:** edema associated with inflammation due to damage to the capillary endothelium. It is localized, nonpitting, red, tender, and warm.

- **Anasarca:** severe, generalized swelling of the whole body indicating a serious systemic problem such as heart failure or renal disease.

- **Lymphedema:** an abnormal accumulation of tissue fluid (potential lymph) in the interstitial spaces. It can be caused by an impairment in the normal uptake of tissue fluid by the lymphatic vessels or by excessive production of tissue fluid caused by venous obstruction (which increases capillary blood pressure). Common clinical causes of lymphedema include neoplastic obstruction of lymphatic flow (such as in metastatic breast cancer), postoperative interference with lymphatic flow (such as in axillary dissection), infectious blockage of lymphatics, and radiation damage to lymphatics (such as post treatment of breast or pelvic cancer).

Lymphedema Classification

- **Subclinical stage (Stage 0):** no visible changes to the limb, but patient may experience feelings of heaviness or tingling in the limb.

- **Stage I:** reversible; an accumulation of protein-rich fluid. Elevation of the affected part can reduce the swelling. The patient may have pitting with pressure.

- **Stage II:** spontaneously irreversible. Proteins stimulate fibroblast formation and proliferation of connective and scar tissue. The patient may have minimal pitting even with moderate swelling.

- **Stage III:** lymphostatic elephantiasis. The dermal tissue becomes hard; the skin has papilloma and elephant-like looks.

Grading of Arterial Pulses

Table 8.19 Grading of Arterial Pulses

0 = no pulse

1+ = weak pulse (difficult to palpate)

2+ = diminished pulse (palpable but not normal)

3+ = normal pulse (easy to palpate)

4+ = bounding pulse (very strong; may imply an aneurysm or other pathological condition)

INTEGUMENTARY INTERVENTIONS

Terms Related to Integumentary Lesions

Table 8.20 **Terms Related to Integumentary Lesions**

- **Blisters** (swellings) are caused by a breakdown between cells and the primary layers of the skin. A blister is a collection of fluid below or within the epidermis. Blisters can be caused by burns, friction, or irritants. They can be elevated (or raised), flat, depressed, ulcer, and fissure.

- **Elevated (raised) blisters** are classified as follows: **papule** (less than 1 centimeter in diameter), **vesicle** (thin walled, filled with fluid, and less than 1 centimeter in diameter), **plaque** (greater than 1 centimeter in diameter), **bulla** (thin-walled, filled with fluid, and larger than 1 centimeter in diameter), **pustule** (filled with pus), **wheal** (irregularly shaped), and **crust** (dried blister with blood or exudate—fluid with high concentration of protein, cells, or solid debris).

- **Flat blisters** are symmetrical with the skin surface. They can be **macules** (spots lighter or darker than the surrounding skin; examples are freckles), **petechiae** (small, purplish, hemorrhagic spots on the skin that may signify platelet deficiency), or **vitiligo** (patchy loss of skin pigment).

- **Depressed blisters** are lower than the skin surface. They can cause excoriation when the epidermis is missing, and the dermis is exposed.

- **Ulcer blisters** are crater-like openings caused by the disintegration of the skin.

- **Fissure blisters** are linear cracks or breaks from the epidermis to the dermis.

- **Urticaria** or **hives** (or wheals) are swollen, raised, red lesions caused by fluid loss from the blood vessels. They are very itchy and usually indicate an allergic reaction. They may appear primarily on the chest, back, face, scalp, or extremities and may last up to 24 hours. Urticaria can be induced by allergic reactions to cold, ice, heat, exposure to sunlight, skin irritation, or certain medications.

- **Rash** is a local redness accompanied by inflammation. It can be caused by allergic reaction, alcoholism, vasomotor disturbance, and skin diseases. It may be accompanied by skin eruption and itching. Examples of skin rashes include diaper rash (contact dermatitis caused by prolonged contact with feces and/or urine) and butterfly rash (on the cheeks and bridge of the nose in systemic lupus erythematosus or seborrheic dermatitis).

- **Pruritus** is skin itching or a skin-burning sensation that prompts a person to scratch or rub. It may be an allergic reaction (caused by excess of bilirubin in the blood, as in jaundice, or by emotional factors).

- **Xeroderma** is excessively dry skin with shedding of the epidermis. It may indicate diabetes or thyroid deficiency.

- **Edema** (swelling of the skin) can be caused by anemia, inflammation, obstruction, circulatory problems, and cardiac or renal decompensation (failure of the heart to maintain adequate circulation; failure of kidneys to work properly).

- **Wrinkles** are creases, crevices, furrows, or ridges in the skin. They occur secondary to aging, dehydration, prolonged sun exposure, cigarette smoking, or prolonged immersion in the water.

- Unusual skin growths include **moles, cysts, nodules** (bumps), and **fibromas** (encapsulated connective tissue tumors that are irregular in shape and slow to grow; they have firm consistency).

Other Integumentary Signs and Symptoms

Table 8.21 Skin Characteristics: Color, Temperature, Perspiration, Soreness, and Growths

- **Changes in skin color:** Red skin may indicate carbon monoxide poisoning. Yellow skin may indicate jaundice, liver disease, or increased carotene intake. Inflammation may not be observed well in dark pigmented skin, therefore in addition to observation, palpation is indicated. The skin is usually warmer in the area and is tight and edematous, and the deeper tissues are hard.

- **Changes in skin color:** Pallor of the skin may indicate lack of sunlight, shock, malnutrition, vasomotor instability, or hemorrhage. For African American patients, skin pallor appears yellow brown for brown-skinned patients (clients) and ashen gray for black-skinned patients (clients). In addition, mucous membranes of African American patients appear ashen, and the lips and nail beds have a similar appearance.

- **Other changes in skin color:** Cyanosis of the skin (blue, gray discoloration) may be caused by lack of oxygen or increased carbon dioxide in the blood system. For African American patients, cyanosis can be seen by close inspection of the lips, tongue, conjunctiva (of the eyelids), palms of the hands, and soles of the feet. For African American patients, one method of testing for cyanosis is by pressing the palms. Slow blood return indicates cyanosis. Another sign is ashen gray lips and tongue.

- For African American patients, **ecchymosis** (superficial bleeding under the skin from trauma) can be detected by swelling of the skin surface.

- **Brown skin with yellow spots** (or liver spots) may be caused by liver malignancies, pregnancy, or aging.

- **Abnormal heat** may indicate a febrile condition, excessive salt intake, or excitement.

- **Abnormal cold** may indicate poor circulation.

- **Increased perspiration** may indicate drug intake, fever, exercise performance, or pulmonary condition.

- **Decreased perspiration** may indicate dehydration.

Clinical Impairments, Activity Limitations, and Participation Restrictions Associated with Integumentary Conditions

Clinical Impairments and Activity Limitations in Wounds/Burns and Ulcerations

Table 8.22 Impairments and Activity Limitations in Wounds/Burns and Ulcerations

- Joint swelling, inflammation, joint stiffness, or contracture
- Increased pain
- Soft-tissue swelling, inflammation, and stiffness
- Decreased gait, locomotion, and balance
- Decreased strength, power, and endurance
- Decreased postural control
- Decreased sensory awareness
- Weight-bearing difficulties
- Decreased ability to perform physical actions, tasks, or activities related to self-care, home management, work (job, school, or play), community, and leisure activities
- Decreased ability to perform activities of daily living (ADLs) or instrumental activities of daily living (IADLs)
- Use of assistive devices and equipment during ADLs or IADLs
- Decreased tolerance of positions and activities

Integumentary Conditions and Impairments (Not Related to Wounds, Burns, or Ulcerations)

Table 8.23 Integumentary Conditions and Impairments (Not Related to Wounds, Burns, or Ulcerations)

- **Dermatitis:** inflammation of the skin characterized by itching, skin lesions (crust, plaque, fibrotic papules and nodules), redness, and skin oozing. It is caused by the following:
  - Allergic reaction (due to chemical, mechanical, or biological agents, sensitivity to sunlight, or ultraviolet exposure)
  - Hereditary cause
  - Psychological disorders
- **Cellulitis:** inflammation of connective tissue or cellular tissue (such as dermis, subcutaneous layers, and tissue spaces) accompanied by infection. Impairments are edema, erythema, skin tenderness, nodules, and skin heat.
- **Herpes:** a group of viral and bacterial infections (herpes simplex; herpes zoster). Impairments caused by herpes include the following:
  - Herpes I (herpes simplex): fever blister or cold sore
  - Herpes II: vesicular genital eruption; newborns may have inflammation of the brain and its meninges
  - Herpes zoster (shingles): pain and tingling; itching of the corresponding dermatome; papules (fluid-filled); malaise; fever; chills; gastrointestinal disturbances; urination difficulty; pain in the affected joints; neuralgia (constant and intermittent)

(continued)

Table 8.23 Integumentary Conditions and Impairments (Not Related to Wounds, Burns, or Ulcerations)   *(continued)*

- **Scleroderma** (systemic sclerosis): immune integumentary disorder; chronic progressive disorder of vessels and connective tissue characterized by hardening or excessive collagen deposition in skin, joints, internal organs (such as the gastrointestinal tract, lungs, kidneys, and heart).
  - Scleroderma can be localized or systemic and can be accompanied by Raynaud's phenomenon (vasospastic disease of small arteries and arterioles; unknown causes; attacks of numbness and sensation of cold; may have throbbing and paresthesia; affects mostly the digits of hands bilaterally).
  - Impairments include pain in the affected areas, joint stiffness, edema of fingers and joints, skin thickening (may be limited to face and distal extremities or may be diffuse to face, whole extremities, and trunk), and contractures.
- **Psoriasis:** immune integumentary disorder; inherited chronic recurrent inflammatory condition accompanied by rash and scaly red or silvery plaques. The rash can be found commonly on the knees, shins, elbows, umbilicus, lower back, buttocks, ears, and hairline. Also, pitting of the nails can occur. The severity of the disease can range from a minimal cosmetic problem to involvement of the total body surface. Precipitating factors for psoriasis include stress, pregnancy, infection, cold weather, smoking, endocrine changes, and anxiety. Impairments include shaded skin areas, skin lesions, thick and scaly skin, and grape-like skin clusters.
- **Eczema:** immune skin disorder; common superficial inflammatory condition characterized by itchy red rash that initially weeps or oozes serum and may become crusted, thickened, or scaly.
  - Causes are allergies, irritating chemicals, drugs, scratching or rubbing the skin, and sun exposure. Eczema may be acute or chronic, and the rash may become infected.
  - Types of eczema: erythematous, herpeticum (from herpes simplex virus), lichenoid (with thickening of the skin), nummular (with coin- or oval-shaped lesions), pustular (follicular, impetiginous such as chronic squamous eczema on soles, legs, scalp), and seborrheic (with excessive secretions from sebaceous glands).
  - Eczema is not treated in physical therapy; however, the physical therapist (PT) or physical therapist assistant (PTA) should be able to recognize the condition and check the patient's (client's) skin before and after applying modalities that use topical substances on the skin.
- **Lupus erythematosus:** immune skin disorder (caused by an autoimmune process); chronic, progressive inflammatory disorder of the connective tissues characterized by remission and exacerbation. The patient (client) may have scaling, red, macular rash.
  - **Systemic lupus erythematosus (SLE):** chronic autoimmune inflammatory disease involving multiple organ systems and marked by periodic acute episodes. The patient has a "butterfly" rash over the nose and cheeks. SLE is most prevalent in women of childbearing age.
  - Impairments include malaise, overwhelming fatigue, polyarthralgia, fever, arthritis, skin rash ("butterfly" rash over face and nose), photosensitivity, hair loss, and Raynaud's disease (vasospastic disease of small arteries and arterioles affecting the digits of the hands bilaterally; the cause is unknown; the patient has intermittent vasospastic attacks in response to cold or emotion).
- **Polymyositis** (dermatomyositis): immune skin disorder; inflammatory disease of the skeletal muscles characterized by symmetrical weakness of the proximal muscles of the extremities; evidence of muscle necrosis on biopsy; skin rash over eyelids or papules over the dorsal surface of the knuckles; rapid and severe etiology; may require ventilator and tube feeding. Impairments include symmetrical weakness of the proximal muscles of the extremities.
- **Skin Lesions:** skin abnormalities that may be suspect for potential skin cancers. According to Skin Cancer.org: "Characteristics are associated with the mnemonic ABCDEs of skin cancer. Unusual lesions may have: **A**symmetrical lesion size; uneven **B**orders; changing **C**olors ranging from hues of tan, brown, black, blue, or reds; **D**iameters greater than 6 millimeters, and **E**volving in reference to any of the aforementioned characteristics."[6]
  - PTAs should report any of these unusual characteristics to the supervising PT for referral to another medical professional.

Figure 8.7 Comparison of normal mole with melanoma.

Table 8.24 Characteristics of Suspicious Skin Lesions Related to Possible Melanomas[6]

PTAs often work with patients in varying levels of disrobe to access specific body regions during treatment, and therefore, PTAs can be valuable in proactive intervention and referral to the appropriate medical profession when suspicious skin lesions are observed.

Table 8.23 provides the PTA with general considerations related to the integumentary system regarding possible suspect skin lesions that coincide with the ABCDEs of melanoma.

Note: one or more characteristics may be observed and any unusual observations warrant consultation with the supervising physical therapist.

Suspicious Characteristics:

- Rapid growth or evolving features that are observed over a few weeks or months
- Lesions with a diameter larger than a pencil eraser (more than 6 millimeters in diameter)
- Changes in color of the lesion ranging from various shades of tans, browns, black, blues, reds
- Inflamed or redness of the margins of the lesion
- Irregular, ragged, jagged border edges
- Weeping from the lesion
- Crusty formation on the lesion
- Bleeding lesions
- Pruritus (pus-like drainage)

Types of Integumentary Interventions

INTEGUMENTARY INTERVENTIONS

Burn Rehabilitation Interventions[1,4]

Table 8.25 General Interventions for Burns

- Burn rehabilitation is a team effort that includes many professionals.[1]
- The PT's goals in the plan of care are devised together with the patient and patient's family. To attain the objectives of optimal long-term function, long-term goals are established at the outset of burn care.
- The PT must consider three general principles: (1) performing ROM exercises, (2) splinting and antideformity positioning, and (3) establishing a long-term relationship with the patient and family members to ensure compliance with therapy goals and to increase the patient's morale for recovery.
- In the intensive care unit, PROM in all planes of motion is performed twice daily considering the patient's pain, anxiety, wound status, extremity perfusion, and security of the patient's airway and vascular access devices.
- In burn care, PROM can be timed to coincide with dressing changes and wound cleansing, thereby minimizing the patient's need for pain medications.
- Burn contractures and prevention interventions follow:
  1. Axillary adduction contractures can be prevented by positioning of the shoulders widely abducted at 90° with axillary splints, padded hanging troughs of thermoplastic material, or a variety of support devices mounted to the bed.
  2. Elbow flexion contractures can be minimized by statically splinting the elbow in extension; elbow splints can be alternated with flexion splints to help retain the full ROM.
  3. Flexion contractures of the hips and knees (particularly common in children) can be prevented by positioning the patient in extension. For contractures of the anterior hip, position the patient supine with hip and knee extended, in external rotation and abduction, with a pillow under the hips for increased extension; the patient can also be positioned prone, although this position is poorly tolerated. For contractures of the posterior knee, the knees must be positioned in extension with the patient in supine without a pillow; a knee immobilizer may also be used.
  4. Equinus deformity (ankle plantarflexed and foot in varus) can be prevented with static splinting of the ankles in neutral position (may use an anterior ankle conformer or an ankle foot orthosis at 90°); use padding on the splints over the metatarsal heads or calcaneus to distribute the pressure evenly.
  5. Anterior neck deformity can be prevented by using a neck conformer that maintains the chin-to-chest distance and by not using a pillow in bed.
  6. Posterior neck deformity can be prevented by using a neck conformer that maintains the length in the posterior neck and by using a pillow in supine position (or a pillow under the chest in prone position).
  7. Hand deformity in an "intrinsic minus position" contracture (metacarpophalangeal (MCP) joints are fixed in hyperextension and proximal interphalangeal (PIP) joints are fixed in flexion) can be prevented by placing the MCP joints at maximum flexion (90°) to maximally stretch the collateral ligaments, the wrist at 30° of extension (some authors indicate only 15° anterior wrist extension or 15° for posterior wrist flexion, depending on the burned area), and the interphalangeal (IP) joints in full extension; the thumb must be fully abducted. With massive burns and patient resuscitation in the first 24–48 hours, the wrist can be elevated (using a volar cock-up splint) at 70° to 80° (pulls the MCP and IP joints in a safe position). The splints need to be inspected at least twice daily to check for poor fit or pressure injury.
- As critical illness is reduced and wounds progressively close, burn interventions concentrate on (1) PROM, (2) AROM, (3) light strengthening exercises, (4) minimizing edema (that contributes to tightness), (5) ADL training, (6) initial scar management, and (7) preparing the patient for work, play, or school.

(continued)

Table 8.25 **General Interventions for Burns**   *(continued)*

- During the wound closure period, the patient may be ready to be discharged from the hospital. The interventions at this point concentrate on (1) progressive PROM, (2) strengthening exercises, (3) specific postoperative therapy after reconstructive operations, and (4) scar management.

- Extreme pruritus may begin shortly after the wound has healed, peak in intensity months after the initial injury, and then gradually subside in most patients. Interventions for this condition include massage, frequent application of skin moisturizers or colloidal baths, vitamin E topical cream, and topical cold compresses. In some cases, pruritus can cause skin excoriation and infections of the wound (with *Staphylococcus aureus* bacteria). In these cases, patients (clients) need to see the physician and receive antibiotics or be admitted to hospital.

- Burn reconstructive surgical methods include incisional release and grafting, excisional release and grafting, Z-plasty, and random flaps (may be used for chest wall or hands burns).

Table 8.26 **Skin Grafts Used for Burns**

- **Split-thickness skin grafts:** used for small burns (especially face burns) and for burns covering less than 40% of the total affected body surface. Split-thickness skin grafts can achieve the best cosmetic outcomes and are preferred to garment pressure therapy because of their decreased healing time.

- **Full-thickness skin grafts with primary closure of donor site:** used for small burns because of their functional and cosmetic outcomes.

- **Skin expansions:** meshing devices that expand the skin. They are used for burns covering more than 40% of the total affected body surface.

- **Cultured and autologous epidermal sheets:** used for burns covering 85–90% of the total affected body surface. Cultured epidermal sheets need 2–3 weeks to grow, are fragile, and can cause hypertrophic scarring.

- **Skin substitutes that contain an epidermal and a dermal component:** used for burn/wound contraction after skin grafting was performed. Types of skin substitutes include the Apligraf bilayer products (made of bovine-collagen–based dermis and Silastic epidermis).

- **Biologic dressings**: biosynthetic, temporary skin substitutes for burns and wounds. Their role is to prevent wound contamination and reduce pain and loss of fluid. Biologic dressings contain epidermal and dermal layers. They can deliver growth factors and matrix proteins. They can decrease infections, speed epithelialization, and minimize scarring. Biologic dressings can be applied in the first 6 hours after the burn occurs.

Elements to Effect Wound Healing

Table 8.27 **Wound Healing Elements**

Oxygen[1]

- Necessary for wound healing; important for granulation, angiogenesis, collagen deposition, and wound contraction; has an antibiotic effect and helps the wound resist pathogens.

- With wounds, oxygen has difficulty reaching tissue especially when edema, necrotic tissue, and peripheral vasoconstriction are present. Interventions such as debridement (to clean necrotic tissue) and compression (to decrease edema) are necessary to decrease the obstruction to wound oxygenation. Vasoconstriction may not always be improved.

(continued)

INTEGUMENTARY INTERVENTIONS

Table 8.27 **Wound Healing Elements** *(continued)*

- Factors contributing to improvement of oxygen levels in the wound include nutrition, hydration, keeping the wound warm, controlling pain and anxiety, avoiding smoking, and possibly using supplemental oxygen.
- Recent studies indicate that oxygen delivered directly to a localized limb chamber (called topical hyperbaric oxygen [THBO]) can improve wound healing.

Moisture[1]

- Necessary for wound healing; represents a newer concept of wound healing.
- Moisture can soften eschar and create autolytic debridement (the body's own enzymes dissolves the eschar under the right conditions).
- Factors contributing to improvement in moisture levels in the wound include providing for wound hydration, using occlusive dressings (such as hydrocolloids, which can be applied over even an infected wound with a systemic antibiotic regimen), limiting fluid loss from the wound surface, controlling heavy exudates, and allowing gaseous exchange.

Nutrition[1]

- Necessary for wound healing.
- Factors contributing to improvement of wound healing through nutrition include increasing levels of iron, vitamin B_{12}, folic acid, vitamin C, zinc, vitamin A, arginine (for healing and immune response), and amino acids (high protein intake) in the blood.

Integumentary Patient Education

Table 8.28 **Patient Education Elements**

- Community resources include support groups (related to the patient's diagnosis)
- Counseling
- Family and/or caregiver participation
- Internet resources
    1. Lymphedema: http://www.lymphnet.org/ (see Appendix D for the patient's copy for lymphedema education)
    2. Wound care: http://www.apwca.org
    3. Burn care: http://www.ameriburn.org
    4. Diabetes: https://www.niddk.nih.gov/health-information
    5. Pressure Injury information: https://npiap.com/
- Education materials such as instructional materials, multimedia information, or self-management information
- Home program
    1. Skin care
    2. Wound care
    3. Prevention: for diabetes—inspect the feet daily; be aware of changes in skin color, visible skin breakdown such as cracks, fissures, blisters, and abrasions; inspect for callus formation; keep dry and flaky skin hydrated with non-perfumed water-based lotions; do not place lotions between the toes; apply lotions after cleaning first with mild soap and warm tap water; test the water temperature with a thermometer or the elbow but never with the fingers

(continued)

Table 8.28 Patient Education Elements *(continued)*

4. Scar management
5. Exercises
6. Compression garment or bandage wear and care
7. Pressure-relieving devices (e.g., beds, mattresses, overlays placed on top of mattress, or special seat cushions)
8. Edema control
9. Foot care for patients with diabetes

Patient Education: Skin Care for Patients with Diabetes

Table 8.29 Skin Care Education for Patients with Diabetes[7]

- After you wash with a mild soap, make sure that you rinse and dry yourself well. Check places where water can hide, such as under the arms, under the breasts, and between the legs and toes.
- Drink lots of fluids (such as water) to keep your skin moist and healthy.
- Keep your skin moist by using a lotion or cream after you wash. Ask your doctor to suggest one.
- Wear all-cotton underwear. Cotton allows air to move around your body better.
- Check your skin after you wash. Make sure you have no dry, red, or sore spots that might lead to an infection.
- Tell your doctor about any skin problems.

Patient Education: Foot Care for Patients with Diabetes

Table 8.30 Foot Care Education for Patients with Diabetes[7]

- Wash your feet in warm water every day. Make sure the water is not too hot by testing the temperature with your elbow. Do not soak your feet. Dry your feet well, especially between your toes.
- Look at your feet every day to check for cuts, sores, blisters, redness, calluses, or other problems. Checking every day is more important if you have nerve damage or poor blood flow. If you cannot bend over or pull your feet up to check them, use a mirror. If you cannot see well, ask someone else to check your feet.
- If your skin is dry, rub lotion on your feet after you wash and dry them. Do not put lotion between your toes.
- File corn and calluses gently with an emery board or pumice stone. Do this after your bath or shower.
- Cut your toenails once a week or when needed. Cut toenails when they are soft from washing. Cut them to the shape of the toe and not too short. File the edges with an emery board.
- Always wear socks or slippers to protect your feet from injuries.

(continued)

Table 8.30 Foot Care Education for Patients with Diabetes *(continued)*

- Always wear socks or stockings to avoid blisters. Do not wear socks or knee-high stockings that are too tight below your knee.
- Wear shoes that fit well. Shop for shoes at the end of the day when your feet are bigger. Break in shoes slowly. Wear them 1–2 hours each day for the first 1–2 weeks.
- Before putting your shoes on, feel the insides to make sure they have no sharp edges or objects that might injure your feet.
- Tell your doctor right away about any foot problems.
- Ask your doctor to look at your feet at each checkup. To make sure your doctor checks your feet, take off your shoes and socks before your doctor comes into the room.
- Ask your doctor to check how well the nerves in your feet sense feeling.
- Ask your doctor to check how well blood is flowing to your legs and feet.
- Ask your doctor to show you the best way to trim your toenails. Ask which lotion or cream to use on your legs and feet.
- If you cannot cut your toenails or if you have a foot problem, ask your doctor to send you to a foot doctor (podiatrist).

Wound Cleansing Methods

Table 8.31 Wound Cleansing Methods

Whirlpool

- A whirlpool[1,8] is rarely used today, except for special situations when the wound needs intensive cleansing or softening of loosely adherent tissue (before sharp, enzymatic, or autolytic debridement) that cannot be done with other methods.
- When the whirlpool is used, minimal agitation of water for 5–10 minutes is necessary to limit the negative effects of temperature and pressure changes. Iodine-povidone or chlorine can be added to the water, but only if infection is present. Also, wounds that need stimulation of peripheral circulation may benefit from the whirlpool.
- When the whirlpool is used with PVD, the temperature should not exceed 1°C (1.8°F) above skin temperature. The whirlpool water temperature ranges from 33.5°–35.5°C (92°–96°F).
- For patients with cardiopulmonary conditions, the whirlpool temperature should not exceed 38°C (100.4°F).
- In general, the whirlpool is contraindicated for clean granulating wounds, epithelializing wounds, migrating epidermal cells, new skin grafts, new tissue flaps, venous ulcers (and venous insufficiency), non-necrotic diabetic ulcers, wound maceration, dry gangrene, and wounds with active bleeding.[1,9]

Pulsatile Lavage with Suction

- Pulsatile lavage with suction (PLWS), also called forceful irrigation, is a technique for cleaning the wound and performing debridement. PLWS can remove the irrigation fluid, wound exudates, and loose debris by using pulsed irrigation and simultaneous suction. PLWS can also deliver antiseptics, topical antibiotics, and antibacterial solutions to the wound and can treat tunneling and undermining wounds (using special cannula tips).
- PLWS is a better method than the whirlpool because it requires less treatment time and less staff and can be performed at the bedside or at the patient's home.

(continued)

Table 8.31 Wound Cleansing Methods *(continued)*

- The patient's family or visitors are not allowed in the room during the procedure.

- The disadvantages of PLWS are risk of trauma to newly formed tissue (because of the plastic tips or the suction) and risk of overuse with clean, granulating wounds.

Nonforceful Irrigation

- Nonforceful irrigation is another form of cleaning the wound using minimal pressure or force. It can be accomplished using packaged saline for wound cleansing, single-dose sterile saline, and spray containers (at gentle pressure) with saline.

- Nonforceful irrigation can be used for infected wounds, clean wounds with new tissue growth (to remove excess fluids or residue from dressings), and necrotic wounds or debris (may need a few sessions of nonforceful irrigation or the PLWS).

Wound Debridement Methods

Table 8.32 General Debridement Methods

Debridement Techniques

- **Debridement:** removal of foreign material and dead or damaged tissue.
- **Nonselective mechanical debridement:** removal of all tissue (necrotic and living tissue). These techniques are used:
  1. Wet to dry dressings: wet gauze applied to the wound bed that debrides the wound by being pulled away when it dries; used for moderate amounts of necrotic tissue; may traumatize healthy or healing tissue; can be painful to the patient. The research is controversial regarding this technique's benefits and disadvantages.
  2. Pulsatile lavage with suction.
  3. Whirlpool: biggest disadvantage is tissue maceration; waterborne pathogens can cause contamination or infection; disinfecting additives may be cytotoxic.[2]
  4. Scrubbing: use of sponge, brush, or gauze with fluid to break up adhered devitalized tissue from the wound bed. Contraindicated for granulating wounds.[1]
- **Chemical (enzymatic) selective debridement:** removal of necrotic tissue (usually in large amounts) and eschar using topical agents containing enzymes. Some enzymatic debriders are selective, and some are not. The dressings are prescribed by a physician. Enzymatic debridement has the following characteristics:
  1. Fast acting
  2. Causes minimal or no damage to healthy tissue with proper application
  3. Expensive
  4. Needs to be applied and performed carefully and only to the necrotic tissue
  5. May require a specific secondary dressing
  6. May cause inflammation or discomfort
- **Autolytic debridement:** a type of enzymatic selective debridement that uses the body's own enzymes and moisture to rehydrate, soften, and liquefy hard eschar and slough. With this type of debridement, only necrotic tissue is liquefied. Types of autolytic debridement dressings are occlusive or semi-occlusive dressings (such as hydrocolloids, hydrogels, and transparent films).

(continued)

Table 8.32 General Debridement Methods *(continued)*

- **Biologic debridement:** uses maggot therapy to promote enzymatic lysis without harming viable tissue and provides a bactericide for MRSA and Strep A and B. This method is seldom used in the United States despite Food and Drug Administration approval in 2004.[2]
  - Advantages[2]
  1. Wound odor is decreased due to the bactericide effect.
  2. Increased granulation may result from removal of devitalized and infected tissue in the wound bed.
  - Disadvantage[2]
  1. It poses psychological stress to the patient because it involves living creatures crawling on the patient in the wound bed.
- **Sharp selective debridement:** a type of debridement in which the clinician uses surgical instruments to remove the necrotic tissue from the wound. In physical therapy, *PTs (as per the American Physical Therapy Association [APTA]) are the only individuals allowed to use sharp debridement (with scalpels, scissors, or forceps) and only in the presence of necrotic tissue (the PTA should check his or her state's practice act).* Surgeons may also use surgery (and laser) to perform this method of debridement. The biggest challenge is to differentiate yellow slough from tendons. Usually, sharp debridement would be recommended for infected wounds with systemic sepsis or necrotizing fasciitis. Caution should be used in patients with clotting disorders and those who are taking anticoagulants (because uncontrolled bleeding may occur). Sharp debridement is painful to the patient and is costly if the operating room and surgery are required.

Two Types of Enzymatic Debriding Agents

- Agent containing papain and urea in a cream base (or in a formulation of chlorophyllin and copper) that may need to be applied once or twice a day application. For example, a proteolytic enzyme dressing uses topical enzymes to digest and liquefy necrotic tissue in the wound bed. The dressing should be left in place for 2–3 days. When it is removed, the wound should be irrigated with normal saline solution to remove liquefied debris. Such dressings require multiple applications but are pain free and less stressful to the patient. They are not appropriate for infected wounds.

- Collagenase in a petroleum base that may need to be applied once daily. The water-soluble proteinase specifically attacks and breaks down collagen; digests undenatured collagen fibers, allowing the necrotic plug to be removed; and is more selective than proteolytic enzyme. Studies[10,11] showed that granulation and epithelialization proceeded faster with collagenase treatment than was expected in chronic dermal lesions (ulcers and pressure injuries). This approach, which is also a good choice for maintenance debridement, decreases bacterial capability.

Biophysical Agents

Table 8.33 Biophysical Agent Interventions[2,9,12]

- **Electrical stimulation:** used adjunctively for wound healing of the infected or noninfected wounds that are chronic or recalcitrant. Electrical stimulation is not to be used on simple, noncomplex or superficial wounds. Specific parameters need to be utilized based on treatment outcomes. Refer to your physical agent publications for specific parameters.

(continued)

Table 8.33 **Biophysical Agent Interventions**   *(continued)*

- **Desired Effects**
1. Increases blood flow
2. Edema reduction
3. Autolysis
4. Fights infections
5. Contributes to galvanotaxis
6. Restores normal electrical skin activity post-tissue insult

- **Precautions**
1. Standard precautions relative to this modality must be considered
2. Lack of sensation associated with some wound pathologies
3. Patient's lack of sensation due to neuropathy

- **Contraindications**
1. Not used on simple, superficial wounds
2. Osteomyelitis
3. No topical agents containing metallic ions[2]
4. Active bleeding

■ **Hyperbaric oxygen treatments:** indicated for hypoxic wounds (chronic or slow healing) that respond favorably to transcutaneous oxygen monitoring tests. Specific parameters need to be utilized based on treatment outcomes. Refer to physical agent publications for specific parameters. Two types: Topical is performed by physical therapists or physical therapist assistants. Systemic (whole body or chamber) is performed by specially trained nurses or respiratory therapists.

- **Desired Effects**
1. Increases healing via increased oxygen concentration gradients
2. Edema reduction
3. Enhances collagen synthesis, angiogenesis, tissue granulation, epithelization, and wound contracture

- **Precautions**
1. Altered sensation of skin where unit is applied

- **Contraindications**
1. Not used on simple, superficial wounds
2. DVT
3. Congestive heart failure (CHF)
4. Severe arterial insufficiency
5. Severe claustrophobia = relative contraindication
6. Chronic obstructive pulmonary disease = relative contraindication
7. Pregnancy = relative contraindication

■ **Light therapies** (Ultraviolet-C, low level laser): indicated for wound healing and tissue repair. Low level laser therapy (LLLT) and Ultraviolet C (UVC) have been shown to have beneficial effects on wound healing when used as part of a wound management program. Studies show an overall decrease in wound healing times with use of LLLT.

- **Desired Effects**
1. Increased collagen synthesis (LLLT)
2. Increase in the tensile strength of healed tissues (LLLT)
3. Inhibit growth of bacteria (UVC)
4. Acceleration of epithelial tissue turnover (UVC)
5. Vasodilation, increase blood flow
6. Increased rate of wound healing

(continued)

Table 8.33 Biophysical Agent Interventions *(continued)*

- **Precautions**
1. Over low back or abdomen during pregnancy (LLLT)
2. Impaired sensation
3. Impaired mentation
4. Photosensitivity or treatment with photosensitizing medications
5. Recent radiation therapy (UVC)

- **Contraindications**
1. Malignancy in general (LLLT), skin cancer (UVC)
2. Within 6 months of receiving radiation therapy (LLLT)
3. Areas of hemorrhage (LLLT)
4. Pulmonary tuberculosis (UVC)
5. Systemic Lupus Erythematosus (UVC)
6. Irradiation over the eyes.

■ **Negative pressure wound therapy (NPWT)/Vacuum assisted wound therapy:** indicated for chronic, slow healing; post-surgical wounds/grafts; and acute wounds. Specific parameters need to be utilized based on treatment outcomes. Refer to your physical agent publications for specific parameters.

- **Desired Effects**
1. Increases local circulation to the wound
2. Decreases edema associated to the wound/periwound
3. Increases tissue granulation to wound bed
4. Facilitates angiogenesis
5. Facilitates epithelization
6. Reduces wound bed bioburden
7. Maintains a moisture-retentive environment

- **Precautions**
1. Actively bleeding wounds
2. Patients on anti-coagulation therapy

*Bleeding may be increased with NPWT—USE CAUTION.

*Reduced pressure should be employed if treatment is to be performed to accommodate for the precautions

- **Contraindications**
1. Dry wounds
2. Necrotic wounds
3. Body cavity wounds
4. Overexposed blood vessels
5. Untreated osteomyelitis

■ **Pneumatic compression therapy**

- **Desired Effects**
1. Edema reduction
2. Increases venous return from distal segments

- **Precautions**
1. Altered skin sensation

(continued)

Table 8.33 Biophysical Agent Interventions *(continued)*

- **Contraindications**
1. Known or suspected DVT or pulmonary edema (PE) in the past 6 months
2. Active cancer
3. Bleeding disorders
4. Should be avoided in cases of arterial insufficiency. Compression bandaging should be considered as an alternative[1]

A. Ultrasound (high and low frequency): used for the healing of chronic or recalcitrant wound healing. Ultrasound is not indicated for simple, noncomplex, or superficial wounds. Specific parameters need to be utilized based on treatment outcomes. Refer to your physical agent publications for specific parameters.

- **Desired Effects**
1. Enhances all three phases of wound healing
2. Wound contraction enhancement
3. Improves granulation, collagen deposition, and angiogenesis
4. Improves pliability of scars

- **Precautions**
1. Standard precautions relative to this modality
2. Patient's lack of sensation due to neuropathy

- **Contraindications**
1. Not to be used on simple, superficial wounds
2. Untreated acute wound infections
3. Osteomyelitis
4. Active bleeding
5. DVT
6. Severe arterial insufficiency
7. Over large areas of necrosis, as eschar may be too thick to allow ultrasound transmission to the underlying tissues

B. Ultrasound (low frequency with saline mist):[2] used to promote improved cellular and protein responses by causing greater acoustical streaming and cavitation to facilitate debridement of fibrin in chronic wound beds.

- **Desired Effects**
1. Enhances wound healing, including: increased collagen production, increased angiogenesis, increased fibrinolysis, increased macrophagic responses, increased nitric oxide levels[2]
2. Augments wound debridement by destroying biofilms, bacteria, viruses, and fungal formation within the wound bed[2]

- **Precautions**
1. Proper personal protective equipment required due to increased possibility of splash injuries or aerosolization from the mist to exposed areas susceptible to microbial exposures (eyes, ears, nose, mouth, superficial cuts in skin)

- **Contraindications**
1. Not to be used on simple, superficial wounds
2. Untreated acute wound infections
3. Osteomyelitis
4. Active bleeding
5. DVT
6. Severe arterial insufficiency
7. Over large areas of necrosis, as eschar may be too thick to allow ultrasound transmission to the underlying tissues

INTEGUMENTARY INTERVENTIONS

Wound Types: Clinical Decision Making and Outcomes

Table 8.34 Wound Type Clinical Decision-Making Pearls[2]

- Draining wounds: require dressing to absorb moisture and protect the periwound.
- Nondraining wounds: require a dressing that allows moisture to evaporate and not allow moisture pooling when covered.
- Granular wounds: require dressings that protect the healing wound bed from any trauma (i.e., friction or shear forces).
- Necrotic wounds: may require debridement.
- Use of the Red-Yellow-Black system may also be beneficial in achieving wound healing goals and choosing the correct dressings.

Red-Yellow-Black System[2]

Wound Color	Wound Characteristics	Wound Healing Goals
Red	Pink, granular tissue	Protect wound; maintain moist environment
Yellow	Moist, yellow slough	Remove debris and exudate; absorb drainage
Black	Black eschar, firmly attached	Debride necrotic tissue

Table 8.35 Wound Types and Outcomes[2]

Wound Type	Dressing Objective	Desired Outcome	PTA Considerations
Granular, nondraining	■ Moisture retentive ■ Wound bed protection	■ Protect and promote normal healing	■ Use proper infection prevention techniques ■ Periwound maceration ■ Nonselective debridement of granular tissue with dressing removal
Granular, draining	■ Moisture absorption ■ Moisture wicking	■ Protect granulation and periwound	■ Use proper infection prevention techniques ■ Excessive drainage: may indicate a silent infection in an immunocompromised patient ■ Nonselective debridement of granular tissue with dressing removal

(continued)

Table 8.35 Wound Types and Outcomes
(continued)

Wound Type	Dressing Objective	Desired Outcome	PTA Considerations
Necrotic, nondraining	■ Moisture retentive (hydrocolloid, occlusive) ■ Enzymatic debridement	■ Eschar needs softening in preparation for removal	■ Use proper infection prevention techniques ■ Use skin sealant on surrounding tissue to deter maceration from moisture-promoting dressings
Necrotic, draining	■ Remove devitalized tissue ■ Absorb excessive moisture ■ Protect surrounding tissues from maceration	■ Debride ■ Absorb ■ Protect	■ Use proper infection prevention techniques ■ Monitor for signs of infection since necrotic tissue has greater susceptibility to infection, and a wet environment may promote microbial proliferation

Wound Dressings and Topical Agents

Table 8.36 Wound Dressings

Wound dressing choice depends on the following wound characteristics: necrosis, drainage, infection, granulation tissue, epithelialization, periwound area, cavities and tunneling, friction, wound odor, and incontinence.

■ **Primary dressing:** applied directly to the wound
■ **Secondary dressing:** dressing applied over the primary dressing

Gauze Dressing

■ Gauze dressing can be used as a secondary dressing, especially if changed frequently. It should not be used as a primary dressing because it leaves contamination fibers, is adherent to the wound, is permeable to bacteria, can cause wound desiccation, releases excessive amounts of bacteria, and causes pain on removal. Gauze ribbon can be used to maintain an opening for drainage in a tunneling wound.

■ Wound cavities should not be packed full to allow flow of oxygen and nutrients to the wound, a place for granulation tissue, and epithelial cells survival.

■ Impregnated gauze (also called petrolatum gauze) can be used as the primary dressing because it does not stick to the wound, is minimally absorptive, can create a greasy wound bed, and offers minimal protection.

Transparent Films

■ Transparent films are made of a transparent membrane with an acrylic adhesive layer. Films do not allow bacteria or moisture into the wound and assist with skin protection from shearing, friction, or contamination (from incontinence). Film removal can cause skin tears (with frail or aging skin).

(continued)

Table 8.36 Wound Dressings *(continued)*

- Films are semiocclusive and trap moisture, allowing autolytic debridement of necrotic wounds and creating a moist healing environment for granulating wounds.
- Films[13] can be used as a protective dressing and as a topical treatment for stage 1 and stage 2 pressure injuries, minimally draining or nondraining surgical wounds, lacerations and abrasions, partial-thickness wounds, noninfected wounds, and wounds with necrosis or slough.

Application of Film Dressings

1. Clip excess hair around the wound site (to ensure proper adhesion).
2. Clean the wound and periwound skin with normal saline solution (or other cleaner).
3. Dry the skin well so that the film can adhere to it.
4. Apply the film dressing over the wound, smoothing it into the place.
5. Remove the film's delivery systems (such as window, frame, or paperback release) before applying it.
6. Do not use tension when applying the film (can tear the skin).
7. Remove the film by following the manufacturer's instructions.

Hydrogels

- Hydrogels can be amorphous (liquid-like gel) or sheets (thin, flexible sheets with 90% water).
- Hydrogels increase moisture [14,15] in a dry wound bed and soften necrotic tissue.
- Hydrogels may require a secondary dressing to be contained in the wound, which feels very soothing for the patient.

Foams

- Foams are highly absorbent pads, sheets, or packing of polyurethane, available with or without adhesive backing. They can be used as primary or secondary dressings.
- Foams create an occlusive environment. They should not be used alone on a dry wound.

Hydrocolloids

- Hydrocolloids are the most occlusive of the moisture-retentive dressings; they are also available as less occlusive or semipermeable dressings and are available in various styles and shapes. Hydrocolloids work best on moderate to mild exudating wounds.
- Three types of hydrocolloids are available: pastes, powders, and sheets. Pastes and powders can be used as wound fillers but should not protrude above the level of the surrounding skin. The hydrocolloid sheets usually cover the pastes and powders.
- Hydrocolloid dressings[15,16] react with wound drainage and may swell or "melt out," leaving a residue in the wound with a malodorous smell (from product breakdown, not necessarily from infection). The residue needs to be removed by cleaning gently with a wound cleanser.

Application of Hydrocolloids

1. Hydrocolloids adhere best at body temperature.
2. To increase adherence, the therapist should place his or her hand over the dressing after applying it to the wound. The heat from the therapist's hand will assist in molding the dressing to the wound and facilitate adherence.
3. Hydrocolloid dressings with thick edges may "roll up" and adhere to the patient's clothing or bed linen, decreasing the dressing's wear time. Thinner hydrocolloid dressings with tapered edges adhere better to the periwound skin without rolling up.
4. When the dressing is removed, be careful with patient's skin (can tear).

(continued)

Table 8.36 **Wound Dressings** *(continued)*

Types of Hydrocolloid Dressings

- DuoDerm
- 3M's Tegasorb

DuoDerm has been shown to be an effective barrier to Methicillin-resistant Staphylococcus aureus (MRSA), urine, stool, hepatitis B, HIV-1, and *Pseudomonas aeruginosa*[2]; the 3M product can be used on wounds at all stages of healing, from black necrotic tissue to epithelializing wounds.

Alginates

- Alginates are fibrous products derived from brown seaweed that are available in nonwoven sheets and ropes. Alginic acid (main component from alginates) is converted into calcium salts (that are water insoluble) and sodium salts (that are water soluble).
- Alginates can be used for wounds with moderate to heavy drainage. They form a gel when they come in contact with wound fluid. The dressing can absorb up to 20 times its weight in fluid.
- Alginates can be used in both infected and noninfected wounds. They should not be used with dry wounds or wounds with minimal drainage because they could dehydrate the wound, thereby delaying the healing process.

Application of Alginate Dressings

1. The alginate dressing is packed into the wound bed as the primary dressing.
2. A secondary dressing is added to hold the alginate in place and maintain the moist healing environment; petrolatum gauzes or foams can secure the alginate and keep it from drying out. If the wound is infected, the secondary dressing should be nonocclusive (so that it will not harbor bacteria and to allow the wound to be monitored).
3. When the secondary dressing is removed, hydration of the alginate should be assessed. If the alginate has absorbed wound exudates [17,18] (as intended), it will be in a gelled state and easy to remove from the wound. If the alginate is difficult to remove or if fibrous material adheres to the wound base, the wound is drying out. In that situation, the alginate may not be needed to maintain hydration, and another dressing appropriate for a wound with little or no exudates may be used.

Composite Dressings

- Composite dressings contain multiple layers and can be used as primary or secondary dressings. They are appropriate for wounds with minimal to heavy exudates, healthy granulation tissue, necrotic tissue (or moist eschar), or a mixture of granulation and necrotic tissue. Some composite dressing cannot be used on infected wounds (check the manufacturer's instructions).
- Composite dressings should be used cautiously if the patient is dehydrated or has fragile skin. Also, some insurers may not reimburse a facility or provider if a composite dressing is used as secondary dressing with a hydrogel or impregnated gauze.
- Most composite dressings have three layers:
  1. A semiadherent or nonadherent layer: touches and protects the wound from adhering to other material, allows dressing to be removed without disturbing new tissue, and when applying an antibiotic ointment, it will not stick to it.
  2. An absorptive layer: wicks drainage and debris from the wound's surface, prevents skin maceration and bacterial growth, maintains a moist healing environment, and helps to liquefy eschar and necrotic debris (autolytic debridement)

(continued)

INTEGUMENTARY INTERVENTIONS

Table 8.36 Wound Dressings *(continued)*

   3. A bacterial layer: outer layer of the composite dressing that allows moisture vapor to pass from the wound to the air, keeps bacteria and particles out, and maintains a moist environment

- Examples of composite dressings include Alldress, Covaderm Plus, Telfa, Ventex, Viasorb, and Tegaderm with absorbent pad.

Bioengineered Tissue

- Bioengineered tissue,[19,20] also known as tissue-engineered biological dressing, can deliver growth factors and extracellular matrix components to a wound. Bioengineered tissue can be used for burns, chronic venous or pressure ulcers, donor-site and other surgical wounds, blisters, and skin desquamation.

- Bioengineered tissue is controversial[17] in wound care because it does not match a treatment modality to an underlying pathology. Its clinical effect is modest[18,19] and not necessarily justifiable from a cost–benefit perspective.

- Examples of bioengineered tissue products include Dermagraft, Apligraf, and Cultured Epidermal Autograft (Epicel, or a newer version called OrCel).

- Research studies[19] indicate that bioengineered tissue such as Dermagraft and Apligraf have suffered commercial setbacks in recent years, although clinical trials have proved the efficacy of these products. The reasons for the setbacks were high costs and restricted healthcare resources. New products such as OrCel and older ones such as AlloDerm acellular dermal matrix and Integra Bilayer Matrix Wound Dressing are finding niche applications where their clinical utility is high and their cost can be defended.

Table 8.37 Wound Dressings and PTA Implications[2]

Type of Wound Dressing	Benefits	Concerns	PTA Considerations
Absorptive Dressings			
Gauze Woven = cotton yarn or thread Can have a loose weave or a nonwoven texture; can come in rolls to be used as a secondary dressing to secure other bandaging; can be absorptive or nonadherent to be used as a primary or secondary dressing *Examples: ■ 2×2s; 4×4s ■ Abdominal (ABD) pads	■ Aids in mechanical debridement (wet to dry) ■ Used with infected or noninfected wounds ■ Provides cushioning if layered ■ Can add more layers if wound is highly draining	■ Fragile new granulation tissue may be dislodged if the gauze dries to the wound bed	■ New granulation tissue may be removed with bandage removal = delayed healing ■ Monitor for adverse reactions to periwound and wound bed ■ Consult with supervising PT with any unexpected changes in the wound integrity
Nonwoven Gauze ■ Synthetic fibers pressed together	■ More absorbency than loose weave	■ Wound bed desiccation may occur if the gauze sticks to the wound bed	■ Same as above ■ Use a topical agent before applying the gauze or use another type of dressing
Gauze Rolls *Examples: ■ Elastomull ■ Kerlix ■ Kling	■ Helps to secure other gauze coverings like 2×2s or 4×4s in place	■ Tourniquet effect ■ Skin allergies to tape used to secure gauze roll covering	■ Use angles during application ■ Instruct patient to remove and reapply if dressing rolls down or wound is exposed to potential contamination
Gauze—Nonadherent Dressings ■ Less likely to stick to wound bed *Examples: ■ Telfa pads	■ Less likely to stick to the wound bed	■ Not very absorptive	■ Use on superficial, nondraining wound types ■ May cause maceration if wound is draining

(continued)

(continued)

Table 8.37 Wound Dressings and PTA Implications

Type of Wound Dressing	Benefits	Concerns	PTA Considerations
<u>Impregnated Gauzes</u> (petroleum, bismuth, or zinc) *Examples:* ■ Adaptic (petroleum) ■ Aquaphor (petroleum) ■ Xeroform (bismuth and petroleum)	■ ↑ occlusiveness of secondary dressing ■ ↓ potential of wound bed damage upon removal of dressings	■ Are not absorptive ■ If highly impregnated, may alter normal wound healing	■ Use with a secondary dressing ■ Monitor for maceration or abnormal tissue healing timelines
Moisture-Retentive Dressings			
<u>Semipermeable Dressings</u> Flexible, thin sheets of transparent polyurethane with adhesive backing *Examples:* ■ BIOCLUSIVE ■ Polyskin ■ Tegaderm	■ Retains moisture ■ ↑autolytic debridement ■ ↓ friction ■ Visualization of wound beds ■ Waterproof ■ Can be left on for 5–7 days ■ Waterproof so patients can shower or be used to cover wounds prior to ultrasound treatment ■ Covers IV catheters Indicated for: ■ Superficial wounds ■ Donor graft sites ■ Red granular or yellow slough covered wounds with minimal drainage	■ Periwound trauma from adhesive ■ Not indicated for significantly draining wounds ■ Not indicated for infected wounds ■ Wrinkles in the dressing may become a portal for contamination or potential infection	■ Not indicated for frail skin ■ Need 1–2-inch border of intact skin around the wound borders to apply the adhesive dressing ■ Inspect periwound for maceration or trauma from adhesive and bandage removal ■ Check for adverse adhesive allergic reactions to intact skin ■ Larger sized dressings may be difficult to apply ■ Change dressing as soon as wrinkles are noted to deter contamination or infection

Table 8.37 Wound Dressings and PTA Implications *(continued)*

Type of Wound Dressing	Benefits	Concerns	PTA Considerations
Hydrogels: Water or glycerin-based dressings that come in sheets, impregnated gauzes (see above) or amorphous gels *Examples:* ■ AQUASORB (sheet) ■ Elasto-Gel (sheet) ■ Carrysyn (amorphous gel) ■ Carrington gel (amorphous gel) ■ SAF-GEL (amorphous gel)	■ Retains moisture ■ ↑ autolytic debridement ■ ↓ pressure ■ Non-adherent Indicated for: ■ Minimal or moderately draining wounds ■ Superficial wounds ■ Partial thickness wounds ■ Pressure injuries ■ Graft donor sites ■ Thermal burns ■ Radiation burns ■ As padding between casts/splints to ↓ shearing/pressure Amorphous gel indications: ■ Coupling agent for ultrasound ■ Soften eschar ■ Provide moisture to dry wounds	■ Not to be used on wounds with significant exudate ■ Not appropriate for bleeding wounds ■ Not appropriate for infected wounds	■ A skin sealant must be used to protect the periwound from maceration ■ Need a secondary dressing to cover the hydrophilic sheet or amorphous gel ■ Watch wound bed for signs of dehydration
Semipermeable Foams Polyurethane foam with a hydrophilic property inside the dressing and hydrophobic outside *Examples:* ■ Allyyen ■ Curafoam ■ Epilock ■ Hydrasorb	■ Moisture retentive ■ Promotes autolytic debridement ■ Thickness varies and may provide cushioning ■ May provide thermal insulation ■ Easy application and removal ■ Adherent and non-adherent types available	■ Unless changed daily, contraindicated for infected wounds ■ Periwound trauma upon removal if adherent type is used ■ Rolling in areas prone to friction	■ Not to be used with dry wound types (arterial ulcers, eschar) ■ Use non-adherent foams with frail skin types ■ Secondary dressing required if non-adherent option is chosen ■ Change daily if wound is infected

(continued)

(continued)

Table 8.37 Wound Dressings and PTA Implications

Type of Wound Dressing	Benefits	Concerns	PTA Considerations
	Indicated for: ■ Moderate to heavy exudate ■ Donor sites ■ Diabetic ulcers ■ Venous insufficiency ulcers ■ Pressure injuries ■ Ostomy sites ■ Minor burns		■ Monitor integrity of periwound if adherent type is used especially in frail skin situations ■ Use skin sealants as barriers for periwound protection
Hydrocolloids: Contain gelatin, pectin, methyl carbon cellulose colloid particles (which are hydrophilic) making this dressing very absorptive *Examples: ■ Cutinova ■ Duoderm (regular, extra thin, controlled gel formula [CGF]) ■ Tegaderm (regular, thin)	■ Moisture retentive ■ Absorbs exudate slowly turning into a gel-like mass ■ Promotes autolytic debridement ■ Moderate absorption ■ Provides thermal insulation ■ Waterproof ■ Beveled edges may discourage edge rolling with friction prone areas Indications: ■ Pressure injuries ■ Burns ■ Venous insufficiency ulcers	■ Periwound trauma upon removal ■ May roll in areas prone to friction ■ Occlusiveness = higher rates of anaerobic infection ■ Occlusiveness = increased risk of silent infections with immunocompromised patients ■ Hypergranulation rates are increased with hydrocolloid use	■ Contraindicated for infected wounds ■ Discontinue use at the first sign of hypergranulation to avoid delayed healing ■ Do not use on dry wounds, bleeding wounds, third-degree burns ■ Do not use on wounds where tendons or fascial tissue is exposed, as it will lead to tissue desiccation ■ Should be secured to a 1-2-inch border of intact skin ■ Use a skin sealant as a barrier to protect periwound from trauma/maceration

Table 8.37 Wound Dressings and PTA Implications *(continued)*

Type of Wound Dressing	Benefits	Concerns	PTA Considerations
<u>Alginates</u> Alginic acid extracts from certain types of brown seaweed that are converted into calcium salts. *Examples: ■ Curasorb ■ Maxorb	■ Moisture retentive ■ Highly absorptive ■ No-adherent ■ Biocompatible Indications: ■ Use with partial-full thickness draining wounds ■ Venous insufficiency ulcers, ■ Diabetic ulcers (neuropathic and/or pressure) ■ Burns ■ Infected wounds	■ Tissue desiccation may occur when used over an exposed tendon, capsule, or bone ■ Periwound trauma	■ Requires secondary dressings ■ Third-degree burns are contraindicated ■ Do not use over highly collagenous structures such as exposed tendon, capsule, and bone ■ Change dressings daily with infected wounds ■ Use alginate swabs over regular cotton tipped swabs when assessing for undermining, tunneling, or wound depth measuring to deter the inflammatory response that may result from wisps being left in the wound bed during the probing process
<u>Composite Dressings</u> Multilayer dressings (most have three layers) that can be used as primary OR secondary dressings. Inner-most layer closest to the wound/skin is non-adherent, protecting granulation tissue upon removal, usually Telfa-like material.	■ Moisture retentive ■ Highly absorptive Indications: ■ Minimal to heavily draining wounds ■ Healthy granulation wounds ■ Mix of necrotic and granular tissue type wounds	■ Prepackaged may mean the clinician cannot customize the dressings to meet the needs of the patient or wound type ■ Cost and storage of these products may prove to be a fiscal concern in some instances	■ Less flexibility for indications for use because of being prepackaged with the three layers

(continued)

Table 8.37 Wound Dressings and PTA Implications *(continued)*

Type of Wound Dressing	Benefits	Concerns	PTA Considerations
Middle layer is moisture absorbing and wicks away excessive moisture from wound edges to prevent maceration. It is usually a hydrogel, semipermeable foam, hydrocolloid, or alginate. Outermost layer serves as a bacterial barrier to keep bacteria out while maintaining a moist environment and creating a moisture vapor to pass from the wound to the air. It is usually a semipermeable film *Examples: ▪ Alldress ▪ Covaderm Plus ▪ Telfa ▪ Tegaderm with absorbent pad ▪ Viasorb			
Other Types of Dressings			
Skin Sealants/Moisture Barriers Provide a protective layer over the skin to deter topical agents, water exposure, or bodily fluids from causing skin breakdown *Examples: ▪ Aloe Vesta ▪ Skin Prep ▪ Sensicare	▪ Moisture barrier ▪ Provides wicking of moisture away from wound Indications: ▪ Prevention of skin breakdown associated with incontinence ▪ Protect periwound when using dressings that will not be changed daily	▪ Creams usually cannot be used with adhesive dressings as the dressing will not stick	▪ Use with moisture-retentive dressings to protect periwound ▪ Use on areas susceptible to maceration ▪ Use on perineum to deter skin breakdown ▪ Observe for any signs of allergic reactions on the skin

Table 8.37 Wound Dressings and PTA Implications

(continued)

Type of Wound Dressing	Benefits	Concerns	PTA Considerations
Bioengineered Tissue/Biologic Dressings Derived from natural tissues that are purported to promote the autolytic debridement process and facilitate granulation in the wound bed *Examples ■ Apligraf ■ Dermagraft ■ Epicel	■ Collagen can adhere to the wound bed, but not the periwound Indications: ■ Can be used on infected and noninfected wounds ■ Burns ■ Chronic venous ulcers ■ Chronic pressure ulcers ■ Donor-sites ■ Blisters ■ Skin desquamation	■ Cost-benefit analysis may dictate use of this as a modality for wound healing [16-18] ■ Contraindicated for patients sensitive to bovine products ■ Contraindicated for patients sensitive to collagen products	■ PTA would need to have the skill set and training to work with this modality, as it falls into a highly specialized area of wound care
Growth Factors[2] Growth promoting materials that are used to increase proliferation of cellular activity for healing *Examples: Regranex (Becaplermin) Oasis (porcine-derived small intestine submucosa)	■ Stimulates migration of inflammatory cells and fibroblasts to wound bed ■ Enhances collagen deposition ■ Promotes granulation tissue formation Indications: ■ Infected/noninfected wounds ■ Diabetic foot ulcers not extending through subcutaneous regions ■ Partial thickness venous insufficiency ulcers ■ Pressure ulcers ■ Diabetic ulcers ■ Surgical debridement ■ Traumatic wounds	■ Contraindicated for patients' sensitive to porcine products ■ Costly if used with delayed healing wounds	■ If significant drainage is present or wound is infected, Oasis must be fenestrated ■ Regranex has showed promise when used in conjunction with pressure relief, debridement and standard wound care

* These examples of dressings and products that are commonly used in the treatment of wounds are a non-exhaustive list, and this author has no affiliation or financial interest in the endorsement of these products.

INTEGUMENTARY INTERVENTIONS

Table 8.38 Common Topical Agents Used in Wound Management[2]

Topical Agent	Purpose/Benefits	Limitations	PTA Considerations
Antibacterial ■ Bacitracin	■ Sulfa-free alternative ■ Gram-negative and gram-positive *cocci* and *bacilli* Indications: ■ Superficial and partial-thickness wounds	■ Delayed hypersensitivity may develop	■ Wound bed may be traumatized if secondary bandaging sticks to wound bed ■ Use a Telfa pad before applying gauze to secure the bandaging ■ Monitor for any adverse reactions to medication
Gentamicin sulfate (Garamycin)	■ Gram-negative bacteria, *Streptococci* and *Staphylococci* Indications: ■ Superficial and partial-thickness wounds	■ Resistance to medication is common ■ Sulfa allergies ■ Ototoxicity ■ Nephrotoxicity	■ Report signs and symptoms of ototoxicity or nephrotoxicity to the supervising PT immediately ■ Ototoxicity may affect balance ■ Monitor for any adverse reactions to medication
Mafenide acetate (Sulfamylon)	■ Gram-negative and gram-positive including *Pseudomonas aeruginosa* Indications: ■ Burn wounds ■ Penetrates wound eschar	■ Potential development of fungal overgrowth ■ Sulfa allergies ■ Rash, itching, hives ■ Metabolic acidosis may develop ■ May result in compromised respiratory function ■ May inhibit epithelization ■ May be more painful than sulfadiazine	■ Monitor patient for respiratory compromise ■ May be used with or without occlusive dressings ■ Penetrates eschar nicely ■ Caution with secondary dressing removal to deter traumatization ■ Monitor for any adverse reactions to medication
Silver sulfadiazine (Silvadene, SSD cream, Thermazene)	■ Gram-negative bacteria including *E. coli, Enterobacter, Klebsiella*; and gram-positive bacteria *S. aureus* and *Candida albicans* Indications: ■ Burns ■ Wounds	■ Sulfa allergies ■ May develop a rash ■ Potential for fungal growth ■ May inhibit epithelization	■ Does not penetrate eschar ■ Film residue left in wound bed must be removed with each dressing change ■ Caution with secondary dressing removal to deter traumatization ■ Monitor for any adverse reactions to medication

Table 8.38 Wound Dressings and PTA Implications *(continued)*

Topical Agent	Purpose/Benefits	Limitations	PTA Considerations
■ Mupirocin (Bactroban)	■ Gram-negative and gram-positive organisms Indications: ■ MRSA	■ Burning and stinging may result	■ Caution with secondary dressing removal to deter traumatization ■ Monitor for any adverse reactions to medication
■ Neomycin sulfate	■ Gram-negative and gram-positive bacteria	■ Sulfa allergies ■ May develop a rash ■ Ototoxicity ■ Nephrotoxicity	■ Report signs and symptoms of ototoxicity or nephrotoxicity to the supervising PT immediately ■ Ototoxicity may affect balance ■ Caution with secondary dressing removal to deter traumatization ■ Monitor for any adverse reactions
■ Triple Antibiotic (Neosporin) *Contains neomycin, Bacitracin, and polymyxin B sulfate	■ May enhance epithelization ■ Broader spectrum coverage against bacteria than each agent individually Indications: ■ Superficial and partial-thickness wounds ■ Facial wounds	■ Sulfa allergies	■ May be open to air or cover with a secondary dressing ■ Wound bed trauma may result if secondary dressing sticks to wound bed ■ Use Telfa pad before gauze application to avoid wound bed trauma ■ Monitor for any adverse reactions
<u>Antifungals</u> ■ Nystatin (Mycostatin)	■ Effective against *candida* Indications: ■ Yeast infections	■ Resistance is possible	■ Monitor for any adverse reactions
■ Miconazole	■ May be used intravenously for severe infections Indications: ■ Tinea	■ Pruritus may be an adverse reaction	■ Monitor for any adverse reactions

(continued)

Table 8.38 Common Topical Agents Used in Wound Management

Topical Agent	Purpose/Benefits	Limitations	PTA Considerations
■ Oxiconazole nitrate (Oxistat)	■ Combats fungal infections on intact skin and nails Indications: ■ Tinea	■ Adverse reactions may include pruritus, burning, dermatitis, maceration	■ Monitor for any adverse reactions
<u>Antiseptics</u> ■ Povidone-iodine (Betadine)	■ Gram-positive and gram-negative bacteria Indications: ■ Pre-surgical scrub on intact skin	■ Adverse reactions may include: sensitization, systemic toxicity with prolonged use on large surfaces, delayed epithelialization	■ Monitor for any adverse reactions

(continued)

For all wound care, the PTA must use proper hand sanitation techniques and sterile fields as warranted by wound type.

Patient Safety Precautions During Wound Interventions

Table 8.39 **Precautions in Wound Interventions**

- Monitor the patient's vital signs at all times. Some facilities may use ankle brachial index (ABI) monitoring, which measures patient's blood pressure (BP) at two sites (the ankle and the brachial artery) at rest and after 5 minutes of treadmill walk; the ABI is calculated by then dividing the highest BP at the ankle by the highest BP at the brachial artery. The normal resting ABI = 1 or 1.1 (the BP at the ankle is the same or greater than the BP at brachial artery; there is no narrowing or blockage of blood flow). A resting ABI of less than 1 is abnormal; an ABI of less than 0.95 indicates narrowing of one or more blood vessels in the legs. Pain in the leg, foot, or buttock during exercises and an ABI of less than 0.8 indicates intermittent claudication with exercise or activity. Compression should not be used with ABI less than 0.5. With an ABI of less than 0.4, the patient exhibits symptoms of claudication at rest. With an ABI of 0.25 or less, severe peripheral artery disease (PAD) is present.

- During wound interventions, be aware of signs and symptoms of infection, and immediately inform the PT (and the nursing staff when necessary) if they are observed. Infection signs and symptoms include (1) an increase or decrease in BP; (2) fever; (3) a decrease in the red blood cell count; (4) an increase in the white blood cell count; and (5) wound development signs such as the appearance and development of odor (or worsening of odor).

- Be aware of excessive wound bleeding that will not coagulate (especially if debridement is included in interventions).

Pressure Ulcers and Interventions

Table 8.40 **Pressure Ulcers and Interventions**

Pressure ulcers: ulcers located at areas of tissue compression and inadequate perfusion.

- Pressure ulcers commonly occur in patients who are bed or chair bound, especially members of the following populations:
  1. Patients with sensory and mobility impairments (such as spinal cord injury, stroke, or coma)
  2. Patients (clients) who are malnourished
  3. Patients with peripheral vascular disease
  4. Older patients who are hospitalized
  5. Nursing home residents
  6. Patients (clients) who are incontinent

- The most common sites of skin breakdown where pressure sores can occur are the bony prominences (such as elbows, scapulae, sacrum, ischial tuberosities, malleoli, greater trochanter, and heels).

- The combination of pressure shearing forces, friction, and moisture may lead to tissue injury and occasionally necrosis.

- The pressure ulcer can progress rapidly from a red patch of skin to erosion into the subcutaneous tissues and extension to muscle or bone.

- Deep ulcers may become infected with bacteria and develop gangrene.

(continued)

INTEGUMENTARY INTERVENTIONS

Table 8.40 Pressure Ulcers and Interventions   *(continued)*

Prevention of Pressure Ulcers

The most important principle of therapy for pressure ulcers is prevention. Assessment of risk in aforementioned populations should be ongoing. Prevention includes the following measures:

1. Regular skin inspection
2. Frequent turning of immobile patients (considering potential areas of breakdown)
3. Application of pressure-relieving devices (PRDs), such as skin protectors to bony body parts, and use of specialized air–fluid beds, waterbeds, or beds with polystyrene beads
4. Cleansing and drying the skin
5. Application of skin lubricants and emollients
6. Maintaining clean, dry linen and clothing
7. Elimination of mechanical forces
8. Encouragement of early ambulation and appropriate use of assistive devices
9. Encouragement of ROM exercises

Interventions for Pressure Ulcers

1. Use interventions that produce minimal skin friction. When the skin becomes ischemic, the reddened areas of the skin should never be massaged because such treatment can damage ischemic deep layers of tissue. Instead, the skin should be thoroughly cleansed, rinsed, and dried, and emollients should be gently applied by minimizing force and friction especially over bony prominences.
2. Patients who are able to sit in a chair should be placed on a low-pressure cushion and helped to shift their weight every 15 minutes. Sitting time should be limited to less than 2 hours to reduce pressure over the ischial tuberosities.
3. Patients who are not able to position themselves need to be repositioned every 1–2 hours to prevent tissue hypoxia (from compression).
4. A turning schedule is necessary.
5. A turning sheet or a pad can be used to turn patients (using minimal skin friction).
6. The head of the bed should not be elevated higher than 30° (except for short periods of time) to reduce shearing forces on the skin and subcutaneous tissues overlying the sacrum.
7. Early ambulation and ROM exercises should be encouraged as well as consumption of high-protein, nutritious meals.
8. Doughnut-type cushions should not be used because they decrease blood flow to tissues resting in the center of the doughnut.
9. When pressure ulcers occur, they need to be cleansed and debrided depending on the institution's protocol (or prescription) and the PT's plan of care.

Other Integumentary Interventions for Lymphedema, Edema, and Wounds

Table 8.41 Other Lymphedema, Edema, and Wound Interventions

Manual Lymphatic Drainage[1]

Manual lymphatic drainage (MLD) is a specialized manual therapy technique that affects primarily the superficial lymphatic circulation. The benefits of MLD are improvement of lymph transport capacity, redirection of lymph flow toward collateral vessels, increased frequency of lymphangion contractions, anastomoses, and mobilization of excess lymph fluid (which might otherwise overwhelm a body is a segment)

(continued)

Table 8.41 Other Lymphedema, Edema, and Wound Interventions *(continued)*

MLD requires specialized education to be able to perform it. MLD should not be used on edema that is related to cardiac or pulmonary dysfunction.

External Compression Pump

An external compression pump (ECP) is indicated for patients who have congenital lymphedema or acquired lymphatic dysfunctions (to prevent pain and infection, decrease possibility of skin breakdown, and increase function).

Other Indications for ECP

- Chronic edema in patients with decreased mobility: creates a pumping effect in patients who have decreased muscle pump capability due to paralysis or weakness
- Venous stasis wounds: can remove edema and prevent venous pooling, allowing the wound to heal
- Residual limb shrinkage: for amputations, to prepare them for prosthetic fitting
- Prevention of thrombophlebitis, tissue healing, and scar management for wounds and burns

Types of ECP[9]

- Intermittent pneumatic compression (IPC) unit (air pump)
- IPC units with additional features (such as the Wright linear pump, the Huntleigh sequential system, the NormaTec pneumatic compression pump,)
- Small, portable units for the home are available for both IPC and compression with cold (Aircast Cryo Cuff unit for ankle, foot, knee, hand, wrist, and elbow injury intervention since it contains a cooling unit)

Contraindications and Precautions to ECP[9]

- Pulmonary edema
- CHF
- Recent or acute DVT
- Obstructed venous or lymphatic vessels
- Unstable fracture
- Acute local infection
- Severe peripheral arterial occlusive disease
- Arterial revascularization
- Significant hypoproteinemia
- Impaired sensation / mentation (precaution)
- Uncontrolled hypertension (HTN) (precaution)
- Cancer (generally considered a precaution, but may be contraindicated in some cases)

ECP Intervention Method Precautions[9]

- Pressure on an upper extremity should not exceed 40–60 mm Hg.
- Pressure on a lower extremity should not exceed 40–80 mm Hg.
- Pressure lower than 30 mm Hg is not recommended.
  - For post-mastectomy lymphedema: pressure should be 30–60 mm Hg; one to two 3-hour treatments per day; 80–100 seconds on and 25–35 seconds off.
- For peripheral edema and venous stasis ulceration: pressure should be 85 mm Hg; one 2.5-hour treatment, three times per week; 80–100 seconds on and 30 seconds off.

(continued)

Table 8.41 Other Lymphedema, Edema, and Wound Interventions *(continued)*

- For lower-extremity edema: pressure should be 40–80 mm Hg; one or two 3-hour treatments per day; 80–100 seconds on and 25–35 seconds off.

Other Lymphedema/Wounds Interventions

- Extremity elevation: to control mild and acute swelling; may be a precursor to, or in conjunction with, a compression pump
- Unna's boot: application of zinc paste–impregnated gauze; good for venous wounds
- Four-layer bandage system (using Profore): for leg ulcers closure; can be left in place for a week; manufacturer claims that it provides 40 mm Hg of pressure at the ankle
- Long stretch and short stretch bandages: for edema control and for lymphedema
- Lymphedema bandaging: highly specialized form of bandaging using multiple layers of unique padding materials and short stretch bandages; the PT/PTA needs to learn different techniques for different body areas.
- Compression garments: garments used to assist venous flow; used for arterial wounds, venous wounds, neuropathic ulcers, lymphedema, and edema; also used for burns and surgical scars; contraindicated for DVT, acute local infection, CHF, acute dermatitis, and cor pulmonale; provide support to venous circulation; prevent re-accumulation of fluid in the lymphedema; should not be used to remove excess fluids from an extremity; should be customized to each individual.

Prevention Interventions

- Positioning: to prevent or support pressure ulcers, wounds, edema, lymphedema, and vascular disorders.
- PRDs: check websites for information and experts on PRDs.
- Exercises: PT/PTA to make a customized exercise prescription for the patient depending on the patient's needs and medical status; recommended exercises/activities include aquatic exercises and ambulation activities.
- Scar management: can use compression garments; stretching exercises; orthotics; positioning; silicone gel sheets; topical oils, creams, and ointments; and specific massage techniques.
- See Appendix D for additional education for patients with lymphedema.

Orthotics

- Resting splints; dynamic splints; total contact cast and posterior walking splints for neuropathic ulcers on plantar surface of foot
- Neuropathic walker made from a removable customized ankle foot orthosis
- Cast shoes or postoperative shoes for wound offloading.
- Extra-depth shoes with room for the toes and a deep sole for shock absorption
- For distal aspects of the foot, wedge shoes (e.g., OrthoWedge)

Electrotherapeutic Modalities

- High-voltage pulsed current (HVPC): used at frequency of 100 pps for 60 minutes, 5 days/week, promotes healing of dermal ulcers. This method involves the application of one electrode over the wound using a saline-moistened gauze interface and the other electrode some distance from the wound. For debridement or epithelialization, use the positive electrode; for all other indications, use the negative electrode.
- Ultrasound (US): pulsed 2 milliseconds on and 8 milliseconds off at a frequency of 1 or 3 MHz depending on the tissue depth, with intensity of 0.5 watt/cm^2 (best for dermal tissue).

Immunocompromised Patients and Infection Control

Table 8.42 Immunocompromised Patients and Infection Control

■ Patients with burns and wounds may have a compromised immune system. The altered immune system can affect the endogenous normal flora, gastrointestinal system, genitourinary system, respiratory system, mucous membrane function, and skin breakdown. Immunocompromised patients vary in their susceptibility to nosocomial infections, depending on the severity and duration of their immunosuppression. They are at increased risk for bacterial, fungal, parasitic, and viral infections from both endogenous and exogenous sources.

■ PTs/PTAs should use standard precautions for all patients and transmission-based precautions for specified patients to reduce the acquisition by these patients of institutionally acquired bacteria from other patients and environments.

■ For Centers for Disease Control and Prevention standard precautions and transmission-based precautions, see Part 2.

■ Infection control strategies during wound/burn interventions:

1. Use proper hand-washing techniques.
2. Use standard precautions.
3. Use clean and sterile techniques when handling wounds or burns.
4. Use masks for respiratory diseases.
5. Sterilize and disinfect equipment used in wound/burn interventions.
6. Maintain the patient's (client's) skin integrity.
7. Remember the modes of transmission of infection: direct transmission (through hands and broken skin), indirect transmission (through tubes, needles, dressings, catheters, and equipment), droplet transmission (cough or sneeze), and vehicle transmission (blood).

■ Infectious agents: exogenous and endogenous bacteria, fungi, and viruses.

■ Opportunistic agents: *Pseudomonas aeruginosa* (bacterial), tuberculosis, *Pneumocystis carinii* pneumonia (protozoan), cytomegalovirus (viral), *Candida albicans* (fungal).

Integumentary Interventions

APTA's Guide to Physical Therapist Practice: APTA's Integumentary Intervention Patterns 7A-7E

Table 8.43 Therapeutic Exercises[21]

1. Strength, power, and endurance training, standardized, programmatic, complementary exercise approaches for task-specific performance training
2. Flexibility exercises: muscle lengthening, range of motion, and stretching to prevent contractures
3. Balance, coordination, and agility training, important with foot and LE dysfunction
4. Body mechanics and postural stabilization: body mechanics training, posture awareness training, postural control training, and postural stabilization activities
5. Gait and locomotion training: developmental activities training; gait training; implement and device training; perceptual training; wheelchair training as applicable
6. Aerobic capacity and endurance conditioning and reconditioning: walking and wheelchair propulsion programs, aquatic programs, and gait and locomotor training

Table 8.44 Functional Training in Self-Care and in Domestic, Education, Work, Community, Social, and Civic Life[21]

1. ADL training: bathing, bed mobility and transfer training, developmental activities, dressing, eating, grooming, and toileting
2. IADL training: caring for dependents, home maintenance, household chores, shopping, structured play for infants and children, and yard work
3. Injury prevention or reduction: injury prevention education related to self-care and home management skills with ADLs and IADLs, with use of devices and equipment related to barrier modification or accommodation, and safety awareness training during work, social, community, or civic integration or reintegration
4. IADL training: community service training involving instruments, school and play activities, training including tools and instruments, and work training with tools
5. Injury prevention or reduction: injury prevention education during work at job, school, play, community, and leisure integration or reintegration; injury prevention or reduction with use of devices and equipment; safety awareness training during work at job, school, play, community, and leisure integration and reintegration

Table 8.45 Assistive Technology: Prescription, Application, and (as Appropriate) Fabrication or Modification of Devices and Equipment[21]

1. Adaptive devices: environmental controls, raised toilet seats, seating systems, and hospital beds
2. Assistive devices: canes, crutches, long-handled reachers, power devices, static and dynamic splints, walkers, and wheelchairs
3. Orthotic devices: braces, shoe inserts, and splints
4. Prosthetic devices: lower-extremity and upper-extremity prostheses
5. Protective devices: braces, cushions, and protective taping
6. Supportive devices: compression garments, corsets, elastic wraps, neck collars, serial casts, slings, and supportive taping

Table 8.46 **Manual Therapy Techniques (Excludes Joint Mobilization)**[21]

1. Massage (such as connective tissue massage and therapeutic massage)
2. Soft-tissue mobilization
3. Manual lymphatic drainage

Table 8.47 **Modalities**[21]

Biophysical Agents

- Cryotherapy: cold pack, ice massage
- Hydrotherapy: pools, whirlpool tanks, and pulsatile lavage
- Ultrasound
- Light agents: laser and ultraviolet
- Negative pressure wound therapy
- Hyperbaric oxygen
- Compression therapies: compression bandaging, taping, contact casting, compression garments, total contact casting, and vasopneumatic compression devices
- Electrical muscle stimulation (EMS), transcutaneous electrical nerve stimulation (TENS), and HVPC

Table 8.48 **Patient/Client-Related Instruction**[21]

- Instruction, education, and training of patients/clients and caregivers regarding the current condition: pathology; pathophysiology—disease, disorder, or condition; impairments, functional limitations, or disabilities
- Prevention strategies
- Risk factors: for pathology; pathophysiology—disease, disorder, or condition; impairments, functional limitations, or disabilities
- Enhancement of performance
- Health, wellness, and fitness

Other Integumentary Intervention Patterns (Not Related to Wounds, Burns, and Ulcerations)

Table 8.49 **Other Integumentary Intervention Patterns for Integumentary Conditions***

Dermatitis Intervention Patterns

- Patient education about the disorder/disease awareness, healthy lifestyle, and risk reduction.
- Patient education on skin care (irritants).
- Patient education on exacerbating factors (precautions should be applied to physical therapy modalities and topical agents containing alcohol that may exacerbate the condition).
- The PTA should monitor patient's skin before and after application of interventions. The PTA should inform the supervising PT if the patient has an adverse reaction to any intervention.

(continued)

INTEGUMENTARY INTERVENTIONS

Table 8.49 Other Integumentary Intervention Patterns for Integumentary Conditions *(continued)*

Cellulitis Intervention Patterns

- Wound care for open wounds
- Muscle-setting exercises
- Positioning

Herpes I (Herpes Simplex), Herpes II, and Herpes Zoster (Shingles) Intervention Patterns

- Relaxation exercises and techniques.
- Ultrasound and heat modalities are contraindicated because of the possibility of increasing symptoms.
- Standard precautions should be followed with therapists who have not had chickenpox (by using extra caution).

Scleroderma (Systemic Sclerosis) Intervention Patterns

- ROM and stretching exercises: to increase skin and joint flexibility and blood flow, to prevent contractures
- Splints and orthotics: for joint contracture and joint protection
- BP monitoring
- Precautions about cryotherapy (because of increased sensitivity to cold), cuff weights (which can increase stress on the joints), and the patient's anxiety (caused by pain)

Psoriasis Intervention Patterns

- Whirlpool baths (with Aveeno or Balnetar bath oil)
- ROM exercises to affected extremities
- Mobility training
- Ultraviolet light therapy (administered by the PT; PTA to check state's practice act)

Lupus Erythematosus Intervention Patterns

- Gradual return of function (after acute exacerbation).
- Patient education about activity pacing.
- Patient education about relaxation exercises and techniques.
- Patient education about the disease, healthy lifestyle, and coping ability.
- Precautions should be applied in the case of side effects of corticosteroid medications (which the patient may be taking), edema, hypertension, weight gain, acne, bruising, increased susceptibility to infection, osteoporosis, diabetes, gastric irritation, low potassium, purplish stretch marks, myopathy, and tendon rupture.

Polymyositis Intervention Patterns

- Heat.
- Whirlpool.
- Gentle massage.
- Graded exercises.
- Aquatic therapy.
- When the patient is in bed and cannot move, he or she needs positioning and splinting to prevent pressure ulcers and contractures. Precautions should be applied regarding not giving the patient too much exercise, and the side effects of corticosteroids.

* The precise interventions depend on the PT's specific recommendations in the plan of care.

Wound Documentation

Wound Documentation Elements[2]

Table 8.50 Wound Documentation Elements and Reimbursement Pearls

Wound Documentation Elements

- **Take wound measurements (in centimeters).** Trace the wound edges on a clear acetate film (plastic sheet) using a fine-point, indelible-ink marker. Measure the length and width of the wound. Depth can be measured by placing a cotton swab into the base of the wound (placed in the wound, withdrawn, and measured with a tape measure). Depth can also be measured by filling a syringe with saline solution, injecting the solution into the wound cavity until filled, and subtracting the volume of liquid remaining in the syringe from the original amount.

- **The wound surface area** can be determined by multiplying the greatest length and width of the wound. If there is access to computer and software, the tracing can be digitized and area computed electronically (very accurate). Measurements (in centimeters) can also be described as linear by the clock position (e.g., 12:00 to 6:00 and 3:00 to 9:00). Photographic assessments can be used in addition to measurements.

- **Describe wound drainage:** nondraining or draining (amount—minimal, moderate, maximum; strike-through of exudates; saturation of dressing; amount of time dressing was in place).

- **Describe types of drainage** (color, viscosity, and amount): sanguineous (bloody), serous (clear), serosanguineous (clear with blood), purulence versus necrotic debris, and liquefied eschar.

- **Describe wound odor:** foul, mild, typical of dressing type, sweet, and none.

- **Describe the wound characteristics:** presence of nonviable tissue (slough or eschar), granulation (or hypergranulation), granulation buds, neoepithelium, skin buds, skin graft, undermining (measured around the area in centimeters, such as 1.2 centimeter at 4:00), tunneling or tracts (depth and direction, such as 5.8 centimeters at 7:00), exposed tendon muscle or bone, and exposed foreign body (fixators, prosthesis, screws, and stitches).

- **Describe wound healing for skin changes:** black (necrotic), pink (sufficient vascular supply), and hard or callus formation (requires debridement).

- **Describe the surrounding tissues:** intact healthy skin; color and pigmentation; scratches, tape injury, or rash; excoriated skin; feel and texture of the skin; neoepithelium; and maceration of the skin.

- **Take edema circumferential measurements.** Measure above and below the wound site using a tape measure; areas where measurements were taken need to be described.

- **Describe the patient's pulses** (taken by palpation or by Doppler ultrasound). Pulses that are commonly assessed include the dorsalis pedis and posterior tibialis.

- **Document progress** in relation to wound size, granulation, and wound drainage.

Reimbursement Pearls[2]

Documentation must reflect the need for continued treatment based on medical necessity. The following bullet points are items that need to be considered when it comes to wound care documentation.

- Follow the plan of care and review goals weekly to provide a clinical picture of improvement.
- Links must be made between wound healing and functional improvement to justify continued medical necessity for wound care in the assessment section of the daily notes.
- Objective measurements may support wound healing necessity.

Examples

Figure of 8 assessment of ankle girth has decreased from 58 centimeters to 55 centimeters resulting in increased right ankle ROM from neutral to 15 degrees dorsiflexion allowing for normalization of heel strike at initial contact phase of gait cycle.

OR

Increased scar pliability over the distal incision status post right TKA has resulted in AROM improvement from 90 degrees to 105 degrees knee flexion.

- Anatomical references should be made without the use of comparison to everyday objects (i.e., the size of a penny).
- Direct wound measurements should be documented in length × width × depth and compared to previous measurements.
- Types of dressings and topical agents; use of brand names is acceptable (see **Table 8.37** and **Table 8.38**).
- Photographic images must be accompanied by some type of encryption process for HIPAA compliance with digital transference of medical information.
- Photographic images must also have some type of measurement tool in the picture to confirm the wound size L × W × D (i.e., long-tipped cotton swab next to a tape measure to illustrate depth of wound).
- Signed releases for photographic transmission of information may need to be obtained per facility policy.
- Consult with the supervising PT to amend goals when appropriate and/or if new or unusual responses are observed a re-evaluation or change in plan of care may be warranted.

References

1. O'Sullivan SB, Schmitz TJ, Fulk GD. *Physical Rehabilitation*. 6th ed. Philadelphia, PA: F.A. Davis Company; 2014.
2. Myers BA. *Wound Management Principles and Practice*. 3rd ed. Upper Saddle River, NJ: Pearson Education; 2011.
3. The National Pressure Injury Advisory Panel–NPIAP. Educational and clinical resources. NPIAP pressure injury stages. https://npiap.com/page/PressureInjuryStages. Updated August 2016. Accessed June 14, 2021.
4. Goodman CC, Fuller KS. *Pathology for the Physical Therapist Assistant*. 2nd ed. St. Louis, MO. Elsevier; 2017.
5. Fruth, SJ. *Fundamentals of the Physical Therapy Examination*. Enhanced ed. Burlington, MA: Jones & Bartlett Learning; 2014.
6. Skin Cancer Foundation. Melanoma warning signs. https://www.skincancer.org/skin-cancer-information/melanoma/melanoma-warning-signs-and-images/#abcde. Updated January 2021. Accessed June 15, 2021.
7. National Institutes of Diabetes and Digestive and Kidney Diseases. Diabetes and foot problems. https://www.niddk.nih.gov/health-information/diabetes/overview/preventing-problems/foot-problems Accessed June 17, 2021.
8. McCulloch J. The integumentary system: Repair and management: An overview. apta.org. http://learningcenter.apta.org/Student/MyCourses.aspx?Type=Course&Mode=completed Updated July 2016. Accessed August 2016.
9. Cameron M. *Physical Agents in Rehabilitation: An Evidence Based Approach to Practice*. 5th ed. St. Louis, MO: Elsevier; 2018.
10. Riley KN, Herman IM.Collagenase promotes the cellular responses to injury and wound healing in vivo. *Journal of Burns and Wounds*. 2005;4:e8.
11. Harvey C.Wound healing. Orthop *Nursing*. 2005;2:24–25.
12. Kloth LC.Electrical stimulation technologies for wound healing. *Advances in Wound Care*. 2014;3(2):81–90. doi:10.1089/wound.2013.0459
13. Sood A, Granick MS, Tomaselli NL. Wound dressings and comparative effectiveness data. *Advances in Wound Care*. 2014;3(8):511–529. doi:10.1089/wound.2012.0401
14. Bishop SM, Walker M, Rogers AA, Chen WY. Importance of moisture balance at the wound dressing interface. *J Wound Care*. 2003;4:12–16.
15. Barnea Y, Weiss J, Gur E. A review of the applications of the hydrofiber dressing with silver (Aquacel Ag®) in wound care. *Therapeutics and Clinical Risk Management*. 2010;6:21–27.

16. Vowden K, Vowden P. Understanding exudate management and the role of exudate in the healing process. *Br J Community Nursing*. 2003;8:4–13.

17. Edwards J.Use of Exu-Dry in the management of a variety of exudating wounds. *Br J Nursing*. 2001;12:10–22.

18. Tricco AC, Antony J, Vafaei A, et al. (2015). Seeking effective interventions to treat complex wounds: An overview of systematic reviews. *BMC Medicine*, 13, 89. http://doi.org/10.1186/s12916-015-0288-5

19. Ehrenreich M, Ruszczak Z. Update on tissue-engineered biological dressings. *Tissue Eng*. 2006;9:12–21.

20. Ehrenreich M, Ruszczak Z. Update on dermal substitutes. *Acta Dermatovernerol Croat*. 2006;3:14–17.

21. American Physical Therapy Association guide to physical therapist practice 3.0. apta.org. https://guide.apta.org /interventions. Updated August 1, 2014. Accessed February 3, 2021.

PART 9

Geriatric Interventions

Geriatric Overview

Theories of Aging

Table 9.1 General Concepts of Aging

- Aging is developmental.
- Aging occurs across the life-span.
- Aging changes are the result of cellular changes. Cells increase in size as a result of fragmentation of the Golgi apparatus and mitochondria. There is also a decrease in cell capacity to divide and reproduce, as well as an arrest of DNA synthesis and cell division.
- In aging, tissue changes occur due to an accumulation of pigmented materials (lipofuscins), an accumulation of lipids and fats, and connective tissue changes. These changes result from decreased elastic content, degradation of collagen, and the presence of pseudoelastins.
- In aging, organ changes cause decreases in functional capacity and homeostatic efficiency.

Table 9.2 Theories of Aging[1]

Functional decline in older adults may be a result of normal aging, but disease can cause functional decline and accelerate the speed at which a person ages. People age at different rates, and there is no universally accepted theory of aging. Some more common theories are presented.

Developmental Genetic Theory[1]

Aging is intrinsic to the organism and is part of the normal and continuous genetic development. Genes are programmed to modulate aging changes, and there is an overall rate of progression. Individuals vary in the expression of aging changes (such as graying of hair and wrinkles). Multiple genes are involved in aging. No one person's genes can modulate the rate of development in all aspects of aging. Premature aging syndromes, such as progeria, provide evidence of defective genetic programming. Some individuals exhibit premature aging changes, such as atrophy and thinning of tissues, graying of hair, and arteriosclerosis.

Hayflick Limit Theory[1]

This aging theory is based on the doubling of the biologic clock. This process occurs in three phases, with the last phase (phase III) showing a complete cessation of cell division. Termination of cell division involves a functional deterioration within cells because of the limited number of genetically programmed cell doublings (cell replication). A person's deterioration in terms of his or her cells does not depend on environmental influences. Cell aging is an intrinsic (built-in) process.

Free Radical Theory[1]

Free radicals are highly reactive and toxic forms of oxygen produced by cell mitochondria. They can have five effects:

1. They can cause damage to cell membranes and DNA cell replication.
2. They can interfere with cell diffusion and transport, resulting in decreased O_2 delivery and tissue death.
3. They can decrease cellular integrity and enzyme activities.
4. They can make cross-linkages such as chemical bonding of elements not generally joined together.
5. They can interfere with normal cell function.

Free radicals can also result in an accumulation of aging pigments (such as lipofuscins) and trigger pathologic changes such as atherosclerosis in blood vessel walls, cell mutations, and cancer. These cell mutations (intrinsic mutagenesis) result from errors in the synthesis of proteins (DNA and RNA). Eventually, cell mutations lead to abnormal proteins and aging changes.

(continued)

Table 9.2   **Theories of Aging**[1]   *(continued)*

Neuroendocrine and Hormonal Theories[1]

Neuroendocrine and hormonal theories of aging suggest that functional declines in neurons and their associated hormones lead to aging changes. According to these theories, the hypothalamus, pituitary gland, and adrenal gland are the primary regulators and timekeepers of aging. Thyroxine is the master rate-controlling hormone of the body for metabolism and protein synthesis. Also, secretion of regulatory pituitary hormones influences the thyroid. The theories also indicate that

1. Decreases in protective hormones such as estrogen, growth hormone, and adrenal dehydroepiandrosterone (DHEA) contribute to aging, and
2. Increases in stress hormones (cortisol) can damage the brain's memory center (i.e., the hippocampus) and destroy immune cells.

Immunity or Immunological Theory[1]

According to this theory, the thymus size decreases after birth, and atrophy is evident in older adults. As a result, T-cell function is diminished. T cells become less able to fight foreign organisms, and B cells become less able to make antibodies. As a result, autoimmune diseases increase with age, and older adults are both more susceptible to infection and have a decreased ability to fight off an infection. This theory is also categorized as a developmental genetic theory.

Environmental Theories (Stochastic or Nongenetic Theories)

According to these theories, aging is caused by an accumulation of insults from the environment. Environmental toxins include ultraviolet and cross-linking agents (e.g., unsaturated fats, toxic chemicals such as the metal ions Mg and Zn, radiation, and viruses). Exposure to these agents can result in errors in protein synthesis and in DNA synthesis/genetic sequences and can cause cross-linkage of molecules, with resultant mutations. Ultimately, the results of these insults are such that the organism reaches a level incompatible with life.

Caloric Restriction Theory (Energy Restriction)[1]

A lifestyle that incorporates a high-nutrient and low-calorie diet, with moderate vitamin and mineral supplementation and a regular exercise regimen, is beneficial. Caloric restrictions may slow down immune system decline. The caloric-restricted diet theorizes a reduction in the aging rate and disease susceptibility. Those events can happen because the immune system is considered the pacemaker of aging.

Telomerase Theory of Aging[1]

This theory evolved as a result of genetic engineering and shows promise for repair of damaged telomeres by utilizing the enzyme telomerase. Telomeres are cellular structures that extend from the ends of chromosomes. The function of a telomere is to maintain chromosomal integrity. This theory embraces use of telomerase inhibition for rebuilding of telomeres, to deter the natural aging process of these cells, which when left alone without intercession will result in cellular demise or cellular death overtime.

Psychological Theories (Stress Theory)

The stress theory speculates that homeostatic imbalances result in changes in the structural and chemical composition of the body. The general adaptation syndrome (described by Selye) postulates that

1. An initial alarm reaction takes place;
2. This reaction progresses to a stage of resistance; and
3. Finally, it goes into a stage of exhaustion (of the body and its organs).

The stress theory is closely linked to the hormonal theory.

(continued)

Table 9.2 Theories of Aging[1]	*(continued)*

Sociological Theories (Jury, Maslow, Levinson, Disengagement Theory, and Continuity and Activity Theories)

These theories focus on life experiences and lifestyle influences on the aging process. The activity theory states that older persons who are socially active exhibit improved adjustment to the aging process. According to this theory, continued role performance is essential for positive self-image and improved life satisfaction. The disengagement theory states that distancing of an individual or withdrawal from society affects aging. There is:

1. A reduction in social roles causing further isolation and life dissatisfaction, and
2. An increase relying on others for meeting physical and emotional needs. The focus of sociological theories is to enhance a person's identity improving the aging process.

Sleep Patterns in Older Persons

Table 9.3 Sleep Patterns in Older Persons[2]

- Transient insomnia: poor sleep over a few nights that may be caused by stress, work, or time zone changes, restless leg syndrome, and sleep apnea syndrome.

- Short-term insomnia: poor sleep over less than 1 month that may be related to acute medical or psychological conditions.

- Long-term insomnia: can present problems falling asleep (of more than 1 month's duration) that may be related to poor sleeping habits, anxiety, medication side effects, changes in activity level, or medical problems. Can also manifest as frequent awakening, which may be related to medication side effects, depression, sleep apnea, changes in activity level, or medical problems.

- Sundowners' syndrome: a neuropsychiatric term associated with the elderly person, with or without dementia, that displays uncharacteristic behaviors at sunset, evening, or night. Typical uncharacteristic behaviors may include agitation, confusion, delirium, unruliness, and outbursts of screaming or yelling. This phenomenon has been most closely observed in individuals with cognitive impairments, dementia, and the hospitalized. This syndrome poses challenges for caregivers, both at home and in institutionalized settings, and also for nursing staff or ancillary providers who work afternoons or night shifts.[2]

Factors Contributing to Malnutrition in Older Persons

Table 9.4 Malnutrition in Older Persons

Malnutrition in older persons is generally considered to reflect inadequate intake of micro and macronutrients and overall reduced caloric intake. However, people can be overweight and still be malnourished if the composition of nutrients in the diet is less than what is needed for the body to function. This condition increases a person's vulnerability to skin breakdown, medication toxicity, infections, gastrointestinal ulcerations, and other illnesses. Many of the symptoms associated with malnutrition, such as muscular weakness and wasting, may be attributed incorrectly to advanced age and underdiagnosed as a result.

(continued)

Table 9.4 **Malnutrition in Older Persons** *(continued)*

Factors Contributing to Malnutrition

1. Alcoholism
2. Chronic infection
3. Cancer
4. Chronic obstructive pulmonary disease
5. Depression
6. Dental or facial pathologies
7. Dysphagia (difficulty swallowing)
8. Excessively low-fat diet
9. Hyperthyroidism
10. Hypercalcemia
11. Impaired sense of taste or smell
12. Inability to gather or prepare food
13. Loneliness
14. Side effects of medications
15. Medication withdrawal
16. Pheochromocytoma—a neuroendocrine tumor that causes hypertension and is difficult to diagnose (patient has palpitations, nausea, sweating, abdominal pain, fainting spells, hyperglycemia, weakness, and anxiety)
17. Poverty
18. Getting full rapidly with a little food

Physical Signs[1] of Malnutrition in Adults

1. Sores at the angles of the mouth
2. Red swollen lingual papillae
3. Glossitis (inflammation of the tongue)
4. Papillary atrophy of tongue
5. Stomatitis (inflammation of the mouth including the lips, tongue, and mucous membranes)
6. Spongy and bleeding gums
7. Edema
8. Muscle tenderness in the extremities
9. Poor muscle tone
10. Skeletal deformity
11. Loss of vibratory sensation
12. Increased or decreased deep tendon reflexes
13. Hyperesthesia of the skin
14. Neuropathies
15. Purpura (rash in which blood cells leak into the skin or mucous membranes; related to blood coagulation)
16. Dermatitis (facial butterfly type, and perineal, scrotal, and vulval dermatitis)
17. Thickening and pigmentation of the skin over bony prominences
18. Poor or delayed wound healing
19. Nonspecific vaginitis
20. Anemia that does not respond to iron
21. Fatigue of visual accommodation
22. Conjunctival changes of the eye
23. Mild dementia, confusion

Thermal Regulation in Older Adults

Table 9.5 Risk Factors for Hyperthermia and Hypothermia[3]

- Hyperthermia in older adults can be a result of infections, brain lesions, impaired sweating mechanism, heavy exercise, or the environment (including exercise outdoors on a hot day).

- Hypothermia in older adults can be a result of diminished activity due to disease, dementia, or general immobility, poor diet including low calorie intake, muscle loss (impaired shivering mechanism), post-surgery due to anesthesia, diseases i.e., hypothyroidism.

- Impaired thermal regulation leading to either hypothermia or hyperthermia can be triggered by many factors:
  1. Alcohol
  2. Medication
  3. Dehydration
  4. Environmental factors
  5. Impaired circulation
  6. Cardiac dysfunction
  7. Cognitive impairment
  8. Impaired vasomotor response
  9. Diminished effectiveness of thermoreceptors in the skin
  10. Economic status

Age-Related Impairments, Activity Limitations, Participation Restrictions, and Suggestions for Interventions

Muscular Impairments, Activity Limitations, and Suggestions for Interventions

Table 9.6 Muscular Impairments

- Muscular impairments and activity limitations are caused mostly by decreased activity levels (hypokinesis) and disuse atrophy rather than by the normal aging process.
- There is a normal loss of muscular strength, which peaks at 30 years old, remains fairly constant until age 50, and then is characterized by accelerating loss. A 20–40% muscular strength loss occurs by age 65 in nonexercising adults.
- A normal loss of muscular power (force/unit time) may be due to losses in the speed of muscle contraction and changes in nerve conduction and synaptic transmission.
- A normal loss of skeletal muscle mass (atrophy) occurs due to a decrease in both the size and the number of muscle fibers. By age 70, there is 33% deficit in the skeletal muscle mass. Changes occur in muscle fiber composition, with a selective loss of type II fibers (fast-twitch fibers), which are important for rapid high force production. There is a proportional decrease in type I fibers (slow-twitch fibers), which are important for low force production.
- Age-related changes in muscular endurance occur as well. Muscles fatigue more readily. There is decreased muscle tissue oxidative capacity and decreased peripheral blood flow, affecting oxygen delivery to the muscles.
- The chemical composition of muscle is altered, with decreased myosin ATPase activity and glycoproteins and contractile protein being noted. Collagen changes include denser collagen (an irregularity because of cross-linkages) and loss of water content and elasticity. These changes affect tendons, bones, and cartilages, such that movements become slower and are accompanied by increased complaints of fatigue.
- The connective tissues become denser and stiffer with age. As a result, there is an increased risk of muscle and tendon strains and ligament sprains.
- As a result of connective tissue changes, a loss of range of motion occurs that is highly variable by joint and by individual, with an accompanying loss in activity level.
- There is an increased tendency to develop fibrous adhesions and contractures.
- Activity limitations occur with decreased functional mobility as a result of movement impairments. Gait changes include the following:
  1. The gait becomes stiffer with fewer automatic movements.
  2. The gait has a decreased amplitude and speed and a slower cadence.
  3. There is evidence of shorter steps, a wider stride, increased double support to ensure safety, and compensation for decreased balance.
  4. Decreased trunk rotation and arm swing are shown. The gait may become unsteady because of changes in balance and strength and the increased need for assistive devices. There is a clinical risk of falls.
- Sarcopenia is age-related loss of muscle strength and power, which leads to frailty and disability. Physical therapy focus is on resistance exercises.[4]

Intervention Strategies to Slow or Reverse Muscular Impairments

1. Make recommendations that the patient (client) will see the physician—to improve his/her medical health. These include correction of medical problems that may cause weakness, such as hyperthyroidism, excess adrenocortical steroids, Cushing's disease, use of steroids, or hyponatremia.
2. Make recommendations that the patient (client) will see the dietician—to improve nutrition, such as by correcting hyponatremia.

(continued)

Table 9.6 Muscular Impairments *(continued)*

3. Make a recommendation to address the possibility of alcoholism.
4. Increase the patient's (client's) levels of physical activity by stressing functional activities and organized activity programs (with a gradual increase in intensity of activity to avoid injury, adequate warm-ups and cool-downs, and appropriate pacing and rest periods).
5. Provide strength training (using isometric and progressive resistive exercise regimes); high-intensity training programs, such as those involving 70–80% of the one-repetition maximum (1 RM), produce quicker and more predictable results than moderate-intensity programs.
6. Improve the patient's (client's) functional abilities—through flexibility and range of motion exercises; use of slow, prolonged stretching, maintained for 20–30 seconds; heating of tissues before stretching; and maintenance of the newly gained range through its incorporation into functional activities.
7. Increase the patient's (client's) mobility activities (gains are usually slower with older adults).

Skeletal Impairments, Activity Limitations, and Suggestions for Interventions

Table 9.7 Skeletal Impairments, Activity Limitations and Interventions

- Skeletal impairments and activity limitations can occur from skeletal age-related changes, such as the cartilage changes that result from decreased water content, with cartilage becoming stiffer, fragmented, and eroding by age 60. More than 60% of older adults have degenerative joint changes and cartilage abnormalities.

- There is a normal loss of bone mass and density. Peak bone mass is reached in the third decade of life. A slow loss of bone begins around age 40 for both males and females.[3] Between the ages of 45 and 70, bone mass decreases (for women, by approximately 25%; for men, by 15%). There is also another 5% decrease of bone mass by age 90.

- There is a normal loss of calcium and bone strength, especially in trabecular bone. Osteoporosis can occur as a pathological manifestation of aging.

- There is a normal decrease in bone marrow red blood cell production.

- The intervertebral disks flatten and become less resilient because of loss of water content. There is a 30% loss by age 65 with loss of collagen elasticity.

- The trunk length and overall height diminish. As a result, postural changes are observed:
  1. Forward head
  2. Kyphosis of the thoracic spine
  3. Flattening of the lumbar spine

- With prolonged sitting, there is a tendency to develop hip and knee flexion contractures.

Intervention Strategies to Slow or Reverse Skeletal Impairments and Activity Limitations

1. Reduce the risk of contractures using positioning, exercises, or orthotics.
2. Reduce the risk of falls through patient/caregiver education.
3. Provide exercises for balance and other fall prevention interventions.
4. Use postural exercises stressing components of good posture.
5. Use weight-bearing (gravity-loading) exercises, which can decrease bone loss in older adults.
6. Use walking, stair climbing, and weight belts (to increase load).
7. Refer the patient (client) to the dietician and social worker (for help with "meals on wheels") to improve nutritional and hormonal status.

Neurologic Impairments, Activity Limitations, and Suggestions for Interventions

Table 9.8 Neurological Impairments and Interventions

- Age-related atrophy of nerve cells in the cerebral cortex causes an overall loss of cerebral mass/brain weight of 6–11% between the ages of 20 and 90. This loss accelerates after age 70.

- Changes in brain morphology include gyrus atrophy, with accompanying narrowing and flattening of the gyri and widening of the sulci; ventricular dilation; generalized cell loss in the cerebral cortex, especially in the frontal and temporal lobes with associated areas of the prefrontal cortex and visual tracts; the presence of lipofuscins (insoluble fatty pigments found in aging cells), senile or neuritic plaques, and neurofibrillary tangles (NFTs); and significant accumulations of plaque associated with Alzheimer's dementia pathology.

- Age-related selective cell loss[1] is found in the basal ganglia (substantia nigra and putamen), cerebellum, hippocampus, and locus coeruleus (depression in the floor of fourth ventricle of the brain). The brain stem is minimally affected.

- A normal decrease in cerebral blood flow and energy metabolism is evident.

- Normal changes in synaptic transmission take place due to decreased synthesis and metabolism of major neurotransmitters (acetylcholine and dopamine).

- Age-related slowing of many neural processes occurs, especially in polysynaptic pathways (multiple synapses' nerve pathways).

- Age-related changes in the spinal cord and peripheral nerves occur as a result of neuronal loss and atrophy. These changes are manifested as a 30–50% loss of anterior horn cells. A 30% loss of posterior roots (sensory fibers) occurs by age 90.

- Normal loss of motorneurons results in an increase in the size of the remaining motor units. Macro motor units develop.

- Slowed nerve conduction velocity is observed, with the slowing effect being greater in sensory fibers than in motor fibers.

- A normal loss of sympathetic nerve fibers may account for diminished autonomic stability and an increased incidence of postural hypotension in older adults.

- Age-related tremors (essential tremors) occur as an isolated symptom, particularly in the hands, head, and voice. These tremors are characterized as postural or kinetic and rarely occur at rest. They are usually benign and slowly progressive, although they may limit function in late stages and are exaggerated by movement and emotion.

- Clinical neurologic impairments affect functions such as the patient's (client's) movement. Overall speed and coordination are decreased, with the individual experiencing increased difficulty with fine motor control. Slower recruitment of motorneurons contributes to loss of strength. Both reaction time and movement time are increased.

- Older adults also experience decreased speed and accuracy of movements. The simpler the movement, the less the change. More complicated movements require more preparation. There are longer reaction and movement times. Faster movements have a decreased accuracy with an increase in movement errors.

- There is a general age-related slowing of neural processing of learning. The memory may be affected. Problems with homeostatic regulation may occur, such that stressors (heat, cold, and excess exercise) can be harmful, even life-threatening.

(continued)

Table 9.8 Neurological Impairments and Interventions   *(continued)*

Intervention Strategies to Slow or Reverse Neurological Impairments and Activity Limitations

1. Make recommendations that the patient (client) will see the physician—for correction of medical problems, such as improving cerebral blood flow.
2. Provide patient education to improve the individual's general health (such as diet and smoking cessation).
3. Increase levels of physical activity (may encourage neuronal branching, slow the rate of neural decline, and improve cerebral circulation).
4. Provide effective strategies to improve motor learning and motor control—to allow for increased reaction and movement time during activities, which will also improve motivation and accuracy of movements; to allow for limitations of memory by avoiding long sequences of movements; to allow for increased cautionary behaviors by providing adequate explanations and demonstrations when teaching new movement skills; and to stress familiar, well-learned skills and repetitive movements. (For more information on basic motor learning strategies, see the "Neurologic Interventions" section, Table 6.44.)

Sensory Visual Impairments, Activity Limitations, and Suggestions for Interventions

Table 9.9 Visual Impairments and Interventions

- Older adults experience a normal loss of function of the senses. This loss alters the quality of life and the ability to interact both socially and with the environment. It may lead to sensory deprivation, isolation, disorientation, and confusion and give the appearance of senility. Such impairments can also strain social interactions and lead to decreased functional mobility. As a result of decreases in sensory function, risk of injury is also increased.

- Visual impairments because of vision changes are the largest sensory impairments in older adults. Depression, functional decline and increased fall risk have all been associated with visual impairment.[3] Visual impairments result in a general decline in visual acuity. There is a gradual decline before the sixth decade of life, and a rapid decline between ages 60 and 90. Visual loss may be as much as 80% by age 90.

- The visual changes include presbyopia,[1] which results in a visual loss in middle-age and older individuals. Presbyopia is characterized by the inability to focus properly and blurred images due to the loss of accommodation and the elasticity of the lens. Presbyopia is also manifested through a decreased ability to adapt to dark and light. There is an increased sensitivity to light and glare, as well as a loss of color discrimination, especially for blues and greens.

- Another visual impairment is decreased sensitivity of the corneal reflex, which is associated with greater proclivity to eye injury or infection. Oculomotor responses are diminished with resultant restricted upward gaze and reduced pursuit eye movements. Ptosis (difficulty or inability to raise the eyelid) may also develop.

- Additional vision impairments may be caused by a visual pathology such as cataracts, in which the lens becomes clouded due to changes in lens proteins, leading to visual opacity. The impairments produced by cataracts can cause a gradual loss of vision—central vision first and then peripheral. There are increased problems with glare, a general darkening of vision, loss of acuity, and accompanying distortion.

- Other impairments, such as early loss of peripheral vision (tunnel vision) that may progress to total blindness, can be caused by glaucoma (which is characterized by increased intraocular pressure, degeneration of the optic disc, and atrophy of the optic nerve). Loss of central vision may progress to blindness if it is caused by senile macular degeneration (age-related degeneration of the macula owing to a decreased blood supply or abnormal growth of blood vessels under the retina).

(continued)

Table 9.9 Visual Impairments and Interventions *(continued)*

- Other central vision impairments are caused by diabetic retinopathy, which is characterized by damage to retinal capillaries, growth of abnormal blood vessels, and hemorrhage leading to retinal scarring and finally retinal detachment.

- A pathological visual impairment (caused by CVA) is homonymous hemianopsia, which results in loss of half of the visual field in each eye (the nasal half of one eye and the temporal half of the other eye). This condition results in an inability to receive information from the right or left side. The defect corresponds to the side of the sensorimotor deficit.

- Side effects of certain medications may also cause vision impairments (such as decreased or fuzzy vision). Medications that may cause such impairments include antihistamines, tranquilizers, antidepressants, and steroids.

Intervention Strategies to Slow or Reverse Sensory Visual Impairments and Activity Limitations

1. Physical therapist will perform an examination and evaluation of visual impairments (such as acuity, peripheral vision, light and dark adaptation, depth perception, diplopia, eye fatigue, and eye pain).
2. Maximize visual function by assessing the use of glasses and need for environmental adaptations.
3. Increase sensory thresholds by allowing extra time for visual discrimination and response.
4. Provide patient (client) education (e.g., to work in adequate light, reduce glare, and avoid abrupt changes in light and when going from light to dark).
5. Ensure that proper communication and interaction are used with the patient or client. For example, the therapist may need to stand directly in front of the patient at the same eye level; assist the patient in color discrimination; use warm colors such as yellow, orange, or red for identification and color coding; and provide other sensory cues when vision is limited, such as verbal descriptions of new environments and touching to communicate that you are listening to the patient.
6. Provide safety education to reduce the risk of falls.
7. Report all new findings to the physical therapist, who can make appropriate changes to the plan of care if warranted.

Sensory Hearing Impairments, Activity Limitations, and Suggestions for Interventions

Table 9.10 Hearing Impairments and Interventions

- Normal aging changes in hearing can occur as early as the fourth decade of life. These changes affect a significant number of older individuals (23% of individuals aged 65–74 have hearing impairments). Forty percent of those older than age 75 have hearing loss. The rate of hearing loss in men is twice the rate in women. Hearing loss in men also typically starts earlier than in women.

- Conductive hearing loss is common in older men. This type of hearing loss (in the outer ear) is a result of buildup of cerumen (ear wax), which then obstructs the external auditory meatus.

- Conductive hearing loss may also take the form of a mechanical hearing loss from damage caused by trauma or disease to the external auditory canal, the tympanic membrane, or the middle ear ossicles. Conductive hearing loss can affect all sound frequencies. Tinnitus (ringing in the ears) may also be present.

(continued)

Table 9.10 **Hearing Impairments and Interventions** *(continued)*

- Hearing changes as a result of aging process can occur in the inner ear as well. These changes may be significant in terms of sound sensitivity, thereby affecting the understanding of speech. Changes may also occur in the vestibular mechanism of the inner ear, affecting equilibrium. The hearing changes may be the result of degeneration and atrophy of cochlear and vestibular structures with an accompanying loss of neurons.

- Sensorineural hearing loss is a (permanent or temporary) loss affecting cochlear and peripheral structures in the inner ear. Causal factors with this type of sensory hearing loss may include noise exposure, acoustic or mechanical trauma, disease, drugs, and arteriosclerosis.

- Presbycusis is a term describing normal loss of hearing due to aging. This type of sensorineural hearing loss is associated with middle-aged and older adults. It is generally characterized by bilateral hearing loss, especially at high frequencies (greater than 3 kHz, affecting reception of consonant sounds in the speech range). It can eventually affect all frequencies pertinent to speech reception. With this condition, there is poor auditory speech discrimination and comprehension, especially in the presence of background noise. Often there is accompanying tinnitus.

- Central hearing loss is a type of hearing loss that results from disorders affecting neural tracts and structures from the cochlea of the inner ear and eighth cranial nerve pathways to the auditory receptors of the brain.

- Another type of hearing loss associated with pathology is otosclerosis, a condition caused by a bony overgrowth immobilizing the stapes (ankylosis of the stapes) in the middle ear with resulting conductive loss. If untreated, otosclerosis may result in eventual intrusion into the otic capsule, affecting the sensory function of the inner ear. When treated early, this pathology is generally amenable to surgical intervention (stapedectomy). Otosclerosis is not necessarily a type of hearing loss related to aging; it can also occur in younger individuals.

- Paget's disease (osteitis deformans) is a pathology of older individuals affecting the middle ear and eventually, if untreated, the inner ear. Paget's disease is characterized by thickening and hypertrophy of the long bones and deformity of the flat bones. It may respond to medical intervention through use of medication.

- Hypothyroidism is another pathology (inadequate levels of thyroid hormone in the body) affecting hearing sensitivity and acuity.

Intervention Strategies to Slow or Reverse Sensory Hearing Impairments and Activity Limitations

1. Recommend professional audiological assessment of hearing to evaluate speech acuity, word discrimination/comprehension, presence of tinnitus, cochlear recruitment, dizziness, vertigo, and pain.
2. Recommend audiological assessment by a professional audiologist and perhaps the use of amplification (hearing aid) to improve speech discrimination and help communication.
3. Improve communication by minimizing auditory distractions.
4. When communicating with a patient exhibiting hearing impairments, the therapist should speak slowly and clearly; be directly in front of the patient at the eye level; use nonverbal communication (such as gestures or demonstration) to reinforce the message; and orient the patient (client) away from topics of conversation he or she cannot hear to reduce feelings of paranoia and isolation.

Vestibular and Balance Sensory Impairments, Activity Limitations, and Suggestions for Interventions

Table 9.11 Vestibular and Balance Impairments and Interventions[1]

- Changes inherently associated with aging affect the mechanism involving control of balance. These include degenerative changes in the otoconia of the utricle and saccule within the vestibular segments of the inner ear located in the temporal bone of the skull. There is a normal age-related loss of vestibular hair-cell receptors and a decreased number of vestibular neurons. This loss is accompanied by a decrease in the vestibular ocular reflex (VOR). This condition begins at age 30, with an accelerating decline noted at ages 55–60, resulting in diminished vestibular sensation. Ultimately, the diminished acuity results in delayed reaction times and longer response times. The reduced function of the VOR affects retinal image stability with head movements and produces blurred vision.

- As a result of altered sensory organization in the inner ear and the eye, older adults depend more on somatosensory inputs for balance.

- Older adults are less able to resolve sensory conflicts when presented with inappropriate visual or proprioceptive inputs due to vestibular losses.

- Postural response patterns for balance are disorganized. This effect is manifested as diminished ankle torque, increased hip torque, and increased postural sway.

- Other vestibular and balance impairments caused by pathology include tinnitus and dizziness, a sensation of fullness in the ear (caused by Meniere's disease), and sensorineural hearing loss (usually low frequency, also caused by Meniere's disease). Severe manifestations of Meniere's disease, if unresolved through medical intervention, may require surgical intervention.

- Benign paroxysmal positional vertigo (BPPV) also causes vestibular and balance impairments characterized by brief episodes of vertigo (less than 1 minute) associated with position change. This effect is the result of degeneration of the utricular otoconia that settle on the cupula of the posterior semicircular canal. This condition is common in older adults.

Intervention to Slow or Reverse Vestibular and Balance Sensory Impairments and Activity Limitations (See Part 4 for additional information on vestibular disorders in the general population.)

1. Improve balance and coordination.
2. Decrease incidence of falls in older adults (see the somatosensory balance interventions in the next section).
3. Provide the patient and patient's family with safety education to identify risks and modify the environment (see the somatosensory balance interventions in the next section).
4. Improve tolerance to activities by performing habituation exercises when warranted.
5. Have the patient review medications with physician to identify any that might be causing dizziness.[3]

Somatosensory Balance Impairments, Activity Limitations, and Suggestions for Interventions

Table 9.12 Somatosensory Balance Impairments and Interventions

- With normal aging changes, there is a decrease in the sensitivity of touch associated with a decline of peripheral receptors and atrophy of afferent fibers. The lower extremities are more affected than the upper extremities.

- Normal proprioceptive losses occur with increased thresholds in vibratory sensibility, beginning around age 50. These losses are greater in the lower extremities than the upper extremities and greater in the distal extremities than in the proximal extremities.

- A loss of joint receptor sensitivity occurs, with losses more evident in the lower extremities. Cervical joints may also contribute to loss of balance.

- Cutaneous pain thresholds are increased, with greater changes being noted in the upper body areas (upper extremities and face) than in the lower extremities. Additional sensation impairment may be caused by pathologies such as diabetes (peripheral neuropathy), CVA (central sensory losses), and peripheral vascular disease (peripheral ischemia).

Intervention Strategies to Slow or Reverse Somatosensory Balance Impairments and Activity Limitations

1. Physical therapist will perform an examination and evaluation for increased thresholds to stimulation and to sensory losses.
2. Allow extra time for the patient's (client's) responses with increased thresholds to stimulation.
3. Use touch to communicate with the patient (client).
4. Maximize proprioceptive inputs by using facilitation interventions such as rubbing and stroking.
5. Highlight and enhance naturally occurring intrinsic feedback during movements by using stretch and tapping.
6. Provide augmented feedback through appropriate sensory channels (e.g., walking on carpeted surfaces may be easier than on smooth floor).
7. Teach compensatory strategies to prevent injury to anesthetic limbs and to prevent falls.
8. Provide assistive devices as needed for fall prevention.
9. Use biofeedback devices as appropriate, such as a limb load monitor, which offers visual load signaling to prevent a fall.

Taste and Smell Impairments, Activity Limitations, and Suggestions for Interventions

Table 9.13 Taste and Smell Impairments and Interventions

- Aging changes in taste and smell comprise a gradual decrease in taste sensitivity and decreased smell sensitivity.

- There is additional loss of sensation (sensitivity) in smokers and persons with chronic allergies and respiratory infections.

- Use of dentures contributes to the loss of taste and smell, as does CVA with involvement of the hypoglossal nerve.

(continued)

Table 9.13 **Taste and Smell Impairments and Interventions** *(continued)*

Intervention Strategies to Slow or Reverse Taste and Smell Impairments and Activity Limitations

1. Provide patient education on compensatory strategies for identification of odors, tastes (sweet, sour, bitter, salty), and somatic sensations (temperature, touch).
2. Provide patient education on the use of taste enhancers (such as herbs and spices) to help with the patient's diet and nutrition (decreased taste and enjoyment of food leads to poor diet and nutrition).
3. Perform an environmental assessment (home or nursing facility) and use safety monitors, especially for home safety (there is a decrease in home safety with a diminished capacity to detect gas leaks or smoke).
4. Provide patient education on making eating an enjoyable social and physical experience.
5. Encourage good oral hygiene and dental care (to deter avoidance of eating due to mouth pain or inability to masticate because of missing teeth or improperly fitting dentures).

Cognitive Impairments, Activity Limitations, and Suggestions for Interventions

Table 9.14 **Cognitive Impairments, Activity Limitations, and Interventions**

- There is no uniform decline in intellectual abilities throughout adulthood.
- Age-related cognitive changes do not typically show up until the mid-60s.
- Significant declines affecting everyday life do not show up until the early 80s.
- The most significant cognitive impairments (in measures of intelligence) occur in the years immediately preceding death. This condition is termed terminal drop.
- Tasks involving perceptual speed show early declines by age 39, when longer times are required to complete tasks.
- Numeric abilities (tests of adding, subtracting multiplying) peak in the mid-40s and are well maintained until the 60s.
- Verbal ability peaks at age 30 and is well maintained until the 60s.
- Memory impairments are typically noted in short-term memory. Long-term memory is retained.
- Memory impairments are task dependent. Deficits are noted primarily with novel conditions and with new learning.
- Persons in all age groups can learn.
- Learning in older adults is affected by increased cautiousness, anxiety, and the pace of learning. Fast pace is problematic. There may also be interference from prior learning.

Intervention Strategies to Slow or Reverse Cognitive Impairments and Activity Limitations

1. Provide patient education to use different strategies for learning. For example, context-based strategies work better than memorization in young adults.
2. Stress the relationship and the importance of learning for functional skills.
3. Improve the patient's (client's) general health by making recommendations to seek care from the appropriate medical personnel and correct medical problems. For example, imbalances between oxygen supply and demand to the central nervous system can be present in cardiovascular disease, hypertension, diabetes, and hypothyroidism.

(continued)

Table 9.14 Cognitive Impairments, Activity Limitations, and Interventions *(continued)*

4. Make recommendations that the patient (client) seek care from the appropriate medical personnel for pharmacological changes (such as drug reevaluation and decreased use of multiple drugs).
5. Monitor the patient (client) for drug toxicity.
6. Recommend reduction or cessation of the use of tobacco and alcohol.
7. Provide recommendations for correction of nutritional deficiencies.
8. Improve physical and mental activity. For example, older adults may keep mentally engaged by playing chess, doing crossword puzzles, and having a high level of reading.
9. Provide patient education on following a lifestyle that stresses social activity through clubs, travel, and work.
10. Make recommendations for cognitive training activities (provide written instruction because the auditory processing may be decreased).
11. Make recommendations for developing a stimulating, "enriching" environment for the patient (client) in familiar environments, because hospitalization or institutionalization may produce disorientation and agitation in some older patients (clients).
12. Make recommendations for counseling and family support (to help to reduce stress).
13. Encourage socialization and group-related activities to stimulate problem solving (i.e., card playing, puzzle, bingo).

Cardiopulmonary System Impairments, Activity Limitations, and Suggestions for Interventions

Table 9.15 Cardiopulmonary Impairments, Activity Limitations, and Interventions

- Age-related impairments and activity limitations of the cardiovascular system are due more to inactivity and disease than aging.
- Cardiovascular pathological changes[1] include degeneration of the heart muscle with accumulation of lipofuscins (characterized by mild cardiac hypertrophy of the left ventricular wall), decreased coronary blood flow, thickening of the cardiac valves, changes in the conduction system (loss of the pacemaker cells in the sinoatrial (SA) node), blood vessel changes (such as thicker and less distensible arteries), slowed exchange in capillary walls and increased peripheral resistance, increased resting blood pressure (systolic is greater than diastolic), decreased blood volume and hemopoietic activity of bone, and increased blood coagulability.
- The following cardiac clinical impairments and activity limitations should be noted during exercises:
  1. Increased systolic blood pressure
  2. Weakened cardiovascular responses to exercise (such as a decrease in heart rate, and heart rate acceleration and decrease in maximal oxygen uptake)
  3. Reduced exercise capacity
  4. Increased recovery time after exercises
- Stroke volume decreases due to decreased myocardial contractility. The maximum heart rate declines with age. The cardiac output decreases 1% per year after age 20 owing to decreases in heart rate and stroke volume.
- Other clinical impairments may include orthostatic hypotension (due to reduced baroceptor sensitivity and vascular elasticity) and increased fatigue.
- Anemia is common in older adults.
- Systolic ejection murmurs are common in older adults. EKG changes may occur with loss of normal sinus rhythm, longer PR and QT intervals, a wider QRS segment, and increased arrhythmias.

(continued)

Table 9.15 Cardiopulmonary Impairments, Activity Limitations, and Interventions *(continued)*

- Age-related impairments and activity limitations affecting the pulmonary system include chest wall stiffness with declining strength of respiratory muscles, which results in increased work of breathing; loss of lung elastic recoil with decreased lung compliance; and changes in lung parenchyma (such as the alveoli become larger and thinner, and fewer capillaries being available for delivery of blood).

- Other impairments relate to the following conditions:
  1. Changes in the pulmonary blood vessels, which become thicker and less distensible
  2. Decreased total lung capacity and vital capacity
  3. Increased residual volume
  4. Decreased forced expiratory volume
  5. Altered pulmonary gas exchange (e.g., the oxygen tension falls with age, at a rate of 4 mm Hg per decade)
  6. Lower partial pressure of oxygen in arterial blood (PaO_2): at age 70, it is 75 mm Hg, versus 90 mm Hg at age 20

- A decrease in the homeostatic response and the immune response is caused by a decrease in ciliary action, which hampers the body's ability to clear secretions and by a decrease in the secretory immunoglobulins and alveolar phagocytic function.

- The following pulmonary clinical impairments and activity limitations should be taken into account during exercises:
  1. Increased ventilatory rate during work
  2. Greater blood acidosis
  3. Increased likelihood of breathlessness
  4. Increased perceived exertion in response to higher-intensity exercises (no impairments with low- and moderate-intensity exercises)
  5. Reduced signs of hypoxia
  6. Impaired cough mechanism
  7. Decreased gag reflex
  8. Increased risk of aspiration

- Recovery from respiratory illness is prolonged in older patients. Significant changes in function are often noted with chronic smoking and exposure to environmental toxic inhalants.

Intervention Strategies to Slow or Reverse Cardiopulmonary Impairments and Activity Limitations

1. Have the physical therapist perform a comprehensive cardiopulmonary assessment before commencing an exercise program.
2. Select the appropriate exercise tolerance testing protocol (ETT). Many older patients cannot tolerate maximal testing, so submaximal testing is commonly used with members of this age group.
3. Testing and exercise training modes should be similar.
4. Have the physical therapist develop an individualized exercise prescription. The choice of training program is based on fitness level, presence or absence of cardiovascular disease, musculoskeletal impairments and limitations, and the patient's goals and interests; the exercise prescription elements should include frequency, intensity, duration, and mode.
5. Have the physical therapist develop an aerobic training program, which may include walking, chair and floor exercises, and modified strength/flexibility calisthenics that are well tolerated by most older patients.
6. Offer pool programs (safer for bone and joint impairments).

(continued)

Table 9.15 Cardiopulmonary Impairments, Activity Limitations, and Interventions *(continued)*

7. Multiple modes of exercise may be used, such as circuit training on alternate days (to reduce the likelihood of muscle injury, joint overuse, pain, and fatigue).
8. Increase the physiologic benefits to the patient from the aerobic training program. These benefits may include decreased heart rate at a given submaximal power, improved maximal oxygen uptake, improved peripheral adaptation and muscle oxidative capacity, improved recovery heart rate, decreased systolic blood pressure, increased maximum ventilatory capacity, and reduced breathlessness.
9. Increase the psychological benefits to the patient of the aerobic training program, such as improved sense of well-being and self-image, and improved functional capacity.
10. Increase the overall daily activity levels for independent living.
11. Provide patient education—about the lack of exercise as an important risk factor in the development of cardiopulmonary diseases and a contributing factor to problems of immobility and disability in the older population.

Integumentary, Gastrointestinal, and Renal Impairments

Table 9.16 Integumentary, Gastrointestinal, and Renal Impairments

Age-Related Integumentary Impairments

- Changes in skin composition include the following:
    1. The dermis becomes thinner with a loss of elastin.
    2. There is a decrease in vascularity.
    3. Vascular fragility results in easy bruising.
    4. There is a decrease in sebaceous activity.
    5. There is a decrease in integumentary hydration.
    6. The skin appears dry, wrinkled, yellowed, and inelastic.
    7. Aging spots—clusters of melanocyte pigmentation that increases with exposure to the sun—appear.
- There is a normal general thinning and graying of the hair because of vascular insufficiency and decreased melanin production.
- Nails grow more slowly and become brittle and thick.
- There is a loss of integumentary efficiency as a protective barrier: The skin grows and heals more slowly; it is less able to resist injury and infection; the skin inflammatory response is slower; there is decreased sensitivity to touch and perception of pain and temperature; there is an increased risk for injury from concentrated skin pressures or excess temperatures.
- Decreased sweat production with loss of sweat glands results in decreased temperature regulation and homeostasis.

(continued)

Table 9.16 Integumentary, Gastrointestinal, and Renal Impairments

Age-Related Gastrointestinal and Renal Impairments

- Decreased salivation, taste, and smell occur and may be exacerbated by inadequate chewing because of tooth loss or poorly fitting dentures.
- A poor swallowing reflex may lead to poor dietary intake and nutritional deficiencies.
- Motility and control of the lower esophageal sphincter decreases, potentially leading to acid reflux and heartburn.
- Hiatal hernia is common in older adults.
- In the stomach, there is reduced motility and control of the lower esophageal sphincter, delayed gastric emptying, decreased levels of digestive enzymes and hydrochloric acid, and decreased digestion and absorption. Indigestion is common in older adults.
- There is decreased intestinal motility, with constipation being common in older adults.
- In the kidneys, there is a loss of mass and total weight with nephron atrophy.
- Both renal blood flow and filtration are decreased. The blood urea rises.
- The kidney's excretory and reabsorptive capacities decrease.

Bladder Impairments and Interventions (for Incontinence)

Table 9.17 Bladder Impairments and Interventions (for Incontinence)

- In the bladder, muscle weakness impairments result in decreased capacity, leading to urinary frequency. There is difficulty with emptying the bladder, which produces increased urinary retention. Urinary incontinence is common, affecting more than 10 million adults. More than half of all nursing home residents and one-third of community-dwelling older persons are affected. Urinary incontinence affects older women with pelvic floor weakness and older men with bladder or prostate disease. There is an increased likelihood of urinary tract infections.

Types of Incontinence[3]

- Urge incontinence—patient cannot get to the bathroom in time when they feel the need to urinate. Commonly linked to overactive bladder but may be found in patients with diabetes, Alzheimer's disease, Parkinson's disease, and multiple sclerosis.
- Stress incontinence—patient experiences loss of urine with cough, strain, laugh, or physical activity. This is most common type of incontinence in middle aged women.
- Overflow incontinence—bladder becomes overfull typically due to an obstruction blocking the outlet. Patient loses small amounts of urine constantly although bladder remains full. Found in patients with diabetes, spinal cord injury, or enlarged prostate.
- Functional incontinence—patient has normal bladder function but has difficulty with mobility and cannot get to the bathroom in time or may have mental confusion and not recognize need to void.

(continued)

Table 9.17 **Bladder Impairments and Interventions (for Incontinence)** *(continued)*

Incontinence Interventions

- Incontinence interventions for older adults include isometric exercises for pelvic floor awareness training and strengthening. These exercises are used to treat or prevent incontinence and a "leaky bladder," which may occur with coughing, sneezing, laughing, or other straining activities. Instruct the patient (client) to use these exercises and to practice sphincter control by attempting to stop urine flow intermittently when using the bathroom.
  1. Supine or side-lying position is the easiest in which to begin; progress to sitting or standing.
  2. Instruct the patient (client) to tighten the pelvic floor as if attempting to stop urine flow.
  3. Ask the patient to hold the contraction for 3–5 seconds and then relax.
  4. The bladder should be empty when performing this exercise.
  5. Biofeedback used in conjunction with pelvic floor exercises helps patients with stress and urge incontinence.[3]

- The pelvic floor muscles are highly fatigable; thus contractions should not be held longer than 5 seconds and a maximum of 10 repetitions performed per session. When these muscles are fatigued, substitution of the gluteals, abdominals, or hip adductors may occur.

- Scheduled voiding may help some patients.

- Management of incontinence typically requires a multidisciplinary approach.

GERIATRIC INTERVENTIONS

Geriatric Disorders/Diseases and Intervention Patterns

Clinical Practice Guidelines

Clinical Practice Guidelines (CPGs), developed by American Physical Therapy Association (APTA) sections, other organizations, societies, and healthcare organizations, are based on a systematic review of the evidence and provide therapists with resources to help guide clinical decision-making. The Academy of Geriatric Physical Therapy, a section of the APTA, provides access to CPGs and other evidence-based resources relevant to the management of older adults. Examples of topics addressed by the Academy of Geriatric Physical Therapy include[5] Physical Therapy Management of Older Adults with Hip Fracture (in conjunction with Academy of Orthopedic Physical Therapy), Management of Falls in Community Dwelling Older Adults, and Determining Risk of Falls in Community Dwelling Older Adults: A Systematic Review and Meta-Analysis Using Posttest Probability. A full listing of practice resources, including links to exercise recommendations and outcome measures useful with older adults can be found at https://geriatricspt.org/practice/.

Osteoporosis: Intervention Goals

Table 9.18 Osteoporosis: Intervention Goals

Osteoporosis[6] is a disease process that results in reduction of bone mass caused by failure of bone formation (osteoblast activity) to keep pace with bone reabsorption and destruction (osteoclast activity). More bone is reabsorbed than is laid down. The skeleton loses some of the strength derived from its intact bone trabeculation. The aging process causes type II osteoporosis (formerly called senile osteoporosis). Type I osteoporosis (also called involutional bone loss) occurs as a result of the protective effects of estrogen on bone; it begins at menopause. Areas commonly affected by osteoporosis include the vertebral column (spine and ribs), femoral neck, distal radius/wrist, and humerus.

The National Osteoporosis Foundation (NOF) estimates that 10 million Americans[6] have osteoporosis. Among these individuals, 8 million are women, and 2 million are men. Eighty percent of individuals affected by osteoporosis are women. Twenty percent of non-Hispanic white and Asian women aged 50 and older are estimated[6] by the NOF to have osteoporosis and 52% to have low bone mass. Seven percent of non-Hispanic and Asian men aged 50 and older are estimated by the NOF to have osteoporosis and 35% to have low bone mass.

Etiologic Factors[6]

- Hormonal deficiency: estrogen in women and testosterone in men
- Nutritional deficiency: inadequate calcium, impaired absorption of calcium, excessive alcohol, and caffeine consumption
- Decreased physical activity: inadequate mechanical loading
- Diseases that affect bone loss: hyperthyroidism, diabetes, hyperparathyroidism, rheumatoid arthritis, liver disease, Paget's disease, and certain types of cancer
- Medications that affect bone loss: corticosteroids, thyroid hormone, anticonvulsants, catabolic drugs, some estrogen antagonists, and chemotherapy
- Additional risk factors: family history, white/Asian race, early menopause, thin/small build, and smoking

(continued)

Table 9.18 Osteoporosis: Intervention Goals *(continued)*

Osteoporosis Characteristics

One-third of individuals affected by osteoporosis will experience major orthopedic problems related to osteoporosis. Bone loss progresses for many years without causing symptoms. Bone loss is approximately 1% per year (starting for women at ages 30–35 and for men at ages 50–55). Accelerating bone loss happens in postmenopausal women (approximately 5% per year for 3–5 years). Structural weakening of bone can take place (decreasing ability to support loads; high risk of fractures; trabecular bone more involved than cortical bone). As a result of bone weakening, fractures, bone pain, and loss of mobility can occur. Also, skeleton deformities such as kyphosis and loss of height occur (especially if vertebral compression fractures take place).

Medications Approved[6] by the FDA to Prevent and/or Treat Osteoporosis

- Alendronate and alendronate plus vitamin D (Fosamax and Fosamax plus D)
- Ibandronate (Boniva)
- Risedronate and risedronate with calcium (Actonel and Actonel with calcium)
- Calcitonin (Miacalcin)
- Estrogens (Climara, Estrace, Estraderm, Estratab, Premarin, and others)
- Estrogens and progestins (Activella, Premphase, Prempro, and others)
- Parathyroid hormone (Teriparatide)
- Raloxifene (Evista)

Physical Therapy Assessments and Reassessment in Osteoporosis

- Dizziness
- Sensory integrity
- Vision
- Hearing
- Somatosensory system
- Vestibular system
- Sensory integration
- Motor function
- Strength
- Endurance
- Motor control
- Range of motion (ROM) and flexibility
- Postural deformity (such as the feet, for hammer toes and bunions leading to antalgic gait)
- Postural kyphosis (forward head position)
- Hip and knee flexion contractures
- Postural hypotension
- Gait and balance

(continued)

Table 9.18 Osteoporosis: Intervention Goals   *(continued)*

Physical Therapy Intervention Goals

1. Exercises and activities to maintain bone mass—weight-bearing exercises; daily walking for at least 30 minutes; stair climbing; use of weight belts during walking to increase loading; resistance exercises for hip and knee extensors and triceps; postural/balance training; postural exercises to reduce kyphosis; and flexibility exercises
2. Functional balance exercises—chair rises; standing/kitchen sink exercises; toe raises; unilateral stance for hip extension and abduction; and partial squats
3. Gait training
4. Safety education and fall prevention
5. Patient education—using proper shoes with thin soles and using flat shoes that enhance balance abilities
6. Assistive devices training—using a cane or a walker as needed
7. Patient education for fracture prevention—counseling on safe activities; avoiding sudden forceful movements; avoiding twisting, standing for too long, bending over, lifting, and performing supine sit-ups

Osteoporosis PTA Pearls

- Choose closed kinetic chain exercises when appropriate.
- Include balance activities to decrease risk of falls and associated fractures.
- Include postural exercises and flexibility exercises to promote more upright posture and eliminate excessive forward trunk flexion outside center of gravity, again, to deter potential fall-related fractures.
- Avoid supine, prone, or side-lying exercises 30–60 minutes after ingestion of bisphosphonate medications to avoid adverse esophageal reflux occurrences.[6]

Common Geriatric Fractures: Interventions

Table 9.19 Common Geriatric Fractures: Interventions

- Fractures: associated with low bone density and multiple risk factors (such as age, comorbid diseases, dementia, and psychotropic medications), especially for older patients/clients

Hip Fractures

Hip fractures are the most common orthopedic problem[3,7] among older adults in the United States. The mortality rate for hip fractures is associated mostly with post-fracture complications. Most hip fractures occur in the femoral neck or intertrochanteric area of the femur. Preoperatively, Buck's traction may be used for a short period of time to alleviate muscle spasms. Most hip fractures are treated surgically using an open reduction internal fixation (ORIF) to realign the bone ends. A femoral prosthesis may be used for femoral neck or femoral head fractures. In older patients, bone healing takes from 6 to 12 weeks.

Interventions for Hip Fractures

- Positioning
- Progressive weight bearing (as per MD/DO order) and gait training
- Assistive devices for ambulation training
- Transfer training
- ROM, strengthening, and conditioning exercises
- Balance activities

(continued)

Table 9.19 **Common Geriatric Fractures: Interventions**   *(continued)*

Hip Fractures PTA Pearls

General Precautions[6]

- Sub-trochanteric fracture precautions: No bridging or straight leg raising for 6 weeks post-surgically or as directed per MD/DO protocol.
- Maintain weight-bearing limitations as per MD/DO protocols.
- Monitor for postsurgical orthostatic hypotension.
- Monitor for deep vein thrombosis (DVT).

Vertebral Compression Fractures

Vertebral compression fractures occur in the lower thoracic and lumbar regions at T8–L3; they may result from routine activities such as bending, lifting, or rising from a chair. The patient's chief complaint is immediate, severe local spinal pain that increases with trunk flexion. Vertebral compression fractures may lead to shortening of the spine, progressive loss of height, and spinal deformity (kyphosis) that can progress to respiratory compromise.

Intervention Goals for Vertebral Compression Fractures

1. Acute phase: patient education for horizontal bed rest (being out of bed for 10 minutes every hour); patient education for proper posture (such as keeping the spine in extension in sitting, standing, or sleeping; bending forward is contraindicated); isometric extension exercises in bed
2. Chronic phase: patient education (extension exercises; avoidance of flexion activities); postural training; modalities and physical agents for pain relief; patient education for safety and modification of the environment; decrease vertebral loading; and the use of soft-soled shoes

Vertebral Compression Fractures PTA Pearls

- Thoracolumbar Sacral Orthosis (TLSO) to be worn as per MD/DO protocol for 12 weeks unless otherwise indicated per physician.
- Monitor areas of skin that may be prone to breakdown while using the TLSO brace.
- Exercises should be performed in neutral spine positions.
- Avoid trunk flexion and extremes of trunk extension; think stabilization exercises.
- Incorporate closed chain weight bearing functional exercises when appropriate.
- Follow postsurgical protocol for Vertebroplasty or Kyphoplasty procedures.

Stress Fractures

Stress fractures are fine, hairline fractures without soft-tissue injury. They are common in the pelvis, proximal tibia, distal fibula, and metatarsal shafts.

Intervention Goals for Stress Fractures

1. Rest
2. Correction of exercise excesses or faulty exercise program
3. Reduction of vertical loading
4. Use of soft-soled shoes

Other Extremity Fractures

Other types of fractures may include upper extremity fractures (e.g., fracture of the humeral head) and Colles' fractures. (For interventions in these types of injuries, see the "Musculoskeletal Interventions" section.)

(continued)

Table 9.19 Common Geriatric Fractures: Interventions *(continued)*

Clinical Implications of Geriatric Fracture Interventions

Fractures heal more slowly in older individuals. Older adults are also prone to complications such as pneumonia and decubitus ulcers. Mental status complications may occur with hospitalization. Rehabilitation may be complicated or prolonged by lack of support systems. Comorbid conditions (such as decreased vision and poor balance) are frequently observed in older adults.

Degenerative Joint Disease: Interventions

Table 9.20 Degenerative Joint Disease: Interventions

Osteoarthritis (OA) is a progressive disorder of joints, typically affecting the shoulders, hips, knees, fingers, and the spine. The incidence of OA increases with age. OA can cause moderate to severe limitations in functional daily activities.

OA Characterization

- Pain, swelling, and stiffness that are worse early in the morning or with overuse
- Knee pain
- Hip pain
- Muscle spasm
- Loss of range of motion
- Mobility deficits
- Crepitus
- Bony deformity
- Muscle weakness secondary to disuse atrophy

OA Intervention Goals[7]

1. Reduction of pain and muscle spasm—using modalities and physical agents, and relaxation exercises
2. Therapeutic exercises and activities—to maintain or improve ROM; correct muscle imbalances; strengthening exercises to support joints; exercises to improve balance and ambulation
3. Aerobic conditioning
4. Walking programs—associated with decreased joint symptoms, improved function, and sense of well-being
5. Aquatic programs—walking in the pool and pool exercises
6. Patient education—about the disease, taking an active role in one's own care, joint protection, and energy-conservation strategies
7. Assistive device and equipment training—for ambulation and activities of daily living (ADLs)
8. Promotion of a healthy lifestyle
9. Weight reduction—to relieve stress on the joints

OA General Physical Therapy Interventions

- Joint protection, modalities, and physical agents for pain control and decreasing edema and adhesions
- Conditioning exercises
- ROM and strengthening exercises

(continued)

Table 9.20 **Degenerative Joint Disease: Interventions** *(continued)*

- Gait training
- Orthotics as necessary
- Assistive devices during ambulation as necessary

For more interventions, see the "Musculoskeletal Interventions" section.

Total Joint Replacements PTA Pearls

Total Hip Arthroplasty[7]

General

- Maintain weight bearing restrictions as per physician protocol.
- Monitor for DVT/pulmonary embolism (PE); incorporate DVT prophylaxis into treatment (compression stockings, ankle pumps).
- Monitor for postsurgical orthostatic hypotension.
- Monitor for signs and symptoms of infection at the incision.
- Monitor prothrombin time -international normalized ratio (PT-INR) values if patient is on Coumadin.
  1. Direct anterior approach
     - No hip extension
     - No hip abduction
     - No combined movements
  2. Anterolateral approach
     - No hip flexion greater than 90 degrees
     - No hip extension
     - No hip adduction
     - No hip external rotation
  3. Posterior approach/posterolateral approach
     - No hip flexion greater than 90 degrees
     - No hip adduction
     - No hip internal rotation
     - No combined movements

Total Knee Arthroplasty[7]

General

- Maintain weight bearing restrictions as per physician protocol.
- Monitor for DVT/PE; incorporate DVT prophylaxis into treatment (compression stockings, ankle pumps).
- Monitor for postsurgical orthostatic hypotension.
- Monitor for signs and symptoms of infections at the incision.
- Monitor PT-INR values if patient is on Coumadin.
  1. Unicompartmental: only the damaged compartment is replaced
     - ROM to avoid arthrofibrosis within the joint capsule
     - No pillows directly under the popliteal fossa to deter development of flexion contractures
     - May need to consider healing of other intra-articular structures if they needed to be repaired
     - Foster edema reduction with gravity-assisted positioning when possible

(continued)

Table 9.20 **Degenerative Joint Disease: Interventions** *(continued)*

- Range of motion benchmarks should follow general guidelines and include the following:

  0–90 degrees within 2 weeks

  0–105 degrees by 3–4 weeks

  0–115 degrees by 6 weeks

- Traditional: complete knee replacement, both medial and lateral compartments are replaced; anterior cruciate ligament (ACL) and/or posterior cruciate ligament (PCL) may or may not be spared
  - ROM to avoid arthrofibrosis within the joint capsule.
  - No pillows directly under the popliteal fossa to deter development of flexion contractures.
  - Foster edema reduction with gravity assisted positioning when possible.
  - Range of motion benchmarks should follow general guidelines and include the following:

    0–90 degrees within 2 weeks

    0–105 degrees by 3–4 weeks

    0–115 degrees by 6 weeks

Total Shoulder Arthroplasty[7]

General

- No weight bearing through the affected arm.
- Monitor for signs and symptoms of infection of incision.
- Use immobilizer or sling use as per physician protocol.
- Monitor for post-surgical orthostatic hypotension.
- Traditional or hemiarthroplasty:
  - No active/passive abduction
  - No active/passive external rotation
  - Flexion and internal rotation motions may be limited per protocol
  - No lifting more than a full coffee cup
  - Include balance interventions as per plan of care since the center of gravity may be altered by immobilizer/sling use, which affects transfers and increases fall risk during ambulation
  - Include balance exercises when appropriate secondary to altered balance/lack of protective extension due to sling use
  - Treatment focus initially = pain management, edema reduction, regaining ROM within the limitations imposed on the patient per the protocol; scapular stabilization, postural re-education, and elbow/wrist complex strengthening; balance training; ADL training
- Reverse total shoulder arthroplasty:
  - No shoulder extension
  - No internal rotation
  - No horizontal adduction
  - Other motions can be performed as per physician protocol
  - No lifting more than a full coffee cup
  - Include balance interventions as per plan of care since the center of gravity may be altered by immobilizer/sling use which may affect transfers and increases fall risk during ambulation
  - Treatment focus initially = pain management, edema reduction, regaining ROM within the limitations imposed on the patient per the protocol; scapular stabilization, postural re-education, and elbow/wrist complex strengthening; balance training; ADL training

* Physician protocol takes precedence over these general guidelines.

Stroke, Traumatic Brain Injury, and Parkinson's Disease: Interventions

Table 9.21 Stroke, Traumatic Brain Injury, and Parkinson's Disease: Interventions

Cerebrovascular Accident (CVA)

- Sudden, focal neurologic deficit resulting from ischemic or hemorrhagic lesions in the brain; most common cause of adult disability in the United States.
- Possible impairments: homonymous hemianopsia, impaired sensory and motor function on the affected side, decreased or lost sensation, hypertonicity, increased reflexes, synergy patterns, hemiplegia or hemiparesis, incoordination, motor programming deficits, speech and language disorders with lesions involving the dominant hemisphere, perceptual disorders with lesions of the parietal lobe of the nondominant hemisphere, cognitive and behavioral changes, bladder and bowel dysfunction, and oral and facial dysfunction.
- Possible activity limitations: decreased mobility skills, impaired gait, impaired postural control and balance, and impaired ADLs and instrumental ADLs (IADLs).

CVA General Physical Therapy Interventions

- Gait training
- Transfers
- Positioning
- Ankle foot orthoses (AFO)
- ROM and strengthening exercises
- Facilitation and inhibition techniques
- Locomotion training
- Balance and coordination training
- Functional electrical stimulation (FES)
- Family and patient education
- For more interventions, see the "Neurologic Interventions" section.

Cerebrovascular Accidents PTA Pearls[8]

General Considerations

- Monitor for changes in arousal, sudden changes in muscle tone, and/or deep tendon reflexes (DTRs) = STOP treatment and seek medical assistance.
- Monitor for DVTs—STOP treatment and seek medical assistance if DVTs are suspected.
- Aspiration precautions apply, use thickened liquids and ask registered nurse (RN) before providing any liquids to patient.
  a. If patient is aspirating seek immediate medical treatment, initiate Heimlich maneuver or CPR if necessary.
- Monitor for skin breakdown due to sensory impairments.
- Use weight bearing to modulate tone.
- Use slow rotational motions away from the synergistic pattern to modulate tone and improve mobility (proprioceptive neurological facilitation (PNF) principles).
- Implement proper shoulder positioning with subluxation.
- Perform ROM for all joints or provide joint protection to maintain ROM and prevent contractures.
- Incorporate facilitatory techniques to increase tone.
- Incorporate inhibitory techniques to decrease tone.

(continued)

Table 9.21 **Stroke, Traumatic Brain Injury, and Parkinson's Disease: Interventions** *(continued)*

Right Hemisphere Lesions

- Contralateral loss of sensation and muscle weakness results in monitoring for integumentary issues.
- Provide sensory stimulation to the involved side.
- Visual field cuts may result in increased risk of falls.
- Patient presents with weakness, paralysis, and sensory impairments on the left side.
- Left sided hemianopsia necessitates cueing for visual scanning strategies to task safely.
- Decreased awareness and poor judgment may result in patient impulsivity and increased fall risk.
- Emotional lability may interfere with staying on task; PTA must redirect the patient.
- Left-sided neglect necessitates increased sensory stimulation toward left side: Utilize cueing strategies to scan left environment to increase safety with tasking.
- Memory deficits warrant mass practice with simple one step commands.
- Decreased spatial orientation and abstract reasoning may result in increased fall risk.

Left Hemisphere Lesions

- Patient presents with weakness, paralysis, and sensory impairments on the right side.
- Possible visual field cuts on the right side result in cueing to scan the environment and cues for the neglected side to increase awareness.
- Broca's aphasia (expressive) may be present necessitating use all types of communication (verbal, written, pictures); however, keep it simple and allow the patient time to respond.[9]
- Wernicke's aphasia (receptive) may be present, necessitating the use of gestures, slowing of your speech; do not give commands from across the room; assign key words to pictures.[10]
- Decreased processing necessitates slow commands and allowance of more time to respond to commands.
- Increased frustration results in the need to speak in calm tones, give simple commands, and allow time to respond.

Brainstem Lesions

- Close monitoring of vital signs in the patient.
- Decreased consciousness may be observed or changes in consciousness warrant reporting to RN.
- Presence of bilateral weakness/paralysis.
- Increased risk of aspiration due to swallowing impairment.

Cerebellar Lesions

- Decreased balance and coordination and presence of ataxia results in increased fall risk/increased safety concerns.
- Patient may experience nausea.
- Nystagmus may be present.
- Challenges with postural adjustment may result in increased fall risk.

(continued)

Table 9.21 **Stroke, Traumatic Brain Injury, and Parkinson's Disease: Interventions** *(continued)*

Parkinson's Disease (PD)

- Chronic, progressive disease of the nervous system.
- Possible impairments: rigidity, bradykinesia, resting tremor, and impaired postural reflexes.
- Possible activity limitations: decreased mobility skills, difficulty initiating movements and freezing episodes, slowed movements, gait deficits (such as shuffling gait, festinating gait, and/or loss of arm swing and reciprocal trunk movements), impaired postural control and balance (such as flexed, stooped posture and impaired balance reactions), impaired speech, oral-motor deficits, impaired handwriting, and deficits in ADLs and IADLs.

PD General Physical Therapy Interventions

- Gait training (without assistive device)
- Stretching exercises
- Breathing exercises
- Relaxation exercises
- Facilitation and inhibition techniques
- Balance and coordination training
- Functional training
- For more interventions, see the "Neurologic Interventions" section.

PD PTA Pearls[8]

- Incorporate ROTATION to break up rigidity.
- Optimize cardiovascular endurance to improve lung expansion and oxygenation to working muscles.
- Enhance flexibility and lower rigidity with deep breathing cues and relaxation strategies.
- Incorporate large amplitude movements for recalibration of the neurosensory system to promote reduction of impoverished movement patterns.[11]
- Swallowing difficulties with disease progression may result in increased aspiration risk or nutrition compromised due to difficulty with chewing and swallowing.

Clinical Implications of Geriatric Neurologic Interventions

- Older adults are prone to complications such as contractures, deformities, decubitus ulcers, and mental status complications.
- Interventions may take more time or be complicated by lack of a support system, comorbidities, sensorimotor deficits, and poor balance.
- The focus should be on the improvement of function.
- Compensatory treatment strategies should be used when impairments cannot be remediated (such as environmental modifications and the use of assistive devices and equipment for the home).

Cognitive Disorders: Intervention Goals

Table 9.22 Cognitive Disorders: Intervention Goals

Delirium

Delirium is an acute, reversible state of agitated confusion, although it may potentially be irreversible. Delirium produces temporary confusion and loss of mental function. It is characterized by acute onset (often at night); intervals of lucidity; hypo-alertness or hyper-alertness; impaired orientation; memory deficits (affecting immediate and recent memory); illusions and/or hallucinations; worst symptoms at night; duration of hours to weeks; disorganized thinking; incoherent speech; and disrupted sleep and wake cycles. Delirium may not necessarily happen in patients 65 years or older. It can be caused by drug and alcohol withdrawal, drug toxicity, systemic illness, oxygen deprivation of the brain (hypoxia), environmental changes and sensory deprivation, recent hospitalization, recent surgery or institutionalization, infections such as sepsis, and electrolyte and acid–base imbalances.

Delirium Intervention Goals

1. Provide supportive care by minimizing unanticipated, frightening, or invasive procedures.
2. Integrate orienting statements into normal conversation.
3. Do not try to convince the patient (client) that his or her perception is distorted.
4. Speak in a calm, clear voice, and maintain eye contact.
5. Encourage patient participation in ADLs.
6. Provide complementary interventions such as music therapy, massage, and shared activities.

Dementia[12]

Dementia is a progressive, irreversible decline in intellectual functions and memory, leading to diminished social, occupational, and intellectual abilities.

Criteria for Dementia Characterization

- Intellectual impairments, such as impoverished thinking, impaired judgment and decision-making, disorientation, confusion, and impaired social functioning
- Higher cortical functions impairments, such as aphasia (language impairment), apraxia (motor skill impairment), and agnosia (perception impairment)
- Learning and memory impairments, such as loss of recent and long-term memory
- Personality impairments, such as alteration or accentuation of premorbid traits and behavioral changes
- Fragmented sleep (alertness may be normal)

Types of Common Dementias

- Reversible dementia
- Alzheimer's disease
- Vascular dementia
- Mixed dementia
- Dementia with Lewy bodies
- Dementia in Parkinson's disease
- Frontotemporal lobar degeneration

(continued)

Table 9.22 Cognitive Disorders: Intervention Goals   *(continued)*

Reversible Dementia

Reversible dementia[1] accounts for 10–20% of all dementias. It has multiple causes:

- Medications such as sedatives, hypnotics, antianxiolytics, antidepressants, antiarrhythmics, antihypertensives, anticonvulsants, antipsychotics, and drugs with anticholinergic side effects
- Nutritional disorders such as vitamin B_6 deficiency, thiamine deficiency, vitamin B_{12} deficiency and pernicious anemia, and folate deficiency
- Metabolic disorders such as hyperthyroidism/hypothyroidism, hypercalcemia, hypernatremia/hyponatremia, hypoglycemia, kidney or liver failure, Cushing syndrome, Addison's disease, hypopituitarism, and carcinoma
- Psychiatric disorders such as depression, anxiety, and psychosis
- Toxins such as air pollution and alcohol ingestion

Primary Dementia Associated with Alzheimer's Disease

Primary dementia associated with Alzheimer's disease accounts for 60–80% of dementias and affects a very large number of individuals. It is very costly, as institutionalization of the patient may be necessary. Etiology includes multiple interacting causes—genetic risk factors (such as evidence of chromosomal abnormalities, family history, or Down syndrome) and environmental agents (such as viruses, traumatic brain injury, aluminum toxicity, or minor strokes).

Two types of primary dementia are distinguished:

- Presenile dementia of the Alzheimer's type (PDAT): starts between 40s and 60s; affects women more than men; has a rapid onset; is less gradual and more severe than SDAT; progresses rapidly; has a poor prognosis; is diffuse and generalized; has a mean survival of 4 years; death may occur and be caused by general systemic failure or infection; patients may have occasional seizures.
- Senile dementia of the Alzheimer's type (SDAT): starts after 60 (average age 75); affects women more than men; onset varies from months to years; mean survival can be between 7 and 11 years; has a gradual onset; can progress slowly or rapidly; prognosis is poor (in moderate to severe cases); death may occur and be caused by general systemic failure or infection; patients may have rare episodes of seizure.

PDAT and SDAT impairments and activity limitations include the following:

- Occasional tremors
- Generalized weakness
- Unsteady gait
- Increased tone
- Rigid postures
- Decreased postural reflexes
- Increased risk of fall
- Repetitive behaviors
- Periods of agitation, restlessness, and wandering

(continued)

Table 9.22 Cognitive Disorders: Intervention Goals   *(continued)*

- Sundowning syndrome (confusion and agitation that increase in the late afternoon)
- Progressive disorientation
- Memory loss
- Impaired cognition
- Impaired judgment
- Impaired abstract thinking
- Visual and spatial deficits
- Apraxia
- Delusions
- Hallucinations
- Disorders of sleep and eating, inappropriate sexual behaviors, and apathy (in late stages)
- Personality changes (such as egocentricity, impulsivity, irritability, and inappropriate social behaviors)

Alzheimer's Disease PTA Pearls[3,12]

- Use a calm voice and keep commands and instructions simple.
- Decreased memory warrants mass practice and simple cues (sensory, verbal, and visual).
- Balance challenges arise as the patient with dementia ages resulting in increased fall risk.
- Educate family/caregivers on sundowning in the evenings.
- Maintain routine and consistency. Treat patient in own environment when possible.
- Build on patient's intact skills during therapy.
- Mirroring techniques may increase patient understanding of what to do (you want the patient to lift the right arm, you face the patient and lift your left arm as they lift their right arm).
- Hand-over-hand facilitation techniques include the PTA manually placing their arm on the patient's limb to be moved taking the patient's arm and moving it into the desired position.
- Task breakdown and chaining techniques are initiated by whole to part to whole observation for a task analysis, and then break the task down into simple segments for movement (i.e., ultimate goal is supine to sit; PTA practices rolling to side lying first, once mastered incorporates side lying to sit and do chain linking to put patterns together to achieve the ultimate goal of the task).
- As disease progresses, keep patient as functional as possible to decrease caregiver burden.
- End stage situations result in caregiver training for transfers, bed mobility, pressure relief, body mechanics for caregiving safety, and provision of resources for assistance and respite if warranted.

Vascular Dementia

Vascular dementia accounts for 15–30% of dementias; it is caused by large and small vascular infarcts in both the gray and white matter of brain, which lead to loss of brain function. Vascular dementia is associated with a history of stroke, hypertension, and cardiovascular disease. It has a sudden onset rather than an insidious course. Deficits have a spotty and patchy distribution; areas of preserved ability may coexist with impairments. Impairments and activity limitations include gait and balance abnormalities, muscular weakness, exaggerated DTRs, and emotional lability.

(continued)

Table 9.22 **Cognitive Disorders: Intervention Goals**   *(continued)*

Dementia Intervention Goals

1. Provision of a safe living environment—to prevent injury, falls, and consequently further dysfunction
2. Patient's safety from wandering—use of safety monitoring devices
3. Provision of a calming environment and reduction of environmental disturbances—reduces agitation and increases the patient's attention
4. Maintaining the patient's remaining functional abilities—by retraining the patient in ADLs; by approaching the patient in a friendly, supportive manner and modeling calm behavior
5. Use of consistent, simple commands and speaking slowly
6. Use of nonverbal communication, such as sensory cues, gesture, and demonstration
7. Reorienting the patient as necessary—by using prompts, calendars, daily schedules, and memory aids
8. Avoidance of stressful tasks and emphasis on familiar, well-learned skills
9. Use of simple learning techniques—repetitions, progressing slowly, and adequate rest time
10. Intellectual stimulation, such as simple, well-liked activities and games
11. Regular physical activity interventions—a walking program; balance activities for fall prevention; activities to promote body awareness and sensory stimulation
12. Family education (team approach to the patient's care)

Depression

Depression is one of several mood disorders characterized by lack of interest or pleasure in activities and living. It is frequently found in older adults living in the community and in institutions.

The U.S. Preventive Services Task Force recommends screening all patients for depression in primary care settings. A simple means of screening for depression is to ask patients two questions: (1) "Over the past 2 weeks, have you felt depressed or hopeless?" and (2) "Over the past 2 weeks, have you felt little interest or pleasure in doing things?"

Predisposing factors for depression may include family history, prior episodes of depression, illness, medications' side effects, hormonal imbalances, chronic conditions, a loss of physical functions, pain (especially after a stroke), loss of vision or hearing, losses among the family or friends (death of the spouse or a close friend), loss of a job, loss of income, loss of independence, social isolation (including lack of family support), and psychological losses (such as memory and/or intellectual functions).

Characteristics of Depression

- Sadness
- Hopelessness
- Tearfulness
- A loss of energy
- Persistent fatigue
- Persistent feelings of guilt or self-criticism

(continued)

Table 9.22 Cognitive Disorders: Intervention Goals   *(continued)*

- Irritability and agitation
- Inability to concentrate
- A decreased interest in ADLs and, consequently, self-neglect
- Changes in appetite or body weight (losing or gaining weight)
- Insomnia or excessive sleep
- Recurrent thoughts of death or suicide
- Local and general body weakness
- Impaired memory
- Indecisiveness
- Withdrawal from family and friends

Depression Intervention Goals

1. The PTA should report a patient's (client's) depression characteristics immediately to the PT.
2. The PT will recommend that the patient receive medical interventions (see a physician, psychotherapist, or behavioral therapist; receive medications; receive adequate nutrition and hydration).
3. The therapist should avoid excessive cheerfulness when working with the patient (client) and provide support and encouragement.
4. The therapist should assist the patient in the adjustment process (for losses).
5. Provide patient education (for coping strategies).
6. The therapist should encourage activities and exercise programs (such as an aerobic training program).
7. The therapist should assist the patient in improving and maintaining independence (through patient education related to independent skills).
8. The therapist should focus on reaching short-term goals (rather than long-term goals).

Depression PTA Pearls[1]

- Positive reinforcement provided in an upbeat manner may result in increased motivation.
- Use humor, empathetic kindness, and nurturing to promote return to a more optimal level of functioning.
- Daily interactions and relationship building may facilitate increased motivation to regain function and potentially break the depressive cycle.

Cardiopulmonary Disorders and Diseases: Intervention Goals

Table 9.23 Cardiopulmonary Disorders and Diseases: Intervention Goals

Hypertension (Blood Pressure (BP) > 130/80 mm Hg)

- Common condition affecting the cardiovascular system; one of the major risk factors for coronary artery disease (CAD), congestive heart failure (CHF), stroke, peripheral vascular disease (PVD), kidney failure, and retinopathy.
- Research shows that controlling hypertension increases longevity and helps prevent cardiovascular illnesses.
- Older patients taking medications for hypertension can have drug-induced side effects such as dizziness, hypokalemia, depression, syncope, and confusion.

Hypertension PTA Pearls

- Elderly adults with BP above 160 mm Hg systolic and 95 mm Hg diastolic may be at an increased risk for CVA, CHF, and renal failure.[1]
- Monitor BP during interventions.
- Monitor for orthostatic hypotension due to renal insufficiency, with drug metabolism or medication side effects.[1]
- Have patients count aloud to decrease breath holding during treatment.
- Look for outward facial signs of redness during activity.
- Act on any complaints of new onset of headaches or increased pressure in the head while exercising.
- Seek immediate medical attention if the patient reports vision changes, slurs words, exhibits facial drooping, or complain of chest discomfort during treatment.

Coronary Artery Disease (CAD)

- Narrowing of the coronary arteries as a result of atherosclerosis.
- CAD accounts for most of the hospital admissions of older persons.
- CAD is characterized by the following:
  1. Angina. Warning: Angina pain is not always a consistent indicator of ischemia in older patients; shortness of breath and other indicators, such as light headedness and dizziness, may be better indicators of ischemia than angina pain.
  2. EKG changes. ST-segment depression may be the most reliable indicator in older patients.
  3. Acute myocardial infarction (MI). The clinical presentation of MI in older adults may differ from that in younger adults; CAD may present with sudden dyspnea, acute confusion, and syncope. The clinical course of MI is often more complicated in older patients, and mortality rates are higher than in younger adults.

Congestive Heart Failure (CHF)

- Inability of the heart to circulate blood effectively and meet the body's metabolic needs.
- Older patients having CHF may present with shortness of breath (because of inadequate oxygen to the heart muscles); marked need for rest even after mild physical activity; rising pulse over the day, with a slow and incomplete recovery during resting periods; difficulty in completing ADLs; dyspnea while lying down to rest (causing the individual to fear going to sleep, thereby increasing fatigue); ankle edema (needs to be distinguished from the deficit in venous return); absence of the normal increase in systemic BP with exercise; and slow recovery of pulse and respiration after cessation of effort.

(continued)

Table 9.23 Cardiopulmonary Disorders and Diseases: Intervention Goals *(continued)*

Peripheral Vascular Disease (PVD)

- PVD may be the result of untreated hypertension, diabetes mellitus, and hypercholesterolemia.
- Atherosclerosis and other forms of peripheral vascular disease can lead to partial or complete obstruction of the main arterial supply to the extremities. This can cause intermittent claudication (cramping or pain in leg muscles) with a small amount of walking and skin lesions (which may lead to amputations).
- In older patients, an acute lack of oxygen to the working muscles (intermittent claudication) is very dangerous and complaints of leg pain with activity must be closely monitored.
- Impaired circulation associated with peripheral arterial disease can lead to complications with minor orthopedic problems such as a hammertoe and can induce an ulcer that may lead to gangrene (due to inadequate blood supply). Immobility, depression, renal complications, and even death (as a result of thrombosis or hemorrhage) are possible consequences of poorly managed PVD.

Chronic Obstructive Pulmonary Disease (COPD)

- Asthma: reversible obstructive airway disease with episodic increases in airway resistance due to spasm and narrowing of airways in response to infection, allergic reaction, and environmental conditions.
- Emphysema: abnormal increase in the size of air spaces distal to the terminal bronchiole and destruction of the alveolar walls.
- Chronic bronchitis: chronic inflammation of the tracheobronchial tree with increased mucus secretion due to cigarette smoking or environmental agents such as asbestos, silica, coal, and dust.
- Older patients (clients) may have comorbid emphysema and chronic bronchitis.
- The impairments caused by COPD in older patients (clients) may present (because of hypoxia or hypercapnia) as shortness of breath (dyspnea), confusion, and fatigue.

Pneumonia

- Pneumonia is an infectious pulmonary disease that requires hospitalization.
- Older patients do not necessarily experience high fever and productive cough (as typical symptoms), but rather show altered mental status (confusion), alteration of sleep and wake cycles, anorexia, tachypnea, and dehydration.
- Early recognition of pneumonia is very important for successful medical interventions.

Valve Diseases of the Heart[1]

- The function of heart valves is to allow blood to flow in one direction.
- Compromise of flow results in valvular diseases.
- There are two types:
  1. Valvular stenosis = narrowing or stenosis of the valve
  2. Valve insufficiency = regurgitation or back flow of blood as the valve does not close completely
- Mitral valve and aortic valves are the two most commonly affected by the aging process.
- Etiology: rheumatic fever for mitral valve stenosis and vascular insufficiency in the elderly.
- Complications include: CHF, cardiac arrhythmias and thromboembolic events.

(continued)

Table 9.23 Cardiopulmonary Disorders and Diseases: Intervention Goals *(continued)*

Cardiopulmonary Intervention Goals

1. Patient education for CAD prevention—reduction or discontinuation of risk factors such as cigarette smoking and controlling hypertension
2. Cardiac and pulmonary interventions (see the "Cardiopulmonary Interventions" section)
3. Cardiac exercise prescription using the exercise tolerance test
4. Maintaining consistency with medications
5. Not exceeding the target heart rate during exercises
6. Increasing the recovery time during cardiac rehabilitation or aerobic exercises
7. Individualizing the warm-up and/or the cool-down periods (to address muscle imbalances, postural deficits, and/or flexibility problems)
8. Increasing the patient's (client's) functional level

PTA Pearls for Cardiac Dysfunctions (CAD, COPD, Angina, PVD)[1]

General Considerations

- Use rate of perceived exertion (RPE's) to monitor patients versus target heart rate as medications may blunt cardiopulmonary responses to exercises.
- Use talk test to monitor cardiovascular response to exercise in conjunction with RPE.
- If dyspnea occurs during exercise, consider positional changes to those of lesser energy expenditure (i.e., if standing, transition to sitting, sitting transition to supine legs elevated).
- Monitor oxygen saturation rates keeping above 90% whenever possible.
- Use deep breathing, ankle pumping, or fisting to try to promote increased venous return if the patent has patent vessels.
- Encourage diaphragmatic breathing for relaxation or to calm anxiousness when appropriate.

COPD/EMPHYSEMA

- All of the above.
- Use pursed lip breathing for COPD as it allows air to stay in lungs longer[13]; cue "smell the roses" (for 2 counts), "blow out the candles" (for 4 counts).[14]

PVD

- All of the above.
- Monitor for skin lesion in PVD such as hammer toes or claw toes as these could lead to potential gangrenous situations due to poor or lack of vascularity in the distal extremities.[1]
- Monitor distal pulses and check for paleness and coolness of the limb to detect changes in vascular perfusion and seek medical intervention if these signs and symptoms are observed in the patient with PVD.

CHF

- All of the above.
- Check with RN for fluid restrictions, bed rest, or daily weighing to determine fluid retention.
- Fluid retention typically is reported by the patient as "shortness of breath," "easily fatigued," or having "heavy limbs."

(continued)

Table 9.23 **Cardiopulmonary Disorders and Diseases: Intervention Goals** *(continued)*

- Focus of treatment is on ADLs and functional tasks incorporating rest breaks, breathing strategies, and relaxation techniques into the treatment session.
- Intermittent compression is not indicated in CHF.
- Elevation of the lower extremities above heart level is not indicated as distal edema interferes with venous return. Consultation with supervising PT or RN is warranted for interventional strategies related to distal edema related to CHF.
- Monitor systolic BP in patients with CHF as it does not rise as expected with the younger client or the patient without CHF.
- Stroke volume decreases versus increase in the patient with CHF.
- Heart rate recovery and ventilation is slow compared to the patient without CHF or younger client.
- Dilated cardiomyopathies may include pulmonary edema and may present with low oxygenation saturation rates, dyspnea, and increased metabolic need for cardiac contraction, warranting the use of Digoxin.
- Lasix may also be used to treat peripheral edema therefore, electrolyte monitoring for imbalances is necessary especially with multi-organ system decline

Valve Disorders (valvular stenosis = "narrowing" and valve insufficiency = "blood regurgitation")

- Exercise is introduced gradually and progressed slowly.
- Allow for rest periods as needed; patients with valve disorders fatigue easily.
- Anti-coagulation is common = increased risk of bleeding/bruising during interventions.
- Skin protection due to blood thinning consequences with anti-coagulation.
- Use RPE to monitor exercise intensities as medication may blunt heart rate responses and latent closing of the valves may impact overall tolerance to active interventions and ADL training.

Integumentary Conditions and Diseases and Intervention Goals for Pressure Ulcers

Table 9.24 **Integumentary Conditions and Diseases and Intervention Goals for Pressure Ulcers**

Pressure (Decubitus) Ulcers

Pressure ulcers (decubitus ulcers) are localized areas of tissue ischemia and ulcer formation; they result from prolonged pressure over an area or damage to the skin by shear forces. These ulcers are potentially fatal in frail older and chronically ill patients.

Risk Factors for Decubitus Ulcers

- Immobility and inactivity
- Sensory impairments
- Cognitive deficits
- Decreased circulation
- Poor nutritional status
- Incontinence and moisture

(continued)

Table 9.24 Integumentary Conditions and Diseases and Intervention Goals for Pressure Ulcers *(continued)*

Bony Prominences That Are Common Sites of Decubitus Ulcer Formation

- Ischial tuberosities
- Sacrum
- Greater trochanter
- Heels
- Ankles
- Elbows
- Scapulae

Assessments and Reassessments for Decubitus Ulcers

- Sensory deficits
- Cognitive impairments
- Hygiene (incontinence)
- Mobility and activity level of patient
- Effective use of pressure-relieving devices
- Pressure sore risk assessment (Norton or Braden Scales)

Decubitus Ulcers Intervention Goals

1. Prevention (paying special attention to potential areas of skin breakdown)
2. Regular skin inspection
3. Patient, family, and medical personnel education about proper skin care—cleansing and drying the skin; applying skin emollients and lubricants; eliminating mechanical forces; maintaining clean, dry linen and clothing
4. Wound care (see the "Integumentary Interventions" section)
5. Pressure relief: frequent positioning changes—every 2 hours or less while lying in bed and every 15 minutes or less while sitting; turning schedules
6. Consistent use of appropriate pressure-relieving devices—air fluid beds, waterbeds, and beds with polystyrene beads; using a log for checking adherence to the pressure-relieving devices schedule
7. Improvement of circulation and healing—physical agents such as electrical current and ultrasound; active ROM; passive ROM; functional mobility training through ambulation and use of assistive devices as necessary
8. Discussion of the patient's nutritional status with the rehabilitation team members

Herpes Zoster (Shingles)

- Herpes zoster (shingles) is the result of an acute viral infection (varicella-zoster or chickenpox virus) and is associated with inflammation of the posterior root ganglia of only a few segments of the spinal or cranial peripheral nerves.
- The patient has intense pain (especially in older patients) and vesicular eruption.
- The virus may cause meningitis or affect the optic nerve or hearing.

Skin Cancer

Malignant skin tumors increase in incidence with age. Types of skin cancers include the following:

- Basal cell carcinoma: most common human cancer; found on the skin exposed to sun or other forms of ultraviolet light. It begins as a small shiny papule and enlarges to form a whitish border around a central depression or ulcer that may bleed.

(continued)

Table 9.24 Integumentary Conditions and Diseases and Intervention Goals for Pressure Ulcers *(continued)*

- Malignant skin tumors increase in incidence with age. Types of skin cancers include the following:
- Basal cell carcinoma: most common human cancer; found on the skin exposed to sun or other forms of ultraviolet light. It begins as a small shiny papule and enlarges to form a whitish border around a central depression or ulcer that may bleed.
- Squamous cell carcinoma: carcinoma that develops primarily from squamous cells; can be found on the skin, mouth, lungs, bronchi, esophagus, or cervix.
- Malignant melanoma: malignant tumor of darkly pigmented cells that often arises in a brown or black mole; it can spread aggressively throughout the body to the brain and other internal organs. This type of skin cancer has higher prevalence in older individuals. Approximately 90% of melanomas occur on the skin; survival depends on the depth of the lesion and whether it is ulcerated and thicker.
- See Part 8, Table 8.23 for ABCDEs of skin cancer detection.

Metabolic Disease Associated with the Aging Process

Table 9.25 Diabetes Mellitus: Intervention Goals

Diabetes Mellitus[3]

- Diabetes mellitus (DM) is a disorder of carbohydrate metabolism characterized by elevated blood sugar (hyperglycemia) and sugar in urine (glycosuria).
- Type 1 DM (insulin-dependent or juvenile-onset diabetes): inadequate production of insulin.
- Type 2 DM (non–insulin-dependent): inadequate utilization of insulin. Type 2 DM results partly from a decreased sensitivity of muscle cells to insulin-mediated glucose uptake and partly from a relative decrease in pancreatic insulin secretion.
- Aging is associated with deteriorating glucose tolerance and type 2 DM (which is caused primarily by obesity and sedentary lifestyles).

Medical Problems Associated with Long-Term Elevation of Blood Glucose

- Neuropathy
- Retinopathy and blindness
- Cardiovascular disease
- Cerebral vascular accident
- Peripheral ulcerations (feet ulcerations)
- Kidney disease
- Reduced resistance to infections
- Erectile dysfunction

(continued)

Table 9.25 Diabetes Mellitus: Intervention Goals *(continued)*

Classic Symptoms of DM

- Frequent urination
- Increased thirst
- Dizziness on arising
- Fatigue
- Nausea
- Weight loss
- Blurred vision

Severe DM can progress to delirium, coma, or death.

DM Intervention Goals

1. A dietary assessment should be recommended for the patient and referral to a dietician.
2. Exercises and activities are important, as they may delay disease onset, improve blood glucose control and circulation, and reduce cardiovascular risks.
3. Exercise testing is recommended prior to exercise because of the patient's increased cardiovascular risk; the exercise prescription should include daily aerobic exercises.
4. The response to exercise depends on the adequacy of disease control.
5. Monitor the patient for exercise/activity-induced hypoglycemia (symptoms: anxiety, confusion, dizziness, unusual fatigue, headache, nausea, and sweating).
6. Provide patient education about exercise/activity-induced hypoglycemia. The patient should recognize symptoms of low blood sugar such as confusion, sweats, and palpitations.
7. Provide patient education about hypoglycemia control, including reducing insulin use or increasing carbohydrate intake prior to or during exercise.
8. Provide patient education about hyperglycemia. The patient should recognize symptoms of high blood sugar such as excessive urination and excessive thirst.
9. Provide patient education on skin care, especially of the legs and feet.
10. Provide patient education on health promotion measures (e.g., to reduce other atherosclerotic risk factors through smoking cessation and control of hypertension).

Diabetes Mellitus (DM) PTA Pearls

- Distal neuropathy may result in increased falls risk.
- Check skin, especially with AFO use.
- Check tops of toes, inferior medial malleoli, heels, and fifth digits for shoe rubbing.
- If using iontophoresis, inquire as to patient's sugar levels as dexamethasone may result in elevated glucose responses.
- Monitor patient for hypoglycemic responses to exercise.
- Request the patient to carry glucose replacement tabs to treatment.
- Observe for adverse responses to glucose metabolism in the diabetic exerciser such as anxiety, chills, confusion, paleness, diaphoresis, headache, nausea, vision changes, shakiness, drowsiness. Action: Consume foods containing sugar.

(continued)

Table 9.25 **Diabetes Mellitus: Intervention Goals** *(continued)*

Hypothyroidism

Hypothyroidism is the underproduction of thyroid hormone. In the aging person, signs and symptoms of this disease process can be subtle and sometimes overlooked as they can mimic normal aging processes. Vague symptoms are often reported and treatment typically involves medication replacement of the thyroid hormone.

Commonly reported symptoms include the following:

- Fatigue
- Weight gain
- Muscle and joint pains
- Lethargy
- Intolerance to cold temperatures
- Constipation
- Dry skin

Hyperthyroidism

Hyperthyroidism is the overproduction of thyroxin. Medication management is also the treatment choice for resolution or management of this condition.

Common clinical characteristics include the following:

- Glucose intolerance (diabetes mellitus)
- Congestive heart failure
- Muscle weakness
- Weight loss
- Atrial fibrillation

PTA Pearls for Hypoparathyroidism/Hyperthyroidism[1]

- Aquatic rehab may be beneficial if complaints of joint pain and muscle aches are predominant.
- Monitor fatigue levels during exercise allowing for rest breaks as needed.
- Ambulation-based functional exercises may promote improved motility for relief with constipation.
- If anticoagulation therapy is used for atrial fibrillation, increased risk for bleeding or bruising may result.

* These medical diagnoses do not typically require physical therapy interventions; however, if the patient has other multisystem dysfunctions that warrant treatment, these conditions may be part of the patient's medical history which may contribute to overall outcomes with treatment. For example, the patient who had a total knee arthroplasty (TKA) with a history of hypothyroidism is coming to PT. The main impairments being treated will relate to the TKA; however, the PTA must consider the impact the hypothyroidism may have on overall tolerance to treatment.

Immobility: Intervention Goals

Table 9.26 Immobility: Intervention Goals

- Impaired mobility and disability can result from a host of diseases and problems; limitations in function increase with age, especially in individuals older than 65 years.
- Immobility can result in additional health problems leading to complications in almost every major organ system:
  - Pressure sores
  - Contractures
  - Bone loss
  - Muscular atrophy
  - General deconditioning
  - Negative nitrogen and calcium balance
  - Impaired glucose tolerance
  - Decreased blood plasma volume
  - Altered drug absorption and metabolism
  - Loss of positive self-image and depression
  - Confusion
  - Dementia secondary to sensory deprivation
  - Egocentricity
  - Loss of independence and dependency

Classification of Immobility

1. Acute immobilization: due to acute catastrophic illnesses such as severe blood loss, burns, and hip fracture
2. Chronic immobilization: due to long-standing problems such as CVA, amputations, arthritis, PD, low back pain, and cardiopulmonary diseases
3. Accidental immobilization: due to accidents caused by the environmental barriers in acute and chronic care settings, such as bed rails accidents, inappropriate chair accidents, or physical restraints accidents
4. Immobilization due to cognitive impairments: such as depression, anxiety, or fear of falling
5. Immobilization due to sensory changes or cancer

Intervention Goals for Immobility

1. Increase the patient's (client's) optimal function through a gradual progression of activities so that the individual can resume ADLs.
2. Prevent further complications or injury.
3. Establish a supportive relationship with the patient and patient's family.
4. Use a team approach with health professionals to address all aspects of the patient's problems (medical, pharmacological, nutrition, psychological, social, religious, physical, occupational, and speech therapy).
5. Include the patient (and patient family) in decision-making.

Falls: Intervention Goals

Table 9.27 Falls: Intervention Goals

Falls and fall injury are a major public health concern for older individuals. For the older individual, a fall may result in increased caution and fear of falling, a loss of confidence about the ability to function independently, reduced motivation and levels of activity, and increased risk of recurrent falls.

Factors That Cause Falls[3]

- Intrinsic factors: age-related factors, including decreased proprioception; slower righting reflexes; increased postural sway; balance disorders; decreased muscular tone and strength; slower gait and lower foot swing height during gait; decreased visual abilities such as depth perception, visual clarity, adaptation to dark, color sensitivity, increased sensitivity to glare, and decreased visual and spatial function; bladder incontinence

- Extrinsic factors: poor lighting; furnishings that are too low or too high; slick or irregular floor surfaces; loose carpets and throw rugs; unsafe stairways; bathroom fixtures that are too low or too high; bathroom fixtures that have no arm support; polypharmacy

Medical Conditions That May Predispose Older Patients to Falls

1. Neurologic conditions: CVA, transient ischemic attack, PD, delirium, seizures, cerebellar disorders, carotid sinus supersensitivity, myelopathy
2. Cardiovascular dysfunctions: MI, orthostatic hypotension, cardiac arrhythmias
3. Musculoskeletal conditions: deconditioning, muscular weakness, decreased ROM, altered postural synergies, foot deformities, arthritis, proximal limb myopathy, corns, calluses, bunions
4. Gastrointestinal problems: diarrhea, bleeding, loss of consciousness during or immediately after a bowel movement (defecation syncope), loss of consciousness following a meal (postprandial syncope)
5. Visual deficits: cataracts, glaucoma, age-related macular degeneration
6. Metabolic dysfunctions: hypoglycemia, hypothyroidism, anemia, dehydration, hypokalemia, hyponatremia
7. Genitourinary problems: incontinence, excessive urination at night (nocturia), loss of consciousness during urination (micturition syncope)
8. Vestibular disorders: Meniere's disease, benign proximal positional vertigo, hearing loss, acute labyrinthitis
9. Proprioception impairments: caused by peripheral neuropathy from diabetes mellitus and vitamin B_{12} deficiency
10. Psychological disorders: depression and anxiety

Medications That May Predispose Older Patients to Falls

1. Analgesics (such as opioids) and antidepressants (such as benzodiazepines) that may cause decreased alertness
2. Antihypertensive medications (such as vasodilators, diuretics, and antiarrhythmics) that may impair cerebral blood perfusion
3. Aminoglycosides (antibiotics that include gentamicin and tobramycin) and high-dose loop diuretics (to treat hypertension, CHF, and edema) that may contribute to vestibular toxicity
4. Phenothiazines (tranquilizers) that may induce extrapyramidal syndromes characterized by tremors, chorea, athetosis, and dystonia

(continued)

Table 9.27 **Falls: Intervention Goals** *(continued)*

Activity-Related Risk Factors for Falls

- Most falls occur during normal daily activities (such as getting up from a bed or chair; turning the head and the body; bending, walking, and ascending and descending stairs).
- Descending stairs is more hazardous in terms of falls than ascending stairs. The first and last steps are the most dangerous when ascending or descending stairs.
- Common sites of outdoor falls are curbs and steps.
- In institutions, the most common sites of falls are by the patient's bedside (during transfers in and out of bed) and in the bathroom.

Standardized Tests and Measures for Functional Balance and Instability[3]

- **Tinetti Performance Oriented Mobility Assessment (POMA):** assesses balance (balance subtest has nine items—four static and five dynamic) and walking (gait subtest has eight items). The maximum score is 28. Patients who score less than 19 are at high risk for falls; patients with scores between 19 and 24 are at moderate risk for falls. The POMA focuses on maintenance of posture, postural response to voluntary movement, postural response to perturbation, and gait mobility.
- **Berg Balance Scale:** assesses functional balance (14 items), including maintenance of position (sitting, standing) and postural adjustment to voluntary movements (such as sitting to standing, standing to sitting, transfers, and stepping up). The maximum score is 56; patients who score less than 36 are at high risk for falls. This test focuses on maintenance of position and postural adjustment to voluntary movement.
- **Functional Reach Test (FR; Duncan):** assesses the maximal distance a person can reach forward beyond arm's length while maintaining a fixed position in standing (single-item test). FR normative values for adults between ages 41 and 69: men, 14.9 ± 2.2; women, 13.8 ± 2.2; adults ages 70 to 87: men, 13.2 ± 1.6; women, 10.5 ± 3.5. The FR test focuses on postural responses related to voluntary upper-extremity movement and examines the limits of stability. An FR score of less than 10 is indicative of increased fall risk.
- **Falls Efficacy Scale (Tinetti Scale):** assesses functional performance in 10 common activities and the patient's (client's) extensive fear of falling that contributes to the functional decline.
- **Activities Specific Balance Confidence Scale**: a 16 item self-report measure that correlates physical functioning with falls in community dwelling older adults.
- **Four Square Step test**: measures dynamic balance in four directions.

Intervention Goals for Falls

1. Eliminate or minimize all fall risk factors by stabilizing the disease process and using medications consistently.
2. Improve functional mobility.
3. Provide exercises to increase strength and flexibility.
4. Provide sensory compensatory strategies, such as using mostly those sensory systems that are not affected instead of the affected ones—for example, using visual system in ambulation instead of proprioception.
5. Provide balance and gait training. Tai chi and evidence-based programs such as the Otago exercise program are beneficial for older adults at risk of falls.[7]
6. Provide functional training, focusing on sit-to-stand transitions, turning, walking, and ascending and descending stairs.

(continued)

Table 9.27 Falls: Intervention Goals (continued)

7. Modify ADLs as necessary for safety, by providing assistive devices and adaptive equipment as needed.
8. Allow adequate time for activities (and provide instruction in gradual position changes).
9. Provide patient safety education (e.g., identify risks, provide instructions in writing, and communicate with the family and caregivers).
10. Modify the environment to reduce falls and instability (use the environmental checklist, ensure adequate lighting, use contrasting colors to delineate hazardous areas, and simplify the environment and reduce clutter).

In Case of Falls

1. Do not attempt to lift the patient by yourself. Instead, get help, provide first aid, and call emergency services.
2. Provide reassurance to the patient.
3. Check the patient for risk factors (which may have preceded the fall).
4. Contact the supervising PT.
5. Write a report after emergency services (or help) arrives and the patient is medically stable.

Environmental Modifications to Reduce Falls

■ **Bathroom Modifications**

- Eliminate slippery surfaces in the bathtub.
- Install grab bars.
- Eliminate unstable towel racks near the tub and the shower.
- Check for adequate room lighting for the bathroom cabinets.
- Check for safe distances while trying to reach objects in the bathroom cabinets.
- Ensure that the medications stored in the bathroom cabinets have correct and legible labeling.

■ **Kitchen Modifications**

- Place kitchen cabinets at proper height so that the person does not need to reach excessively.
- Eliminate slippery surfaces in the kitchen.
- Make sure appliances of adequate size so that the patient can read all the controls.
- Ensure that kitchen tables have stable legs.
- If the kitchen table has curved legs, check that they do not impede the walking path.
- Ensure that kitchen chairs are sturdy with arms and without leg rollers.
- Move hard-to-reach items in upper cabinets from higher shelves to lowest shelf and from lower cabinets to counter tops.

■ **Stairs Modifications**

- Ensure that the step height on the stairs should be 6 inches or less.
- Provide handrails for stairs.
- Use nonskid stair surfaces.
- Provide proper lighting in stairways.
- If there are inclines on the stairs, ensure that they are not too long to be managed by the person, and that there are places where someone can rest.

(continued)

Table 9.27 **Falls: Intervention Goals** *(continued)*

- **Other Environmental Considerations**
    - Properly position electrical cords so they do not impede walking.
    - Eliminate unstable furniture.
    - Arrange furniture to minimize obstacles.
    - Ensure a comfortable temperature in the house or room.
    - Eliminate throw rugs that may impede walking.
    - Use hallway lighting at night.
    - Watch for pets under foot.
    - Keep hallways clear of clutter.

Table 9.28 **Polypharmacy and Multipharmacy**[1]

Polypharmacy is the use of multiple drugs for the same condition (i.e., taking more than one glucose-lowering medication).

Multipharmacy is the use of multiple drugs used to treat multiple pathologies related to aging.

Polypharmacy and multipharmacy includes the use of over-the-counter medication in addition to prescribed medications.

PTA Pearls

- Medical complexity of the aging patient may result in polypharmacy and multipharmacy.
- Older adults often see multiple doctors who may be unaware of drugs prescribed by other providers. Educate the patient to take a list of current medications to every doctor's visit.
- Aging renal system or aging effects of digestive system or liver may affect medication metabolism.
- Adverse drug events are more frequent in older adults.
- Polypharmacy and multipharmacy may exacerbate medication metabolism and may increase fall risks due to adverse responses such as orthostatic hypotension, increased confusion, agitation, cognitive dysfunction.
- Ototoxicity may result from medications.
- Include balance and coordination/habituation exercises and vestibular rehabilitation exercises for ototoxicity.

Reimbursement Overview

Medicare Reimbursement

Table 9.29 Medicare Reimbursement[3,15,16]

- Medicare is the largest provider of health services in the United States. This program was established in 1965 by the U.S. Congress as Title XVIII of the Social Security Act to provide medical coverage and healthcare services to individuals 65 years old or older and younger adults with certain disabilities or end stage renal disease. It is administered by the Centers for Medicare and Medicaid Services (CMS).
- Medicare funding comes from the Social Security payroll deductions of employees, the Social Security Act contributions of persons who are self-employed, and the Social Security contributions of employers.
- Medicare provides medical coverage and healthcare services to individuals 65 years or older, persons younger than 65 years who have a long-term disability, persons younger than 65 years who have chronic renal disease, and widows 50 years or older who are eligible for disability payments.
- The fee-for-service Medicare program has two major parts: Medicare Part A and Medicare Part B. Medicare Part A is the hospital insurance part; Medicare Part B is the medical insurance part. Medicare Part A requires no premiums if an individual or his or her spouse paid Medicare taxes while working. If a beneficiary does not get premium-free Medicare Part A, the person may be able to buy it (under certain conditions). If individuals have limited income and resources, their state may help them pay for Part A. Medicare Part B requires premiums because it is considered a supplemental medical insurance program that is purchased separately by the beneficiary. The beneficiary must pay a monthly premium to acquire Medicare Part B coverage. In addition, every Medicare beneficiary (Part A and Part B) must pay deductibles and coinsurance.

Medicare Part A Coverage

1. Most inpatient hospital services and supplies
2. Skilled nursing facility services (including rehabilitative services, albeit only after a 3-day inpatient hospital stay for a related illness or injury and only for a limited time; does not cover long-term care)
3. Certain home health agency services such as home health aide services, physical therapy, occupational therapy, and speech and language pathology ordered by a physician and provided by a Medicare certified home health agency
4. Hospice care (for people with a terminal illness, defined as having less than 6 months to live; care is usually given in the patient's home, including in a nursing facility if that is the person's home)

Medicare Part B Coverage

Covers medically necessary services and supplies (i.e., those services or supplies ordered by a physician). Covers some preventive and screening services (see examples below).

1. Physician visits (but not routine physical exams except for the one-time "Welcome to Medicare" physical exam within 6 months of being a Medicare beneficiary)
2. Outpatient hospital services as part of a physician's care, including outpatient physical therapy, occupational therapy, and speech and language pathology services
3. Outpatient laboratory tests and X-rays, MRIs, CT scans, EKGs, and other diagnostic tests
4. Prosthetic and orthotic items
5. Surgical dressings for treatment of a surgical or surgically treated wound
6. Certain home health services, limited to reasonable and necessary part-time or intermittent skilled nursing care and home health aide services as well as physical therapy, occupational therapy, and speech and language pathology services that are ordered by a physician and provided by a Medicare-certified home health agency
7. Home health services such as medical social services, durable medical equipment (such as wheelchairs, hospital beds, oxygen, and walkers), and medical supplies for use at home
8. Kidney dialysis services and supplies (in a facility or at home)

(continued)

Table 9.29 **Medicare Reimbursement**[3,15,16] *(continued)*

9. Hearing and balance exam (if ordered by a physician); hearing aids and exams for fitting hearing aids are not covered
10. Influenza, pneumococcal, and Hepatitis B shots (for people with Medicare who are at high or medium risk for hepatitis B)
11. Mammogram screening (to check for breast cancer once every 12 months)
12. Medical nutrition therapy services (for people who have diabetes or renal disease and for people who have kidney disease but are not on dialysis)
13. Mental health care (with certain limits)
14. Smoking cessation counseling (if ordered by a physician)
15. Cardiac rehabilitation programs

Medicare Part C Coverage/Medicare Advantage

A health insurance policy (HMO or PPO) administered by a private healthcare entity that is contracted by Medicare to provide optional plans for Medicare beneficiaries; associated with in-network and out-of-network rates for services.

■ Must be eligible for Medicare A and Medicare B to qualify for this program. Medicare Advantage plans provide complete Part A and Part B coverage and some things not covered in original Medicare i.e., vision, hearing, and dental.

■ Patients with end-stage renal disease are not eligible for Part C.

■ Must enroll in a Medicare Advantage Plan that serves the region where you reside.

■ Beneficiaries must subscribe and enroll in Medicare Part C, and they offer different options and price points for coverage.

■ Most Medicare Advantage plans include drug coverage.

Medicare Part D Coverage

■ Must be enrolled in Medicare A and Medicare B to qualify for this program.

■ Medicare Part D is Medicare's Prescription Drug Coverage program.

■ Medicare Part D is optional for beneficiaries.

■ Has two options:

1. Stand-alone optional policy that can be purchased by the Medicare beneficiary
2. Medicare Advantage (HMO or PPO) prescription coverage that is part of the Part C option, so all benefits are attached to one plan

Medicare Special Concerns for the PTA—Skilled Maintenance (APTA Guidance)[17]

■ Medical necessity is still required for skilled maintenance.

■ Skilled maintenance therapy under Medicare does not require the potential for improvement.

■ Improvement is not expected and should not determine coverage.

■ Consideration for coverage is to be based on individualized assessment of the patient's condition.

■ Consideration for coverage is based on need for skilled care to carry out a safe and effective maintenance program.

■ Skilled maintenance therapy is covered in cases in which needed therapeutic interventions require the skills and judgment of a physical therapist due to the high level of complexity related to the patient's diagnosis. Documentation should reflect that skilled services were provided.

■ The disease does not have to be chronic or progressive in nature to be considered maintenance therapy.

(continued)

Table 9.29 Medicare Reimbursement[3,15,16]   *(continued)*

PTA and Skilled Maintenance Provision of Services[17]

- Skilled nursing, Medicare Part B patients—PTA may provide treatment for skilled maintenance.
- Skilled nursing, Medicare Part A patients—PTA may provide both maintenance and/or rehabilitative treatment.
- Home health care, Medicare A patients—the PTA may provide skilled maintenance.

Table 9.30 Medicare Guidelines for PTA Supervision During Interventions[18]

	Supervision	Direct Supervision	General Supervision
Home Health			X
In-Patient Hospital	X		
Out-Patient Hospital	X		
Physician's Office		X	
Private Practice		X	
Skilled Nursing Facility			X

Supervision: when there is no specific delineation of the type of direction required, the provider must defer to his or her physical therapy state practice act to safely and effectively perform services only by or under the supervision of a qualified PT.
Direct supervision: At the time the service is performed, the supervising private practice therapist must be present in the office suite.
General Supervision: requires the initial direction and periodic inspection of the actual activity. However, the supervisor need not always be physically present or on the premises when the assistant is performing services, but the supervising therapist must be readily available.

References

1. Bottomley JM. *Geriatric Rehabilitation: A Text Book for the Physical Therapist Assistant.* Thorofare, NJ: SLACK Incorporated; 2010.

2. Khachiyants N, Trinkle D, Son SJ, Kim KY. Sundown syndrome in persons with dementia: An update. *Psychiatry Investigation*, 2011;8(4): 275–287. http://doi.org/10.4306/pi2011.8.4.275.

3. Kauffman TL, Scott R, Bar JO, Moran ML, Wolf SL. *A Comprehensive Guide to Geriatric Rehabilitation.* 3rd ed. St. Louis, MO: Elsevier; 2014.

4. Morley, JE. Sarcopenia in the elderly. *Family Practice.* http://fampra.oxfordjournals.org/content/29/suppl_1/i44.long Published July 29, 2011. Accessed July 2016.

5. Academy of Geriatric Physical Therapy. Practice Resources. https://geriatricspt.org/practice/. Accessed July 12, 2021.

6. Manske RC. *Fundamental Orthopedic Management for the Physical Therapist Assistant.* 4th ed. St. Louis, MO: Elsevier; 2016.

7. Kisner C, Colby L. *Therapeutic Exercise Foundations and Techniques.* 6th ed. Philadelphia, PA. F.A. Davis Company; 2012.

8. Umphred D, Lazaro RT. *Neurorehabilitation for the Physical Therapist Assistant.* 2nd ed. Thorofare, NJ: SLACK Incorporated; 2014.

9. American Heart Association. Types of aphasia. http://www.strokeassociation.org/STROKEORG/LifeAfterStroke/RegainingIndependence/CommunicationChallenges/Types-of-Aphasia_UCM_310096_Article.jsp#Aphasia. Updated March 8, 2013. Accessed July 2016.

10. 6 strategies to help comprehension with Wernicke's aphasia. theaphasiacenter.com. http://www.theaphasiacenter.com/2013/12/6-strategies-help-comprehension-wernickes-aphasia/. Updated 2014. Accessed July 2016.

11. Fox C, Ebersbach G, Ramig L, Sapir S. LSVT LOUD and LSVT BIG: Behavioral treatment programs for speech and body movement in Parkinson disease. *Parkinson's Disease.* 2012. doi:10.1155/2012/391946

12. American Physical Therapy Association. Clinical summary: Dementia. https://www.apta.org/patient-care/evidence-based-practice-resources/clinical-summaries/dementia. Accessed July 12, 2021.

13. Cleveland Clinic. Pursed lip breathing. http://my.clevelandclinic.org/health/diseases_conditions/hic_Understanding_COPD/hic_Pulmonary_Rehabilitation_Is_it_for_You/hic_Pursed_Lip_Breathing. Accessed July 2016.

14. How to breathe when you are short of breath. medlineplus.gov. https://www.nlm.nih.gov/medlineplus/ency/patientinstructions/000053.htm. Reviewed February 2, 2016. Accessed July 2016.

15. Centers for Medicare and Medicaid Services. Medicare information. https://www.cms.gov/Medicare/Medicare. Accessed July 13, 2021.

16. Medicare. Medicare coverage. https://www.medicare.gov/what-medicare-covers. Accessed July 13, 2021.

17. American Physical Therapy Association. Medicare coverage: Skilled maintenance. https://www.apta.org/your-practice/payment/medicare-payment/coverage-issues/skilled-maintenance-therapy-under-medicare. Accessed July 13, 2021.

18. American Physical Therapy Association. Supervision under Medicare. Use of physical therapist assistants (PTAs) under Medicare. https://www.apta.org/your-practice/payment/medicare-payment/supervision-under-medicare/ptas-under-medicare. Accessed July 13, 2021.

Pediatric Interventions

Pediatric Overview

Pediatric Screening Tests

Table 10.1 Pediatric Screening Tests[1,2]

Test	Age Range	Characteristics
Apgar	At 1 and 5 minutes after birth	Screening test performed by physicians or nurses; administered to a newborn infant twice, at 1 and 5 minutes after birth. The Apgar test measures the newborn's heart rate, breathing function, color, muscle tone, and response to stimulation. The results determine the immediate care necessary for the newborn. A score of 7–10 is normal. A score of less than 7 indicates that the baby needs assistance (e.g., to assist in breathing).
Neonatal Behavioral Assessment Scale (NBAS)	3 days to 4 weeks	Assesses interactive behavior, infant competence, and neurologic status. The NBAS is an effective predictor of future neurologic problems and a good tool for teaching parents about infant behaviors.
Test of Infant Motor Performance (TIMP)	Birth to 4 months	A 42-item assessment of posture and selective motor control of movement in infants from birth to 4 months.[2]
Neurological Evaluation of the Newborn and Infant	Birth to 12 months	Measures reflexes and muscle tone and provides range of motion expectations.
Movement Assessment of Infants	Birth to 12 months	Assesses muscle tone, reflexes, automatic reactions, and purposeful movement.
Alberta Infant Motor Scale	Birth to age of walking	An observational tool that identifies the components of motor development. It differentiates atypical development from small increments that may be attributed to maturation or intervention.
Milani-Comparetti Motor Development Screening Test	Birth to 2 years	Measures functional movement, related reflex, and automatic responses. This screening test assesses motor development in infants and young children, alerts clinicians to deviations in motor development, and provides an overview of gross motor status by examining the integration of primitive reflexes and the emergence of purposeful movement.
Hawaii Developmental Charts (formerly Hawaii Early Learning Profile)	Birth to 3 years	Used to demonstrate approximate age ranges in motor, cognitive, language, self-help, and social skills. It is intended for use in planning intervention programs, documenting progress, and monitoring achievement of individual objectives.
Revised Gesell and Amatruda Developmental Neurological Exam	1 month to 5 years	Assesses four areas of development: motor, adaptive, language, and personal–social.

(continued)

Table 10.1 Pediatric Screening Tests[1]   *(continued)*

Test	Age Range	Characteristics
Bayley Scales of Infant Development II	Birth to 42 months	Includes a mental scale, motor scale, and behavioral record. It is scored as a developmental index and incorporates data on special populations (such as children with prematurity, Down syndrome, HIV, and developmental delays).
Denver Developmental Screening Test	2 weeks to 6 years	Measures four domains: personal–social, fine motor adaptive, language, and gross motor. Screens children for delays and determines the need for further evaluation.
Peabody Developmental Motor Scales	Birth to 83 months	Includes gross and fine motor scales. Standard scores and age-equivalent scores are provided. The test also identifies emerging skills. The child does not need to understand verbal language to be scored on this test.
Gross Motor Function Measure (GMFM)	Birth to 12 years	A 66-item observational tool that measures change in motor function over time in children with cerebral palsy.[2]
Pediatric Evaluation of Disability Inventory	6 months to 7.5 years	Assesses functional skills: designed for use in rehabilitation programs. It includes self-care, mobility, and social skills. Scores are based on function, amount of assistance required, and need for equipment or modification.
Miller Assessment for Preschoolers	2 years, 9 months to 5 years, 8 months	Identifies children with mild to moderate developmental delays. It combines the sensory-motor and cognitive domains and uses a developmental approach.
Tufts Assessment of Motor Performance— Pediatric Clinical Version	3 years and older	Measures functional and motor performance skills to monitor a child's response to treatment and to determine whether treatment goals were met. Measurements include proficiency of skill and time to complete skill.
Bruininks-Oseretsky Test of Motor Performance	4.5–14.5 years	Assesses gross and fine motor function to be able to make educational and therapeutic placement decisions. Scores are given as age equivalents.
Purdue Perceptual Motor Survey	6–10 years	Identifies children lacking the perceptual motor abilities needed to acquire academic skills. It includes balance and postural flexibility, body image and differentiation, perceptual–motor match, ocular control, and visual achievement forms.
Test of Motor Impairment	5–13 years	Detects motor dysfunction problems indicative of possible neurological dysfunction. It is divided into five areas: balance, upper-limb coordination, whole-body coordination, manual dexterity, and simultaneous movement.
School Function Assessment (SFA)	6–12 years	A 316-item assessment of student participation, need for support and performance of functional tasks related to ability to function in the school environment.[2]

PEDIATRIC INTERVENTIONS

Infant Reflexes and Possible Effects When Reflexes Persist

Table 10.2 Infant Reflexes and Possible Effects When Reflexes Persist[1]

Primitive Reflex	Possible Negative Effects If Persistent
Galant Reflex Stimulus: touch to the skin along the spine from shoulder to hip Response: lateral flexion of the trunk to the side of the stimulus Normal age of response: 30 weeks of gestation to 2 months	Interferes with ■ Development of sitting balance ■ Can lead to scoliosis
Positive Support Reflex Stimulus: weight placed on balls of feet when upright Response: stiffening of legs and trunk into extension Normal age of response: 35 weeks of gestation to 2 months	Interferes with ■ Standing and walking ■ Balance reactions and weight shift in standing ■ Can also lead to contractures of ankles into plantarflexion
Walking (Stepping) Reflex Stimulus: supported upright position with soles of feet on a firm surface Response: reciprocal flexion/extension of the legs Normal age of response: 38 weeks of gestation to 2 months	Interferes with ■ Standing and walking ■ Balance reactions and weight shift in standing ■ Development of smooth, coordinated reciprocal movements of lower extremities
Rooting Reflex Stimulus: touch on cheek Response: turning head to same side with mouth open Normal age of response: 28 weeks of gestation to 3 months	Interferes with ■ Oral–motor development ■ Development of midline control of the head ■ Optical righting, visual tracking, and social interaction
Palmar Grasp Reflex Stimulus: pressure in palm on ulnar side of hand Response: flexion of fingers, causing a strong grip Normal age of response: birth to 4 months	Interferes with ■ Ability to grasp and release objects voluntarily ■ Weight bearing on open hand for propping, crawling, and protective responses
Moro Reflex Stimulus: head dropping into extension suddenly for a few inches Response: arms abduct with fingers open, then cross trunk into adduction; cry Normal age of response: 28 weeks of gestation to 5 months	Interferes with ■ Balance reactions in sitting ■ Protective responses in sitting ■ Eye–hand coordination ■ Visual tracking

(continued)

Table 10.2 Infant Reflexes and Possible Effects When Reflexes Persist[1]   *(continued)*

Startle Reflex Stimulus: loud, sudden noise Response: similar to Moro response but elbows remain flexed and hands closed Normal age of response: 28 weeks of gestation to 5 months	Interferes with ■ Sitting balance ■ Protective responses in sitting ■ Eye–hand coordination ■ Visual tracking ■ Social interaction, attention
Asymmetrical Tonic Neck Reflex (ATNR) Stimulus: head position turned to one side Response: extension of arm and leg on face side; flexion of arm and leg on scalp side; spine may curve with convexity toward face side Normal age of response: Birth to 6 months.	Interferes with ■ Feeding ■ Visual tracking ■ Midline use of hands ■ Bilateral hand use ■ Rolling ■ Development of crawling If ATNR persists, it can also lead to skeletal deformities such as scoliosis, hip subluxation, and hip dislocation.
Tonic Labyrinthine Reflex (TLR) Stimulus: position of labyrinth in inner ear—reflected in head position Response: In the supine position, body and extremities are held in extension; in the prone position, body and extremities are held in flexion Normal age of response: birth to 6 months	Interferes with ■ Ability to initiate rolling ■ Ability to prop the body on the elbows with extended hips when prone ■ Ability to flex the trunk and hips to come to a sitting position from the supine position ■ Often causes full body extension, which interferes with balance in sitting or standing
Symmetrical Tonic Neck Reflex (STNR) Stimulus: head position, flexion, or extension Response: When head is in flexion, arms are flexed and legs are extended; when head is in extension, arms are extended and legs are flexed Normal age of response: 6–8 months	Interferes with ■ Ability to prop the body on the arms in prone position ■ Crawling reciprocally ■ Sitting balance when looking around ■ Attaining and maintaining hands and knees position ■ Use of hands when looking at the object in hands (in sitting)
Plantar Grasp Reflex Stimulus: pressure to base of toes Response: toe flexion Normal age of response: 28 weeks of gestation to 9 months	Interferes with ■ Ability to stand with feet flat on a surface ■ Balance reactions and weight shifting in standing

PEDIATRIC INTERVENTIONS

Impairments and Functional Limitations of Tonic Reflexes When Reflexes Persist

- When TLR in supine position persists, the child may have the following impairments: contractures, limited visual field, and abnormal vestibular input. Functional limitations may include rolling from supine to prone position, sitting, coming to sit, and reaching in supine position.
- When the TLR in prone position persists, the child may have the following impairments: contractures, abnormal vestibular input, and limited visual field. Functional limitations may include rolling from prone to supine position, sitting, and coming to sit.
- When STNR persists, the child may have the following impairments: contractures, deficiency in trunk rotation, and deficiency in upper- and lower-extremity dissociation. Functional limitations may include creeping, walking, and kneeling.
- When ATNR persists, the child may have the following impairments: contractures, trunk asymmetry, hip dislocation, and scoliosis. Functional limitations may include reaching, segmental rolling, and bringing the hand to the mouth.

Other Reflexes and Postural Reactions

Table 10.3 **Other Reflexes and Postural Reactions**

Babinski Reflex[3]

- Stimulus: stroking the lateral aspect of the plantar surface of the foot.
- Response: extension and fanning of the toes.
- Normal age of response: birth to 12 months.
- If the reflex persists, the child will have difficulty with balance in standing and weight bearing on his or her feet.

Flexor Withdrawal Reflex

- Stimulus: noxious stimulus (using pressure or causing pain) to the sole of the foot or the palm of the hands.
- Normal age of response: birth to 2 months.
- If the reflex persists, the child may have hypersensitivity to sensory stimuli.

Sucking Reflex

- Stimulus: object in mouth.
- Normal age of response: 28 weeks of gestation to 2 months.
- If the reflex persists, the child may have difficulty developing more mature oral motor patterns. It is similar to the rooting reflex.

Traction Response

- Stimulus: traction on the upper extremities as in pull to sit.
- Normal age of response: 1–5 months.
- If the reflex persists, the child may have difficulty grading the upper-extremity response to traction.

(continued)

Table 10.3 Other Reflexes and Postural Reactions *(continued)*

Landau Reflex

- Stimulus: In a prone position, when passively flexing the head forward, the child's body flexes.
- Normal age of response: 3–18 months.
- If the reflex persists, the child may have difficulty developing various body movements.
- The Landau reflex is absent in children with cerebral palsy and gross motor retardation.

Neonatal Neck Righting (Neck on Body [NOB])

- Stimulus: head turned to the side.
- Response: body turns to the side following the head.
- Normal age of response: birth to 6 months.

Optical Righting

- Stimulus: body tilted with respect to upright position.
- Response: head orients to upright position.
- Normal age of response: 1 month through adulthood.

Body Righting on Head (BOH)

- Stimulus: body contact with solid horizontal surface.
- Response: head orients to upright position.
- Normal age of response: 2 months through 5 years.

Body Righting on Body (BOB)

- Stimulus: body in contact with solid horizontal surface.
- Response: The body orients itself to gravity.
- Normal age of response: 4 months to 5 years.

Labyrinthine Righting

- Stimulus: body tilted with respect to upright with eyes blindfolded.
- Response: head orients to upright position.
- Normal age of response: 1 month through adulthood.

Tilting Reactions

- In prone (start at 5–7 months), supine (start at 7–9 months), sitting (start at 8–11 months), quadruped (start at 9–12 months), and standing (start at 12–18 months) positions.
- Stimulus: instability at the base of support.
- Response: abduction of arm, leg, and concavity of the spine toward the upward side.
- Normal age of response: 5 months through adulthood.

Protective Reactions in Sitting

- Forward at 6 months; lateral at 7 months; backward at 9 months.
- Stimulus: loss of equilibrium.
- Response: extension of the arm to support the body and keep from falling.

(continued)

Table 10.3 Other Reflexes and Postural Reactions   (continued)

Protective Reactions in Standing

- Staggering response at 15–18 months.
- Stimulus: loss of equilibrium.
- Response: placement of lower extremities to reestablish equilibrium.

Downward Parachute (or Visual Placing or Protective Extension Downward)

- Stimulus: downward momentum toward a solid surface.
- Response in the upper extremities: extension of shoulders and elbows to support self.
- Response in the lower extremities: extension of hips and knees to support self.
- Normal age of response: 4 months through adulthood.

Reflexes and Developmental Reactions of Childhood

Table 10.4 Reflexes and Developmental Reactions of Childhood

Reflexes and Developmental Reactions[1]	Effects on Development of Motor Skills
Birth to 1 Month	
Reflexes: sucking and swallowing; palmar grasp; plantar grasp; asymmetrical tonic neck; tonic labyrinthine; Galant; Moro; startle; positive support. Developmental reactions: head righting.	Infant learns vertical orientation to the world. Infant is beginning to strengthen postural muscles. Infant can lift head in prone position to clear airway.
2–3 Months	
Reflexes: traction response of arms in pull to sit is stronger. Sucking and swallowing reflexes are weaker. Galant reflex is inhibited. Stepping reflex is inhibited. Developmental reactions: optical and labyrinthine head righting develops.	Infant is able to hold head up when held at the shoulder. Infant holds head up to 90 degrees briefly in prone position, head bobbing upright in supported sitting position, and chest up in prone position with some weight through forearms.
4–5 Months	
Reflexes: integration of ATNR; integration of palmar grasp reflex. Developmental reactions: equilibrium reactions in prone position develop; protective extension forward in sitting position develops; Landau response becomes stronger.	Infant rolls from prone to supine position, pivots in prone position, bears weight through extended arms in prone position, uses forward propping beginning in sitting position, sits alone briefly, and grasps and releases toys.
6–7 Months	
Reflexes: STNR develops; Moro reflex inhibited. Developmental reactions: protective extension sideward in sitting position; equilibrium reactions in supine position.	Infant rolls from supine to prone position, holds weight on one hand to reach for toy, gets to sitting position without assistance, and stands holding on.

(continued)

Table 10.4 **Reflexes and Developmental Reactions of Childhood**   *(continued)*

Reflexes and Developmental Reactions[1]	Effects on Development of Motor Skills
8–9 Months	
Reflexes: inhibition of plantar grasp and STNR. Developmental reactions: protective extension backward develops in sitting position.	Infant gets into hands-and-knees position, moves from sitting to prone position, sits without hand support, creeps on hands and knees, and cruises along furniture.
10–11 Months	
Developmental reactions: equilibrium responses emerge in quadruped position.	Infant stands briefly without support and pulls to stand using half-kneel intermediate position.
16–24 Months	
Developmental reactions: protective extension sideways and backward in standing position.	Infant squats in play, kicks ball, and propels ride-on toys.

Pediatric Development of Gross and Fine Motor Skills

Table 10.5 **Gross and Fine Motor Skills[1]**

Newborn to 1 Month

- Gross motor skills
    1. Prone: physiological flexion, lifts head briefly, head to side
    2. Supine: physiological flexion, rolls partly to side
    3. Sitting: head lag in pull to sit
    4. Standing: reflex standing and walking
- Fine motor skills: regards objects in direct line of vision, follows moving object to midline, hands fisted, jerky arm movements, movements may be purposeful or random

2–3 Months

- Gross motor skills
    1. Prone: lifts head 90 degrees briefly, chest up in prone position with some weight through forearms, rolls prone to supine.
    2. Supine: strong ATNR influence, kicking legs reciprocally, head to side preference
    3. Sitting: variable head lag in pull to sitting position, needs full support to sit, upright but bobbing head
    4. Standing: poor weight bearing, hips in flexion, held behind shoulders
- Fine motor skills: can see farther distances, hands open more, visually follows through 180 degrees, reflexive grasp, uses palmar grasp

(continued)

Table 10.5 Gross and Fine Motor Skills[1]   *(continued)*

4–5 Months

- Gross motor skills
    1. Prone: bears weight on extended arms, pivots in prone to reach toys
    2. Supine: rolls from supine to side position, plays with feet to mouth
    3. Sitting: head steady in supported sitting position, turns head in sitting position, sits alone for brief periods
    4. Standing: bears all weight through legs in supported stand
- Fine motor skills: grasps and releases toys and uses ulnar–palmar grasp

6–7 Months

- Gross motor skills: radial-palmar grasp and "rakes" with fingers to pick up small objects
- Fine motor skills: voluntary release to transfer objects between hands

8–9 Months

- Gross motor skills
    1. Prone: gets into hands-and-knees position
    2. Supine: does not tolerate supine position
    3. Sitting: moves from sitting to prone position, sits without hand support for longer periods, pivots in sitting position
    4. Standing: stands at furniture, pulls to stand at furniture, lowers to sitting position from supported stand
    5. Mobility: crawls forward, walks along furniture (cruising)
- Fine motor skills: develops active forearm supination and radial-digital grasp, uses inferior pincer grasp, extends wrist actively, points and pokes with index finger, more refined release of objects, takes objects out of container

10–11 Months

- Gross motor skills
    1. Standing: stands without support briefly, pulls to stand using half-kneel intermediate position, picks up object from floor from standing with support
    2. Mobility: walks with both hands held, walks with one hand held, creeps on hands and feet (bear walk)
- Fine motor skills: fine pincer grasp developed, puts objects into container, grasps crayon adaptively

12–15 Months

- Gross motor skills—mobility: walks without support, fast walking, walks backward, walks sideways, bends over to look between legs, creeps or hitches upstairs, throws ball in sitting position
- Fine motor skills: marks paper with crayon, builds tower using two cubes, turns over small container to obtain contents

16–24 Months

- Gross motor skills: squats in play, walks upstairs and downstairs with one hand held and both feet on step, propels ride-on toys, kicks ball, throws ball forward, picks up toy from floor without falling
- Fine motor skills: folds paper, strings beads, stacks six cubes, imitates vertical and horizontal strokes with crayon on paper, holds crayon with thumb and finger

(continued)

Table 10.5 Gross and Fine Motor Skills[1] *(continued)*

2 Years

- Gross motor skills: rides tricycle, walks backward, walks on tiptoe, runs on toes, walks downstairs alternating feet, catches large ball, hops on one foot
- Fine motor skills: turns knob, opens and closes jar, buttons large buttons, uses child-sized scissors with help, does 12- to 15-piece puzzles, folds paper or clothes

Preschool Age (3–4 Years)

- Gross motor skills: throws ball 10 feet, hops 2 to 10 times on one foot, jumps distances of up to 2 feet, jumps over obstacles up to 12 inches, throws and catches small ball, runs fast, and avoids obstacles
- Fine motor skills: controls crayons more effectively, copies a circle or cross, matches colors, cuts with scissors, draws recognizable human figure with head and two extremities, draws squares, may demonstrate hand preference

Early School Age (5–8 Years)

- Gross motor skills: skips on alternate feet, gallops, can play hopscotch, can balance on one foot, is able to control hopping and squatting on one leg, jumps with rhythm and control (jump rope), bounces large ball, kicks ball with greater control, faster growth in limbs than trunk (allowing greater speed and leverage)
- Fine motor skills: evident hand preference, prints well, starting to learn cursive writing, able to button small buttons

Later School Age (9–12 Years)

- Gross motor skills: mature patterns of movement in throwing, jumping, running; competitiveness increases, enjoys competitive games; improved balance, coordination, endurance, attention span; (boys) possible preadolescent fat spurt; (girls) possible prepubescent and pubescent changes in body shape (hips, breasts).
- Fine motor skills: develops greater control in hand usage, learns to draw, handwriting is developed

Adolescence (13 Years)

- Gross motor skills: rapid growth in size and strength, boys more than girls; puberty leading to changes in body proportions: center of gravity rising toward shoulders for boys, lowering to hips for girls
- Fine motor skills: balance skill, coordination, eye–hand coordination, endurance plateauing during growth spurt; develops greater dexterity in fingers for fine tasks (knitting, sewing, art, crafts)

Social, Language, Cognitive, and Adaptive Skills of Childhood

Table 10.6 Social, Language, Cognitive, and Adaptive Skills of Childhood

Age	Social	Language	Cognitive	Adaptive
Newborn to 1 month	Eye contact; molds body when held; relaxes when held; regards the face	Crying to indicate needs; monotonous nasal cry; makes comfort sounds	Quiets when picked up; responds to voice; consoles self by sucking	Opens and closes mouth in response to food; beginning coordination of sucking, swallowing, and breathing

(continued)

Table 10.6 Social, Language, Cognitive, and Adaptive Skills of Childhood *(continued)*

Age	Social	Language	Cognitive	Adaptive
2–3 months	Watches speaker's eyes and mouth; responds with smile when socially approached; enjoys social play; vocalizes pleasure/displeasure	Coos open-vowel sounds; cries vary in pitch and volume to indicate different needs; laughs; squeals	Searches with eyes for sound; shows active interest in person or object for 1 minute; inspects and plays with own hands	Brings hand to mouth—better coordination of sucking, swallowing, and breathing; stays awake longer periods during the day; sleeps for longer periods at night
4–5 months	Socializes with strangers/anyone; lifts arms to mother; enjoys social play; vocalizes pleasure/displeasure	Reacts to music; reacts to own name; babbles consonant chains "bababa"; babbles to people	Looks for hidden voice; plays for 2 to 3 minutes with one toy; finds partially hidden object; works to obtain object out of reach	Holds bottle; eats pureed or strained foods; drinks from cup; naps two to three times per day; sleeps up to 12 hours at night
6–7 months	Smiles at self in mirror; does not like to be separated from mother; recognizes mother visually; anxious about strangers; yells to get attention; loves vigorous play	Babbles double-consonant "baba"; waves bye-bye; produces more consonant sounds when babbling	Looks for family members when named; shakes toys to hear sound; plays peek-a-boo; plays with paper; imitates simple gestures	Mouths solid food; feeds cracker to self; bites and chews toys
8–9 months	Lets only mother meet needs; explores environment enthusiastically; enjoys social games	Babbles single consonant "ba"; adult pattern of inflection in babbling; says "dada" or "mama" nonspecifically	Responds to simple verbal requests ("come here," "give mommy"); throws and drops objects; looks at pictures when named	Finger-feeds self; chews using munching pattern; sleeps up to 14 hours at night
10–11 months	Tests parental reactions; extends toy to show, not give	Babbles monologue when alone; says "dada" or "mama" specifically; repeats sounds or gestures if laughed at; unable to talk while walking	Enjoys looking at pictures in books; stacks and unstacks rings; guides action toy manually; dances	Holds spoon; extends arm or leg for dressing

(continued)

Table 10.6 Social, Language, Cognitive, and Adaptive Skills of Childhood *(continued)*

Age	Social	Language	Cognitive	Adaptive
12–15 months	Displays tantrum behaviors; acts impulsively; enjoys imitating adult behaviors; says "no" and resists adult control; distractible	Uses exclamatory sentences ("uh-oh," "no-no"); uses words or word approximations to express self; has one- to three-word vocabulary; says "no" meaningfully; speech may plateau as child learns to walk	Enjoys messy activities such as finger painting, feeding self; recognizes individuals outside family; helps turn pages	Brings spoon to mouth; holds cup and drinks with some spilling; indicates discomfort over dirty diaper; shows pattern of elimination behavior
16–24 months	Expresses affection; plays alone for short times; gets frustrated easily; displays wide range of emotions, including jealousy of a family member; parallel play; interacts with peers using gestures and vocalizations	Imitates environmental sounds; uses two-word sentences; attempts to sing songs; expressive vocabulary up to 50 words; uses own name to refer to self; uses jargon mixed with intelligible words	Can put things away; names six body parts; matches sounds to pictures of animals; sorts objects	Feeds self with spoon, with some spilling; uses rotary jaw movements to chew food; removes shoes; plays with food; helps with washing hands; turns knob to open doors; begins toilet training
2 years	Talks loudly; becomes bossy and demanding; obeys simple rules; has trouble with changes; separates easily from mother in familiar surroundings; may have tantrums; may develop fears of unfamiliar things such as animals or clowns	Child gains language quickly, up to four words per day; uses three-word sentences; frustrated when not understood; tells full name; recites simple nursery rhymes; sings phrases of songs	Matches shapes; completes a three- to four-piece puzzle; understands concept of "one"; understands concept of "two"; plays house; loves being read to; sorts colors, matches some colors	Undresses/dresses with help; uses spoon and fork; uses napkin; washes and dries hands; uses toilet consistently; places clothes up on hook; blows nose with help; insists on doing things without help
Preschool-aged child (3–4 years)	Enjoys making friends; plays cooperatively; needs praise and guidance from adults; enjoys helping with adult activities (shopping, setting table); enjoys imitating adult behavior; fears of unfamiliar things may continue	Child talks to self at play and rest; uses rhythmic language; uses language actively; has expressive vocabulary of up to 1,000 words; learns entire songs and nursery rhymes; loves to talk	Identifies colors and shapes; able to do a 30-piece puzzle; identifies money, coins; enjoys books; has vivid imagination; may confuse fantasy with reality	Dresses/undresses independently except for back buttons; uses toilet without help; uses utensils (fork, spoon) independently; brushes teeth with supervision; may be very modest with dressing, toileting, and bathing

PEDIATRIC INTERVENTIONS

(continued)

Table 10.6 Social, Language, Cognitive, and Adaptive Skills of Childhood

Age	Social	Language	Cognitive	Adaptive
Early school-aged child (5–8 years)	Prefers to play with peers rather than adults; refines social skills of giving, sharing, and receiving; cares deeply what others think of him or her; likes to impress peers	Uses plurals, pronouns, and tenses correctly; recites or sings rhymes, television commercials, and songs; interested in new words; has a vocabulary of 2,000 to 4,000 words	Learns to read; learns basic math skills of addition and subtraction; learns concept of conservation; learns to write (printing)	May have stomachaches related to school attendance; knows likes and dislikes with food; learns to use knife for spreading and cutting; learns to tie shoes
Late school-aged child (9–12 years)	Increased interest in group activities; spirit of adventure high; interested in organized sports and sees athletes as heroes; interested in practicing skills to gain social approval and develop skills	Increasing vocabulary and maturity of language skills	Enjoys table games; able to think more abstractly; increased attention span; intellectually curious; reads greater variety of materials, including nonfiction	Can bathe independently, wash hair with supervision; independent in daily care activities; learns to cook; takes role in household tasks
Adolescent (13–18 years)	Peer-oriented; self-conscious; interest in opposite sex; increase in social maturity	Expressive writing skills improve	Can develop hypotheses and theories; increased attention span; interests expand beyond self to environment, those less fortunate, and so on	Takes on greater household roles (laundry, cooking, cleaning); learns to drive

Juvenile Idiopathic Arthritis[4]

Juvenile idiopathic arthritis (JIA) is the name given to a group of arthritic disorders of unknown cause that manifest in children before the age of 16 years. JIA was formally known as juvenile rheumatoid arthritis (JRA). JIA is similar to adult rheumatoid arthritis (RA) in that an autoimmune element is present leading to damage to joints, organs, and other inflammatory responses both locally and systemic. Management includes medication (see section on pharmacology in pediatrics, **Table 10.31**) and conservative care involving physical and occupational therapy and patient and family education.

Table 10.7 Subcategories of JIA[4]

- Pauciarticular JIA—generally affects four or fewer joints, often in an asymmetric pattern. Girls are affected more often than boys.
- Polyarticular JIA—affects five or more joints usually in a symmetric pattern. Girls are affected more often than boys.
- Systemic onset JIA (Still's disease)—Affects boys and girls equally. Has most severe extra-articular signs and symptoms, often starting with a fever and rash, followed by joint involvement.
- Psoriatic JIA—patients present with psoriasis in addition to arthritis.

Scoliosis Classification

Table 10.8 Scoliosis: Onset, Curve, and Location

Age of Onset	Magnitude of Curve	Direction	Location	Curve
Congenital: birth to 3 years Juvenile: 3 years to puberty Adolescent: during or after puberty	Mild: 0°–20° Moderate: 20°–40° Severe: ≥ 40°	Right or left apex	Cervical, cervicothoracic, thoracic, thoracolumbar, or lumbar curves	Minor or major curve Single or double curve

Table 10.9 Types of Scoliosis

- **Functional (postural, nonstructural):** no structural changes; correctable with bending or postural correction; may be related to poor posture; may be related to musculoskeletal anomalies.
- **Structural:** changes in vertebrae and supporting tissues; decreased flexibility. Usually rotation of vertebrae is present; related changes occur to the rib cage, pelvis, and hips. Structural scoliosis has a fixed rotational component. Vertebral bodies rotate toward the convexity of the curve. The rotation results in a posterior rib hump in the thoracic region on the convex side of the curve. Structural scoliosis can be treated with bracing and surgery.
- **Congenital:** malformation of vertebrae at 3–5 weeks of gestation.
- **Neuromuscular (paralytic):** associated with neuromuscular diseases (such as cerebral palsy, muscular dystrophy, or myelomeningocele) and diseases with orthopedic manifestations (such as arthrogryposis and osteogenesis imperfecta).
- **Idiopathic:** cause is unknown. There may be a familial tendency for scoliosis. The prognosis varies with age of onset (variable). Idiopathic scoliosis is the most common form of scoliosis.
- **Traumatic onset:** associated with spinal fractures, irradiation, tumors, or metabolic disorders (rickets).

PEDIATRIC INTERVENTIONS

Common Surgical Procedures for Scoliosis

Table 10.10 Common Surgical Procedures for Spinal Stabilization

- **Dwyer anterior fusion:** requires resection of a rib and cutting through the diaphragm to expose the vertebrae. Screws are applied to each vertebra, with wires connecting them to stabilize the spine. Dwyer anterior fusion is used only for low curves in thoracolumbar or lumbar areas. All procedures use bony fusion of spine with instrumentation to stabilize fusion. Most require post-surgical orthosis. Newer procedures allow children to get up within the first few days of surgery and increase their activities gradually over the first year after surgery.

- **Zielke anterior fusion:** same as Dwyer anterior fusion, but a newer procedure with better screws used with rods to stabilize segments. It is used only for low curves in thoracolumbar or lumbar areas. Physical therapy post-operative interventions include teaching the child and family to use post-surgical orthosis.

- **Harrington rod posterior instrumentation:** an older procedure that is rarely used today. Two rods are attached by hooks to posterior spinal segments—a distraction rod on the concave side of the curve and a compression rod on the convex side. This technique cannot control sagittal plane correction, and it always requires post-surgical immobilization of spine. Formerly, it was a standard procedure for spinal stabilization. The Harrington procedure is infrequently used now because of the long rehabilitation time needed and its poor correction in the sagittal plane. Physical therapy post-operative interventions include teaching the child and family body about mechanics and functional skills, including getting in and out of bed, transfers, dressing, and ambulation.

- **Cotrel-Dubousset posterior instrumentation:** two rods with compression and distraction hooks are attached to pedicles or lamina of the vertebrae. Normal spinal curves in the sagittal plane can be obtained by contouring the rods. Children who have idiopathic scoliosis with good correction may not need spinal orthosis after surgery. This surgery is commonly used for idiopathic scoliosis and neuromuscular scoliosis. Physical therapy post-operative interventions include the following: teaching general range of motion and strengthening exercises, emphasizing the importance of early ambulation, monitoring the fit and the use of spinal orthosis (post-operative), monitoring neurologic signs, and monitoring the patient's skin for stability of instrumentation.

- **Luque procedure (posterior):** two L-shaped rods are attached to each level with wiring. This technique provides good stabilization and allows for lumbar lordosis and pelvic stability. It is a good choice for children with poor bone, skin, or muscle quality. The Luque procedure is associated with a high risk of neurologic deficit.

Types of Developmental Dysplasia of the Hip in Infancy

Table 10.11 Developmental Dysplasia of the Hip in Infancy

Dysplasia is a hip disorder in which the acetabulum may be shallow or small with poor lateral borders. Acetabular dysplasia may occur alone or with any level of femoral deformity or displacement. Physical therapy considerations with all types of dysplasia include the general rule that the hip be kept abducted and flexed, with the femoral head centered in the acetabulum. In this position, the acetabulum will continue to deepen, maintaining a correct shape, and the ligaments and joint capsule will tighten to provide extra joint stability.

(continued)

Table 10.11 Developmental Dysplasia of the Hip in Infancy *(continued)*

- **Subluxable dysplasia:** The femoral head can be partially displaced to the rim of the acetabulum. It slides laterally, but not all the way out of the socket.
- **Dislocatable dysplasia:** The femoral head is in the socket, but it can be displaced completely outside the acetabulum with manual pressure.
- **Dislocated dysplasia:** The femoral head lies completely outside the hip socket but can be reduced with manual pressure.
- **Teratologic dysplasia:** The femoral head lies completely outside the hip socket and cannot be reduced with manual pressure. Deformity of the joint surfaces is significant; it is usually related to another severe developmental anomaly, such as arthrogryposis or myelomeningocele. Surgery will be needed to reconstruct the joint. After surgery, the child may have pain with some hip movements and will probably have significant limitation in range of motion (ROM), most likely in abduction and extension.

Slipped Capital Femoral Epiphysis

Table 10.12 Slipped Capital Femoral Epiphysis (SCFE) Classification

- **Chronic slip SCFE:** gradual onset with progression of symptoms for 3 weeks or more; most common type of onset.
- **Acute slip SCFE:** sudden onset of severe pain; precipitated by trauma.
- **Acute on chronic slip SCFE:** symptoms build up gradually over a period of time; a traumatic episode then causes severe symptoms.

Grades of Slippage for SCFE

- Preslip: exhibits mild changes on X-rays, including a widened growth plate.
- Grade I: mild slip; femoral head slipped less than one-third the width of the femoral neck.
- Grade II: moderate slip; femoral head slipped between one-third and one-half the width of the femoral neck.
- Grade III: severe slip; femoral head slipped more than one-half the width of the femoral neck.

Signs and Symptoms of SCFE

- The child has an intermittent limp and pain in the groin, buttock, or thigh. A mild strain (such as jumping off a step) or severe strain (such as falling off a bicycle) may start the pain.
- The child may lean toward the side of the pain and ambulate with an antalgic (painful) gait. The child may also exhibit a Trendelenburg gait (of the unaffected side) because of weakness of the abductor musculature on the affected (involved) side. The leg may be held in external rotation. Also, when attempting to flex the hip, the child will exhibit external rotation.
- Range of motion limitations may be found in hip internal rotation, abduction, and flexion.

Common Surgical Procedures for the Hip in Children

Table 10.13 Common Surgical Hip Procedures[1]

Type of Surgery	Disorder/Disease	Surgical Procedure
Myotomy	Cerebral palsy (CP)	Soft-tissue releases, usually of the adductor muscles, can reduce abnormal pressures that cause subluxation and potential dislocation of the femoral head.
Fixation in situ	Slipped capital femoral epiphysis	A pin is driven through the femoral neck into the femoral head to stabilize the head on the neck.
Proximal femoral derotation osteotomy	CP	The femoral head is rotated to decrease the angle of anteversion. This procedure is usually done with a varus osteotomy.
Proximal femoral varus osteotomy	Developmental hip dysplasia: Legg-Calvé-Perthes disease; CP	A wedge is cut out of the femoral neck so that the neck-to-shaft angle is reduced (the neck sticks out more from the shaft). This procedure increases the stability of the femur.
Innominate pelvic osteotomy	Developmental hip dysplasia: Legg-Calvé-Perthes disease; CP	If the acetabulum faces more anteriorly and laterally than normal, the hip is not stable in a normal weight-bearing position. This procedure rotates the acetabulum so that it faces more downward and provides more stability for the femoral head during weight bearing.
Pemberton pelvic osteotomy	Developmental hip dysplasia: Legg-Calvé-Perthes disease; CP	The acetabulum is deepened and rotated downward to provide more stability to the femoral head. This procedure is used for the younger child with shallow, dish-shaped acetabulum.

Spina Bifida Classification and Functional Skill Levels

Table 10.14 Spina Bifida Classification and Functional Skill Levels

Types of Spina Bifida and Innervations	Functional Skills
Occulta (Not Visible)	
No tissue protruding from nonfused spinous processes; no disability results from this disorder.	Functional abilities: excellent; usually no neurologic or orthopedic problems.
Cystica (Visible)	
Meningocele: Cerebrospinal fluid and superficial tissue protrudes from the spine in a sac. Although tissue protrudes in a sac, neurologic tissue is rarely involved. The patient has no disability.	Functional abilities: excellent; usually no neurologic or orthopedic problems.

(continued)

Table 10.14 **Spina Bifida Classification and Functional Skill Levels** *(continued)*

Types of Spina Bifida and Innervations	Functional Skills
Myelomeningocele: The meninges and parts of the spinal cord protrude from the abnormally formed spine in a sac; abnormal neural elements are part of the protruding sac. The patient may have disability depending on the involvement level. Types of myelomeningocele: thoracic; high lumbar (L1–L2); mid-lumbar (L3–L4); low lumbar (L4–L5); and sacral.	
■ Myelomeningocele thoracic levels: The innervated muscles are the neck, upper limbs, shoulder girdle, and trunk musculature.	No volitional lower limb movements are present. For lesions below T10, lower trunk muscles may be weak. The patient will need to use a wheelchair for mobility (power wheelchair, reciprocating gait orthosis, standing frame) and is likely to develop hydrocephalus; there is no bowel or bladder control.
■ High lumbar myelomeningocele: L1–L2 levels. Innervated muscles are the same as for the thoracic levels. In addition, the patient has hip flexors but has weak hip flexion—may develop dislocated hips; is at risk for hip flexion contracture.	The patient may ambulate for short distances with assistive devices and orthoses but will need wheelchair for longer distances. There is no bowel and bladder control. The patient is likely to develop hydrocephalus.
■ Mid-lumbar myelomeningocele: L3–L4 levels. Innervated muscles are the same as for the L1–L2 levels. In addition, the patient has hip adductors, knee flexors and extensors, and some innervations in ankle dorsiflexion (L4), but has no sensation in the lower legs or feet.	The patient will need orthoses and crutches for household and short-distance community ambulation and a wheelchair for longer distances. There is no bowel and bladder control. The patient is likely to develop hydrocephalus.
■ Low lumbar myelomeningocele: L4–L5 levels. Innervated muscles are the same as for the L2–L3 levels. In addition, the patient has hip extension (weak) and abduction (weak) and weak plantarflexion against gravity with eversion. Sensation is impaired in the lower legs and feet. The patient may have some active knee flexion and ankle dorsiflexion with stronger knee extension.	The patient has weak hip extension and abduction and good knee flexion against gravity. The weak plantarflexion with eversion and strong dorsiflexion with inversion may lead to foot deformities. The patient can walk without orthoses but needs aids for fatigue; he or she can ride a bicycle but may need to use a wheelchair for long community distances. There is no bowel and bladder control. The patient is less likely to develop hydrocephalus.
■ Sacral myelomeningocele: has the same innervated muscles as low lumbar myelomeningocele. In addition, the patient has increased strength in ankle plantarflexion and dorsiflexion and more control of intrinsic foot muscles. Sensation is impaired in the feet. The patient has good hip strength and function.	Improved hip stability leads to independent walking without support (except ankle-foot orthosis). Weakness in hip abductors and plantarflexors leads to gait deviations. The patient has good ambulation with weak push-off and decreased stride length with rapid movement. He or she may have impaired bladder and bowel control.

PEDIATRIC INTERVENTIONS

Cerebral Palsy Classifications

Table 10.15 CP Classifications[5]

By Muscular Tone and Severity	By Motor Involvement	By Brain Involvement
Muscular Tone Classification ■ Hypotonic CP: low muscle tone; floppy, rag doll; weak deep tendon reflexes (DTRs); weak primitive reflexes; overweight; impaired speech; gait deficits such as wide base of support, short stride; poor balance ■ Ataxic CP: poor balance; gait deficits such as wide base of support; poor visual tracking; weak DTRs; weak primitive reflexes ■ Athetoid or dystonic CP: writhing movements; fluctuating tone; high DTRs; persistence of ATNR, STNR, and TLR; impaired speech; thin; poor balance; excessive movements in gait ■ Hypertonic CP: high muscle tone; tight muscles; spastic, stiff, and rigid; contractures in hip adduction, internal rotation (IR), and flexion, knee flexion, and ankle dorsiflexion (DF); thin; impaired speech; poor muscle control in gait; poor balance ■ Mixed CP: hypertonicity and athetosis or hypotonicity and ataxia, or hypertonicity and ataxia **Severity Classification** ■ Mild CP: development of independent functional skills and some language skills ■ Moderate CP: development of independent mobility—crawling, walking with support; may develop a few words of language ■ Severe CP: needs help for most function including mobility and feeding; has no language skills	**Body Involvement Classification** ■ Monoplegia: one extremity involved. ■ Diplegia: both lower extremities affected; may have less involvement of trunk and arms. ■ Hemiplegia: one arm and one leg on the same side affected. ■ Quadriplegia or tetraplegia: all four extremities and trunk affected. ■ Triplegia: both legs and one arm are affected.	**General Classification** ■ Extrapyramidal (including basal ganglia) ■ Pyramidal (including motor tracts and multiple areas) ■ Cerebellar

Common Causes of Cerebral Palsy

Table 10.16 Common Causes of CP

Prenatal (Before Birth) Causes	Perinatal* Causes	Postnatal (After Birth) Causes
■ Genetic ■ Viruses (e.g., herpes, cytomegalovirus, rubella)	■ Prematurity ■ Low birth weight ■ Severe jaundice	■ Infection ■ Trauma ■ Motor vehicle accident

(continued)

Table 10.16 **Common Causes of CP**   *(continued)*

Prenatal (Before Birth) Causes	Perinatal* Causes	Postnatal (After Birth) Causes
<ul><li>Infections (e.g., toxoplasmosis)</li><li>Drugs</li><li>Alcohol</li><li>Prescription and nonprescription drugs with teratogen effects (adversely affecting normal cellular development in the embryo or fetus)</li></ul>	<ul><li>Intraventricular hemorrhage</li><li>Poor nutrition (of the mother)</li><li>Asphyxia</li><li>Prolonged labor</li><li>Breech birth</li><li>Prolapsed cord</li></ul>	<ul><li>Child abuse</li><li>Shaken baby syndrome</li><li>Asphyxia</li><li>Head injury</li><li>Near drowning</li><li>Cardiac arrest</li><li>Cerebral vascular accident</li><li>Brain tumor</li><li>Lead exposure</li><li>Thrombosis</li><li>Sickle cell anemia</li></ul>

* Perinatal = from 28 weeks' gestation to 28 days after birth.

Table 10.17 **Clinical Signs of Hypotonic, Hypertonic, and Athetoid CP**

	Hypotonic CP	Hypertonic CP	Athetoid CP
Characteristics	Low tone, floppy, "rag doll"	High tone—spastic, stiff, or rigid	Fluctuating tone, writhing, constantly moving
Distribution	Generalized, symmetrical	Generalized, often asymmetrical	Generalized, can be asymmetrical
Range of motion	Excessive, too much joint movement, stiffness caused by lack of movement in older children	Limited, contractures developing with age	Full range of motion resulting from constantly moving through range
Risk of contractures and deformities	Risk of dislocation (jaw, hip, atlantoaxial joint), risk of contractures caused by lack of movement in older children	Risk of contractures (flexor muscles), dislocation (hip joint), and deformities (scoliosis, kyphosis)	Risk of deformities (scoliosis, lordosis), risk of joint contractures if spasticity is present in addition to athetosis
DTRs	Weak	Abnormally strong	Abnormally strong
Integration of primitive reflexes	Weak display of reflexes, sometimes delayed integration	Often delayed integration of reflexes	Often delayed integration of reflexes
Achievement of motor milestones	Delayed (amount of delay correlates with severity of hypotonicity)	Delayed (amount of delay correlates with severity of hypertonicity)	Delayed (amount of delay correlates with severity of tone deviations)

Table 10.17 **Clinical Signs of Hypotonic, Hypertonic, and Athetoid CP** *(continued)*

	Hypotonic CP	Hypertonic CP	Athetoid CP
Body position influence	Tone remains the same	Tone fluctuates with change in body position	Tone fluctuates with change in body position
Muscle consistency	Soft, doughy	Hard, rock-like	Stringy, elastic
Respiratory problems	Shallow breathing, choking because of weakness in pharyngeal muscles	Decreased thoracic mobility, limited inspiration and expiration	Decreased thoracic mobility and shallow breathing related to poor control of respiratory muscles
Speech problems	Shallow breathing, difficulty with sustaining voice sounds	Dysarthria (difficulty with motor speech) secondary to hypertonicity in oral muscles	Dysarthria secondary to poor motor control in oral muscles
Feeding problems	Weak gag reflex, open mouth and protruding tongue, poor coordination of swallowing and breathing	Abnormally strong gag reflex, tongue thrust, bite reflex, rooting reflex	Abnormally strong gag reflex, tongue thrust, poor coordination of oral muscles for chewing and swallowing

Genetic Disorders

Table 10.18 **Genetic Disorders[6]**

Chromosome Abnormalities (Deviation in the Number of Chromosomes)

- Down syndrome—trisomy 21: facial features include flat occiput, flat face, and upward-slanting eyes; hypotonicity; broad, short feet and hands; protruding abdomen; mental retardation; possible cardiac anomalies
- Edwards syndrome—trisomy 18: small stature; long, narrow skull; low-set ears; hypotonicity; rocker-bottom feet; scoliosis; profound mental retardation
- Patau syndrome—trisomy 13: microcephaly (abnormally small head); cleft lip and palate; polydactyly of hands and feet (having more than five fingers per hand or toes); severe to profound mental retardation

Sex Chromosome Abnormalities

- Turner syndrome—XO syndrome: congenitally webbed neck caused by fetal lymphedema; growth retardation; ptosis of upper eyelids (drooping of the upper eyelids); lack of sexual development; congenital heart and kidney disease; scoliosis; low normal intelligence
- Klinefelter syndrome—XXY: long limbs; tall and slender build until adulthood when obesity becomes a problem (if no testosterone replacement therapy); small penis and testes; low average to mild mental retardation; tremors, behavior problems

(continued)

Table 10.18 Genetic Disorders[6] *(continued)*

Partial Deletion Syndrome

Partial deletion of chromosome 9, partial monosomy 9p, or partial deletion of the short arm of chromosome 9 are rare pediatric diseases.

- Cri du chat syndrome 5p—caused by a DNA mutation of chromosome 5: high-pitched, catlike cry in infancy; microcephaly; low-set ears; hypotonicity; severe mental retardation; scoliosis; club feet; dislocated hips

- Prader-Willi syndrome 15—caused by absence of chromosomal material: low tone with feeding disorder in infancy; insatiable appetite that develops in toddlerhood; moderate mental retardation; hyperflexibility; obesity; characteristic facial features including almond-shaped eyes; small stature; small hands and feet; small penis

- Williams-Beuren syndrome—caused by a chromosomal deletion near the elastin gene on chromosome 7: syndrome-characteristic facial abnormalities, including prominent lips, medial eyebrow flare, and open mouth; mild microcephaly; mild growth retardation; short nails; mild to moderate mental retardation; cardiovascular anomalies

Specific Gene Defects: Autosomal Dominant

- Neurofibromatosis: areas of hyperpigmentation or hypopigmentation of skin, including "café au lait" spots or axillary "freckling"; tumors along nerves, in connective tissue, eyes, or meninges; macrocephaly (abnormally large head); short stature; skeletal abnormalities including scoliosis, bowing of long bones, and dislocations

- Tuberous sclerosis—rare genetic disease that causes benign tumors to grow in the brain and on other vital organs such as the kidneys, heart, eyes, lungs, and skin; causes seizures and mental retardation; skin lesions on cheeks, around nose; "café au lait" spots; cyst-like areas in bones of fingers; kidney and teeth abnormalities

- Osteogenesis imperfecta—brittle bone disease (See **Table 10.19** for details)

Specific Gene Defects: Autosomal Recessive

- Spinal muscular atrophy: progressive muscle atrophy and weakness; normal intelligence; normal sensation; weakness may begin before birth, in early childhood, or in later childhood

- Sickle cell disease: a group of diseases characterized by blood disorders related to hemoglobin defects; mostly seen in people of African or infrequently of Mediterranean descent; sickle-shaped red blood cells cause anemia, and possibly blockages in veins, causing a variety of conditions including leg ulcers, arthritis, acute pain, and problems in major organ systems such as the spleen, liver, kidney, bones, heart, and central nervous system; children may exhibit weakness, pain, or fever and may have growth retardation

- Hurler syndrome: normal or rapid growth during the first year with deterioration during the second year; coarse facial features characterized by full lips, flared nostrils, thick eyebrows, low nasal bridge, and prominent forehead; stiff joints; small stature; small teeth, enlarged tongue; kyphosis, short neck; claw hand, hip dislocation, and other joint deformities; mental retardation

- Phenylketonuria: children cannot metabolize the amino acid phenylalanine; causes mental retardation, growth retardation, hypertonicity, seizures, pigment deficiency of hair and skin if left untreated; can be successfully treated by limiting the amount of phenylalanine in the diet

- Cystic fibrosis—most common single-gene disorder in whites; abnormal secretions of body fluids including unusual sweat and a thick mucus that prevents the body from properly cleansing the lungs; the mucus interrupts vital organs' function, leading to infections

- Tay-Sachs disease: fatal disorder (by early childhood for infantile onset or teens with juvenile onset) causes a progressive degeneration of the central nervous system; caused by an absence of the enzyme beta-hexosaminidase A that builds up nerve cells in the body

(continued)

PEDIATRIC INTERVENTIONS

Table 10.18 **Genetic Disorders**[6]   (continued)

Sex-Linked Disorders (Affecting Only Boys)

- Fragile X syndrome: one of the most common causes of mental retardation in boys; characteristic facial features including elongated face, large ears, and prominent jaw; develop enlarged testicles in adulthood and prolapse of the mitral valve in the heart; mental retardation usually in the severe range, sometimes with aggressive behaviors; poor coordination and hypotonia in some boys

- Duchenne muscular dystrophy: progressive muscular weakness beginning between 2 and 5 years of age. Often first noticed when a child exhibits Gower's sign (child uses hands on thighs to push up into standing due to weakness of gluteal and lumbar muscles) when getting up from the floor or chair[4]; characteristic gait disturbances, including toe walking, abducted gait, lordosis, and waddling gait; progressive weakness leads to wheelchair use, decreased independence in all areas, and finally death from respiratory or cardiac failure

- Lowe syndrome: X-linked genetic trait and symptoms caused by a lack of the enzyme phosphatidylinositol 4,5-biphosphate, 5-phosphatase; also known as oculocerebrorenal syndrome; rare inherited metabolic disease; characterized by lack of muscle tone (hypotonia), multiple abnormalities of the eyes and bones, the presence at birth of clouding of the lenses of the eyes (cataracts), mental retardation, short stature, multiple kidney problems, protrusion of the eyeball from the eye socket, failure to gain weight and grow at the expected rate, and weak or absent deep tendon reflexes

- Lesch-Nyhan syndrome: inherited metabolic disease that produces an excess of uric acid because of the absence of an enzyme essential to the body's purine metabolism; moderate to severe mental retardation, hypertonicity leading to dislocated hips, club foot, growth retardation, movement disorders including chorea, ballistic movements, and tremor; self-mutilating behaviors including lip-biting and fingertip-biting

Osteogenesis Imperfecta

Table 10.19 **Osteogenesis Imperfecta (OI) Classification**[4,6]

Osteogenesis imperfecta is a genetic disorder characterized by fragile bones that break easily (often without apparent causes), low bone density, and scoliosis. The characteristics of OI vary from person to person, and not all characteristics are evident in each case.

- **Type I:** most common and the mildest type of OI. The collagen structure is normal, but the amount of collagen is less than normal. The child may have a triangular-shaped face and thin and smooth skin. The sclera of the eyes have a blue, purple, or gray tint. The teeth may be brittle. Hearing loss may begin in the patient's teens or 20s. Bones fracture easily, with most fractures occurring before puberty. The joints are loose, and the muscles are weak; bone deformity is absent or minimal.

- **Type II:** less common; the most severe form. Collagen is improperly formed, such that the patient experiences numerous fractures and severe bone deformity. Newborns with OI can get a fracture before birth and may die shortly after birth (because of respiratory problems). Children who live with this type of OI have small stature and undeveloped lungs.

- **Type III:** least common; very severe form. Collagen is improperly formed, such that fractures are present at birth and X-rays reveal healed fractures that occurred before birth. The child has short stature, loose joints, and poor muscle development; he or she has a progressive deformity of the long bones, the skull, and the spine. The child may have a barrel-shaped rib cage; dental problems; respiratory difficulties because of severe kyphosis and scoliosis (both); and hearing loss.

(continued)

Table 10.19 Osteogenesis Imperfecta (OI) Classification[4,6]

- **Type IV:** between type I and type III in severity. Collagen is improperly formed. The child has loose and easily overstretched joints, dental problems, fairly short stature, a triangular-shaped face, barrel-shaped rib cage, and possibly hearing loss. The child may be able to ambulate.

- **Type V:** clinically similar to type IV. The bone has a "mesh-like" appearance (when viewed under the microscope); X-rays show a dense band adjacent to the growth plate of the long bones. The fracture sites (or surgical procedure sites) have unusually large hypertrophic calluses, where new bone is laid down as part of the healing process. The membranes between the radius and ulna in the forearm are calcified, restricting the forearm supination and pronation. The child has normal teeth but white sclera of the eyes.

- **Type VI:** can be determined by a blood test and a bone biopsy (to diagnose this type with certainty). The bone appearance under the microscope has a "fish-scale" look. Very few people are identified with this type, but patients are moderately to severely affected. They have normal white or slightly blue sclera of the eyes; the teeth are not affected. Patients also have slightly elevated levels of the alkaline phosphatase enzyme, which is important in bone formation.

Torticollis (Congenital Muscular Torticollis [CMT])

Table 10.20 Torticollis[4]

- Contracted sternocleidomastoid (SCM) resulting in head tilt to affected side and chin rotation to opposite side.

- Ultrasonography provides evidence of some degree of fibrosis within the affected SCM.

- Causes include possible trauma during birth; restrictive space in utero; poor muscle tone; cervical vertebral abnormalities.

- Can result in plagiocephaly (flattening of the head from lying on the affected side), progressive head tilting and elevated shoulder girdle on the affected side.

- CMT usually resolves with conservative treatment with the first 12 months, although a small percentage may require surgery.

Pediatric Interventions

Screening for Scoliosis

Table 10.21 Scoliosis Screening

Standing

The child is standing and facing away from examiner.

1. Assess symmetry of the shoulders. The shoulder may be elevated on the convex side.
2. Assess symmetry of the scapulae and posterior rib cage. The scapula may be high, and the rib cage may be prominent on the convex side of the curve.
3. Assess symmetry of the waist and gluteal folds. The waist may appear fuller on the convex side of the curve. Gluteal folds may be symmetrical.
4. Assess symmetry of the hips. One hip may protrude.
5. Drop a plumb line from the occiput to assess trunk alignment. The plumb line may fall lateral to the gluteal crease. If it falls over the gluteal crease, check for a compensatory curve.
6. Assess symmetry of the spinous processes.

Bending Forward

7. The child bends forward from the waist as if to touch the ground. The arms should swing freely.
8. As the child bends forward, assess symmetry of the rib cage. The rib hump may appear posteriorly on the convex side.

Pediatric Mobility Interventions

Table 10.22 Mobility Interventions: Ambulation with Assistive Devices[1]

Gaining the confidence of the young children before getting them up to learn to walk on crutches is important. This can be achieved by the following:

- Have the child be medicated prior to activity (if the child has pain post-surgery).
- Gain the confidence of parents or caregivers whom the child trusts.
- Sit and talk or play with the child for a few minutes before getting the child up.
- Tell the child in an honest and simple way what you are planning to do and why.
- Be firm with your expectations, yet considerate of the child's feelings.
- Use toys, games, or music to engage the young child during the activity.
- Use appropriate safety equipment including a gait belt (for the child's safety and control).

Use appropriate assistive devices or equipment to help the child learn the skills.

- For example, a child younger than 5 years will probably not be able to learn to use crutches; thus a pediatric-sized, front-rolling, or pickup walker may be most appropriate.
- The crutches and walker should be fitted before getting the child up.
- For a child with significant pain or fears, progressing from parallel bars to a walker to crutches may be the most effective method to learn to use the assistive device.

(continued)

Table 10.22 Mobility Interventions: Ambulation with Assistive Devices[1] *(continued)*

Involve the parent or guardian in mobility interventions as much as possible.

- Teach the parent or guardian how to help the child get to a sitting position on the side of the bed and how to help the child stand up using the crutches or walker.

- The parent should be able to guard the child while walking on flat surfaces, uneven surfaces, and up and down stairs using crutches.

- The therapist needs to demonstrate the skills with the child and then observe the parent doing the skills. It is very important that the parent be successful in learning these skills because the child may need help for several days after discharge (from the hospital) until the skills are mastered.

- If the child is frightened and uncooperative with the therapist, teaching the parent, grandparent, or sibling to help the child learn the skill is an alternative strategy.

Measuring the Crutches or Walker

- The height of the crutches should be two finger-widths shorter than the child's axillae. The height can be estimated and then fine-tuned when the child first stands.

- The hand pads of the crutches should be placed so that the child's elbows are slightly bent when standing with the crutches. Then, when the elbows are extended fully, the child will be able to lift himself or herself up off the ground slightly.

- The walker height should be between the child's waist and the hip level. The walker's height will depend on the child's skills and confidence.

Teaching Ambulation Skills on Even Surfaces

- Standing up and sitting down in a chair should be the first skill that is learned.
  - From a sitting position, a child should hold the walker or crutches in one hand and place the other hand on the armrest or seat of the chair.
  - Weight should be placed through the uninvolved leg while the arm pushes off the chair. The arm holding the crutches or walker should be used for balance only.
  - Sitting down should be accomplished using the same steps in reverse. Put the crutches or walker in one hand, reach back for the chair with the other hand, and gently lower to sitting.

- Teach how to walk on flat surfaces first. The weight-bearing status of the child should be considered before walking is attempted.
  - The child should firmly grasp the crutches with both hands. Elbows should be held close to the sides to stabilize the crutch tops against the ribs. Weight should not be borne through the axillae, but rather through the arms from the hands.
  - The child needs to move the crutches forward, push down through the crutches, and swing the body either to the crutches or through the crutches for a longer stride.
  - Guarding should be done from diagonally behind or next to the child.
  - One hand (of the therapist) is on the child's shoulder closest (to the therapist), and the other hand is on the gait belt.
  - The priority is to help the child regain balance before a fall (not to catch the child once a fall is imminent).

(continued)

Table 10.22 **Mobility Interventions: Ambulation with Assistive Devices[1]** *(continued)*

Teaching Ambulation Skills Up and Down Stairs

- In going up or down stairs, the therapist or the parent should guard the child diagonally from behind or next to the child in the same manner as on flat surfaces.
- Standing on a lower step in front of the child when the child descends (as for adults) is not safe enough for children.
- The involved leg and the crutches always move together.
- The child should go up with the "good" and down with the "bad."
- During ascent of stairs, the uninvolved leg moves up before the crutches and the involved leg and the crutches follow.
- During descent of stairs, the involved leg and the crutches move down first together. They should move only one step at a time.
- The therapist should not attempt to have the child take longer strides on the stairs.

Pediatric Orthotic Interventions

Table 10.23 **Splints: Indications and Precautions**

Indications for Splints	Precautions for Splints
Prevent joint stress caused by excess motion	Avoid unnecessary restriction of movement; interference with sensory input; pressure or friction over bony prominences or at the splint edges; nerve compression; incorrect angle of pull; misalignment between the movable splint axis and the actual joint axis; improper size of splint
Prevent of correct contractures and deformity	Observe for stressing or overstretching of a joint; developing stiffness in a splinted joint; impaired circulation; and muscular weakness
Maintain range of motion gains achieved by casting, manipulation, or surgery	
Rule out undesirable joint motion	
Support joints in the optimal functional position	
Simplify patterns of coordination	
Facilitate muscle activity	
Decrease agonist spasticity	

Table 10.24 **Pediatric Hand and Wrist Orthotics**

Static Splints

- Indications for dorsal resting hand splints and volar resting hand splints: CP; head injury; arthrogryposis; limb deficiency; juvenile rheumatoid arthritis; burns; trauma.
- Benefits: Lightweight; durable; attractive; comfortable; broad contact area (decreased pressure); can be easily remolded.
- Precautions: Splint fit must be monitored as the child grows to prevent skin breakdown. Prolonged use can produce joint stiffness.
- Indications for static thumb index web space splint: CP, head injury, spasticity, and fisted thumb.
- Benefits: Inhibits spastic muscles; maintains range for thumb opposition; places thumb in a functional position.
- Precautions: Monitor splint edges around the thumb because this can be area of increased pressure.

Semi-Dynamic Splints

- Types: Sof-Splint; Joe Cool thumb splint; Good Samaritan splint; Neoprene web space splint; and Benik Corporation Thumb abduction splint.
- Indications: Marked thumb adduction; CP; web space tightness; increased tone in hand; limited active use of thumb; excessive thumb joint mobility.
- Benefits: Controlled arc of motion; stable and functional position of thumb; quick and easy to fabricate; inexpensive; allows sensory exposure of hand; elasticity to prevent too much pressure.
- Precautions: Not to be used with fixed deformity, bony changes, or strong flexion pattern at wrist; with Neoprene web space splint, skin needs to be monitored closely because it has poor ventilation.

Dynamic Splints

- Indications for orthokinetic wrist splints and MacKinnon splints: Spastic cerebral palsy; hemiplegia with fixed posture of upper extremity; to inhibit spastic flexor muscles; to facilitate extensor muscles; to encourage bilateral hand use.
- Precautions: Not recommended for children with fisted hands, cortical thumb, or severe radial or ulnar deviation.

Table 10.25 **Pediatric Lower-Extremity Orthotics**

Dynamic Ankle–Foot Orthosis (DAFO)

- Indications: neuromuscular disorders.
- Benefits: contoured to produce even pressure distribution; has varying degrees of ankle support; holds forefoot and hind foot in alignment.

(continued)

Table 10.25 Pediatric Lower-Extremity Orthotics   (continued)

- The DAFO is tolerated more easily than conventional plastic bracing, even in cases of extreme and difficult-to-manage spasticity. Allowing some sensation of "give" to the brace reduces the tendency of the child to "hold" forcefully against any portion of the brace. Because it provides for total contact, pressures are distributed much more evenly throughout the brace, reducing the tendency for skin breakdown. Skin breakdown problems are essentially nonexistent in a well-fitting DAFO, even in cases of repeated breakdown and fit problems with conventional ankle-foot orthoses.
- Precaution: Splint fit must be monitored as the child grows to prevent skin breakdown.

DAFO with Free Plantar Flexion

- Indications: mild or severe abnormal lower extremity tone.
- Benefits: allows dorsiflexion and plantarflexion; allows maximal lower-leg contact during crawling; does not interfere with balance reactions.
- Precautions: Splint fit must be monitored as the child grows to prevent skin breakdown.

Solid-Back DAFO

- Indications: children who are unable to do "foot flat" voluntarily during the stance phase of gait.
- Benefits: may eliminate hyperextension of the knee; keeps the heel down in the splint; can prevent shortening of calf muscles.
- Precautions: Observe for redness and poor skin tolerance.

Floor Reaction AFO

- Indications: crouch gait caused by weakness (secondary to myelodysplasia).
- Benefits: blocks ankle dorsiflexion; easy donning and doffing; encourages hip and knee extension.
- Precautions: poor intrinsic foot control; does not work well for children with crouch gait because of high tone (spastic diplegia).

Resting Splints for Night Use

- Indications: plantar flexion contracture not managed by daytime splinting.
- Benefits: prolonged stretch on soft tissues; worn at night; good for static standing.
- Limitations: not for ambulation.

Foot Orthotics Indicated for Hypotonicity and Hypermobility of Feet with Good Control of Muscle Activity

- Types of foot orthotics
  1. UCBL MOD: for hypermobile, flexible, pronated feet with severe transverse plane subluxation and calcaneal eversion
  2. Gait plates for in toe and out toe: functional orthotics for fourth and fifth metatarsal heads
  3. Robert Whitman: for children with excessive—but not severe—pronation at midfoot
  4. Kiddythotics: prefabricated for beginning walkers through 4 or 5 years old depending on shoe size; for moderate pronation
- Benefits: supports weight-bearing surface of the foot; helps with balance; improves mild discrepancy in alignment
- Limitations: does not control spastic foot; does not help with foot that fixes into a poorly aligned position

Other Types of Pediatric Physical Therapy Interventions

Table 10.26 Other Pediatric Interventions

- **Stretching exercises:** used for minor deformities or to supplement orthotics; stretching to be done to counter the deformity (such as for ankle plantarflexion, stretch the ankle into dorsiflexion); when stretching the gastrocnemius or soleus, be careful not to tear the midfoot ligaments.
- **Promotion of normal developmental skills through play:** using creeping; rolling; cruising; pulling to stand; standing; walking.
- **Sensory input stimulation:** rubbing using textured material; sand playing; water playing; massage; weight bearing.
  - To increase muscular tone (for hypotonicity): firm handling; tapping; vibration; brushing; quick movements; deep pressure; spinning; bouncing; swinging.
  - To decrease muscular tone (for hypertonicity or athetosis): rocking; rhythmic movements; firm touch; stroking; slow movements; singing; warm water; relaxing music; wrapping or swaddling; gentle handling.
  - To maximize function, position the child to facilitate visual access; use of arms; child's attention; mobility.
- **Positioning for hypertonicity**
  - Facilitate symmetrical posture: aligned trunk, pelvis, and extremities; head in midline to minimize persistent primitive reflexes.
  - Position hips and knees at 90 degrees.
  - Position hips and knees at more than 90 degrees if the child has a strong extensor tone.
  - Use the posterior tilt in space position: to help trunk and head upright alignment using gravity.
  - Use static standing positioning: improves weight bearing through long bones; improves visceral function such as bowel and bladder elimination, respiration, and venous return; decreases or prevents lower-extremity flexion contractures.
  - Use dynamic positioning: using supports; facilitates mobility; increases dynamic postural control; promotes weight bearing.
- **Improvement of functional skills:** elongate shortened muscle groups; inhibit primitive reflexes; facilitate dynamic mobility; facilitate optimal muscular tone; promote weight-bearing activities; improve balance; increase muscular strength (and tone); educate the child (and the parent to help the child) to learn new skills.
- **Positioning for contractures:** facilitate positions to prevent or minimize joint deformities (especially for hip flexion contractures); see the positioning for hypertonicity.

Pediatric Wheelchair Positioning Components

Table 10.27 Wheelchair Components*

- Head support provides posterior, lateral, or anterior support for head and provides safety during transportation.
- Lateral trunk supports provide postural support for upright positioning and can be used for trunk support in patients with scoliosis.

(continued)

Table 10.27 Wheelchair Components* *(continued)*

- Lateral hip guides promote neutral positioning of the lower extremities and pelvis.
- Medial thigh supports provide for neutral positioning of the thighs. Should not be used as a weight-bearing surface for the groin (to keep the pelvis back in the chair).
- Foot supports support the lower extremities and provide for neutral positioning of the lower extremities.
- Wheelchair accessories
  - Lap tray: provides upper-extremity positioning and support; assists with trunk extension; provides a surface for the upper-extremity activities
  - Pelvic belt: maintains pelvic positioning in the chair and provides for the patient's safety by preventing falling
  - Butterfly strap: provides a broad surface to promote anterior chest support and facilitates upright positioning
  - Chest strap: maintains trunk positioning and prevents falling forward; can be used as a supplement to a posterior and lateral positioning aid
  - Thigh strap: promotes pelvic alignment in sitting and can be a supplement to the pelvic belt

* For more postural support components, see Section 4.5 Wheelchair Management.

Pediatric Disorders and Diseases: Intervention Patterns

Clinical Practice Guidelines

Clinical Practice Guidelines (CPGs), developed by American Physical Therapy Association (APTA) sections, other organizations, societies, and healthcare organizations, are based on a systematic review of the evidence and provide therapists with resources to help guide clinical decision-making. The Academy of Pediatric Physical Therapy, a Section of the APTA, provides access to CPGs relevant to the management of pediatric patients.[7] Examples of topics addressed by the Academy of Pediatric Physical Therapy include Congenital Muscular Torticollis Clinical Practice Guideline and Resources and Developmental Coordination Disorder Clinical Practice Guideline and Resources. A full listing and links to the published CPGs can be found at https://pediatricapta.org/clinical-practice-guidelines/.

Pediatric Spondyloarthropathies: Intervention Patterns

Table 10.28 Pediatric Spondyloarthropathies: Intervention Patterns[1]

Spondyloarthropathies	Age of Onset	Characteristics and Interventions
Ankylosing spondylitis	Adolescence (boys > girls)	May begin with pauciarticular arthritis in childhood or back pain in adolescence, and can lead to general arthritis and, in severe cases, to ankylosis or fusion of the spine. Medical interventions include medications (similar to those used in juvenile idiopathic arthritis) to decrease inflammation. Physical therapy interventions include swimming and gentle exercise to maintain range of motion and strength.
Psoriatic arthritis	9–10 years (girls > boys)	Arthritis that involves primarily the distal joints of the hands with psoriasis. It is usually a mild disease but may lead to general joint destruction. Management is similar to that of other forms of arthritis.
Reactive arthritis	Variable	Also known as Reiter's syndrome. The syndrome includes urethritis, ocular disturbances, and arthritis. It may be a brief illness with complete recovery or, alternatively, may have long-term sequelae.
Inflammatory bowel disease	Variable	Arthritis may be the presenting complaint in children with ulcerative colitis or Crohn's disease. Abdominal cramping, diarrhea, weight loss, unexplained fever, and pauciarticular arthritis are common symptoms. Septic joints, especially the hip, can occur. Interventions vary according to symptoms.

Pediatric Orthopedic Disorders and Diseases: Intervention Patterns

Table 10.29 Pediatric Orthopedic Disorders and Diseases: Intervention Patterns

Developmental Dysplasia of the Hip (DDH)[4]

- Abnormal development of the hip joint resulting in hip instability and dislocation.
- Etiology: develops in the last trimester of pregnancy. It is believed to have some relationship to hormonal changes (affected by the female hormone called relaxin) during pregnancy or trauma at birth (improper and tight positioning in utero and breech positioning at birth).
- Affects girls six times more often than boys.
- If the hip dysplasia is not recognized by the age of 18 months, more complications will occur (contractures).
- Clinically, the child has asymmetrical hip abduction in flexion, asymmetrical groin or buttock skinfolds, the affected hip moving in and out of the socket with manual traction, and apparent femoral shortening on the affected side.

Physical Therapy Tests

- Ortolani test: feeling a hip click with passive movement of adducted and flexed hip into abduction with traction.
- Barlow test: feeling a hip click with manual movement of the flexed hip from abduction to adduction.
- X-rays: subluxation or dislocation of the hip.

Medical Interventions

Surgical or manual repositioning of the femur into the acetabulum with stabilization (using plaster spica cast from 6–18 months) of the surrounding structures.

Physical Therapy Interventions

- Bracing or splinting of affected hip in flexion and abduction (measuring and fitting the brace).
- Parent education about brace application, proper positioning of hips (in abduction and flexion), and lifting and carrying the baby while maintaining the hips in flexion and abduction.
- Interventions involving sensory and motor input to promote normal growth pattern.
- Strengthening exercises: encouraging kicking in infants; encouraging movement transitions such as sit to hands and knees or pulling to stand; encouraging mobility interventions such as creeping or cruising.
- ROM and stretching exercises: to maintain and increase ROM.
- Promotion of developmental skills.

Post-Surgery Interventions for Dysplasia

Initiated after surgery and cast removal:

- Strengthening exercises.
- Stretching exercises.
- Family education.

(continued)

Table 10.29 **Pediatric Orthopedic Disorders and Diseases: Intervention Patterns** *(continued)*

Osteogenesis Imperfecta (OI)[4]

- A connective tissue disorder affecting the formation of collagen during bone development (fragile bones that break easily); genetic disorders causing problems with the amount and quality of collagen in the body.
- Equal likelihood in boys or girls.
- The child may have low bone density or scoliosis, as well as fractures, contractures, and deformity.

Physical Therapy Interventions

- In general, must address treatment and prevention of fractures, contractures, and deformity.
- Parent education for infants about positioning and transfer (infants and young children need to be supported at the head and trunk, not the long bones; when rolling the child for diaper change, not to hold the infant at the ankles).
- Orthotics: splints; lower-extremity orthotics; body jackets for protection.
- Strengthening exercises: against gravity; low-impact endurance activities such as swimming and walking; for type IV OI, may use weight training with light weights.
- Active ROM or gentle stretching (not passive stretching due to risk of fractures and joint subluxation).
- Avoidance of rotational forces to the long bones due to fracture risk.
- Positioning.
- Mobility training with assistive devices (walkers or crutches).
- Activities of daily living: dressing, bathing, and training for reaching device.

Skeletal Fractures

- May result from genetic OI (during formation and development of bone), trauma, motor vehicle accidents, and child abuse.
- The characteristic of fractures in children is rapid healing (because of thicker bone periosteum and better bone blood supply than adults). In a newborn, a femur fracture can heal in 3 weeks; in an 8-year-old, it takes 8 weeks to unite the bones.
- Signs and symptoms of fractures: redness, pain, swelling, heat, and deformity of the extremity, muscle spasm, the child not using the extremity, and the child crying.

Most Common Types of Fractures

- Buckle fracture: compression of long bone on one side of the bone.
- Greenstick fracture: on one side of the long bone is compression, while on the other side is distraction.
- Epiphyseal fracture: involves the epiphyseal plate (growth plate).
- Spiral fracture: caused by twisting forces on the long bone.

Medical Interventions

- Immobilization: plaster casts, splints, internal/external fixation.
- Medications: analgesics.

(continued)

Table 10.29 **Pediatric Orthopedic Disorders and Diseases: Intervention Patterns** *(continued)*

Physical Therapy Interventions

- Pain control (using modalities).
- Patient education for mobility training with assistive devices: crutches or walker (for children younger than age of 5).
- Strengthening and endurance exercises of the uninvolved extremity before cast removal and of the involved extremity after cast removal.
- Balance/coordination and endurance (conditioning with treadmill, bike) exercises.

Osgood-Schlatter Disease (Jumper's Knee)

- Common in athletic children from osteochondritis of the epiphysis of the tibial tubercle (degenerative changes in the epiphyseal plate of bone during periods of rapid growth).
- May result in aseptic necrosis of bone or gradual healing and repair of the bone.
- Site of pathology: patellar tendon insertion into the tibial tuberosity (partial separation of bone). Patient cannot kneel on the tibia.

Physical Therapy Interventions

- Acute stage: splint (felt bar, athletic tape, elastic support, or cast) and decreased loading of the knee (no jumping, running); RICE; isometric quad exercises.
- Later interventions: patellar tendon taping; mobility training (using crutches); ROM exercises.
- Parent education: not to allow the child to jump or run.

Legg-Calvé-Perthes Disease[4]

- Osteochondrosis of the femoral head—the most common and most serious avascular condition in children; due to disturbances in the blood supply to the femoral head.
- Causes: genetic predisposition, trauma, anatomical variations, and generalized disorder of epiphyseal cartilage.
- Age of onset: 4–8 years. Boys have a five times greater incidence than girls (may develop in older girls—between 9 and 16 years).
- Necrosis of the epiphyseal plate occurs with collapse of subchondral bone. The head of femur flattens, and healing is slow (because it has less blood supply).
- The child will initially develop a limp and mild pain in the groin, medial knee, or thigh. Later the child will have limitation in gait in hip flexion, abduction, and external rotation (called psoatic limp); Trendelenburg gait (pelvis drops on one side due to opposite-side gluteus medius weakness); limb length discrepancy; and thigh, calf, or buttock atrophy.
- X-ray shows bony crescent sign.

Medical Interventions

- Immobilization in abduction in plaster cast or splints (young child of 5 years old).
- Femoral surgery (osteotomy for older child).

(continued)

Table 10.29 Pediatric Orthopedic Disorders and Diseases: Intervention Patterns   *(continued)*

Physical Therapy Interventions

- Gait deviation corrections.
- Contracture prevention.
- Patient and parent education: gait training, ROM, strengthening exercises, transfers, and functional skills.
- Mobility training with assistive device on even/uneven surfaces and stairs.
- Consulting with teachers and classroom staff to encourage and support the child and mobility in school.
- Strengthening exercises.
- ROM exercises.
- Functional skills.

Scheuermann's Disease (Osteochondrosis of Thoracic Spine)

- Spinal deformity with an autosomal dominant inheritance, occurring mostly in early adolescence.
- The child has a marked thoracolumbar kyphosis (round back).
- Symptoms: complaints of back pain in the affected area and complaints of poor posture or fatigue avascular necrosis of three to four thoracic vertebrae.
- The child presents with rounded shoulders while in school.

Physical Therapy Interventions

- Thoracic lumbar sacral orthosis (Milwaukee brace) and postural awareness exercises.
- Pain control (modalities).

Operative interventions are reserved for children with significant deformity and those individuals who have stopped growing.

Juvenile Idiopathic Arthritis (JIA)[4,8]

- Inflammation of connective tissue presenting with painful and inflamed joints.
- Etiology: autoimmune response triggered by environmental factors or bacterial or viral infection in children with a genetic predisposition.
- Presentation: inflammation of joints and muscles, and pain and stiffness caused by an autoimmune response (when the body's own immune system cannot distinguish normal cells from infectious or destructive antigens). The result of the disease is destruction of healthy tissue causing ankylosis of the joint.
- There are several types of JIA. Half of all patients have four to five joints affected, and the onset age is 10 years old (girls are affected more frequently than boys in most types of JIA). Complications of JIA include iridocyclitis with vision impairment or blindness and growth problems resulting in problems with bone development.
- Patients can have periods of exacerbation and remission.
- Seventy percent of patients with systemic onset JIA (also called Still's disease) experience remission before 16 years old.

(continued)

Table 10.29 Pediatric Orthopedic Disorders and Diseases: Intervention Patterns   *(continued)*

Physical Therapy Interventions

- Maintain ROM and prevent deformities: splinting of hands and fingers in extension; splinting of knee in extension.
- Stretching exercises: to maintain soft-tissue flexibility; stretching of hamstrings (HS), biceps, finger flexors.
- Patient/family education: stretching; avoidance of joint trauma especially during inflammation flare-ups.
- Strengthening and endurance exercises.
- Developmental interventions: facilitation of appropriate development depending on the patient's developmental skills and age, such as movement transitions from floor to standing, cruising, walking, or running.

Idiopathic Scoliosis

- Abnormal lateral curvature of the spine, consisting of two curves: the original abnormal curve and a compensatory curve in the opposite direction. Normal curves of the spine are cervical and lumbar lordosis and thoracic kyphosis.
- Types of scoliosis: structural (irreversible) and nonstructural (reversible; may also be functional or habitual).
- Nonstructural scoliosis: caused not by actual spinal deformity but by another condition such as a leg-length discrepancy or a habitually improper posture or position.
- The scoliosis curvature is classified based on the convexity of the curve. The most common is the "S" curve, right thoracic, left lumbar. A curvature greater than 10 degrees requires physical therapy interventions.

Physical Therapy Interventions

- Bracing (donning and doffing the brace).
- Strengthening exercises.
- Orthotic management for the shoe, such as a shoe lift (if there is a leg-length discrepancy).
- Electrical stimulation.
- Stretching exercises of the tight muscles on the concave side of the curve (in prone, side-lying, or heel-sitting positions).
- Strengthening exercises of the weak muscles on the convex side of the curve.
- Core strengthening
- Trunk axial elongation: stretching vertically by "walking up the wall" with both hands or hanging by both arms from an overhead bar.

Slipped Capital Femoral Epiphysis (SCFE)

- Signs and symptoms: intermittent limp and pain in the groin, buttock, or thigh; Trendelenburg gait; trauma due to pain and weakness (jumping off a step or falling off a bicycle); leg held in external rotation (also when trying to flex hip goes in external rotation); and limited internal rotation and abduction.
- Also called coxa vara or epiphyseal hip fracture; hip deformity related to the slippage of the femoral epiphysis.
- Etiology: hormonal influences (interaction between sex and growth hormones) and genetic predisposition.
- Populations with greatest prevalence: boys (two to three times more often than girls); tall children with delayed skeletal maturity (obese) near the puberty (9–16 years old); African American or Polynesian children (less common in white children).

(continued)

PEDIATRIC INTERVENTIONS

Table 10.29 **Pediatric Orthopedic Disorders and Diseases: Intervention Patterns**   *(continued)*

Physical Therapy Interventions

- For children without slippage: nonweight bearing with crutches (and dietary changes to lose weight—by dietician); gait or mobility interventions (crutches).
- Post-surgery: wheelchair training; strengthening exercises; home evaluation for wheelchair accessibility; consultation with teachers regarding school mobility; parent education for home exercises, transfers, and mobility.

Arthrogryposis Multiplex Congenita

- Nonprogressive neuromuscular disorder; present at birth; may be associated with the mother having a fever during the first trimester of pregnancy.
- Generally includes severe joint contracture and lack of muscular development; may affect the foot, hip, knee, shoulder, elbow, and wrist (one joint or all joints). Subluxed or dislocated hips are common.
- Children with distal arthrogryposis may be able to ambulate in the community.
- Children with involvement in all joints may use wheelchair and ambulate only at home.

Physical Therapy Interventions

- Parent instruction for stretching (daily) and positioning to maintain and increase ROM.
- Strengthening exercises (of neck, trunk, and extremity muscles) using developmental activities: prone on elbows; reaching for toys; sitting; rolling; kneeling and standing.
- Orthotics: upper- and lower-extremity use of splints and orthoses; promotion of function with orthoses; maintaining ROM.
- Maintenance of posture and prevention of scoliosis (using braces).
- Functional mobility training: rolling; crawling; scooting; wheelchair training (power wheelchair).
- Mobility training with assistive devices: crutches, walkers, parapodium, standers, adapted strollers.
- Quads and hamstrings stretching to prevent contractures (later when the child is developmentally walking). The patient may also need surgery for club foot (when the child is developmentally ready to stand) or for contractures of the knee.

Congenital Muscular Torticollis (CMT)[4]

- Contracted SCM resulting in head tilt to affected side and rotation to opposite side
- Typically resolves within 12 months with conservative care.
- Child may require helmet to help with shaping of skull and prevent flattening due to head position when resting.

Physical Therapy Interventions

- Passive ROM to stretch shortened muscles.
- Soft-tissue massage.
- Family education for positioning.
- Tasks and activities that encourage the child to move out of the position of deformity.

Other Pediatric Disorders and Diseases: Intervention Patterns

Table 10.30 Other Disorders and Diseases: Intervention Patterns[4]

Duchenne Muscular Dystrophy

- X-linked recessive degenerative disease of muscle tissue; inherited by boys; carried by recessive gene from the mother.
- Results in destruction of muscle cells and deposits of collagen adipose tissue (laid down in calf muscles, deltoids, quadriceps, and tongue muscles), leading to pseudohypertrophy.
- Begins around 2–3 years of age with progressive weakness from proximal to distal and can end with death in late adolescence or early adulthood. By age 4 (and up to age 5), the child exhibits Gower's sign: When the child pushes up from the floor on his or her hands, the child walks hands up his or her legs to be able to stand (because of weakness of knee and hip extensors).

Physical Therapy Interventions

- Maintain ROM: stretching of contractures such as heel cords, hamstrings, hip flexors, and tensor fascia latae (TFL); splinting; positioning in standing.
- Maintain ambulation and standing as long as possible: using braces, crutches, standing frames, parapodium, or dynamic standers; involve the child in motivating activities.
- Maintain cardiorespiratory function and strength as long as possible: encourage recreational activities such as swimming; encourage functional activities.
- Maintain functional skills including mobility: use assistive devices as possible; wheelchair mobility in power wheelchair; teach energy conservation techniques.

Down Syndrome (Trisomy 21)

- Chromosomal abnormality caused by breakage and translocation of the 21 chromosome.
- Types of Down syndrome: nondisjunction (more than 90% of children have this type); translocation; and mosaic (the degree of disability depends on the percentage of cells with abnormal characteristics).
- Patient can have hypotonia and decreased strength, heart defects, visual and hearing losses, feeding difficulties, speech and articulation deficits, developmental delays, cognitive deficits, and vertebral instability at the C1–C2 joints (can cause C1–C2 dislocation or subluxation). Atlantoaxial dislocation is a medical emergency. If C1–C2 instability, teach the child and family to avoid diving, tumbling, headstands, contact sports such as tackle football, and other activities that could cause hyperflexion injury to the neck. Other musculoskeletal problems (i.e., hip dislocation, patellar dislocation, scoliosis) can also occur as a result of overall hypotonia and soft-tissue laxity.

Physical Therapy Interventions

- Facilitate gross motor skills: using positioning, feeding, and motivation—teach parents.
- Provide activities to support oral-motor skills: facilitating lip closure; inhibiting tongue protrusion.
- Teach energy conservation of small children: providing frequent small feedings.

Cerebral Palsy

- Nonprogressive perinatal encephalopathy due to hemorrhage of ventricles in the brain, hypoxic encephalopathy, malformations, and trauma of central nervous system.
- CP can be spastic (high tone, lesion of motor cortex), athetoid (fluctuating muscle tone with lesion of basal ganglia), and ataxic (decreased balance with lesion of cerebellum).

(continued)

Table 10.30 Other Disorders and Diseases: Intervention Patterns[4] *(continued)*

Physical Therapy Interventions

- Physical therapy interventions are individualized.

- Hypotonia: support all limbs to prevent injury, prevent hyperextension at elbows and knees; use active ROM and passive ROM to stimulate increased muscle output; and promote active weight bearing.

- Hypertonia: provide positioning of hips and knees greater than 90 degrees of flexion (to inhibit reflexive extension); use midline symmetrical positioning (to inhibit abnormal reflexes); and promote active weight bearing.

- Athetosis: encourage midline symmetrical posture; use gentle rhythmic movements (to encourage controlled motor output); and allow abnormal movements if they contribute to functional skills.

- Ataxia: encourage midline symmetrical positioning; provide sensory input (to help with orientation in space); increase proprioceptive feedback (use weighted belts or vests); and use assistive devices with weights for balance.

Myelodysplasia/Spina Bifida

- Defective closure of vertebral column.

Physical Therapy Interventions

- Family education: for positioning to prevent and minimize joint deformities, especially hip flexion contracture; for support of the flaccid lower extremities and to reduce risk of fracture; to use assistive devices to promote optimal development; to be aware of potential shunt malfunctions causing irritability, headache, lethargy, vomiting, fever, change in behavior or seizure activity—medical emergency.

- Maximizing functional skills: strengthening through play activities; stretching tight joints and muscles; use of assistive devices to promote mobility and upright positioning—dynamic or static stander, scooter or cart, wheelchair, power mobility.

- Use of orthotics: hip knee ankle foot orthosis (HKAFO), rollator walker, standing frame, crutches, and reciprocal gait orthosis—for L1–L2 lesions; Knee ankle foot orthosis (KAFO), AFO, walker, forearm crutches, and wheelchair for long distances—for L3–L4 lesions; AFO and crutches—for L4–L5 lesions; AFO—for sacral myelodysplasia.

Cystic Fibrosis

- Genetic disorder of exocrine mucus-producing glands, including those in the respiratory tract, pancreas, and intestinal tract.

- Leads to frequent lung infection and loss of pulmonary function over time.

- Malabsorption of nutrients leading to weight loss and poor nutrition is linked to gastrointestinal tract changes.

- Decreased bone mineral density is common.

- May require lung or lung heart transplant to address severe disease.

Medical Interventions

- Antibiotics.
- Nutrition.
- Enzyme replacement.
- Surgery.

(continued)

Table 10.30 Other Disorders and Diseases: Intervention Patterns[4] *(continued)*

Physical Therapy Interventions

- Chest physical therapy: airway clearance techniques including percussion and postural drainage.
- Light-graded exercise program.
- Adapted devices as needed.
- Aerobic activity (can help to mobilize secretions).

Brachial Plexus Injury

- Traction or compression injury to the unilateral brachial plexus during the birth process or due to a cervical rib abnormality.
- Types: Erb's palsy, involving C5–C6 upper-arm paralysis; Klumpke's palsy, involving CT1 lower-arm paralysis; and total plexus injury involving the whole arm.
- In Erb's palsy, the child has the upper extremity in adduction, extension, and internal rotation of the shoulder with extension of the elbow.
- In Klumpke's palsy, the child has weakness or flaccidity of the wrist and finger flexors and extensors and the intrinsic muscles of the hand.
- There is a variable recovery from traction injuries.
- Medical interventions: surgery to repair avulsion injuries.

Physical Therapy Interventions

- Partial immobilization of the limb across the upper abdomen for 1–2 weeks (swaddle infant with arm across upper abdomen).
- Gentle ROM to prevent contractures (after initial recovery).
- Facilitated awareness of the involved extremity: joint approximation, stroking, and weight bearing.
- Strengthening of muscles: hand-over-hand activities and reaching for toys.

Autism Spectrum Disorder (ASD)[9]

- ASD is a developmental disorder resulting in social, behavioral, and communication challenges.
- ASD now includes pervasive developmental disorder (PDD), autism, pervasive developmental disorder not otherwise specified (PDD-NOS), and Asperger syndrome.
- Characterized by communication impairments, especially in expressive and receptive language skills and nonverbal communication; echolalic speech (involuntary repetition of words spoken by others); flat and monotonous or high-pitched and loud voice; appearance of not hearing at times; socialization problems; lack of imagination; and abnormal relationships with objects and events.

- May present with difficulty adapting to new situations.
- Often avoid eye contact and will not look at objects when pointed out to them.
- May repeat actions over and over again.
- The presentation of signs and symptoms in someone with ASD is highly variable. The learning, thinking, and problem-solving abilities of people with ASD can range from gifted to severely challenged. Some people with ASD need a lot of help in their daily lives; others need less.

(continued)

Table 10.30 Other Disorders and Diseases: Intervention Patterns[4]   (continued)

Physical Therapy Interventions

- Use familiar objects and routines.
- Use daily activities to strengthen and for functional skills (such as climbing stairs or running on the playground).
- Prepare the child for changes in routine.
- Sensory integration therapy.
- Use of Picture Exchange Communication Systems to promote conversation by use of pictures and symbols.
- Include breaking tasks down into small tasks and affirm success, but ignore incorrect responses.

Sickle Cell Anemia

- Autosomal recessive genetic trait in people of African and Mediterranean backgrounds.
- Abnormal shape of red blood cells (sickle shaped) means they cannot pass through capillaries and cause blockages, resulting in poor oxygen to some tissues. Sickle cells break faster than normal cells, causing jaundice; lack of adequate red cells causes anemia.
- Children have fatigue caused by anemia, organ enlargement, necrosis, scarring, and pain caused by occluded blood vessels in spleen, liver, bones and kidneys; they may also have strokes and skin ulcers.

Physical Therapy Interventions

- Physical therapy interventions are dependent on the needs of the child and are a team effort.
- Orthopedic interventions for children with fractures due to osteoporosis.
- Wound care, including debridement for children with skin ulcers.
- General conditioning exercises (to increase strength).
- Apply caution with use of ice for pain as this may further narrow blood vessels.

Respiratory Distress Syndrome (RDS) or Hyaline Membrane Disease

- Caused by atelectasis (collapsed lungs) owing to insufficient surfactant in premature lungs (in premature babies). Interventions: oxygen supplement and physical therapy positioning.
- Bronchopulmonary dysplasia of newborn: chronic lung disease from using mechanical ventilation or O_2 because RDS. Interventions: respiratory support and positioning.

Postnatal Complications/Disorders: Periventricular Leukomalacia or Periventricular Hemorrhage

- Necrosis of white matter of the brain and bleeding of the brain, respectively, resulting in CP
- Retinopathy: due to low birth weight and high oxygen levels, can have detached retina and blindness
- Necrotizing enterocolitis: infected bowel (feeding problems)
- Physical therapy interventions in neonatal care: positioning

Table 10.31 Medications for Common Pediatric Conditions[8,10,11]

*Classes of Drugs	Purpose of Medication	*Common Side Effects	Physical Therapist Assistant Implications
JIA Medications NSAIDs (nonsteroidal anti-inflammatory) ■ Aspirin ■ Naproxen ■ Ibuprofen ■ Indomethacin	■ Pain reliever ■ Inflammation reduction	■ Stomach irritation ■ Reye's Syndrome (aspirin only) ■ Rashes ■ Headaches ■ Dizziness ■ Renal toxicity ■ Edema	■ Monitor exercise intensities, especially if medications are taken before treatment as they may mask pain
SAARDs (slow-acting antirheumatic drug) ■ Sulfasalazine (azulfdine) ■ Methotrexate (Trexall)	■ Slow the progression of the disease process ■ Suppresses immune system	■ Thrombocytopenia ■ Rash ■ Renal problems ■ Nausea/vomiting ■ Headache ■ Dizziness ■ Drowsiness/fatigue	■ Fall risk if dizzy/drowsy or dehydrated from vomiting ■ Increased risk of infections so wear personal protection equipment (PPE) if appropriate
Tumor necrosis factor blockers ■ Etanercept (Enbrel) ■ Adalimumab (Humira)	■ Pain reduction ■ Morning stiffness reduction ■ Controls joint swelling	■ Pancytopenia ■ Reaction at injection site (both meds) ■ Anemia/fatigue if RBC's ↓ ■ Headaches (Humira) ■ Rash (Humira)	■ Increased risk of infections so wear PPE if appropriate ■ ↑ bleed/bruise if ■ ↓ platelets ■ Monitor during exercise for undue fatigue
Immune suppressants ■ Abatacept (Orencia) ■ Anakinra (Kineret) ■ Rituximab (Rituxan)	■ Suppress the immune response for inflammation	■ ↑ risk of infections ■ Headaches ■ Nausea/vomiting ■ Runny/stuffy nose ■ Diarrhea ■ Injection site reaction ■ Cough ■ Insomnia	■ Wear PPE when appropriate to protect patient from infections
Corticosteroids ■ Prednisone (medrol dose pack) ■ Dexamethasone	■ Systemic anti-inflammatory agent	■ ↑ risk of infections ■ Osteoporosis ■ Weight gain ■ Sterility growth suppression in long-term use with children	■ Wear PPE when appropriate to protect patient from infections ■ If osteoporotic, caution with exercises

PEDIATRIC INTERVENTIONS

(continued)

Table 10.31 Medications for Common Pediatric Conditions[8,10,11] *(continued)*

*Classes of Drugs	Purpose of Medication	*Common Side Effects	Physical Therapist Assistant Implications
Musculoskeletal Injuries (Sprain, Strains, Tendinitis) NSAIDs ■ Aspirin ■ Naproxen ■ Ibuprofen	■ Pain reliever ■ Inflammation reduction	■ Stomach irritation ■ Reye's Syndrome (aspirin only) ■ Rashes ■ Headaches ■ Dizziness ■ Renal toxicity ■ Edema	■ Monitor exercise intensities, especially if medications are taken before treatment as they may mask pain
Cystic Fibrosis[11] Digestive medications ■ Pancreaze ■ Creon	■ Replacement of pancreatic enzymes	■ Flatulence ■ Stomach pains ■ Diarrhea	
Inhaled or nebulized medications ■ Albuterol ■ Pulmozyme ■ Tobi	■ Bronchodilator ■ Deter mucous plugs in the respiratory system	■ Anxiety ■ Tremors ■ Headaches ■ Rapid heart rate ■ Rash ■ Sore throat ■ Voice alteration ■ Tinnitus	■ Hand washing for infection control; cystic fibrosis patients at higher risk for pulmonary infections ■ Chest physical therapy should be done 30 minutes to 1 hour after nebulizer treatments to allow for best airway clearance ■ Encourage secretion clearance throughout interventions ■ Utilize breathing techniques throughout treatment ■ Monitor vitals during exercise

(continued)

Table 10.31 Medications for Common Pediatric Conditions[8,10,11]   *(continued)*

*Classes of Drugs	Purpose of Medication	*Common Side Effects	Physical Therapist Assistant Implications
Antibiotics ■ Augmentin ■ Bactrim ■ Cipro	■ Treat bacterial infections in the lungs	■ Nausea/vomiting ■ Diarrhea ■ Arthralgias ■ Tendinopathies	■ Hand washing for infection control; cystic fibrosis patients at higher risk for pulmonary infections ■ Monitor for joint pain/gait abnormalities/tendinopathies ■ Encourage secretion clearance throughout interventions ■ Utilize breathing techniques throughout treatment
Corticosteroids ■ Prednisone (inhaled)	■ Anti-inflammatory agent for lungs	■ ↑ risk of infections ■ Osteoporosis ■ Weight gain ■ Sterility ■ Growth suppression in long-term use with children	■ Wear PPE when appropriate to protect patient from infections ■ If osteoporotic, caution with exercises ■ Encourage secretion clearance throughout interventions ■ Utilize breathing techniques throughout treatment

*Brand names associated with classes of medications and side effects found within this table are not representative of an all-inclusive list. It is incumbent on the clinician to research an appropriate drug information resource to obtain complete information about medications that patient may use while attending rehabilitation.

PEDIATRIC INTERVENTIONS

References

1. Ratliffe KT. *Clinical Pediatric Physical Therapy*. St. Louis, MO: Mosby; 1998.
2. Shirly Ryan Ability Lab. Rehab measures database. https://www.sralab.org/rehabilitation-measures. Accessed July 14, 2021.
3. Rothstein JM, Scalzitti DA, Mayhew TP. *The Rehabilitation Specialist's Handbook*. 3rd ed. Philadelphia, PA: F.A. Davis Company; 2005.
4. Goodman CC, Fuller KS. *Pathology for the Physical Therapist Assistant*. 2nd ed. St. Louis, MO: Elsevier; 2017.
5. Martin ST, Kessler M. *Neurologic Interventions for Physical Therapy*. 2nd ed. Philadelphia, PA: W.B. Saunders Elsevier Company; 2007.
6. Genetic and Rare Diseases Information Center. nih.gov.. http://www.rarediseases.info.nih.gov. Accessed November 17, 2021.
7. Academy of Pediatric Physical Therapy. Clinical practice guidelines and resources. https://pediatricapta.org/clinical-practice -guidelines/. Accessed July 15, 2021.
8. Mayo Clinic. Disease and conditions juvenile idiopathic arthritis. https://www.mayoclinic.org/diseases-conditions/juvenile -idiopathic-arthritis/diagnosis-treatment/drc-20374088. Accessed July 19, 2021.
9. Center for Disease Control. Autism spectrum disorder. https://www.cdc.gov/ncbddd/autism/index.html. Accessed July 15, 2021.
10. Ciccone CD. *Pharmacology in Rehabilitation*. 4th ed. Philadelphia, PA: F.A. Davis Company; 2007.
11. Anne and Robert Lurie's Children's Hospital of Chicago. Common CF medications. https://www.luriechildrens.org/en /specialties-conditions/cystic-fibrosis-program/ongoing-care-health-maintenance/common-cystic-fibrosis-medications/. Accessed July 19, 2021.

PART 11

Acute Care: Interventions for Select Medical and Surgical Conditions

Interventions for Select Acute Medical and Surgical Conditions

General Guidelines for Physical Therapist Assistants in the Acute Care Setting[1]

In addition to information in this section, refer to Part 2 to review "Safety in the Clinical Environment."

Table 11.1 General Guidelines for the Physical Therapist Assistant (PTA) Working in the Acute Care Setting

---

The Academy of Acute Care Physical Therapy has established a list of core competencies for the entry-level PTA working in acute care. This document can be found at https://www.apta.org/for-educators/curriculum-resources/acute-care. Select points are summarized here, but detailed description of PTA competencies in acute care should be reviewed from the document.

- In the acute care setting, there are constant changes in patient status. The PTA must be able to recognize and respond appropriately. The PTA must be able to accurately use knowledge and skills to make clinical decisions regarding patient status.
- Collaboration with other healthcare professionals is an essential component of acute care physical therapy.
- The PTA must have the knowledge and skills to assist the physical therapist (PT) in management of patients in the acute care setting, recognizing the PTA's own limits and abilities.
- The PTA should recognize the need for ongoing communication with the supervising PT. (See Appendix A for the problem-solving algorithm utilized by PTAs in patient/client interaction to help identify key points for communication with the PT.)
- The PTA should review the medical chart for pertinent information prior to seeing the patient. Information to review includes past medical history and current medical status, including PT evaluation and plan of care (POC), lab values, and medications.
- The PTA should integrate findings from the chart review, patient's subjective report, vital sign assessment, and interprofessional team communications when determining appropriateness of physical therapy services on any given day.
- Significant changes in the patient's condition should be reported to the PT and documented.

Significant Factors for Patients with Endocrine Diseases and Disorders

---

Table 11.2 Significant Factors for Patients with Diabetes Mellitus

---

- Patient's safety: Observe the patient for ischemia symptoms in the lower extremities while ambulating (excruciating pain in the limb, leg pallor, leg coolness, and absence of palpable pulses); observe the patient for symptoms of angina (nausea, vomiting, dizziness, and shortness of breath); observe the patient for postural hypotension (have adequate warm-up and cool-down).
- Peripheral neuropathic pain: The pain comes and goes and can last for months or years. It may occur mostly in the hands and feet; the patient may lose complete sensation (deep pressure can be preserved the longest). The patient has muscle weakness, especially during gait activities. The patient can also have foot drop (plantarflexion of the foot; dragging of the foot or toes while walking).

(continued)

Table 11.2 Significant Factors for Patients with Diabetes Mellitus   *(continued)*

- Peripheral vascular disease can cause peripheral nerve damage.
- Visual acuity needs to be assessed from a functional perspective. It is important for the patient to see any skin changes such as blisters or erythema, especially in the initial phase of acquiring a wound. Patients with retinopathy of the eyes should avoid isometric exercises, Valsalva maneuver, and positioning the head down (such as in Trendelenburg positioning) due to risk of excessive pressure on blood vessels and the possibility of hemorrhage. Activities that increase the systolic blood pressure to more than 170 mm Hg should be avoided.
- Wound infections are common in patients with diabetes mellitus.
- Charcot foot develops when glucose levels are elevated for a long time. The blood decreases in the bone, causing the bone to become softer and fracture easily. The clinical signs of Charcot foot are diffuse foot pain, mild edema, and possibly erythema.
- Hypoglycemia: The patient can have low blood glucose levels of 70 mg/dL or less. This can occur because of late meals, timing of insulin administration, and the increased insulin-like effects of exercises. Severe hypoglycemia causes dizziness, fatigue, confusion, palpitations, weakness, headaches, abnormal behavior, vision abnormalities, inability to concentrate, seizures, and coma. Prolonged hypoglycemia can lead to permanent brain damage.

Significant Factors for Patients with Gastrointestinal Diseases and Disorders

Table 11.3 Symptoms of Abdominal Disturbances in Need of Monitoring or Discontinuation of Physical Therapy

- Characteristics of abdominal pain: burning pain (can be peptic ulcer—in the lining of the duodenum, at the lower end of the esophagus, or in the stomach); cramping pain (can be gastroenteritis—inflammation of the stomach and intestinal tract); knifelike pain (pancreatitis—inflammation of the pancreas); pain with a gradual onset (infection).
- Anatomic locations of pain: liver, gallbladder, duodenum, pancreas, portion of kidneys, ureter, adrenal gland, cecum, pancreas, mesentery, colon (transverse, descending or sigmoid), stomach, or spleen.
- Referred pain from the liver and gallbladder might manifest as intrascapular pain or pain in the right shoulder, upper trapezius, or right subscapular pain. Referred pain from the kidneys may lead to pain in the flank.
- Hematemesis: bloody vomitus (may be red blood or dark; may have "coffee-ground" appearance); can be caused by duodenal or gastric ulcers, esophageal varices, esophagitis, gastritis, or duodenitis.
- Melena: black tarry feces caused by the digestion of blood in the gastrointestinal tract; in adult patients, may be caused by gastrointestinal bleeding from the esophagus, stomach, or proximal small intestine.
- Abdominal distention: can be caused by intestinal obstruction.
- Ascites: abnormal accumulation of fluid in the peritoneal cavity; from gastrointestinal perspective can be liver disease, cirrhosis, or portal hypertension; can also be caused by congestive heart failure or obstruction in the vena cava.
- Local abdomen tenderness: can be caused by intestinal obstruction, appendicitis, cholecystitis, or diverticulitis.

ACUTE CARE: INTERVENTIONS FOR SELECT MEDICAL AND SURGICAL CONDITIONS

(continued)

Table 11.3 **Symptoms of Abdominal Disturbances in Need of Monitoring or Discontinuation of Physical Therapy** *(continued)*

- Rebound of abdomen: abdominal tenderness that increases with palpation; can be caused by peritoneal inflammation or duodenal ulcers.
- Abdominal rigidity: involuntary contraction of the abdominal muscles due to peritoneal inflammation, gastric/duodenal ulcers, intestinal obstruction, hepatomegaly (enlarged liver), or liver atrophy.
- Bowel sounds: can be caused by hunger, gastroenteritis, diarrhea, or diverticulitis.
- Absent bowel sounds: indicative of peritoneal inflammation or paralytic obstruction of ileus.
- Abdominal bruit: indicative of aortic aneurysm.

Table 11.4 **Types of Physical Therapy Interventions for Patients with Gastrointestinal Diseases and Disorders**

1. Mobility training: log-rolling and bracing with a pillow; transfer training and gait training (may use splinting of the incision with a pillow and/or abdominal binder).
2. Breathing exercises: deep breathing; directed coughing; incentive spirometry; chest percussion or chest vibration.
3. Post-surgery patient education: abdominal protection and activity restriction (no driving, swimming, or active abdominal exercises for 4–6 weeks); minimizing lifting (more than 5–10 pounds; PT/PTA should consult with the surgeon); lifestyle modifications; and ostomy (surgery connecting a portion of the intestine to the exterior of the body); care regarding the stoma (enterostomal care); and irrigation of the bowel (done with the multidisciplinary team).
4. Pain assessment and pain control (with the multidisciplinary team).
5. Discharge planning (with the multidisciplinary team).

Significant Factors for Patients with Genitourinary Diseases and Disorders

Table 11.5 **Dialysis**

- Dialysis is a process of diffusing blood across a semipermeable membrane to remove toxic materials and to maintain fluid, electrolyte, and acid–base balance in case of impaired kidney function (or absence of kidneys).
- Indications: management of renal failure (a disorder in which fluids, electrolytes, acids, and medications are eliminated in the urine); hyperkalemia; uremia; acidosis; and uremic pericarditis.
- Effects: dehydration; hypovolemia (decreased blood volume); hypotension; fatigue.
- Hemodialysis: circulates the patient's blood through an arterial-venous fistula, arteriovenous graft, or central venous catheter.
- Peritoneal dialysis: uses the peritoneum through an implanted catheter; typically is an alternative to hemodialysis.

Table 11.6 **Considerations When Applying Physical Therapy to Patients on Dialysis**

- Mobilization activities are contraindicated during dialysis; therapeutic exercises and airway clearance are indicated.
- Fluid and electrolyte status should be assessed by the PT prior to physical therapy interventions.
- The PT or PTA must monitor the patient's cardiovascular system for blood pressure, pulse, mental status, urinary output, intracardiac pressure changes, and cardiac output (to avoid the potential for hypovolemia and electrolyte imbalances).
- The blood pressure cuff should not be placed over the arteriovenous fistula.

Table 11.7 **Terminology Related to the Examination/Evaluation of the Genitourinary System**

Refer to Table 9-17 for review of types of incontinence and management.

- **Urinary urgency:** strong urge to urinate. Can be related to inflammation of the bladder, urethra, or prostate or to infection.
- **Nocturia:** excessive or frequent urination after going to bed at night. Can be caused by excessive fluid intake, congestive heart failure, uncontrolled diabetes mellitus, urinary tract infection, diseases of the prostate, impaired renal failure, or use of diuretics.
- **Dysuria:** painful or difficult urination. May indicate other conditions such as cystitis, urethritis, infection in the urinary tract, ulcerated prostate in men, pelvic peritonitis, or urethral stricture.
- **Hematuria:** blood in the urine.
- **Proteinuria:** loss of proteins (such as albumin or globulins) in the urine. Can be a sign of underlying kidney disease or systemic illness. Excessive loss of protein in the urine can cause peripheral edema (secondary to decreased osmotic pressure and excessive water retention in the blood vessels of the extremities).
- **Pyelonephritis:** inflammation of the kidneys and renal pelvis. Can be a result of a bacterial infection that started in the urinary bladder.
- **Urethritis:** inflammation of the urethra.
- **Vaginitis:** inflammation of the vagina. Can be caused by overgrowth or invasion of microorganisms such as gonococci, staphylococci, streptococci, viruses (such as herpes), and fungi, or detergents or chemicals.
- **Herpes:** vesicular eruption caused by a virus. Genital herpes is a recurring eruption of the genital or anorectal skin or mucous membrane caused by the herpes simplex virus type II. This sexually transmitted disease affects mostly adolescents and young adults and is spread by intimate contact.
- **Epididymitis:** inflammation of the epididymis (an organ resting on and beside the posterior surface of a testicle).
- **Renal calculus:** kidney stone.
- **Prostatitis:** inflammation of the prostate gland as a result of infection (most often an acute bacterial infection).
- **Hernia:** the protrusion of an anatomical structure (such as the bladder or fatty tissue or the stomach) through the wall that normally contains it. There are several types of hernias: abdominal; acquired (developed any time after birth); bladder; congenital (existing from birth); cystic (bladder); indirect inguinal (protrusion of a hernia sac containing intraperitoneal contents at the superficial inguinal ring); direct inguinal (protrusion of the hernia sac through the abdominal wall at the area bounded by rectus abdominis, inguinal ligament, and inferior epigastric vessels).
- **Testicular cancer:** malignancy of the testicles.

Significant Factors for Patients with Oncological Diseases and Disorders

Table 11.8 Oncological Diseases and Disorders: Types and Physical Therapy Interventions

Breast Cancer

- Most common type of cancer in American women. Breast cancer occurs most frequently in the ducts or lobes of the breast.
- Stages of breast cancer:
  - Stage I: localized disease
  - Stage II: axillary node involvement
  - Stage III: advanced regional disease with metastasis
  - Stage IV: distant metastases
- Medical interventions (depend on the stages): biopsy (sentinel node biopsy); lumpectomy or partial mastectomy for patients with Stage I and Stage II (tumor smaller than 4 centimeters); mastectomy (if tumor is larger than 4 centimeters or for multiple tumors).
- Mastectomy can be simple, modified radical, skin sparing, or radical. Breast reconstruction with implants is an elective surgery. The surgeon dictates the acute care PT for implants.
- Post-surgery physical therapy interventions: shoulder range of motion (ROM) exercises (all planes of motion); postural exercises; lymphedema education.

Leukemia

- Hematological disorder classified by the type of cells and the stage of cancer.
- Medical interventions: chemotherapy.

Lymphoma (Hodgkin's or Non-Hodgkin's)

- Hematological disorders of the lymphoreticular system. Can be slow-growing, indolent, or fast-growing tumors.
- Stages of Hodgkin's disease:
  - Stage I: one area of lymph node involvement
  - Stage II: two or more areas of lymph node involvement above the diaphragm
  - Stage III: two or more areas of lymph node involvement both above and below the diaphragm
  - Stage IV: widespread disease
- Medical interventions: chemotherapy and stem-cell transplantation.
- Physical therapy in acute care must consider prevention of impairments that may be caused by the disease and/or medical interventions.

Skin Cancers

- Can include melanoma and nonmelanoma skin cancers.
- Medical interventions: surgery (excision); radiotherapy; immunotherapy; hormonal therapy.
- Physical therapy considerations: the patient's function, especially in cases involving metastasis to the brain and bone; lymphedema (due to lymph node excision).

(continued)

Table 11.8 **Oncological Diseases and Disorders: Types and Physical Therapy Interventions** *(continued)*

Radical Hysterectomy

- Removal of the uterus, uterosacral and uterovesical ligaments, pelvic lymph nodes, and upper third of the vagina.
- Potential side effects of surgery: bladder and sexual dysfunctions, lymphedema, and sexual stenosis.
- Salipingo-oophorectomy: removal of the ovary and fallopian tube.
- Medical interventions: radiation therapy.
- Potential side effects of medical interventions:[4] peripheral neuropathy; pelvic pain; urinary incontinence; lymphedema; sexual dysfunction; muscular fibrosis; dyspareunia (pain with sexual intercourse); urinary incontinence; stress incontinence; overflow incontinence; urge incontinence.
- Physical therapy interventions: ROM and flexibility exercises for hip and abdominal muscles; pelvic floor reeducation and exercises (Kegel exercises); biofeedback; vaginal cones exercises; electrical stimulation for the pelvic floor.

Lung Cancer

- Types: small cell lung cancer (worst prognosis) and non-small cell lung cancer.
- Medical interventions: surgical resection; chemotherapy; radiation therapy.
- Physical therapy interventions: splinted coughing (post-surgery); shoulder ROM; posture training; breathing exercises; musculoskeletal conditioning exercises.

Prostate Cancer

- Physical therapy (post-radical prostatectomy): splinted coughing; mobility training; patient education regarding erectile dysfunction and urinary incontinence.

Table 11.9 **Types of Surgical Procedures and Postsurgical Physical Therapy for Oncological Diseases and Disorders[2]**

- **Debulking:** surgery to remove a large portion of a tumor (when complete removal is not possible).
- **Biopsy:** surgery to remove a sample from the patient's body for microscopic examination to establish a diagnosis. Biopsy can also be done through aspiration (when tissue removal is done with a needle and syringe, such as from a cyst or the bone marrow).
- Surgery to remove a precancerous lesion (growth that is not yet, but probably will become, cancerous).
- **Tumor resection:** cutting off or cutting out an abnormal mass that may be benign or malignant.
- Surgical correction of life-threatening conditions caused by cancer: palliation—surgery to reduce the effects of a cancerous tumor (to decrease some problematic aspects of the cancer, such as for reduction of pain and suffering).
- Common post-surgery physical therapy procedures: early mobilization; pulmonary hygiene (deep and diaphragmatic breathing; splinted coughing); postural education; gait training; training in activities of daily living as necessary (such as in amputations).

Table 11.10 Tumor Terminology[3]

- Benign—usually harmless tumor that does not spread or invade other tissue but can grow quite large if untreated.
- Malignant—cancerous tissue with the ability to spread or metastasize to other tissues.
- Tumors whether benign or malignant are classified by cell type of origin.
  1. **Epithelial tissue**—Benign: Papilloma, adenoma, nevus. Malignant: Squamous cell carcinoma, adenocarcinoma, malignant melanoma.
  2. **Connective tissue/muscle**—Benign: Fibroma, chondroma, osteoma, rhabdomyoma. Malignant: Fibrosarcoma, chondrosarcoma, osteosarcoma, rhabdomyosarcoma.
  3. **Nerve tissue**—Benign: Neuroma, neurilemoma, meningioma. Malignant: Glioma, neurilemic sarcoma, meningeal sarcoma.
  4. **Lymphoid tissue**—Malignant: Lymphoma.
  5. **Hematopoietic tissue**—Malignant: Leukemia, multiple myeloma.

Table 11.11 Side Effects of Radiation Therapy[3]

- Fatigue: cumulative over the course of radiation therapy; either resolves when radiation is complete or can last 6 months to 1 year post-radiation.
- Immunosuppression: increased risk of infection.
- Decreased platelet and white blood cell counts.
- Fibrosis.
- Burns.
- Diarrhea, nausea.
- Hair loss.
- Ulcers and delayed wound healing.
- Avascular necrosis of the hip: loss of blood supply and necrosis of the femoral head of the hip joint (can cause fractures and bone collapse). The patient may have pain with weight bearing, ache in the groin and anterior thigh areas, and minimal relief of pain while resting.

Table 11.12 Side Effects of Chemotherapy[3]

- Fatigue
- Diarrhea, constipation, nausea, and vomiting
- Anorexia
- Mucositis (mouth sores)
- Damage of various internal organs such as the liver, heart, or kidneys
- Hair loss (alopecia)
- Anemia, bone marrow suppression, leukopenia, neutropenia, and increased risk for infection
- Sterility
- Peripheral neuropathy (sensory and motor changes due to damage of myelin covering of peripheral nerves; patients may have motor weakness as well as pain, numbness, or burning in the feet)
- Muscle weakness
- Other sensory symptoms: sensation of pins and needles; cold extremity; sharp type of shooting pain
- Autonomic nervous system symptoms: orthostatic hypotension; tachycardia; feeling flushed

Table 11.13 Evidence-Based Physical Therapy for Oncological Diseases and Disorders[4-8]

- Aerobic training (such as walking on a treadmill) increases hemoglobin concentration, reduces fatigue, and decreases psychological distress.
- Exercises may help with treatment-related complications, especially when the patient was administered high doses of chemotherapy and radiotherapy.
- Patients with terminal cancer who receive therapy consisting of aerobic exercises have reduced physical limitations.
- Patients who exercise during cancer medical interventions have less fatigue, more energy, and less emotional distress.
- The best exercises are home exercise programs designed in collaboration with the patient and the patient's family.
- When designing exercise programs, the PT and PTA need to consider the patient's physiological impairments and functional limitations, which may depend on the type of cancer:
  - Reduction of total lung capacity
  - Changes in pulmonary architecture due to surgical treatment
  - Loss of muscle mass and severe myopathy (due to high doses of corticosteroids and cyclosporine)
  - Reduced protein and calorie intake as a consequence of anorexia and nausea
  - Impaired absorption after gastrointestinal surgery, which can lead to a catabolic state that impairs exercises
  - Decreased oxygen transport
  - Damaged bone marrow and production of red blood cells
  - Myocardial damage and decreased cardiac output

Table 11.14 Administration of Exercises in Oncology

- Exercises should be personalized.
- Exercises must begin slowly.
- Exercises must build up gradually.
- Exercises must be selected with the patient, after considering the patient's activity choices.
- Exercises must be learned together with a friend or a family member.
- Patients must keep an exercise journal.
- Patients must have an alternative exercise plans for days when they are ill.
- Exercises must be immediately modified if patients have pain.
- The patient's hemoglobin level must be monitored for anemia.
- Patients must be educated not to exercise if they have an infection.
- Patients must be educated not to use exercise equipment and crowded gyms and to avoid swimming. When weights are used, they should be light weights.

SECTION 11-2

Laboratory Tests, Values, and Implications for the Physical Therapist Assistant

General Guidelines for Laboratory Tests and Values[9]

- Reference ranges vary between laboratories; thus, different hospitals and healthcare organizations will have different upper and lower limits. Always review the test results as most are marked if high or low.
- The PTA needs to be aware of normal reference values for common laboratory tests.
- The PTA should recognize when lab values are outside of normal ranges and consult with the supervising PT to discuss whether to hold, modify, or continue with the plan of care.
- Patients in a hospital are more likely to exhibit abnormal or less-stable vital signs, and the risk for adverse events is high. More frequent measurement of vital signs is indicated. (Refer to Part 2 for normal values.)
- Vital signs should be assessed continuously during physical therapy interventions with patients in the intensive care unit.
- The PTA needs to be aware of medications taken by the patient and how these might impact vital signs at rest and during activity or exercise.

Complete Blood Count

Table 11.15 Complete Blood Count[3,10]

	Reference Values	Possible Causes	Implications for the PTA
White Blood Cells (WBC)	4,500–11,000 cells/mm^3 (4.5–11.0 × 10^9/L)	Decreased: infection, bone marrow suppression, i.e., due to radiation, chemotherapy, autoimmune disease. Increased: infection, leukemia, stress, trauma, inflammation.	<1,000 cells/mm^3 requires use of mask and other personal protective equipment to prevent risk of infection. Exercise is not permitted. <5,000 cells/mm^3 or 10,000 with a fever—no exercise permitted. Absent fever, then light exercise. Elevated WBC—patient may have compromised exercise tolerance and symptoms-based approach is indicated.
Red Blood Cells (RBC)	Males: 4.5–5.3 million cells/mm^3 (4.5–5.3 × 10^{12}/L) Females: 4.1–5.1 million cells/mm^3 (4.1–5.1 × 10^{12}/L)	Decreased: anemia, blood loss, chemotherapy, multiple myeloma, systemic lupus erythematosus (SLE). Increased: dehydration, polycythemia vera, chronic heart disease, pulmonary fibrosis.	See hematocrit and hemoglobin.

(continued)

Table 11.15 Complete Blood Count[3,10]

	Reference Values	Possible Causes	Implications for the PTA
Platelets	150,000–400,000 cells/mm³ (150–400 × 10⁹/L)	Decreased: anemia, medications (i.e., anti-inflammatories, steroids), infection, radiation, chemotherapy, liver disease. Increased: inflammation, infection, cancer, trauma, splenectomy.	With low counts is a risk of easy bruising and/or hemorrhage. Use fall risk precautions. < 20,000 cells/mm³ restricted to activities of daily living and walking with doctor approval. ⩾ 30,000 cells/mm³ active ROM, moderate exercise, walking as tolerated. ⩾ 50,000 cells/mm³ progressive resistive exercises (PREs) as tolerated, swimming cycling. Elevated count can put patient at risk for venous thromboembolism.
Hemoglobin (Hbg)	Male: 13–18 g/dL Female: 12–16 g/dL	Decreased: hemorrhage, sickle cell disease, lymphoma, SLE, some medications i.e., aspirin, severe burns Increased: congestive heart disease, severe dehydration, chronic obstructive pulmonary disease (COPD), living at high altitude, polycythemia vera.	< 8g/dL—no exercise permitted 8–10 g/dL—light exercise permitted >10 g/dL resisted exercise permitted Patients with low Hgb levels will have decreased activity tolerance and may present with tachycardia and orthostatic hypotension. Use a symptoms-based approach. Elevated Hgb levels can lead to blockage in capillaries. Treatment requires consultation with the interdisciplinary team.
Hematocrit (HCT)	Male: 42–52% Female: 37–47%	Decreased: anemia, hemorrhage, leukemia, bone marrow failure, hyperthyroidism, dietary deficiency (i.e., folate, iron, B12). Increased: severe dehydration, burns, erythrocytosis, COPD, cor pulmonale.	Patient will have decreased endurance with lower HCT levels. Use a symptoms-based approach. < 25% no exercise permitted; consult with interprofessional team for activity/mobilization. >25% light exercise; 30%–32% add resistive exercise as tolerated. Elevated levels >60% can result in spontaneous blood clotting.

* Reference values are presented in standard units followed by SI units in parenthesis. Values listed are for the adult population unless specified.

ACUTE CARE: INTERVENTIONS FOR SELECT MEDICAL AND SURGICAL CONDITIONS

Lipid Profile

Table 11.16 Lipid Profile[3,10]

Lipid / Lipoprotein	Expected Values	Abnormal values	Comments
High-density lipoprotein (HDL)	Males ⩾ 40 mg/dL Females ⩾ 50 mg/dL		Often referred to as "happy" or "good" cholesterol. Higher levels are considered beneficial and can lead to a reduction in incidence of heart disease.
Low-density lipoprotein (LDL)	< 100mg/dL	Borderline high: 130–159 mg/dL High: 160–189 mg/dL Very high: ⩾ 190 mg/dL	Often referred to as "bad" or "lousy" cholesterol. Elevated LDL is a strong predictor of cardiovascular disease. LDL deposits cholesterol in arteries.
Triglycerides	< 150 mg/dL	Borderline high: 150–199 mg/dL High: 200–499 mg/dL Very high: > 500mg/dL	Elevated triglycerides are usually found along with elevated cholesterol.
Total cholesterol	< 200 mg/dL	Borderline high: 200–239 mg/dL High: >240 mg/dL	

Kidney Function

Table 11.17 Kidney Function[3,10]

Test	Reference Value	Possible Causes	Implications for the PTA
Blood Urea Nitrogen (BUN)	10–20 mg/dL	Decreased: Hepatic disease, malnutrition. Increased: Renal failure, CHF, GI bleed, high protein diet, fever.	Elevated BUN leads to decreased tolerance to activity. Patient may present with hypertension (HTN) and fatigue easily.
Serum Creatinine	Male: 0.6–1.2 mg/dL Female: 0.5–1.1 mg/dL	Decreased: low muscle mass, age, low protein diet, pregnancy. Increased: Renal disease, rhabdomyolysis, dehydration, muscular dystrophy.	Elevated serum creatinine results in decreased tolerance to activity. Patient may present with fatigue, low fever, headache, and confusion.

Hemostasis

Table 11.18 Hemostasis (Blood Clotting)[3,10]

Test	Normal Range	Other Factors for the PTA to Consider
International Normalized Ratio (INR)	0.9–1.1	Therapeutic range for deep vein thrombosis, pulmonary embolus (PE), atrial fibrillation: 2.0–3.0. Therapeutic range for mechanical heart valves: 2.5–3.5. Values > 3.6 place patient at higher risk for bleeding.
Prothrombin Time	11–13 seconds	> 25 seconds puts patient at a high risk for bleeding. Discuss with interprofessional team before therapy. Therapy may be contraindicated.
Activated Partial Thromboplastin Time (aPTT)	21–35 seconds	> 70 seconds indicates spontaneous bleeding.

Intracranial Pressure

Table 11.19 Intracranial Pressure[9]

- Normal range for intracranial pressure (ICP): 7–15 mm Hg
- Risk occurs when ICP is elevated higher than 20 mm Hg.
- ICP pressure should be maintained below 22 mm Hg in patients with traumatic brain injury.

Additional Laboratory Tests and Values

Refer to Part 2, Section 2-3, for additional values and information relevant to the PTA on blood glucose levels, electrolytes, and acid–base balance.

ACUTE CARE: INTERVENTIONS FOR SELECT MEDICAL AND SURGICAL CONDITIONS

References

1. American Physical Therapy Association. Core competencies for entry-level physical therapist assistants in acute care. https://www.apta.org/for-educators/curriculum-resources/acute-care. Accessed July 20, 2021.

2. Malone D, Lindsay K, eds. *Physical Therapy in Acute Care: A Clinician's Guide*. Thorofare, NJ: SLACK; 2006.

3. Goodman CC, Fuller KS. *Pathology for the Physical Therapist Assistant*. 2nd ed. St. Louis, MO: Elsevier; 2017.

4. Bower JE. Cancer-related fatigue: Mechanisms, risk factors, and treatments. *Nature reviews. Clinical Oncology*. 2014;11(10):597–609. doi:10.1038/nrclinonc.2014.127

5. Mishra SI, Scherer RW, Snyder C, Geigle PM, Berlanstein DR, Topaloglu O. Exercise interventions on health-related quality of life for people with cancer during active treatment. *Cochrane Database Syst Rv*. 2012 Aug. 15;(8): CD008465. doi10.1002/14651858. CD008465.pub2

6. Bergenthal N, Will A, Streckmann F, Wolkewitz KD, Monseff I, Engert A, Elter T, Skoetz N. Aerobic and physical exercise for adult patients with haematological malignancies. *Cochrane Database Syst Rev*. 2014 Nov 11;(11):CD009075. doi: 10.1002/1465185. CD009075.pub2

7. Thorsen L, Skovlund E, Stromme SB, Hornslein K, Dahl AA, Fossa SD. Effectiveness of physical activity on cardiorespiratory fitness and health-related quality of life in young and middle-aged cancer patients shortly after chemotherapy. *J Clin Onc*. 2005;23(10):2378–2388.

8. Boyette-Davis JA, Walters ET, Dougherty PM. Mechanisms involved in the development of chemotherapy-induced neuropathy. *Pain Management*. 2015;5(4):285–296. doi: 10.2217/pmt

9. Academy of Acute Care Physical Therapy. Adult vital sign interpretation in acute care guide 2021. https://www.aptaacutecare.org/page/ResourceGuides. Accessed May 21, 2021.

10. Academy of Acute Care Physical Therapy. Laboratory values interpretation resource. https://cdn.ymaws.com/www.aptaacutecare.org/resource/resmgr/docs/2017-Lab-Values-Resource.pdf. Accessed June 2, 2021.

Appendix A

American Physical Therapy Association Algorithms for Physical Therapist Assistant Practice

Problem-Solving Algorithm Utilized by PTAs in Patient/Client Intervention

This algorithm, developed by the APTA's Departments of Education, Accreditation, and Practice, is intended to reflect current policies and positions on the problem-solving processes utilized by physical therapist assistants in the provision of selected interventions. The controlling assumptions are essential to understanding and applying this algorithm (see **Figure A-1**). (This document can be found in *A Normative Model of Physical Therapist Assistant Education: Version 2007*.)

Figure A-1 Controlling assumptions.
Issued by Advisory Panel of Physical Therapist Assistant and adopted by the American Physical Therapy Association Board of Directors, January 2011. Reprinted from http://www.apta.org, with permission of the American Physical Therapy Association. Copyright (c) 2015 American Physical Therapy Association. APTA is not responsible for the translation from English.

- The physical therapist integrates the five elements of patient/client management—examination, evaluation, diagnosis, prognosis, and intervention—in a manner designed to optimize outcomes. Responsibility for completion of the examination, evaluation, diagnosis, and prognosis is borne solely by the physical therapist. The physical therapist's plan of care may involve the physical therapist assistant to assist with selected interventions. This algorithm represents the decision making of the physical therapist assistant within the intervention element.
- The physical therapist will direct and supervise the physical therapist assistant consistent with the APTA House of Delegates positions, including Direction and Supervision of the Physical Therapist Assistant (HOD P06-05-18-26); APTA core documents, including Standards of Ethical Conduct for the PTA; federal and state legal practice standards; and institutional regulations.
- All selected interventions are directed and supervised by the physical therapist. Additionally, the physical therapist remains responsible for the physical therapy services provided when the physical therapist's plan of care involves the physical therapist assistant to assist with selected interventions.
- Selected intervention(s) includes the procedural intervention, associated data collection, and communication, including written documentation associated with the safe, effective, and efficient completion of the task.
- The algorithm may represent the thought processes involved in a patient/client interaction or episode of care. Entry into the algorithm will depend on the point at which the physical therapist assistant is directed by the physical therapist to provide selected interventions.

- Communication between the physical therapist and physical therapist assistant regarding patient/client care is ongoing. The algorithm does not intend to imply a limitation or restriction on communication between the physical therapist and physical therapist assistant (see **Figure A-2**).

Figure A-2 Problem-solving algorithm utilized by PTAs in patient/client intervention.
*See controlling assumptions.

PTA Direction Algorithm

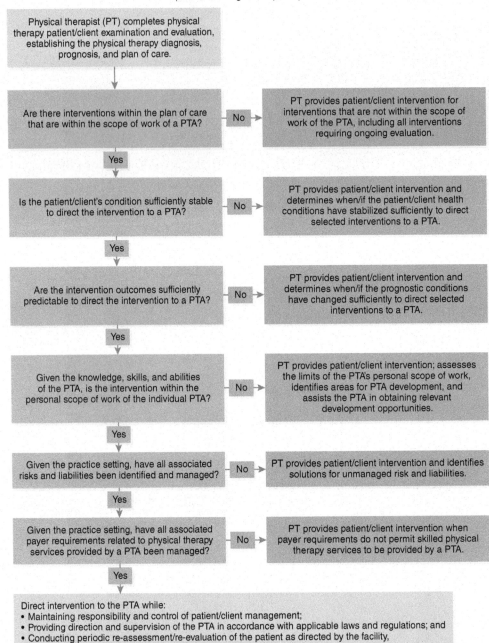

PTA Direction Algorithm
(See Controlling Assumptions)

Physical therapist (PT) completes physical therapy patient/client examination and evaluation, establishing the physical therapy diagnosis, prognosis, and plan of care.

Are there interventions within the plan of care that are within the scope of work of a PTA? — **No** → PT provides patient/client intervention for interventions that are not within the scope of work of the PTA, including all interventions requiring ongoing evaluation.

Yes

Is the patient/client's condition sufficiently stable to direct the intervention to a PTA? — **No** → PT provides patient/client intervention and determines when/if the patient/client health conditions have stabilized sufficiently to direct selected interventions to a PTA.

Yes

Are the intervention outcomes sufficiently predictable to direct the intervention to a PTA? — **No** → PT provides patient/client intervention and determines when/if the prognostic conditions have changed sufficiently to direct selected interventions to a PTA.

Yes

Given the knowledge, skills, and abilities of the PTA, is the intervention within the personal scope of work of the individual PTA? — **No** → PT provides patient/client intervention; assesses the limits of the PTA's personal scope of work, identifies areas for PTA development, and assists the PTA in obtaining relevant development opportunities.

Yes

Given the practice setting, have all associated risks and liabilities been identified and managed? — **No** → PT provides patient/client intervention and identifies solutions for unmanaged risk and liabilities.

Yes

Given the practice setting, have all associated payer requirements related to physical therapy services provided by a PTA been managed? — **No** → PT provides patient/client intervention when payer requirements do not permit skilled physical therapy services to be provided by a PTA.

Yes

Direct intervention to the PTA while:
• Maintaining responsibility and control of patient/client management;
• Providing direction and supervision of the PTA in accordance with applicable laws and regulations; and
• Conducting periodic re-assessment/re-evaluation of the patient as directed by the facility, federal and state regulations, and payers.

Figure A-3 PTA direction algorithm.

PTA Supervision Algorithm

Figure A-4 PTA supervision algorithm.

Appendix B

Standardized Tests

Berg Balance Scale
Performance Oriented Mobility Assessment
Functional Reach Test
Timed Up and Go Test

Berg Balance Scale

1. Sitting to Standing
   Patient instruction: Please stand up. Try not to use your hands for support.
   - ❑ 4, able to stand without using hands and stabilizes independently
   - ❑ 3, able to stand independently using hands
   - ❑ 2, able to stand using hands after several tries
   - ❑ 1, needs minimal aid to stand or stabilize
   - ❑ 0, needs moderate to maximal assist to stand

2. Standing Unsupported
   Patient instruction: Please stand for 2 minutes without holding on to anything.
   - ❑ 4, able to stand safely for 2 minutes
   - ❑ 3, able to stand for 2 minutes without supervision
   - ❑ 2, able to stand for 30 seconds unsupported
   - ❑ 1, needs several tries to stand unsupported for 30 seconds
   - ❑ 0, unable to stand for 30 seconds without support

3. Sitting with Back Unsupported but Feet Supported on Floor or on a Stool
   Patient instruction: Please sit with arms folded for 2 minutes.
   - ❑ 4, able to sit safely and securely for 2 minutes
   - ❑ 3, able to sit for 2 minutes with supervision
   - ❑ 2, able to sit for 30 seconds
   - ❑ 1, able to sit for 10 seconds
   - ❑ 0, unable to sit without support for 10 seconds

4. Standing to Sit
   Patient instruction: Please sit down.
   - ❑ 4, sits safely with minimal use of hands
   - ❑ 3, controls descent by using hands
   - ❑ 2, uses back of legs against the chair to control descent
   - ❑ 1, sits independently, but has uncontrolled descent
   - ❑ 0, needs assistance to sit

5. Transfers
   The physical therapist assistant (PTA) arranges chairs for a pivot transfer. The PTA can use either two chairs (one with arms and one without armrests) or a bed/mat and a chair (with armrests). The patient is asked to transfer one way toward a seat without armrests and one way toward a seat with arms.
   - ❑ 4, able to transfer safely with minor use of hands
   - ❑ 3, able to transfer safely with definite need of hands
   - ❑ 2, able to transfer with verbal cuing and/or supervision
   - ❑ 1, needs one person to assist
   - ❑ 0, needs two people to assist or supervise to be safe

6. Standing Unsupported with Eyes Closed

   Patient instruction: Please close your eyes and stand still for 10 seconds.
   - ❑ 4, able to stand for 10 seconds safely
   - ❑ 3, able to stand for 10 seconds with supervision
   - ❑ 2, able to stand for 3 seconds
   - ❑ 1, unable to keep eyes closed for 3 seconds but stands safely
   - ❑ 0, needs help to keep from falling

7. Standing Unsupported with Feet Together

   Patient instruction: Place your feet together and stand without holding on to anything.
   - ❑ 4, able to place feet together independently and stand safely for 1 minute
   - ❑ 3, able to place feet together independently and stand with supervision for 1 minute
   - ❑ 2, able to place feet together independently but unable to hold for 30 seconds
   - ❑ 1, needs help to assume the position but can stand for 15 seconds, feet together
   - ❑ 0, needs help to assume the position and unable to stand for 15 seconds

8. Reaching Forward with Outstretched Arm While Standing

   Patient instruction: Please lift your arm to 90 degrees. Stretch out your fingers and reach forward as far as you can.

   The PTA places a ruler at the tips of the patient's outstretched fingers—the patient should not touch the ruler when reaching. The distance recorded by the PTA is from the patient's fingertips (with the patient in the most forward position). The patient should use both hands when possible to avoid trunk rotation.
   - ❑ 4, can reach forward confidently 20–30 centimeters (10 inches)
   - ❑ 3, can reach forward safely 12 centimeters (5 inches)
   - ❑ 2, can reach forward safely 5 centimeters (2 inches)
   - ❑ 1, reaches forward but needs supervision
   - ❑ 0, loses balance when trying, requires external support

9. Pick Up Object from the Floor from a Standing Position

   Patient instruction: Please pick up the shoe (or slipper) that is in front of your feet.
   - ❑ 4, able to pick up the shoe safely and easily
   - ❑ 3, able to pick up the shoe but needs supervision
   - ❑ 2, unable to pick up the shoe, but reaches 2–5 centimeters (1–2 inches) from the shoe and keeps balance independently
   - ❑ 1, unable to pick up and needs supervision while trying
   - ❑ 0, unable to try and needs assistance to keep from losing balance (or falling)

10. Turning to Look Behind over Your Left and Right Shoulders While Standing

    Patient instruction: Please turn and look directly behind you over the left shoulder. Repeat to the right.

    The PTA, standing in the back of the patient, may pick up an object looking at the object directly. This will prompt the patient to turn around.
    - ❑ 4, looks behind from both sides and weight shifts well
    - ❑ 3, looks behind one side only; other side shows less weight shift
    - ❑ 2, turns sideways only but maintains balance
    - ❑ 1, needs close supervision or verbal cuing
    - ❑ 0, needs assistance while turning

11. Turn 360 Degrees

Patient instruction: Please turn completely around in a full circle, pause, and then turn in a full circle in the other direction.

❑ 4, able to turn 360 degrees safely in 4 seconds or less
❑ 3, able to turn 360 degrees safely, one side only, 4 seconds or less
❑ 2, able to turn 360 degrees safely, but slowly
❑ 1, needs close supervision or verbal cuing
❑ 0, needs assistance while turning

12. Place Alternate Foot on Step or Stool While Standing Unsupported

Patient instruction: Please place each foot alternately on the step stool. Continue until each foot has touched the step stool four times.

❑ 4, able to stand independently and safely and complete 8 steps in 20 seconds
❑ 3, able to stand independently and complete 8 steps in more than 20 seconds
❑ 2, able to complete 4 steps without aid with supervision
❑ 1, able to complete more than 2 steps but needs minimal assistance
❑ 0, needs assistance to keep from falling (or is unable to try)

13. Standing Unsupported, One Foot in Front

PTA needs to demonstrate the action to the patient.

Patient instruction: Please place one foot directly in front of the other. If you feel that you cannot place your foot directly in front, try to step far enough ahead that the heel of your forward foot is ahead of the toes of your other foot.

To score 3 points (at number 3), the length of the step should exceed the length of the other foot, and the width of the stance should approximate the patient's normal stance width.

❑ 4, able to place foot tandem independently and hold 30 seconds
❑ 3, able to place foot ahead of the other independently and hold 30 seconds
❑ 2, able to take a small step independently and hold 30 seconds
❑ 1, needs help to step but can hold 15 seconds
❑ 0, loses balance while stepping or standing

14. Standing on One Leg

Patient instruction: Please stand on one leg as long as you can without holding on to anything.

❑ 4, able to lift leg independently and hold for longer than 10 seconds
❑ 3, able to lift leg independently and hold for 5–10 seconds
❑ 2, able to lift leg independently and hold for 2 seconds (or longer)
❑ 1, tries to lift leg but unable to hold for 3 seconds—patient remains standing independently
❑ 0, unable to try or needs assistance to prevent fall

Maximum Total Score = 56

Score Interpretation—Older Adults

48–56—low fall risk
40–47—medium fall risk
< 39—high fall risk

References

1. Shirley Ryan Ability Lab. Berg balance scale. Last updated June 30, 2020. Accessed August 2, 2021. https://www.sralab.org/rehabilitation-measures/berg-balance-scale. Last updated June 30, 2020
2. Muir SW, Berg K, Chesworth B, Speechley M. Use of the Berg balance scale for predicting multiple falls in community dwelling elderly people: A prospective study. *Phys Ther* 2008; 88(4):449-459.

Functional Balance Test: Performance-Oriented Mobility Assessment (Tinetti-POMA)

Data from Tinetti ME, Williams TF, Mayewski R. Fall risk index for elderly patients based on number of chronic disabilities. *Am J Med.* 1986:80:429–434.

Client's Name:_____

Initial Instructions: Subject is seated on a hard, armless chair. The following maneuvers are tested. Total assessment time is between 10 and 15 minutes.

Score Interpretation:

< 19 = High Fall Risk   19–24 = Moderate Fall Risk   25–28 = Low Fall Risk

Tinetti Assessment Tool: Balance

Task	Description of Balance	Possible	Score
1. Sitting Balance	Leans or slides in chair	0	
	Steady, safe	1	
2. Rises from Chair	Unable without help	0	
	Able, uses arms to help up	1	
	Able without using arms	2	
3. Attempts to Rise from Chair	Unable without help	0	
	Able, requires more than one attempt	1	
	Able to rise in one attempt	2	
4. Immediate Standing Balance (first 5 seconds)	Unsteady (swaggers, moves feet, trunk sways)	0	
	Steady but uses walker or other support	1	
	Steady without walker or other support	2	

Task	Description of Balance	Possible	Score
5. Standing Balance	Unsteady	0	
	Steady but wide stance (heels 4 inches apart) and uses cane or other support	1	
	Narrows stance without support	2	
6. Nudged (subject at max position with feet as close together as possible, examiner pushes lightly on subject's sternum with palm of hand three times)	Begins to fall	0	
	Staggers, grabs, catches self	1	
	Steady	2	
7. Eyes Closed (at max position—see 6 above)	Unsteady	0	
	Steady	1	
8. Turning 360 Degrees	Discontinuous steps	0	
	Continuous steps	1	
	Unsteady (grabs, swaggers)	0	
	Steady	1	
9. Sitting Down	Unsafe (misjudged distance, falls into chair)	0	
	Uses arms or not a smooth motion	1	
	Safe, smooth motion	2	
	BALANCE SCORES:		/16

Tinetti Assessment Tool: Gait

Client's Name:_____

Initial Instructions: Subject stands with examiner, walks down the hallway or across the room, first at "usual" pace, then back at "rapid but safe" pace. Use usual walking aid.

Task	Description of Balance	Possible	Score
10. Initiation of Gait (immediately after told to "go")	Any hesitancy or multiple attempts to start	0	
	No hesitancy	1	

Task	Description of Balance	Possible	Score
11. Step Length and Height	RIGHT swing foot does not pass left stance foot with step	0	
	RIGHT foot passes left stance foot	1	
	RIGHT foot does not clear floor completely with step	0	
	RIGHT foot completely clears floor	1	
	LEFT swing foot does not pass right stance foot with step	0	
	LEFT foot passes right stance foot	1	
	LEFT foot does not clear floor completely with step	0	
	LEFT foot completely clears floor	1	
12. Step Symmetry	RIGHT AND LEFT step length not equal (estimate)	0	
	RIGHT AND LEFT step appear equal	1	
13. Step Continuity	Stopping or discontinuity between steps	0	
	Steps appear to continue	1	
14. Path (estimated in relation to floor tiles, 12-inch diameter; observe excursion of 1 foot over about 10 feet of the course)	Marked deviation	0	
	Mild/moderate deviation or uses walking aid	1	
	Straight without walking aid	2	

Task	Description of Balance	Possible	Score
15. Trunk	Marked sway or uses walking aid	0	
	No sway—but flexion of knees or back, or spreads arms out while walking	1	
	No sway, no flexion, no use of arms, and no use of walking aid	2	
16. Walking Stance	Heels apart	0	
	Heels almost touching while walking	1	
	Score: Gait:		/12
	Score: Balance:		/16
	Score: Balance and Gait Combined:		/28

References

1. https://www.leadingagemn.org/assets/docs/Tinetti-Balance-Gait--POMA.pdf Accessed November 18, 2021
2. Shirley Ryan Ability Lab. Tinetti performance oriented mobility assessment. Accessed May 8, 2021. https://www.sralab.org/rehabilitation-measures/tinetti-performance-oriented-mobility-assessment

Functional Reach

General Information: The functional reach test can be administered while the patient is standing (functional reach) or sitting (modified functional reach).

Functional Reach (standing instructions):

The patient is instructed to stand next to, but not touching, a wall to which a yardstick has been attached, and position the arm that is closer to the wall at 90 degrees of shoulder flexion with a closed fist.

The assessor records the starting position at the third metacarpal head on the yardstick.

Instruct the patient to "Reach as far as you can forward without taking a step or touching the wall."

The location of the third metacarpal at the end of the reach is recorded.

Scores are determined by assessing the difference between the start and end position. This is the reach distance, usually measured in inches.

Three trials are done and the average of the last two is noted.

Age-Related Normative Values for the Functional Reach Test

Age Group	Female	Male
20–40 years	14.6 (+/– 2.2) inches	16.7 (+/– 1.9) inches
41–69 years	13.8 (+/– 2.2) inches	14.9 (+/– 2.2) inches
70–87 years	10.5 (+/– 3.5) inches	13.2 (+/– 1.6) inches

References

1. Shirley Ryan Ability Lab. Functional reach test. Accessed May 8, 2021. https://www.sralab.org/rehabilitation-measures/functional-reach-test-modified-functional-reach-test
2. Fruth SJ, Fawcett C. *Fundamentals of Tests and Measures for the Physical Therapist Assistant*. Burlington, MA: Jones and Bartlett Learning; 2020.

Timed Up and Go Test (TUG)

- Place a chair (approximately 46 centimeters [18 inches] in height) against a wall or a firm object to prevent it from sliding backward (for the patient's safety). Place a cone on the floor exactly 3 meters (9.8 feet) away. The distance to place the cone must be measured from the edge of the chair to the back of the cone. Ensure there is clearance beyond the cone to allow for turning room. The PTA needs a stopwatch.
- Starting position: The patient is seated in the chair with hands on thighs and feet on the floor.
- Testing: The patient is instructed that on the signal of "Go," he or she will rise from the chair, walk "as quickly as possible" around the cone, and return to a seated position in the chair. While rising from the chair, the patient is permitted to push off of the thighs or the chair.
- The patient is told that he or she will be timed and should walk as quickly as possible but not to run.
- The PTA demonstrates the action to the patient. The patient is allowed one practice trial, followed by two test trials.
- Scoring: The PTA begins the timer when the "Go" signal is given (even if the patient has not begun to move) and stops the time at the exact instant that the patient's buttocks contact the chair after the walk segment.
- The scores of both test trials must be recorded, but the faster of the two trials is documented on the assessment form. Results from this test may be compared with age-related normative values.
- Assistive device used in testing: Permitted if required. The type of assistive device needs to be included in the assessment form. If an assistive device was used, the result of the test (the score) cannot be compared with age-related normative values.

Normative Values for the TUG Test

A cut-off score of 13 seconds for older community dwelling adults places the individual at increased risk for falls

Mean Scores by Age and Gender for the TUG Test

Patient Age	60–69	70–79	80–89	90–101
Mean (SD) scores for men (in seconds)	7.3	6.8 (1.1)	13.5 (6.3)	23.4 (9.2)
Mean (SD) scores for women (in seconds)	8.1 (0.9)	8.5 (2.8)	13.6 (5.5)	17.0 (5.3)

References

1. Lusardi MM. Functional performance in community living older adults. *J Geriatr Phys Ther.* 2004;26(3):14–22.
2. Shirly Ryan Ability Lab. Timed UP and Go Test. https://www.sralab.org/rehabilitation-measures/timed-and-go Accessed November 18, 2021

Appendix C

Borg Scale of Rating of Perceived Exertion

Patient Instructions For Use of The Borg Rating Scale

- While doing exercises or physical activity, we want you to rate your perception of exertion. This feeling should reflect how heavy and strenuous the exercise feels to you, combining all sensations and feelings of physical stress, effort, and fatigue.
- Try to appraise your feeling of exertion as honestly as possible without thinking about what the actual physical load is. Your own feeling of effort and exertion is important, not how it compares with other people's feelings.
- Nine (9) corresponds to "very light" exercises. For a healthy person, it is like walking slowly at his or her own pace for a few minutes.
- Thirteen (13) on the scale is "somewhat hard" exercise, but it still feels okay to continue.
- Seventeen (17), which is "very hard," is a very strenuous exercise. A healthy person can still go on, but the person needs to push himself or herself. It feels very heavy, and the person is very tired.
- Nineteen (19) on the scale is an extremely strenuous exercise level. For most people, this is the most strenuous exercise that they have ever experienced.

6	No exertion at all
7	Extremely light
8	
9	Very light
10	
11	Light
12	
13	Somewhat hard
14	
15	Hard (heavy)
16	
17	Very hard
18	
19	Extremely hard
20	Maximal exertion

Appendix D

Skin Care for Lymphedema

Education on Skin Care for Patient's with Lymphedema

- Avoid trauma and injury to the skin of your limb(s).
- Wear loose-fitting clothing and no jewelry. Wear proper, well-fitting footwear.
- Avoid prolonged sitting, standing, or crossing your legs.
- When traveling by air, ask for a seat with adequate leg room (for lower limb lymphedema).
- Get up every 30–60 minutes and walk up and down the aisle of the plane.
- Obtain a note from your doctor for security (related to your bandages or compression garment).
- Increase your water intake during the air travel because the cabin is dry and your body can get dehydrated.
- Obtain assistance for carrying, lifting, and transporting your luggage.
- Wear a lymphedema alert bracelet especially when traveling out of the country.
- Obtain a prescription for antibiotics from your doctor and fill it before leaving the country (in case an infection occurs while you are away).
- Consultation with your doctor is recommended before travel.
- If you are wearing compression garments, make sure that they are well fitting. For strenuous activity (such as prolonged standing or sitting), support your affected limb with a compression garment (that fits well).
- Avoid exposure to extreme temperatures (such as cold or heat). Do not expose your limb to hot tubs or saunas or water temperature greater than 102°F.
- Apply moisturizer daily to prevent chapping and chaffing of skin (especially during cold weather).
- Keep your limb clean and dry.
- Do not cut your cuticles.
- Use care with razors to avoid nicks and skin irritation and to prevent infection.
- Protect exposed skin with sunscreen and insect repellant.
- Avoid punctures of your skin (if possible), such as injections and blood draws.
- Wear gloves while doing activities that might cause skin injury, such as gardening, working with tools, or using chemicals (such as detergents).
- If scratches or punctures of your skin occur, wash them with soap and water, apply antibiotic (ointment), and observe for signs of infection such as redness.
- If a rash, itching, redness, pain, increased skin temperature, fever, or flu-like symptoms occur, contact your doctor immediately.

Appendix E

Documentation Examples

SOAP Note 1—Acceptable note
SOAP Note 2—Acceptable note
SOAP Note 3—Unacceptable note

SOAP Note 1

Patient name: Jane Doe   Date of birth: 02/06/1960
Diagnosis: Generalized OA, R TKA 11/2/2020
Date: 12/10/2020
Time: 11:00 am
S: Pt reports that she is now able to sleep upstairs in her own bed, but limits going up stairs to once a day as she still finds the stairs tiring and fears falling when coming downstairs in the morning. Reports current pain 2/10 R Knee, worst pain since last visit has been 5/10 after sitting for too long.

O: Vitals: BP 130/78, HR R radial pulse 76 BPM, RR 16
Sx scar R knee healing, steri strips no longer present over scar. Mild redness and localized warmth distal scar. PT notified of finding at 11:15 am
R Knee girth: 44 cm, decreased from 47 cm last visit
R knee: AROM: flex 95 deg, ext -5 deg
            PROM: flex 100 deg, ext 0 deg
Intervention: stationary bike with seat raised, no resistance x 10 min
Inf patellar mobilization Gr II 3X10, patient in long sitting.
Minisquats at // bars 2X10, standing resisted terminal knee ext with red T/band 3X8, Step ups on 2" block at // bars for support forward, backward and lateral with focus on inc R knee flexion and dec R hip circumduction. Hold relax to inc R hamstring flexibility 3X30 secs, R calf stretch on slant board at wall 3X 45 sec. Gait reed on levels and stairs with straight cane and verbal and tactile cues to facilitate improved knee flexion on swing phase and knee extension on stance phase of gait. Cold pack R knee X 15 mins patient in long sitting.

A: Patient continues to make progress in all areas of PT. Knee ROM has increased by 10 deg since start of care and patient is now doing stairs unassisted, using straight cane and rail. Continue PT to achieve Knee ROM goals of 110 deg flex and 0 deg ext, RLE overall strength of 5/5 and safety on stairs with normal gait pattern.

P: PT to see patient next visit for reevaluation prior to MD visit.
Sally Brown PTA 12/10/20 12:15 pm

SOAP Note 2

Patient name: Fred Doe   Date of birth: 01/06/1950
Diagnosis: Parkinson's Disease, Unsteady gait
Date: 12/10/2020
Time: 10:00 am
S: Pt and caregiver report that patient is now getting out of bed with supervision only. Pt reports that he is able to walk to bathroom with RW alone, caregiver verifies that patient amb around

house with RW independently during the day but is unsteady and needs assist if he has to go to the bathroom at night. Both parties note benefit from physical therapy. Patient denies pain.

O: Vitals: BP 128/74, HR R radial pulse 80 BPM, RR 16
Posture and gait: Patient exhibits kyphotic posture in sitting and standing and episodes of freezing during gait. Gait reed with RW and SBA over level surfaces 20'x3. Patient exhibits festinating gait and needs frequent cues to take larger steps.
Functional activities to improve bed mobility and transfers: rolling right <-> left, supine to sit and sit to stand from mat table. Verbal and tactile cues provided to direct arm and leg placement during supine to sit and sit <-> stand. Patient now Ind in rolling was Min A. Practiced sit <->stand with mat table at varying heights. Patient requires CGA with table at lower height. Therex Interventions: Stepping activities over low objects on floor within // bars: forward backward and lateral with emphasis on inc. step height and length X 8 mins. Pectoral stretching against corner walls of room in standing 3X30 secs. Exs on mat table for trunk rotation in Hook Lying 3X10, Bridging 3X10. Stationary bike 10 mins. Caregiver educated in trunk rotation and bridging exs for HEP. Provided good return demonstration.

A: Patient continues to make progress in all areas of PT. Patient easily distracted when in PT gym and requires frequent redirection on task. Bed mobility has improved since initial eval as patient now rolling independently and sit to stand improved from Min A to Sup/CGA based on height of seat. Continue with PT to improve safety during gait on even and uneven surfaces and to acheive LTG of Ind and safe transfers.

P: Next visit focus on transfer training and static and dynamic balance in standing. Speak with PT about plans for discharge.
Sally Brown PTA 12/10/20 11:10 am

SOAP Note 3

Patient name: John Brown
Date: 12/10/2020
DX: R fracture humerus
S: Patient reports pain 4/10. Patient states pain keeps him awake at night.
O: Wand exs R shoulder 3X10. AROM R elbow and wrist. Putty exs R hand. Ice pack R shoulder 15 minutes. Patient given written HEP to do every day.
A: Patient tolerated treatment well. ROM improving.
P: Cont per plan next visit.
Jane Smith PTA

Index

G

P

X

Y

Z